Clinical Orthodontics

Clinical Orthodontics

Edited by **Regina Stuart**

hayle
medical

New York

Published by Hayle Medical,
30 West, 37th Street, Suite 612,
New York, NY 10018, USA
www.haylemedical.com

Clinical Orthodontics
Edited by Regina Stuart

International Standard Book Number: 978-1-63241-396-3 (Hardback)

Printed in China.

Contents

Preface

Orthodontics refers to that area of dentistry which deals with the malocclusion i.e. the improper positioning of teeth and jaws. It uses tools like braces, plates, headgears, etc. to treat the problematic teeth. The treatments covered in this area are reduction of teeth gaps, aligning the teeth, improving oral functioning, etc. This book explores all the important aspects related to orthodontics and its clinical applications. Most of the topics introduced here in cover new techniques and advances in this area. This book will provide comprehensive knowledge to anyone interested in this subject. It will also help readers in keeping pace with the rapid changes in this field. Therefore, this book will prove to be a beneficial source of knowledge for the students as well as professionals engaged in the area of orthodontics.

This book is a comprehensive compilation of works of different researchers from varied parts of the world. It includes valuable experiences of the researchers with the sole objective of providing the readers (learners) with a proper knowledge of the concerned field. This book will be beneficial in evoking inspiration and enhancing the knowledge of the interested readers.

In the end, I would like to extend my heartiest thanks to the authors who worked with great determination on their chapters. I also appreciate the publisher's support in the course of the book. I would also like to deeply acknowledge my family who stood by me as a source of inspiration during the project.

Editor

1

An *in vitro* study on the effect of an oscillating stripping method on enamel roughness

Stefan Baumgartner[1*], Anna Iliadi[2], Theodore Eliades[1] and George Eliades[2]

Abstract

Background: The aim of the present study was to assess the changes in enamel roughness parameters before and after stripping with an oscillating diamond strip system.

Methods: Sound premolars extracted for orthodontic reasons were embedded up to their cervical area in a polyvinylsiloxane putty, creating four groups of four teeth with three interproximal areas each (mesial/distal). The same regions of interproximal enamel surfaces were studied by 3D optical interferometric profilometry before and after stripping with the Ortho-Strips system (Intensiv Dental SA, Montagnola, Switzerland) (n teeth = 16, n contact points = 12, n sites measured = 24). The roughness parameters tested were the amplitude parameters Sa and Sz, the hybrid parameter Sdr, and the functional parameters Sci and Svi. The parameter differences (ΔSa, ΔSz, ΔSdr, ΔSci, ΔSvi) were calculated per region and statistically analyzed by one-sample Mann-Whitney rank sum test ($a = 0.05$).

Results: High statistically significant differences were found in ΔSa, ΔSz, and ΔSvi median values (0.453, 3.870, and 0.040 μm, respectively); a significant difference in ΔSdr median value (1.514%); and no statistically significant difference in ΔSci (0.110 median value).

Conclusions: Under the conditions of the present study, the Ortho-Strips system seems to significantly increase the amplitude parameters Sa and Sz; the hybrid parameter Sdr, associated with the developed interfacial area ratio; and the functional parameter Svi, which depicts the volume of the deepest valleys. Under the conditions of the present study, the Ortho-Strips seems to significantly increase four of five measured roughness parameters.

Keywords: Stripping; Enamel roughness; 3D profilometry

Background

Interproximal stripping, defined as the removal of interproximal enamel, is routinely used in orthodontics to eliminate Bolton tooth-size discrepancies between teeth of the maxillary and mandibular anterior and posterior arch [1,2], treat mild or moderate crowding [3], prevent relapse [4,5], and improve aesthetics [5]. This procedure, also known as interdental enamel reduction, interdental polishing, enamel approximation, or slenderizing [6], may have a favorable effect on treatment duration and allows transverse arch dimensions and anterior inclinations to be maintained.

Stripping may have a variable extent, and although in most cases it entails a 1- to 2-mm mesiodistal reduction, removal of as high as 50% in enamel width has been reported, which in radical cases can generate 7 mm of space [7]. If the anterior dentition also is included, an additional gain of 2.5 mm can be achieved [8]. At the moment, most authors suggest about 0.3 to 0.5 mm per tooth surface as the maximum amount of stripping without severely affecting tooth structure [9], or up to half of the enamel thickness [8]. It has been recommended that reduction should not exceed 0.3 mm of the width of maxillary incisors, 0.6 mm in maxillary premolars and molars, 0.2 mm in the mandibular incisors, and 0.6 mm in the mandibular premolars and molars [10].

Despite its advantages, enamel reduction has attracted the concern of investigators, owing to enamel tissue removal. In operative dentistry, it is crucial to maintain contact points in the posterior teeth to allow for proper self-cleaning and avoid the retention of plaque, although in orthodontic treatment, the interdental tooth enamel is ground down therapeutically. Adequate polishing of

* Correspondence: stefan.baumgartner@zzm.uzh.ch
[1]Clinic for Orthodontics and Paediatric Dentistry, Center of Dental Medicine, University of Zurich, Plattenstr. 11, 8032 Zürich, Switzerland
Full list of author information is available at the end of the article

the stripped teeth is essential for a good long-term prognosis, since scratches and furrows remaining on the enamel surface facilitate plaque accumulation and possibly caries development [11-13]. A number of researches have focused not only on the orthodontic aspects but also on the cariogenic and periodontal implications associated with this procedure since it has been shown that changes in enamel integrity may be considered as a predisposing factor for caries and periodontal disease [11,12]. After grinding, the tooth surface seems to become rougher, with a significantly greater plaque accumulation capacity [3,12,14,]. Although the results of a recent systematic review [15] were inconclusive regarding enamel roughness after interdental stripping *in vitro*, the meta-analysis of the *in vivo* results did not find that interdental enamel reduction was a predisposing factor for caries development.

Proximal enamel reduction entails a wide array of mechanical, automatic, rotating, or translatory devices. Recently, oscillating mechanisms have been introduced, claiming a smooth enamel topography following stripping. The aim of this *in vitro* study was to quantitatively assess the changes in enamel roughness after interproximal stripping with oscillating diamond strips. The null hypothesis was that stripping does not increase the amplitude, hybrid, and functional roughness parameters of the enamel.

Methods

Sample preparation

Sixteen premolars devoid of caries, enamel cracks, fluorosis, or abrasion under stereomicroscopic inspection (M80, Leica, Wetzlar, Germany) at ×10 magnification were used in the study. The teeth had been extracted for orthodontic reasons, cleaned, and stored in distilled water with 0.5% sodium azide at 8°C.

In order to simulate intraoral stripping conditions, four teeth were embedded up to their cervical region in an addition-type polyvinylsiloxane putty impression material (Aquasil Putty, Dentsply/Detrey, Konstanz, Germany), creating thus an arch with three interproximal contact areas. Four equal setups were used (n teeth = 16, n contact points = 12, n sites measured = 24). Before embedding, the roughness parameters of the proximal untreated surfaces were measured and served as reference.

Grinding was performed according to the manufacturer's instructions under water cooling by one operator (SB). The three interproximal areas per setup were ground on both sides (mesial/distal) using the Ortho-Strips system (Intensiv Dental SA, Montagnola, Switzerland) employing two-sided flexible diamond-coated strips of three different grit sizes (40 μm for contouring, 25 μm for finishing, and 15 μm for polishing). New devices were used for each stripping session. The strips used were attached to a micromotor (Eva Intra Lux Prophy head 61 LRG KaVo, Biberach, Germany, 7,500 rpm) operated for 20 s per grit size. Under these conditions, a 0.25-mm interproximal enamel reduction was achieved as checked by a steel ligature. The roughness parameters of the stripped areas were measured again under the same conditions.

Roughness parameter measurements

Roughness analysis was performed by optical interferometric profilometry. A 3D optical profiler was used (Wyko NT 1100, Veeco, Santa Barbara, CA, USA) under the following conditions: vertical scanning mode, Mirau lens, ×20.3 magnification (231.1 × 303.8 μm^2 analysis area), tilt correction, 5-μm Gaussian high-pass filter, and 0.2 μm (x, y) and 0.1 nm (z) resolution. Three measurements were performed per specimen and averaged representing surface roughness before and after stripping at the same region per tooth. The roughness parameters tested were the following:

a) The amplitude parameters Sa (the absolute profile deviation versus the average over a 3D surface) and Sz (the ten-point height over the complete 3D surface representing the average difference between the five highest peaks and five lowest valleys)
b) The hybrid parameter Sdr (the developed interfacial area ratio, expressed as the percentage of additional surface area contributed by the texture as compared to an ideal plane of the same size)
c) The functional parameters Sci (the core fluid retention index, a measure of the volume the surface would support from 5% to 80% of the bearing ratio) and Svi (valley retention index, the volume the surface would support at the valley zone, 80% to 100% of the bearing ratio)

The differences (Δ: after-before stripping) of the individual roughness parameters were calculated per tooth and region [16].

Statistical analysis

The results of ΔSa, ΔSz, ΔSdr, ΔSci, and ΔSvi were statistically analyzed by one-sample Mann-Whitney rank sum test [17] at a 95% confidence level ($a = 0.05$).

Results

Representative 3D profilometric images of interproximal enamel margins before stripping are illustrated in Figure 1a,b. At the beginning, the enamel surface is smooth with no specific features, apart from the appearance of a prismatic structure in some domains (Figure 1b). After stripping (Figure 2a,b), the same regions presented a rough texture with polishing grooves produced from the grinding direction of the strips.

The results of the differences in the surface roughness parameters (Δ: paired values of the same region after-before stripping) and the results of the statistical analysis

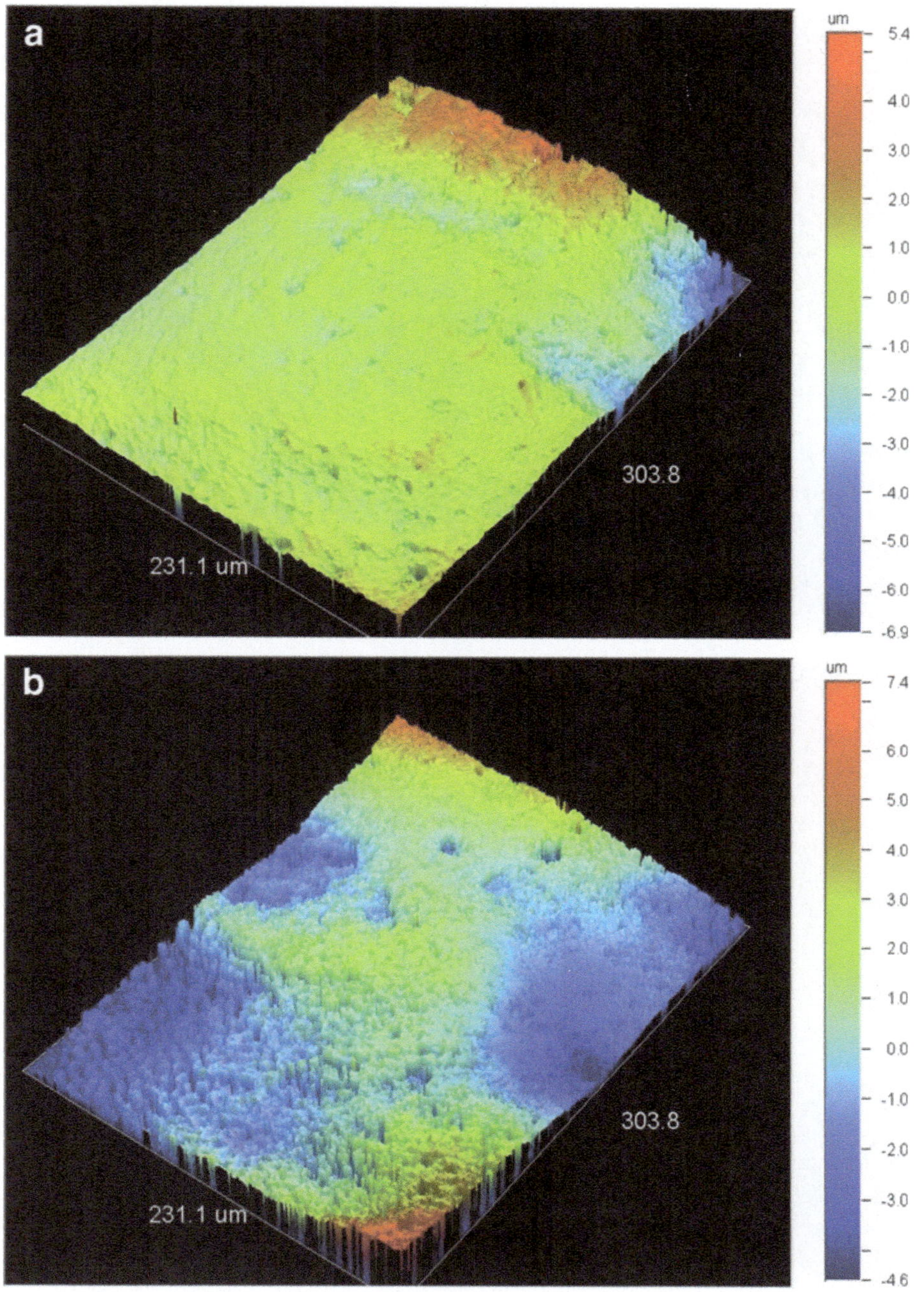

Figure 1 3D profilometric images of enamel interproximal areas before stripping (×20.3). (a) Area with a smooth topography; **(b)** distal area revealing a prismatic structure at the left/front region of the image.

are presented in Table 1. The Mann-Whitney rank sum test showed very high statistically significant differences ($p < 0.001$) in ΔSa, ΔSz, and ΔSvi; a statistically significant difference ($p < 0.05$) in ΔSdr; and no statistically significant difference ($p > 0.05$) in ΔSci.

Discussion

Interdental stripping is a commonly used technique in orthodontics that provides important clinical advantages, but with several limitations. Enamel reduction may impair tooth resistance against the aggressive intraoral environment and may lead to sensitivity [18] or caries development due to plaque accumulation [11-13].

Controversial evidence has been reported so far on the effect of stripping on enamel morphology and roughness. SEM studies [19,20] showed that perforated diamond-coated disks with less than 30-μm grain size minimized grinding defects, whereas subsequent polishing with fine and extra-fine alumina disks (Sof-Lex, 3M ESPE, St. Paul, MN, USA) produced smooth surfaces, equally to

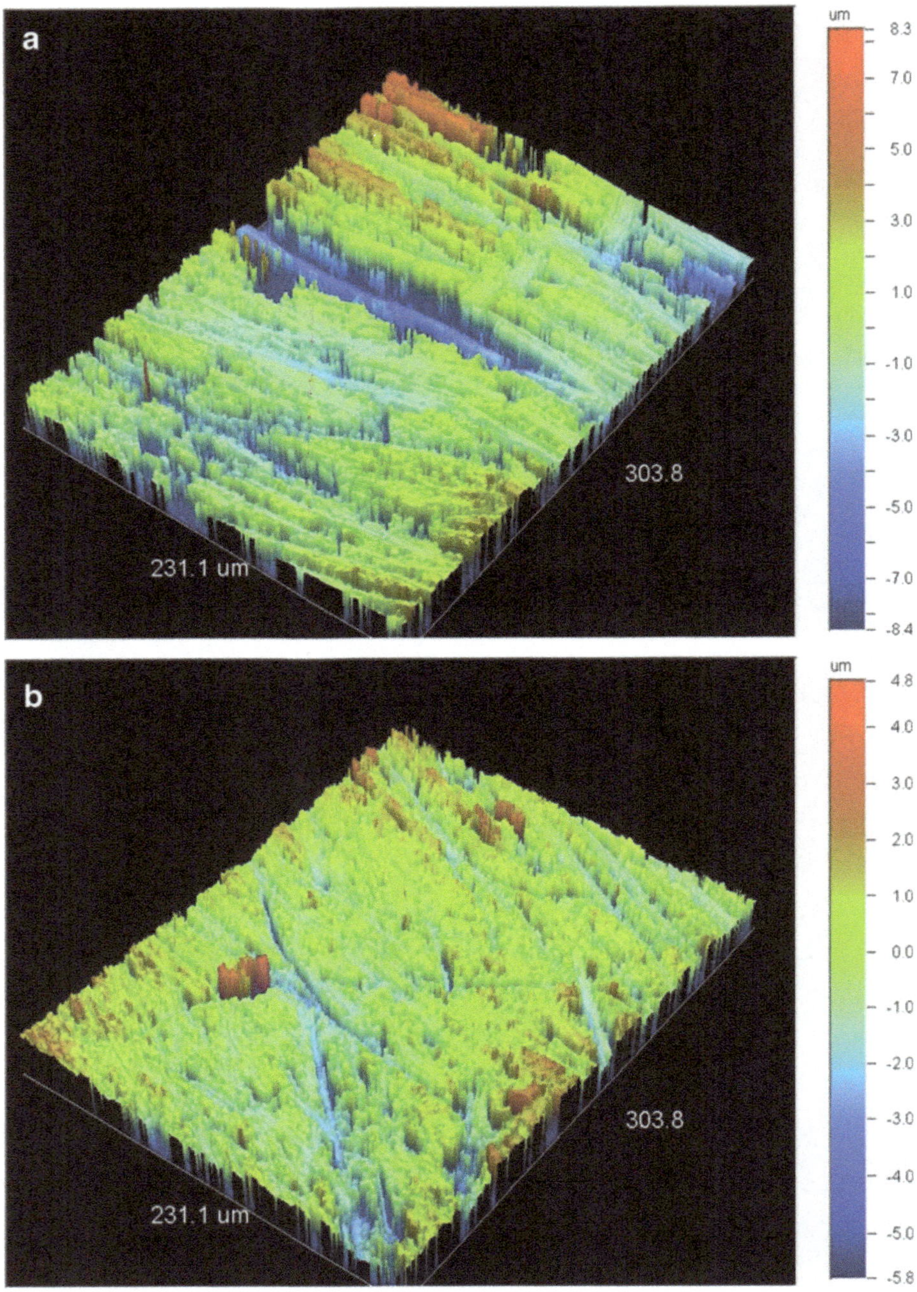

Figure 2 3D profilometric images of enamel interproximal areas after stripping (×20.3). (a) Mesial and **(b)** distal areas of the same teeth as in Figure 1. Both images reveal increased roughness. Note the orientation of the grooves produced from the grinding direction of the strips.

Table 1 Statistics for the five roughness parameters tested

	Median value	25th percentile	75th percentile	Range	Max	Min	*T* statistics	*p* value
ΔSa (μm)	0.453	0.075	0.710	2.940	2.000	−0.940	756	<0.001
ΔSz (μm)	3.870	0.340	5.500	17.720	11.320	−6.400	420	<0.001
ΔSdr (%)	1.514	−0.155	2.640	11.770	8.200	−3.500	708	0.014
ΔSci	0.110	−0.145	0.325	2.030	1.450	−0.580	648	0.219
ΔSvi	0.040	0.08	0.060	0.130	0.100	−0.030	768	<0.001

or smoother than untreated enamel. Nevertheless, the results of this study were mainly based on subjective qualitative assessment of enamel morphological characteristics. On the other hand, qualitative assessment by SEM and quantitative assessment of the amplitude parameter Ra by in-line stylus profilometry [21] showed that stripping disks and diamond-coated metal strips followed by fine Sof-Lex disks produced significantly rougher surfaces in comparison with the intact enamel of permanent and deciduous teeth. Qualitative (scanning electron microscopy) and quantitative (surface roughness test) measurements by Gupta et al. [22] also showed that the enamel after stripping with diamond disks and different polishing methods was significantly rougher than untreated control teeth. To improve the reliability of quantitative analysis, 3D optical profilometry was used to determine the Ra values by scanning sample areas rather than performing in-line analysis on enamel areas [23]. The results showed that grinding and polishing with automatic oscillating systems, including Ortho-Strips, resulted in equally smooth surfaces with untreated enamel, or even better. These systems are considered to provide better results than other common stripping techniques, where enamel defects have been observed [12,14,24].

The results of the present study failed to confirm the findings of the aforementioned studies for the Ortho-Strips system regarding the Sa amplitude parameter (the 3D equivalent to Ra). Moreover, all the parameters tested in the present study (amplitude, hybrid, functional) showed significantly increased values after stripping, except for Sci. Therefore, the null hypothesis should be partially rejected.

As previously considered [23], only the quantitative assessment of roughness parameters allows direct comparisons among surface treatments, without the subjective assessment bias of the SEM techniques. Since optical interferometric profilometry is a non-destructive technique, it may be sequentially used on the same specimens before and after stripping. In such experimental designs, as in the present study, measurements are taken at the same region of the same tooth before and after stripping, the values before stripping serving as controls. Therefore, the variability in roughness values of a separate control group is neutralized by expressing the difference (Δ) induced in surface roughness parameters at the same region of each individual specimen and compares the difference versus the zero value [17]. To further standardize the procedure, a ×20.3 magnification was used to analyze more enamel areas, whereas three regions were measured and averaged per surface and treatment to assure reproducibility. This experimental design provided a total number of 24 measurements for each condition and parameter, which resulted in an equal number of roughness value differences for evaluation.

An important issue, frequently overlooked, is that for the reason of comparison with previous literature, roughness parameters are limited only to Ra (in 2D) or Sa (in 3D) measurements. Although popular, Ra and Sa quantify the 'absolute' height or amplitude of the surface peaks or valleys (all considered as peaks) and are insensitive to their spatial distribution [16,25]. This is the reason for including three types of roughness parameters that were evaluated: amplitude, hybrid, and functional. In the amplitude parameters, besides the common Sa, the Sz was also included. Sz can discriminate between peaks and valleys, being more sensitive to Sa when studying wear effects, just like the stripping-induced effects on enamel. Sdr is related to slope sizes and provides information on the additional surface area produced from the surface texture in comparison with an ideal plane surface of the same size. Sci is associated with the relative retention of fluid the core surface structure provides, and Svi is linked to fluid retention at deepest valleys [16].

The results of the present study showed statistically significant differences in ΔSa, ΔSz, ΔSdr, and ΔSvi and no difference in ΔSci. The statistically significant difference found in the amplitude parameters Sa and Sz implies that the enamel surface left after stripping has higher peaks or/and deeper valleys in comparison with its native reference (intact enamel surface). This was clearly observed in the 3D profilometric images. Since increased amplitude heights (positive or negative) affect the peak and valley slopes, the enamel surface area is increased, a fact confirmed by the statistically significant difference found in ΔSdr. The absence of statistically significant differences in ΔSci implies that the core surface structure of enamel after stripping (excluding the 5% of the shallowest and the 20% of the deepest valleys as per Sci definition) provides the same fluid retention capacity as the intact control. However, in the Svi index, where the contribution of the 20% of the greatest valleys at the bearing ratio is taken into account, a statistically significant difference was found which could substantially increase the plaque retention capacity.

The differences in the profilometric methodology of the present study from the previous were as follows: a) The same surfaces of the specimens used as controls (intact enamel) were scanned before and after stripping (sequential treatment mode). This provides important advantages over the use of another series of specimens as a control group, since the same region is tested before and after in the sequential mode. b) More roughness parameters were tested to better characterize the enamel surfaces. The need for further polishing became evident from the results of the study. However, it is extremely difficult to use other types of interproximal polishing when the proximal reduction is 0.25 mm. Hand-operated finishing strips (i.e., for composite restorations) with a thickness of 0.10 to 0.15 mm may be used, but fail to fully adapt to the curved surface. Common Sof-Lex disks (stiff, urethane-backed/3M

ESPE) have a greater thickness than the proximal reduction (approximately 0.28 vs 0.25 mm of the reduction) and therefore cannot be used. Extra-thin Sof-Lex disks (flexible, polyester-backed/3M ESPE) may fit, but they are very flexible and need a high speed for final polishing, putting at risk the integrity of marginal soft tissues. The results highlight the finding that the surface left after stripping with the Ortho-Strips system is rougher than native enamel, contrary to what has been stated in the literature so far.

Application of stripping in clinical conditions involves teeth, which have the ability to move as the pressure applied by the machine is partially absorbed by the periodontal ligament displacement. Therefore, the lack of stiffness of the system may reduce the amount of enamel tissue ground. The design of the present study included embedding of teeth in a silicone substrate for limited tooth movement in an attempt to simulate the clinical condition.

It has long been established that amplitude parameters alone cannot properly describe the roughness of a surface [26]. Actually, for a complete characterization of the roughness of a surface, 15 parameters are required, including 4 amplitude, 4 spatial, 4 hybrid, and 3 functional [16]. Therefore, there is a need for a concise characterization of the enamel surface roughness parameters including amplitude, spatial or hybrid, and functional parameters. Such an approach would make comparisons among treatments more feasible and establish a basis for explanation of the biological responses.

Conclusions

Summarizing the results of the present study, enamel surfaces after interproximal grinding and polishing with the Ortho-Strips system showed statistically significant increase in Sa, Sz, Sdr, and Svi roughness parameters from their native intact controls, but no statistically significant differences in Sci.

The statistically significant difference found in the amplitude parameters Sa and Sz implies that the enamel surface left after stripping has higher peaks or/and deeper valleys in comparison with its native reference.

Competing interests

The authors declare that they have no competing interests.

Authors' contributions

SB, TE, and GE developed the study protocol. SB performed the stripping procedures. AI and GE made the measurements. AI, TE, and GE performed the statistical analysis and interpreted the data. SB wrote the manuscript. AI, TE, and GE revised the manuscript. All authors read and approved the final manuscript and have given the final approval of the version to be published.

Author details

[1]Clinic for Orthodontics and Paediatric Dentistry, Center of Dental Medicine, University of Zurich, Plattenstr. 11, 8032 Zürich, Switzerland. [2]Department of Dental Biomaterials, School of Dentistry, University of Athens, 2 Thivon Str, 115 27, Goudi, Athens, Greece.

References

1. Zachrisson BU, Mjor IA. Remodeling of teeth by grinding. Am J Orthod. 1975;68(5):545–53.
2. Rossouw PE, Tortorella A. A pilot investigation of enamel reduction procedures. J Can Dent Assoc. 2003;69(6):384–8.
3. Sheridan JJ. Air-rotor stripping. J Clin Orthod. 1985;19(1):43–59.
4. Betteridge MA. The effects of interdental stripping on the labial segments evaluated one year out of retention. Br J Orthod. 1981;8(4):193–7.
5. Zachrisson BU. JCO/interviews Dr. Bjorn U. Zachrisson on excellence in finishing. Part 2. J Clin Orthod. 1986;20(8):536–56.
6. Rossouw PE, Tortorella A. Enamel reduction procedures in orthodontic treatment. J Can Dent Assoc. 2003;69(6):378–83.
7. Stroud JL, English J, Buschang PH. Enamel thickness of the posterior dentition: its implications for nonextraction treatment. Angle Orthod. 1998;68(2):141–6.
8. Sheridan JJ. Air-rotor stripping update. J Clin Orthod. 1987;21(11):781–8.
9. Jarjoura K, Gagnon G, Nieberg L. Caries risk after interproximal enamel reduction. Am J Orthod Dentofac Orthop. 2006;130(1):26–30.
10. Fillion D. Vor- und Nachteile der approximalen Schmelzreduktion. Inf Orthod Kieferorthop. 1995;27:64–90.
11. Arends J, Christoffersen J. The nature of early caries lesions in enamel. J Dent Res. 1986;65(1):2–11.
12. Radlanski RJ, Jager A, Schwestka R, Bertzbach F. Plaque accumulations caused by interdental stripping. Am J Orthod Dentofac Orthop. 1988;94 (5):416–20.
13. Tuverson DL. Anterior interocclusal relations. Part I. Am J Orthod. 1980;78 (4):361–70.
14. Joseph VP, Rossouw PE, Basson NJ. Orthodontic microabrasive reproximation. Am J Orthod Dentofac Orthop. 1992;102(4):351–9.
15. Koretsi V, Chatzigianni A, Sidiropoulou S. Enamel roughness and incidence of caries after interproximal enamel reduction: a systematic review. Orthod Craniofac Res. 2014;17(1):1–13.
16. Stout KJ, Blunt L. Three dimensional surface topography. 2nd ed. London: Penton Press; 2000.
17. Kirkwood B, Sterne J. Essential medical statistics. 2nd ed. Oxford: Blackwell Publishing Ltd; 2006.
18. Dummer PM, Harrison KA. In vitro plaque formation on commonly used dental materials. J Oral Rehabil. 1982;9(5):413–7.
19. Zhong M, Jost-Brinkmann PG, Radlanski RJ, Miethke RR. SEM evaluation of a new technique for interdental stripping. J Clin Orthod. 1999;33(5):286–92.
20. Zhong M, Jost-Brinkmann PG, Zellmann M, Zellmann S, Radlanski RJ. Clinical evaluation of a new technique for interdental enamel reduction. J Orofac Orthop. 2000;61(6):432–9.
21. Arman A, Cehreli SB, Ozel E, Arhun N, Cetinsahin A, Soyman M. Qualitative and quantitative evaluation of enamel after various stripping methods. Am J Orthod Dentofac Orthop. 2006;130(2):131 e7–14.
22. Gupta P, Gupta N, Patel N, Gupta R, Sandhu GS, Naik C. Qualitative and quantitative evaluation of enamel after various post-stripping polishing methods: an in vitro study. Aust Orthod J. 2012;28(2):240–4.
23. Danesh G, Hellak A, Lippold C, Ziebura T, Schafer E. Enamel surfaces following interproximal reduction with different methods. Angle Orthod. 2007;77(6):1004–10.
24. Piacentini C, Sfondrini G. A scanning electron microscopy comparison of enamel polishing methods after air-rotor stripping. Am J Orthod Dentofac Orthop. 1996;109(1):57–63.
25. Gadelmawla ES, Koura MM, Maksoud TMA, Elewa IM, Soliman HH. Roughness parameters. J Mater Process Tech. 2002;123(1):133–45.
26. Wennerberg A, Albrektsson T. Suggested guidelines for the topographic evaluation of implant surfaces. Int J Oral Maxillofac Implants. 2000;15(3):331–44.

2

Evaluation of crown-root angulation of lateral incisors adjacent to palatally impacted canines

Georgios Kanavakis[1*], Karen M Curran[2], Kevin C Wiseman[2], Nicholas P Barone[2], Matthew D Finkelman[3], Sreedevi Srinivasan[4], Moonyoung B Lee[1] and Caroll-Ann Trotman[1]

Abstract

Background: The objective of this study is to explore differences in crown-to-root angulation between lateral incisors adjacent to palatally impacted canines (PICs) and lateral incisors adjacent to normally erupted canines (NECs).

Methods: Orthodontic records of 100 subjects (51 with PICs and 49 with NECs) were reviewed. Crown-to-root angulations of all lateral incisors were measured manually on the final panoramic radiographs. Also, three experienced orthodontists were asked to visually inspect the morphology of the lateral incisors on the panoramic radiographs. A mixed model was used to test the difference in crown-to-root angulation of the lateral incisor between the experimental and the control groups. The association between the examiners' observations and the presence of a canine impaction was assessed by means of a chi-square test. All analyses were performed at the 0.05 level of statistical significance.

Results: A significant ($p = 0.009$) difference of 2.3° in crown-to-root angulation was found between groups. Also, 66.7% of the lateral incisors that were identified as "abnormal" by the panel of orthodontists were adjacent to a PIC. A percentage of 65.2 of lateral incisors that were identified as "normal" were located adjacent to NECs.

Conclusions: The root of lateral incisors adjacent to PICs is angulated more mesially compared to lateral incisors adjacent to NECs. In addition, clinicians are somewhat able to predict if a canine is palatally impacted by visually observing the crown-to-root angulation of the adjacent lateral incisor. Evaluating the crown-to-root angulation of a lateral incisor on a panoramic image might facilitate an early diagnosis of palatally impacted canines.

Keywords: Palatally impacted canines; Panoramic images; Lateral incisor morphology; Crown-to-root angulation

Background

Impacted canines are a frequently encountered problem in orthodontics, and the maxillary canines are the second most frequently impacted teeth after the third molars with a prevalence rate that ranges between 1% and 3% [1-4]. Canines can be impacted labially or palatally, and in non-Hispanic white populations, palatally impacted canines are at least twice as prevalent as labially impacted canines [5,6]. Moreover, palatal canine impactions are more common in females than in males with a 2:1 ratio [7], and their occurrence is bilateral in 19% to 45% of all cases [8-10]. While labial canine impactions are most often associated with the presence of maxillary crowding [6,11], 82% to 85% of palatal impactions occur in the absence of crowding.

There are two primary theories for the development of palatally impacted canines: the guidance theory and the genetic theory. The guidance theory suggests that the eruption of the canine is influenced by local factors such as a retained primary canine and/or absence, underdevelopment, or malpositioning of the maxillary lateral incisor [9,12-14]. Conversely, the genetic theory suggests that the impaction is due to a genetic predisposition; it is supported by evidence revealing an association between palatally impacted canines and other phenotypic dental variations of genetic origin such as small lateral incisor crown size [5,15,16], agenesis of lateral incisors [5,16], aplasia of premolars [16] and third molars [17], distal displacement of mandibular second premolars [18], and tooth transposition [5]. Thus, although

* Correspondence: gkanavak@gmail.com
[1]Department of Orthodontics and Dentofacial Orthopedics, Tufts University, School of Dental Medicine, 1 Kneeland Street DHS#1145, Boston, MA 02111, USA
Full list of author information is available at the end of the article

there is no consensus about the exact etiology of palatally impacted canines, it appears that the adjacent lateral incisor demonstrates an important role, either because its eruption and dimensions are controlled by the same genes that control the eruption of the canine (genetic theory) or because its position in the arch influences the eruption path of the canine (guidance theory).

To this end, the primary aim of this retrospective, observational study was to explore the difference in the morphology of lateral incisors, specifically their crown-to-root angulation, when they are adjacent to palatally impacted canines compared with the morphology of lateral incisors adjacent to canines with a normal eruptive pattern. It was hypothesized that lateral incisors adjacent to palatally impacted canines will present with greater deviations in the crown-to-root angulation compared to lateral incisors adjacent to normally erupted canines. A secondary aim was to explore whether a subjective visual evaluation of the crown-to-root angulation of a lateral incisor on a panoramic radiograph could aid the clinician in predicting the presence of an adjacent palatally impacted canine.

Methods

Study population

Upon approval by the Institutional Review Board at (...) (IRB #10242), a comprehensive search of all patient electronic records was conducted at (...) using the keywords "palatally impacted canine" or "palatally impacted cuspid." In order to be included in the study, subjects had to have at least one palatally impacted canine and have complete initial and final orthodontic records including digital pre- and posttreatment panoramic radiographs. Subjects were excluded if they had one or more missing lateral incisors, a labially impacted canine, or poor-quality radiographs. The search resulted in 51 subjects who met the inclusion criteria for the study group. The control group was composed of 49 subjects, selected consecutively from the electronic archives (2005 to 2011) of the orthodontic clinic at (...), with normally erupted maxillary canines and who had completed orthodontic treatment with full initial and final records. Prior to data collection, records were de-identified and no patient information was revealed. All panoramic X-rays were taken with the same orthopantomogram (Planmeca ProMax®, Planmeca Inc, Roselle, IL, USA).

The primary focus of this study was to evaluate the morphology of lateral incisors next to palatally impacted canines, and thus, each maxillary canine was considered as an individual sample. Therefore, if a subject had two palatally impacted canines, there were two study samples. Similarly, in a subject with normally erupted canines, there were two control samples. In those subjects with a unilateral palatal canine impaction, there was one study sample - the contralateral side was not regarded as a control because genetic predisposition could influence the morphology of the lateral incisor. As a result, there were a total of 175 canines (77 impacted, 98 normal). Subsequently, seven additional canines were excluded due to unclear root morphology of the adjacent lateral incisor on the panoramic radiograph. Therefore, the final study sample consisted of 168 canines (70 impacted, 98 normal).

Methodology

All final (posttreatment) digital panoramic radiographs were de-identified, printed, and given a random code in order to eliminate examiner bias. Only one investigator (SS) had access to the identified subject information and was not part of the data collection or analysis.

Measurement of the crown-to-root angulation of the lateral incisor

Manual measurements of the angle (degree measurement) between the long axis of the crown and the long axis of the root of all maxillary lateral incisors were performed on the final panoramic radiographs (Figure 1) by two investigators (KC, KW), separately. When defining the long axis of the lateral incisor root, dilaceration at the root apex was not considered so as to obtain a better representation of the direction of the long axis (Figure 2). When the long axis of the root was angulated mesially compared to that of the crown, a positive degree measurement was recorded, and when the angulation was distal, a negative measurement was recorded (Figure 3). In order to reduce random error, measurements from both examiners were averaged into a single value.

Visual evaluation of maxillary lateral incisors

Hard copies of all de-identified final panoramic radiographs were randomized and evaluated separately by three orthodontists (CC, CP, and DC), each of whom had at least 20 years of clinical experience. Each asked

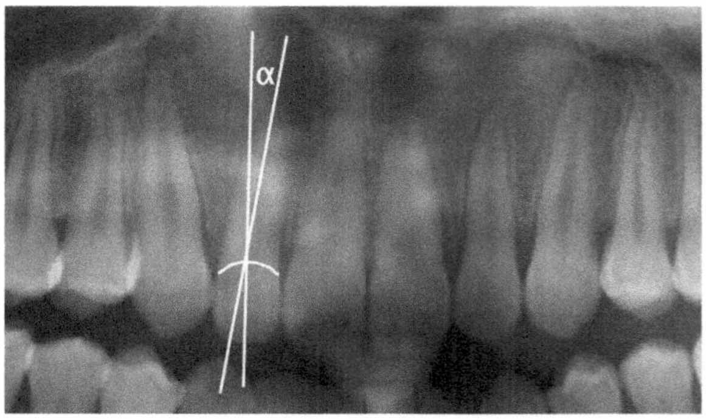

Figure 1 Angle "α" was used to measure mesio-distal crown to root angulation of the lateral incisors.

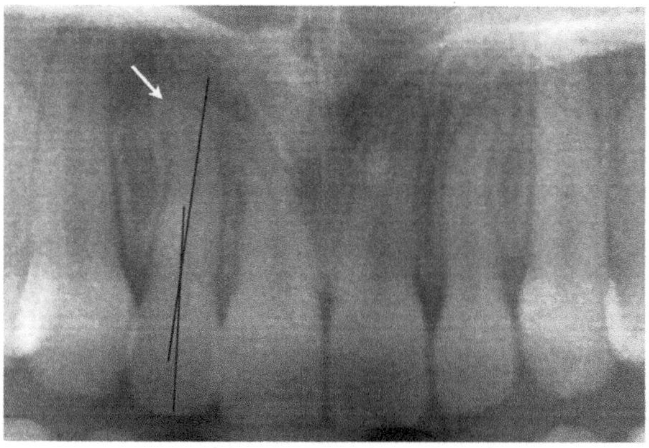

Figure 2 Dilacerations at the root apex were not regarded when defining the long axis of the root.

to visually evaluate all maxillary lateral incisors and determine whether the crown-to-root angulation appeared "normal" or "abnormal." The orthodontists were blinded to the purpose and the details of this investigation.

Statistical analysis

A power calculation was conducted using nQuery Advisor (Version 7.0). In order to assess the power of the study, a pilot study was performed using data from 18 subjects who were not included in the final sample population. Based on the results of the pilot study, the estimated mean difference between the two groups was 4°, with a common standard deviation of 3.5°. Using these estimated values, a sample of 49 subjects with lateral incisors adjacent to normal canines and 51 subjects with at least one lateral incisor adjacent to a palatally impacted canine was adequate to obtain a type I error rate of 5% and a power > 99%.

For the crown-to-root angulation measurement, inter-rater reliability between the two operators (KC, KW) was assessed via the method of Bland-Altman [19] prior to using the averaged measurements.

To test for potential differences in crown-root angulation between lateral incisors adjacent to palatally impacted canines and lateral incisors adjacent to normally erupted canines, a mixed model was used. The dependent variable of the mixed model was the angular measurement; the presence or absence of palatal impaction was defined as a fixed effect, and the subject was defined as a random effect. This model was selected in order to account for the dependency of results within a given subject.

To evaluate the visual assessment of the three orthodontists, their individual answers were combined into a single binary variable based on majority agreement. A chi-square test was used to evaluate the association between the examiners' visual observations of the lateral incisor and the actual presence of a palatally impacted canine. In addition, the relationship between the examiners' observations and the crown-to-root angulation of lateral incisors was assessed via Student's *t* test for independent samples. All statistical analyses were performed at the 0.05 level of significance.

Results

The results for the Bland-Altman plot for inter-rater reliability are presented in Figure 4. The average difference in measurement between the two investigators was 3°; however, in a few instances, this difference was as high as 12°. In order to reduce random error, the average measurement of the two investigators was used for all statistical analyses.

Descriptive statistics (mean and standard deviation) for crown-root angulation of lateral incisors are shown in Table 1. Overall, the results revealed that the roots of lateral incisors were on average 2.30° ($p = 0.009$) more mesially angulated when the lateral incisor was adjacent to a palatally impacted canine (Table 1).

Results for the secondary outcome of this study revealed that when experienced orthodontists described a lateral incisor as "abnormal", its adjacent canine was palatally impacted in 66.7% (24/36) of cases. In cases when a lateral incisor was described as "normal" by the orthodontists, the adjacent canine had erupted normally in 65.2% (86/132) of the cases. The association between the

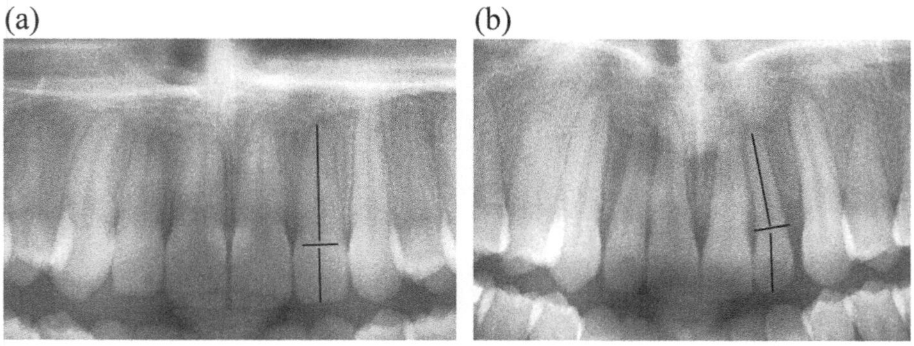

Figure 3 Examples of (a) a "normal" (α-angle = 0) and (b) medially angulated lateral incisor (α-angle > 0).

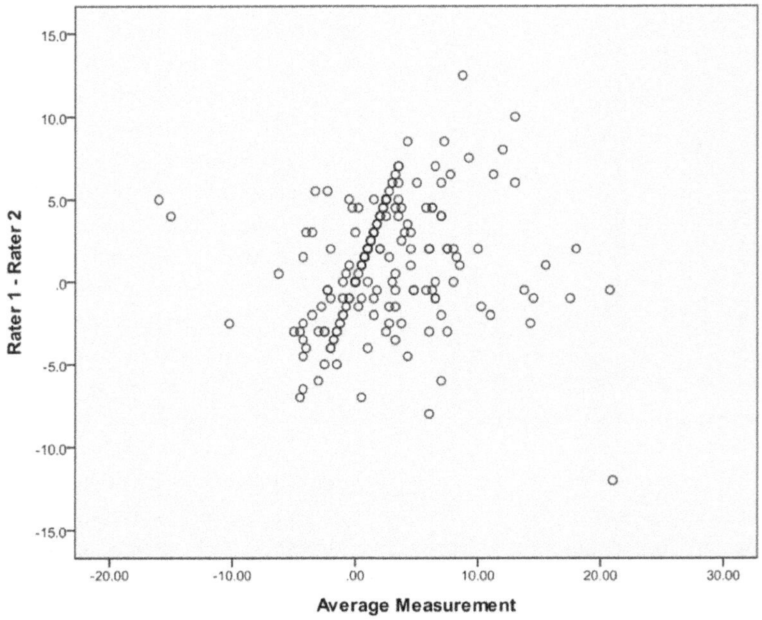

Figure 4 Bland-Altman graph displaying the inter-rater reliability in measurements.

orthodontists' observations and the actual presence of a palatally impacted canine was statistically significant ($p = 0.001$). Detailed results for this comparison are displayed in Figure 5. Furthermore, the mean crown-to-root angulation was significantly higher when the lateral incisors were considered to be "abnormal" by the orthodontists, compared to lateral incisors considered to be "normal" ($p = 0.002$) (Table 2).

Discussion

The present investigation tested the assumption that the crown-to-root angulation of lateral incisors adjacent to palatally impacted canines differs compared to lateral incisors adjacent to normally erupted canines. The results indicated that when a canine is palatally impacted, the long axis of the adjacent maxillary lateral incisor tends to be angulated more mesially by approximately 2.5° when compared to lateral incisors with normal adjacent canines. This difference was found to be statistically significant.

Furthermore, a close look at the data reveals a trend in the morphology of lateral incisors adjacent to palatally impacted canines. In subjects where the root of the lateral incisor was angulated more than 6° mesially to the crown, 48% (20/42) of the adjacent canines were palatally impacted. This percentage increased to 68% (15/22) when the crown-to-root angulation was greater than 7.5°. In three cases with extreme crown-to-root angulation of the maxillary lateral incisor (greater than 18°), the adjacent canine was always (100%) palatally impacted. These observational findings suggest that there might be a diagnostic value to the crown-to-root angulation of the maxillary lateral incisor.

Previous studies have reported significant associations between the morphology of lateral incisors and the presence of a palatally impacted canine. Liuk et al. [20] compared the dimensions of lateral incisors in cases with palatally impacted canines to normal controls using cone-beam-computed tomography (CBCT) and revealed that the former exhibited significantly smaller crown and root dimensions. Morphologically abnormal maxillary lateral incisors have been associated with palatally impacted canines by numerous investigators [5,8,10,15,21,22]; however, there is no consensus regarding the scientific reasoning for this observation. Some tend to support that an abnormally shaped, peg, or missing lateral incisor will cause the adjacent canine to impact by not guiding it into the correct position in the arch [6,12,23,24]. On the other hand, there are numerous studies suggesting that abnormally shaped lateral incisors and palatally impacted canines are both phenotypic expressions of specific genes and therefore tend to occur concomitantly [7,17,21,25]. Results from the present investigation could potentially be used to support either of the two prevailing theories. In support to

Table 1 Comparison of impacted and non-impacted canines in terms of the adjacent lateral incisor's crown-root angulation

	Canine impaction	*N*	Mean	SD	*p* value
Crown/root angulation (°)	Not impacted	98	1.30	4.39	0.009
	Impacted	70	3.60	5.99	

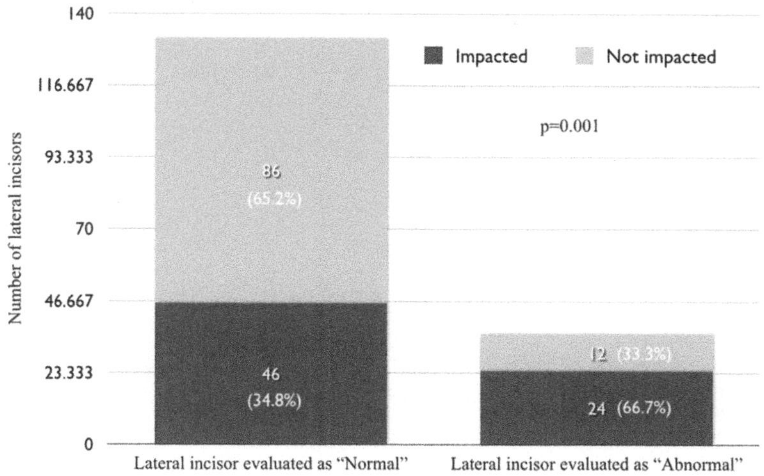

Figure 5 Direct comparison of examiners' opinions and actual presence of canine impaction.

the guidance theory, it could be assumed that a mesially angulated root would not provide appropriate guidance for the eruption of the adjacent canine. At the other end of the spectrum, the same morphological discrepancy could also be considered a developmental abnormality of genetic origin.

This study also found that orthodontists tended to be able to "predict" the presence of a palatally impacted canine by observing the adjacent lateral incisor. When the lateral incisor was considered to be "abnormal," 66.7% of the adjacent canines were palatally impacted. Similarly, in 65.2% of normally erupted canines, the consensus of the orthodontists dictated that the adjacent lateral incisor appeared "normal" (Figure 5). In addition, the description of a lateral incisor as "abnormal" was significantly associated with an increased mesial angulation of its root (Table 2). These findings suggest that the crown-to-root angulation of lateral incisors, as seen on a panoramic radiograph, might have a predictive value when a clinical decision has to be made regarding possible palatal displacement of the adjacent canine. As suggested previously, early diagnosis can lead to prevention of future palatal impaction, if appropriate treatment modalities are used [2,4,26].

Table 2 Comparisons between the examiners' evaluations and the lateral incisor crown-root angulation measurements

	Examiners' consensus		Mean	SD	*p* value
Crown/root angulation (°)	Normal lateral incisor	132	1.21	3.22	0.002
	Abnormal lateral incisor	36	6.08	8.51	

A limitation of the present study is associated with the use of panoramic radiographs to determine crown-to-root angulation of lateral incisors. Previous research has suggested that measurements on panoramic radiographs tend to overestimate the mesial angulation of lateral incisors when compared to a three-dimensional image (CBCT) [27]. In addition, there is an inherent error in using a two-dimensional image to depict three-dimensional structures since the bucco-distal tooth angulations might influence mesio-distal measurements on the panoramic radiographs [28]. Possible gender and age dimorphism in lateral incisor crown-to-root angulation could have also impacted the results of this investigation. This could be a question for future epidemiological research projects. Despite these limitations, there still is substantial clinical value to the findings of this study, especially because the panoramic radiograph is still the most commonly used radiograph in dentistry. Future investigations using computed tomography should be conducted to further clarify the findings of this investigation.

Conclusions

1. When measured on a panoramic radiograph, the root of maxillary incisors adjacent to palatally impacted canines is more mesially angulated to the crown, compared to lateral incisors adjacent to normally erupted canines.
2. Experienced orthodontists are able to "predict" the presence of a palatally impacted canine in two out of three cases, by observing the maxillary lateral incisor.

Competing interests

The authors declare that they have no competing interests.

Authors' contributions

GK conceived the study idea, co-designed the study and wrote the manuscript. KC and KW performed the manual measurements and collected the data. NB collected the data from the orthodontists who performed visual observation of the images and wrote a first draft of the methodology section. MF performed the statistical analysis and wrote a first draft of the Results section. SS de-identified and randomized the sample and critically reviewed and revised the manuscript. ML co-designed the study and critically revised and reviewed the manuscript. CAT supervised the preparation of the paper and critically reviewed and revised the final manuscript. All authors read and approved the final manuscript.

Author details

[1]Department of Orthodontics and Dentofacial Orthopedics, Tufts University, School of Dental Medicine, 1 Kneeland Street DHS#1145, Boston, MA 02111, USA. [2]Private Practice, Boston, USA. [3]Department of Academic Services, Tufts University School of Dental Medicine, Boston, MA, USA. [4]Department of Orthodontics, University of Iowa, Iowa City, IA, USA.

References

1. Grover PS, Lorton L. The incidence of unerupted permanent teeth and related clinical cases. Oral Surg Oral Med Oral Pathol Oral Radiol Endod. 1985;59(4):420–5.
2. Ericson S, Kurol J. Early treatment of palatally erupting maxillary canines by extraction of the primary canines. Eur J Orthod. 1988;94:503–13.
3. Ericson S, Kurol J. Radiographic examination of ectopically erupting maxillary canines. Am J Orthod Dentofacial Orthop. 1987;91(6):483–92.
4. Baccetti T, Leonardi M, Armi P. A randomized clinical study of two interceptive approaches to palatally displaced canines. Eur J Orthod. 2008;30(4):381–5.
5. Mercuri E, Cassetta M, Cavallini C, Vicari D, Leonardi R, Barbato E. Dental anomalies and clinical features in patients with maxillary canine impaction. Angle Orthod. 2013;83(1):22–8.
6. Jacoby H. The etiology of maxillary canine impactions. Am J Orthod Dentofacial Orthop. 1983;84(2):125–32.
7. Peck S, Peck L, Kataja M. The palatally displaced canine as a dental anomaly of genetic origin. Angle Orthod. 1994;64(4):249–56.
8. Peck S, Peck L, Kataja M. Prevalence of tooth agenesis and peg-shaped maxillary lateral incisor associated with palatally displaced canine (PDC) anomaly. Am J Orthod Dentofacial Orthop. 1996;110(4):441–3.
9. Becker A, Smith P, Behar R. The incidence of anomalous maxillary lateral incisors in relation to palatally displaced cuspids. Angle Orthod. 1981;51 (1):24–9.
10. Zilberman Y, Cohen B, Becker A. Familial trends in palatal canines, anomalous lateral incisors, and related phenomena. Eur J Orthod. 1990;12:135–9.
11. Thilander B, Jakobsson S. Local factors in impaction of maxillary canine. Acta Odontol Scand. 1968;26:145–68.
12. Becker A. Palatal canine displacement: guidance theory or an anomaly of genetic origin? A letter to the editor from Adrian Becker, with a response from Sheldon and Leena Peck, and Matti Kataja. Angle Orthod. 2004;65 (2):95–102.
13. Stellzig A, Basdra EK, Komposch G. On the etiology of upper canine impaction - a space analysis. J Orofac Orthop. 2014;55(3):97–103.
14. Becker A, Sharabi S, Chaushu S. Maxillary tooth size variation in dentitions with palatal canine displacement. Eur J Orthod. 2002;24(3):313–8.
15. Sacerdoti R, Baccetti T. Dentoskeletal features associated with unilateral or bilateral palatal displacement of maxillary canines. Angle Orthod. 2004;74 (6):725–32.
16. Anic-Milosevic S, Varga S, Mestrovic S, Lapter-Varga M, Slaj M. Dental and occlusal features in patients with palatally displaced maxillary canines. Eur J Orthod. 2009;31(4):367–73.
17. Peck S, Peck L, Kataja M. Concomitant occurrence of canine malposition and tooth agenesis: evidence of orofacial genetic fields. Am J Orthod Dentofacial Orthop. 2002;122(6):657–60.
18. Baccetti T, Leonardi M, Giuntini V. Distally displaced premolars: a dental anomaly associated with palatally displaced canines. Am J Orthod Dentofacial Orthop. 2010;138(3):318–22.
19. Bland JM, Altman DJ. Statistical methods for assessing agreement between two methods of clinical measurement. Lancet. 1986;8:307–10.
20. Liuk IW, Olive RJ, Griffin M, Monsour P. Maxillary lateral incisor morphology and palatally displaced canines: a case-controlled cone-beam volumetric tomography study. Am J Orthod Dentofacial Orthop. 2013;143(4):522–6.
21. Baccetti T. A controlled study of associated dental anomalies. Angle Orthod. 2002;68(3):267–74.
22. Mossey PA, Campbell HM, Luffingham JK. The palatal canine and the adjacent lateral incisor: a study of a west of Scotland population. Br J Orthod. 1994;21:169–74.
23. Miller BH. The influence of congenitally missing teeth on the eruption of the upper canine. Dent Pract Dent Rec. 1963;13:497–504.
24. Chaushu S, Zilberman Y, Becker A. Maxillary incisor impaction and its relationship to canine displacement. Am J Orthod Dentofacial Orthop. 2003;124(2):144–50.
25. Pirinen S, Arte S, Apajalahti S. Palatal displacement of canine is genetic and related to congenital absence of teeth. J Dent Res. 1996;75(10):1742–6.
26. Baccetti T, Mucedero M, Leonardi M, Cozza P. Interceptive treatment of palatal impaction of maxillary canines with rapid maxillary expansion: a randomized clinical trial. Am J Orthod Dentofacial Orthop. 2009;136(5):657–61.
27. Bouwens DG, Cevidanes L, Ludlow JB, Phillips C. Comparison of mesiodistal root angulation with posttreatment panoramic radiographs and cone-beam computed tomography. Am J Orthod Dentofacial Orthop. 2011;139(1):126–32.
28. Garcia-Figueroa MA, Raboud DW, Lam EW, Heo G, Major PW. Effect of buccolingual root angulation on the mesiodistal angulation shown on panoramic radiographs. Am J Orthod Dentofacial Orthop. 2008;134(1):93–9.

3

An evaluation of two types of nickel-titanium wires in terms of micromorphology and nickel ions' release following oral environment exposure

Abdul Razzak A. Ghazal[1], Mohammad Y. Hajeer[2*], Rabab Al-Sabbagh[1], Ibrahim Alghoraibi[3] and Ahmad Aldiry[4]

Abstract

Background: This study aimed to compare superelastic and heat-activated nickel-titanium orthodontic wires' surface morphology and potential release of nickel ions following exposure to oral environment conditions.

Methods: Twenty-four 20-mm-length distal cuts of superelastic (NiTi Force I®) and 24 20-mm-length distal cuts of heat-activated (Therma-Ti Lite®) nickel-titanium wires (American Orthodontics, Sheboygan, WI, USA) were divided into two equal groups: 12 wire segments left unused and 12 segments passively exposed to oral environment for 1 month. Scanning electron microscopy and atomic force microscopy were used to analyze surface morphology of the wires which were then immersed in artificial saliva for 1 month to determine potential nickel ions' release by means of atomic absorption spectrophotometer.

Results: Heat-activated nickel-titanium (NiTi) wires were rougher than superelastic wires, and both types of wires released almost the same amount of Ni ions. After clinical exposure, more surface roughness was recorded for superelastic NiTi wires and heat-activated NiTi wires. However, retrieved superelastic NiTi wires released less Ni ions in artificial saliva after clinical exposure, and the same result was recorded regarding heat-activated wires.

Conclusions: Both types of NiTi wires were obviously affected by oral environment conditions; their surface roughness significantly increased while the amount of the released Ni ions significantly declined.

Keywords: NiTi wires; Superelasticity; Heat activation; Surface morphology; Nickel release; Scanning electron microscopy; Atomic force microscopy; Atomic absorption spectrophotometer

Background

Introducing nickel-titanium (NiTi) alloys has made a revolution in orthodontic wires industry [1] and made the dream of applying continuous and constant forces almost true [2]. Many improvements were applied in manufacturing austenite active (superelastic) and martensite active (heat-activated) NiTi wires to benefit from the extraordinary superelasticity and shape memory properties of NiTi alloys [3]. Unfortunately, the development of producing NiTi orthodontic wires did not prevent them from corrosion especially when exposed to corrosive conditions [4, 5].

Corrosion resistance of NiTi wires is a very important factor that affects surface roughness [6, 7] and chemical stability [8]. NiTi wires' performance in the oral cavity has been a big concern for researchers [9–12] because it is the environment in which they are intended to function. Extreme temperatures, pH variations, and complex oral flora have made the oral environment a unique media [13] that cannot be simulated in experimental conditions [8].

Surface integrity may affect friction resistance [7]. On the other hand, instable chemical structure causes Ni ions' release and may affect biocompatibility [14–17].

NiTi wires are usually used in the aligning and leveling stage [2], so they have to deal with complex forces that cannot be identical in all cases and vary between cases due to individual factors and the type of malocclusion.

* Correspondence: myhajeer@gmail.com
[2]Department of Orthodontics, University of Damascus Dental School, Damascus, Syria
Full list of author information is available at the end of the article

Many researchers have evaluated and compared "as received" and "retrieved" superelastic and heat-activated NiTi wires. Those studies were performed either in unreliable circumstances (in vitro or animal studies) [2, 18–22] or involved mixed types of orthodontic NiTi wires (different manufacturer and/or composition and/or diameters) or even evaluated corrosion resistance without proper standardization of orthodontic forces (different classes of malocclusion, different inter-bracket distances, dental crown dimensions, and bone response) [6, 11, 23, 24]. Oral conditions of the in vivo studies were also not coincident, i.e., different masticatory forces, different oral hygiene status, different types of foods and drinks, mouth temperature, oral flora, and pH variations among patients [6, 10, 11, 25, 26].

Although the oral environment is a corrosive place in which superelastic and heat-activated NiTi wires are supposed to survive, it seems that there is no published data that compare between both types of NiTi wires with regard to their roughness and potential Ni ions' release following clinical exposure in assorted in vivo conditions apart from any orthodontic forces.

Methods

Two types of orthodontic nickel-titanium archwires were included: NiTi Force I (superelastic archwires) and Therma-Ti Lite (heat-activated archwires). Twelve archwires from each type were randomly selected from different packets with different batches of the same manufacturer (American Orthodontics, Sheboygan, WI, USA) and have the same chemical composition (Ni 55 %, Ti 45 %) and the same arch dimensions 0.019 × 0.025 in. Using a sterilized plier, two 20-mm-length segments of each archwire were cut from the terminal ends of both types of archwires (Fig. 1). As a result, 48 segments (24 distal cuts of NiTi Force I wires and 24 distal cuts of Therma-Ti Lite wires) were kept in self-closed sterilizing plastic bags.

The control and the ex vivo groups

The control group consisted of 12 segments of NiTi Force I wires and 12 segments of Therma-Ti Lite wires that were left unused ("as received" state), whereas the ex vivo group consisted of 12 segments of NiTi Force I wires and 12 segments of Therma-Ti Lite wires. Each segment of the ex vivo group was passively tied using elastomeric ligatures (American Orthodontics, Sheboygan, WI, USA) to a triple set of the first lower premolar brackets, (Standard Edgewise, American Orthodontics, Sheboygan, WI, USA) extraorally. Then, sets were carefully bonded in each two lower semi arches of the volunteers from the first premolar to the first molar, as shown in Fig. 2. Each volunteer had two sets, one of them carrying superelastic NiTi segment, while the other one carries the heat-activated NiTi segment. The allocation of the side of the mouth receiving the superelastic or the heat-activated NiTi segments was based on computer-generated random sequence (Minitab® 15, Minitab Inc., State College, PA, USA).

Volunteers' recruitment

Prior to volunteers' recruitment for this research project, ethical approval was obtained from the University of Al-Baath Dental School Local Ethics Committee (UBDS-1022-2012-PG). Consent forms were obtained for the volunteers following detailed explanation of the intended research work orally and in a written format.

The sample of possible candidates was derived from 186 fourth- and fifth-year dental students from the University of Al-Baath Dental School, Hama, Syria, depending on the following criteria: dental and skeletal class I malocclusion, age range between 21 and 24 years, healthy status with no syndromes or chronic diseases, good oral hygiene assessed by the plaque index and the

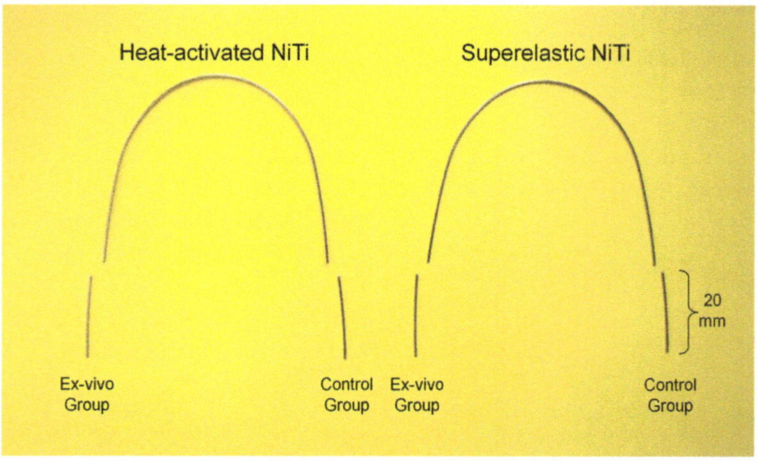

Fig. 1 The method of constructing the control and the ex vivo wires' groups

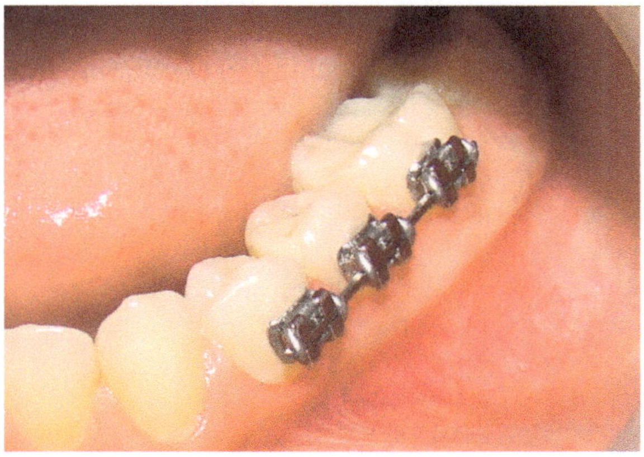

Fig. 2 Experimental set after bonding

gingival index of Löe and Silness [27], no significant dental caries causing significant destruction of one tooth surface, no metallic restorations, and if these had been observed, they were replaced with composite ones, no history of orthodontic treatments, good oral seal and no signs of oral breathing habits, no smoking or intake of liquid drugs and absence of chewing disorders (e.g., unilateral chewing).

Thirty-two students (12 males, 20 females) met the inclusion criteria, and only 27 (10 males, 17 females) of them accepted to participate in this research. Disproportionate stratified random sampling was employed to obtain a group of 12 volunteers (6 males, 6 females), and they were given instructions regarding maintaining good oral hygiene and keeping normal eating habits with no special dietary requirements.

After 30 days of wires' placement in the oral environment, wires were collected and cleaned with 95 % ethanol to remove any precipitation, rinsed with ultrapure water to detach any loose bound deposits, then dried, and saved again in their self-closed sterilizing plastic bags.

The occlusal surface (6 mm from the end) of the wires' segments ("as received" and "retrieved") was tested to evaluate surface morphology and then immersed in artificial saliva to determine the amount of released nickel ions.

Analyzing surface morphology

The surface morphology and roughness of the wires were determined by using scanning electron microscopy (SEM; Quanta 200, FEI™, Hillsboro, OR, USA) and atomic force microscopy measurements (AFM; Nanosurf®, easyScan2, Liestal, Switzerland). Wires were set on the SEM chamber platform, and ×1600 magnification micrographs were obtained to give initial evaluation of wires' surface roughness (Fig. 3).

For further analysis of surface morphology, AFM measurements were performed in a tapping mode in air at room temperature ranged between 26° and 28°. Silicon

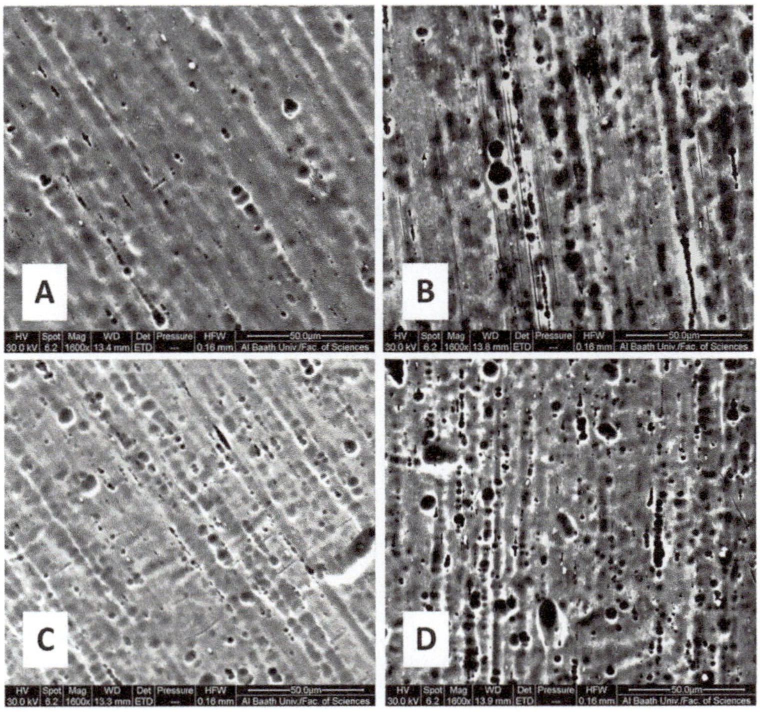

Fig. 3 Scanning electron micrographs at ×1600 magnification of **A** as received superelastic NiTi wires, **B** retrieved superelastic NiTi wires, **C** as received heat-activated NiTi wires, and **D** retrieved heat-activated NiTi wires

cantilevers (Tap190 Al-G, NanoSensors™, Neuchatel, Switzerland) with 30-nm-thick aluminum reflex coating were used. According to the producer's datasheet, the cantilever spring constant was in the range of 1.5–15 N/m and the resonance frequency was 15–500 kHz. The tip radius was less than 10 nm. The scan rate was set at 0.7 Hz, and the scanning size was 10 × 10 μm. The two-dimensional images were captured in the medium mode in a JPEG format (Fig. 4). Each image was processed using AFM Software (Nanosurf Report Expert 5.0 Nano Surf®, Liestal, Switzerland), and three-dimensional images (Fig. 5) were reconstructed using Nanosurf Report Expert 5.0 (Digital Surf, Nano Surf®, Liestal, Switzerland). The area of the roughness profile, Sa, is the parameter that was recorded to evaluate average surface roughness [24, 28, 29].

Nickel ions' release measurement

After analyzing surface morphology, both types of the wire samples ("as received" and "clinically exposed") were placed in polypropylene vessels containing 2 mL of modified Fusayama artificial saliva with the following composition [19, 20]: NaCl (400 mg/L), KCl (400 mg/L), $CaCl_2{\cdot}2H_2O$ (795 mg/L), $NaH_2PO_4{\cdot}H_2O$ (690 mg/L), KSCN (300 mg/L), $Na_2S{\cdot}9H_2O$ (5 mg/L), and urea (1000 mg/L) prepared using ultrapure water (WT 100 Millipore, Qamato, Japan), and then adjusted to a pH of 2 using HCl and maintained at 37 °C for 30 days.

Artificial saliva samples were treated with 5 % nitric acid [30], and standard solutions of nickel (Merck®, Germany) were prepared in the following concentrations: 0, 5, 10, and 25 particle per billion (ppb). Then, released nickel ions in artificial saliva were measured benefiting from standard solutions' light absorption by using a graphite furnace atomic absorption spectrophotometer (GF-AAS) (AA-6800, Shimatzu®, Kyoto, Japan) that was programmed in advance according to the device manufacturer's instructions to detect nickel ions depending on its wavelength (232.0 nm), and the following thermal program was successively applied on the samples: 120 °C for 20 s, 250 °C for 10 s, 800 °C for 10 s, 800 °C for 3 s, and 2500 °C for 3 s.

Statistical analysis

Minitab® 15 (Minitab Inc, State College, PA, USA) was used to perform the statistical analysis. With alpha set at 5 %, paired *t* tests were applied to evaluate intragroup changes ("as received" vs after "clinical exposure" in the same group), whereas two-sample *t* tests were employed to examine intergroup differences (superelastic vs heat-activated in the same wire state).

Results

Micromorphology

Scanning electron microscope (SEM) provided two-dimensional black and white micrographs of NiTi wires.

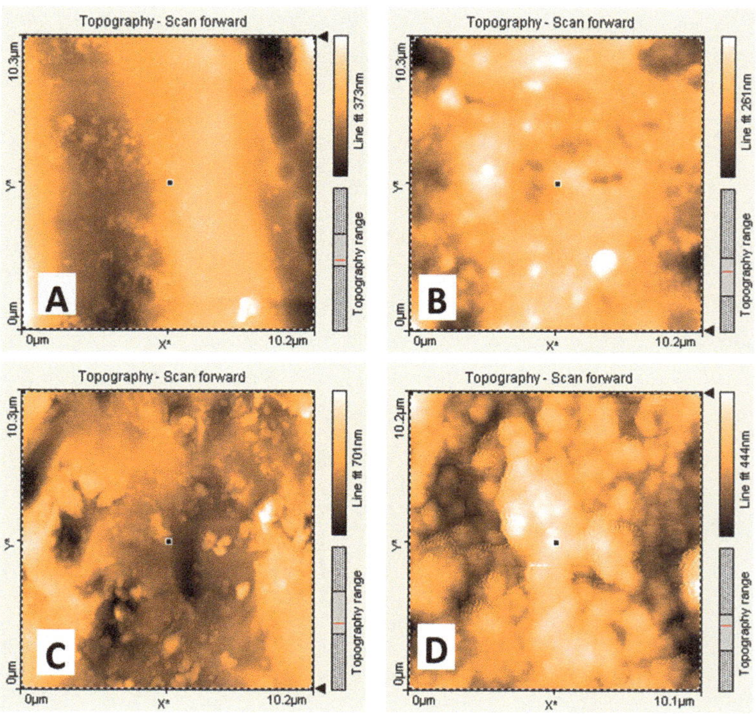

Fig. 4 Atomic force two-dimensional micrographs (10 × 10 μm) of **A** as received superelastic NiTi wires, **B** retrieved superelastic NiTi wires, **C** as received heat-activated NiTi wires, and **D** retrieved heat-activated NiTi wires

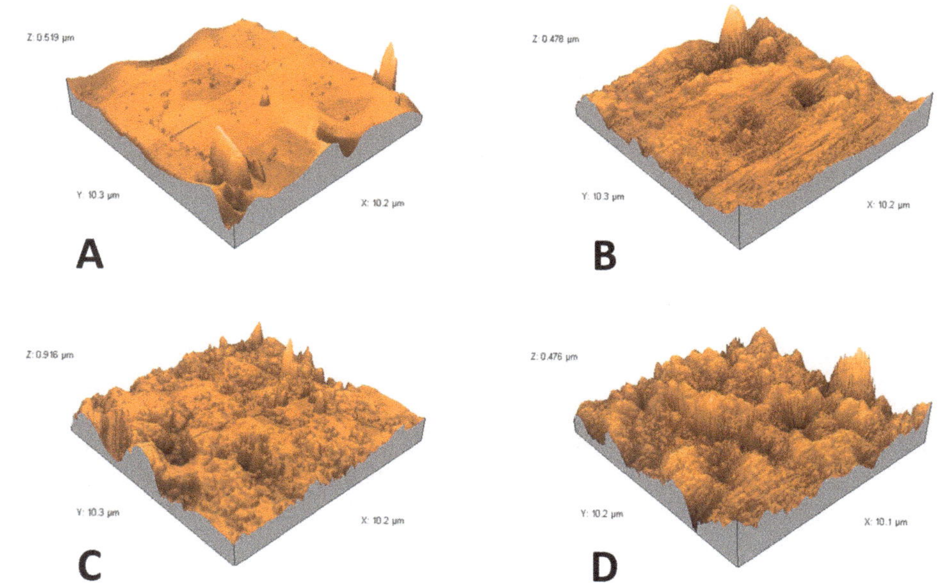

Fig. 5 Atomic force three-dimensional reconstructed micrographs (10 × 10 μm) of **A** as received superelastic NiTi wires, **B** retrieved superelastic NiTi wires, **C** as received heat-activated NiTi wires, and **D** retrieved heat-activated NiTi wires

Some SEM micrographs are shown in Fig. 3. SEM images demonstrated surface textures for each type of wires in the "as received" state, with an apparent greater surface roughness for the heat-activated wires. It was felt that more complicated surface textures were seen after clinical exposure for each of the two types of wires.

AFM analysis provided microscopic information on the surface structure that plot topographies representing the wires' surface relief. Figures 4 and 5 show the 2D and 3D AFM microphotographs, respectively. The results of AFM surface analyses are given in Table 1.

In the control group "as received" superelastic wires showed less average surface roughness (55.73 nm) than heat-activated ones (86.05 nm) and the difference was statistically significant ($P < 0.001$). Following clinical exposure, the average surface roughness of superelastic and heat-activated wires significantly increased to become 81.47 ($P < 0.001$) and 98.68 nm ($P = 0.020$), respectively.

Though less rough surfaces were recorded for the superelastic wires after clinical exposure as compared with heat-activated wires ($P = 0.002$), the mean increase of roughness for the superelastic wires (+25.74 nm) was statistically greater than that of the heat-activated ones (+12.63 nm; $P < 0.001$).

Nickel ions' release

As shown in Table 2, the mean nickel release from "as received" heat-activated wires (8.36 ppb) was insignificantly less than that of the "as received" superelastic wires (7.92 ppb; $P = 5.556$). Following clinical exposure, less nickel ions were released from superelastic wires (5.81 ppb) compared to the same wires in the "as received" state ($P = 0.005$). A similar result was observed for the heat-activated wires (5.65 ppb; $P = 0.008$). Less nickel ions were released from the heat-activated wires after clinical exposure as compared with superelastic wires with no significant difference ($P = 0.837$).

Discussion

This study seems to be the first cross-over ex vivo study that compares superelastic and heat-activated NiTi wires apart from orthodontic forces. Wire segments were placed without inducing any actual tooth movement in a similar way to what was proposed by Marques et al. [12].

Table 1 Average surface roughness of the superelastic NiTi group and the heat-activated NiTi group before ("as received") and after ("retrieved") clinical exposure

Average surface roughness, nm	Superelastic NiTi group ($n = 24$)			Heat-activated NiTi group ($n = 24$)			*P* value between the two groups
	Mean	SD	*P* value in the same group	Mean	SD	*P* value in the same group	
"as received"	55.73	14.04	<0.001	86.05	13.58	0.020	<0.001
"retrieved"	81.47	10.11		98.68	13.38		0.002
Difference between "as received" and "retrieved"	+25.74	10.50		+12.63	8.80		<0.001

SD standard deviation

Table 2 Average nickel ions' release from the superelastic NiTi group and the heat-activated NiTi group before ("as received") and after ("retrieved") clinical exposure

Average nickel ions' release, ppb	Superelastic NiTi group ($n = 24$)			Heat-activated NiTi group ($n = 24$)			*P* value between the two groups
	Mean	SD	*P* value in the same group	Mean	SD	*P* value in the same group	
"as received"	8.36	1.81	0.005	7.92	1.89	0.008	NS
"retrieved"	5.81	2.14		5.65	1.6		NS
Difference between "as received" and "retrieved"	−2.55	1.54		−2.27	1.10		NS

SD standard deviation, *NS* not significant

Neither volunteers nor researcher nor data analyzer knew the wire type in each side (triple blindness) in order to increase the validity of the conducted work.

Similar to previous reports, SEM micrographs revealed only descriptive characteristics of wires' surfaces, whereas AFM images provided us with numeric values of the surface roughness and reconstructed three-dimensional images suitable for quantifying different aspects of micromorphology [23, 31, 32].

More rough texture was found in the non-used heat-activated NiTi wires when compared with superelastic ones. This could be attributed to the different procedures applied on heat-activated wires during manufacturing or tumbling and pickling stage. Other papers that reported the opposite finding [23, 24] compared the two types of wires but from different manufacturers with different chemical compositions.

Surface integrity of both types of NiTi wires were affected by oral environment conditions, i.e., temperature and pH variations, flora, masticatory and brushing forces, etc. The data from AFM showed an increase of 25.74 nm in superelastic NiTi wires' roughness (i.e., 46.2 % increase) and an increase of 12.63 nm in heat-activated NiTi wires' roughness (i.e., 14.7 % increase). This confirms the fact that crevice corrosion happened or calcified protein capsule was formed on the retrieved wires [6]. Other studies which demonstrated that there was no effect of clinical use on the NiTi roughness either used optical microscopy and/or SEM only [6, 11] or applied multiple disinfection procedures on wires before AFM measurements [25] that may have affected the accuracy of their results.

This study showed that heat-activated NiTi wires withstood oral conditions to a greater extent and the increase in their surface roughness was less than that recorded in the superelastic ones. This could be due to the fact that heat-activated NiTi wires used in this study had been originally fabricated to express all memory shape properties in 35 °C, whereas the superelastic archwires were not constructed to react favorably against different oral temperature variations. However, both types of wires maintained an acceptable degree of fine surface topography after clinical exposure based on the classification of Bourauel et al. [28], due to the fact that all Sa values were less than 200 nm at the final assessment.

Several factors that may have changed the current picture of results were not included in this study. The period of clinical use in our study was 30 days only, and this duration might be considered relatively short by some authors. The attached wires to braces were set neutrally and did not apply any active forces to the teeth. In addition, there were no big molecular changes on the archwire structure since superelastic wires were not exposed to stress and heat-activated wires were not exposed to cooling.

Though nickel is considered a toxic and cariogenic element, it is an essential component of orthodontic wires [15]. This made the biocompatibility of NiTi wires an important issue for researchers [11, 15, 33]. It is difficult to determine the exact amount of released nickel from NiTi wires in the oral cavity. So, in order to measure the potential release of nickel from NiTi wires in artificial saliva, a GF-AAS was used which is considered a reliable device in detecting released ions in a liquid sample by particle per billion [33–35].

An interaction was recorded between the nickel-titanium alloy and the surrounding environment (i.e., the artificial saliva) and both new superelastic and heat-activated NiTi wires released nickel ions. This is a support to the notion that this alloy is not an inert one [19]. Only tiny amounts of Ni ions were detected when evaluating unused superelastic and heat-activated NiTi wires (8.36 and 7.92 ppb, respectively). This may be because of the redundant Ni ions on the wires' surfaces [19], those Ni ions unlinked to Ti in both types of wires ("used" and "unused") could be easily released in artificial saliva. Kuhta et al. [36] found that superelastic NiTi wires released more Ni than heat-activated NiTi wires, but they studied wires from different manufacturers and immersed them in a different artificial saliva than that used in the current study.

After clinical exposure, GF-AAS detected less Ni ions released in artificial saliva from both types of wires with decrease of 2.55 ppb from superelastic NiTi wires that equals to −30.5 % and with decrease of 2.72 ppb from heat-activated NiTi wires that equals to −28.6 % that indicates a partial damage of the titanium oxide protecting layer causing the release of other alloy components [20]. This is the same result that Gil et al. [37] found after incurring NiTi wires to thermal sterilization treatments.

They attributed the decline of released nickel in the reused archwires to depletion of nickel matrix caused by the precipitation of Ti_3Ni_4.

In order to understand this decrease in the Ni released ions from clinically exposed NiTi wires in the current study, it should be noted that the breaking of titanium oxide layer usually occurs in high rates in the first day of exposure to a corrosive conditions because of the attack from the oral environment conditions [11, 26]; while after 30 days of clinical exposure, a regrowth of passive film takes place [4, 26, 38]. Probably, the release of nickel ions from the surface oxide film on NiTi completed during clinical exposure and the composition of the oxide film changed with a less content of nickel. Since only small preexisted surface defects were detected on the wires' surface, this may have helped in the regrowth process of the oxide layer to take place [18].

Fortunately, both types of NiTi wires released very small concentrations of Ni ions which were below the toxic levels [15, 39] that would impair the chemotaxis of leukocytes and motivate neutrophils to become aspherical and move slowly [40]. Ni ion concentrations were also below the critical value necessary to induce allergy [18, 41], and the current results go in line with the results of other researchers who have considered the NiTi alloy a safe and biocompatible material when used in the oral cavity [20, 41–43].

Conclusions

This study showed that new heat-activated NiTi wires had more rough surfaces than superelastic NiTi wires, whereas both types released almost the same tiny amounts of Ni ions in the artificial saliva. NiTi wires' surface roughness significantly increased after clinical exposure, whereas the amount of their released Ni ions in the artificial saliva decreased; an increase of surface roughness was observed to a greater extent in superelastic NiTi wires compared to the heat-activated ones, whereas the difference between them regarding the decrease of Ni ions' release following oral exposure was not significant.

Competing interests

The authors declare that they have no competing interests.

Authors' contributions

AAG was the principal researcher, who carried out volunteers' requirement, bonding the experimental set intraorally, participated in the sequence experiments, performed the statistical analysis, and drafted the manuscript. MYH participated in coordinating the study project and helped in drafting and revising the written work. RA was the principal research supervisor and participated in the study design. IA carried out the wires' morphology assessment. AA carried out the nickel ions' release assessment. All authors read and approved the final manuscript.

Authors' information

AAG is an orthodontist and a clinical lecturer at University of Hama Dental School, Hama, Syria. MYH is an associate professor of orthodontics, Department of Orthodontics, University of Damascus Dental School, Damascus, Syria. RA is a professor of orthodontics, Department of Orthodontics, University of Hama Dental School, Hama, Syria. IA is an associate professor of nanotechnology, leader of the nanotechnology activity, Physics Department, Faculty of Sciences, University of Damascus, Damascus, Syria. AA is a PhD student and a supervisor of the Modern Chemistry Lab, Faculty of Veterinary, University of Hama, Syria.

Author details

[1]Department of Orthodontics, University of Hama Dental School, Hama, Syria. [2]Department of Orthodontics, University of Damascus Dental School, Damascus, Syria. [3]Nano Technology Lab, Physics Department, Faculty of Sciences, University of Damascus, Damascus, Syria. [4]Modern Chemistry Lab, Faculty of Veterinary, University of Hama, Hama, Syria.

References

1. Andreasen GF, Hilleman TB. An evaluation of 55 cobalt substituted nitinol wire for use in orthodontics. J Am Dent Assoc. 1971;82(6):1373–5.
2. van Leeuwen EJ, Maltha JC, Kuijpers-Jagtman AM. Tooth movement with light continuous and discontinuous forces in beagle dogs. Eur J Oral Sci. 1999;107(6):468–74.
3. Eliades G, Brantley WA. Instrumental techniques for study of orthodontic materials. In: Brantley WA, Eliades T, editors. Orthodontic materials: scientific and clinical aspects. Stuttgart, Germany: Thieme Medical Publishers; 2001. p. 50–74.
4. Eliades T. Orthodontic materials research and applications: part 2. Current status and projected future developments in materials and biocompatibility. Am J Orthod Dentofac Orthop. 2007;131(2):253–64.
5. House K, Sernetz F, Dymock D, Sandy JR, Ireland AJ. Corrosion of orthodontic appliances—should we care? Am J Orthod Dentofac Orthop. 2008;133(4):584–92.
6. Eliades T, Eliades G, Athanasiou AE, Bradley TG. Surface characterization of retrieved NiTi orthodontic archwires. Eur J Orthod. 2000;22(3):317–26.
7. Iijima M, Endo K, Ohno H, Yonekura Y, Mizoguchi I. Corrosion behavior and surface structure of orthodontic Ni-Ti alloy wires. Dent Mater J. 2001;20(1):103–13.
8. Eliades T, Athanasiou AE. In vivo aging of orthodontic alloys: implications for corrosion potential, nickel release, and biocompatibility. Angle Orthod. 2002;72(3):222–37.
9. Wichelhaus A, Geserick M, Hibst R, Sander FG. The effect of surface treatment and clinical use on friction in NiTi orthodontic wires. Dent Mater. 2005;21(10):938–45.
10. Zinelis S, Eliades T, Pandis N, Eliades G, Bourauel C. Why do nickel-titanium archwires fracture intraorally? Fractographic analysis and failure mechanism of in-vivo fractured wires. Am J Orthod Dentofac Orthop. 2007;132(1):84–9.
11. Petoumeno E, Kislyuk M, Hoederath H, Keilig L, Bourauel C, Jäger A. Corrosion susceptibility and nickel release of nickel titanium wires during clinical application. J Orofac Orthop. 2008;69(6):411–23.
12. Marques IS, Araújo AM, Gurgel JA, Normando D. Debris, roughness and friction of stainless steel archwires following clinical use. Angle Orthod. 2010;80(3):521–7.
13. Oshida Y, Sachdeva RCL, Miyazaki S. Microanalytical characterization and surface modification of TiNi orthodontic archwires. Biomed Mater Eng. 1992;2(2):51–69.
14. Faccioni F, Franceschetti P, Cerpelloni M, Fracasso ME. In vivo study on metal release from fixed orthodontic appliances and DNA damage in oral mucosa cells. Am J Orthod Dentofac Orthop. 2003;124(6):687–93.
15. Ortiz AJ, Fernández E, Vicente A, Calvo JL, Ortiz C. Metallic ions released from stainless steel, nickel-free, and titanium orthodontic alloys: toxicity and DNA damage. Am J Orthod Dentofac Orthop. 2011;140(3):e115–22.
16. Mikulewicz M, Chojnacka K, Woźniak B, Downarowicz P. Release of metal ions from orthodontic appliances: an in vitro study. Biol Trace Elem Res. 2012;146(2):272–80.
17. Galeotti A, Uomo R, Spagnuolo G, Paduano S, Cimino R, Valletta R, et al. Effect of pH on in vitro biocompatibility of orthodontic miniscrew implants. Prog Orthod. 2013;1:14–5.

18. HUANG HH, CHIU YH, LEE TH, Wu SC, Yang HW, Su KH, et al. Ion release from NiTi orthodontic wires in artificial saliva with various acidities. Biomaterials. 2003;24(20):3585–92.
19. Arndt M, Brück A, Scully T, Jäger A, Bourauel C. Nickel ion release from orthodontic NiTi wires under simulation of realistic in-situ conditions. J Mater Sci. 2005;40(14):3659–67.
20. Mikulewicz M, Chojnacka K. Release of metal ions from orthodontic appliances by in vitro studies: a systematic literature review. Biol Trace Elem Res. 2011;139(3):241–56.
21. Mikulewicz M, Chojnacka K, Wołowiec P. Release of metal ions from fixed orthodontic appliance: an in vitro study in continuous flow system. Angle Orthod. 2014;84(1):140–8.
22. Mikulewicz M, Wołowiec P, Janeczek M, Gedrange T, Chojnacka K. The release of metal ions from orthodontic appliances: animal tests. Angle Orthod. 2014;84(4):673–9.
23. D'Antò V, Rongo R, Ametrano G, Spagnuolo G, Manzo P, Martina R, et al. Evaluation of surface roughness of orthodontic wires by means of atomic force microscopy. Angle Orthod. 2012;82(5):922–8.
24. Perinetti G, Contardo L, Ceschi M, Antoniolli F, Franchi L, Baccetti T, et al. Surface corrosion and fracture resistance of two nickel-titanium-based archwires induced by fluoride, pH, and thermocycling. An in vitro comparative study. Eur J Orthod. 2012;34(1):1–9.
25. Alcock JP, Barbour ME, Sandy JR, Ireland AJ. Nanoindentation of orthodontic archwires: the effect of decontamination and clinical use on hardness, elasticmodulus and surface roughness. Dent Mater. 2009;25(8):1039–43.
26. Liu JK, Lee TM, Liu IH. Effect of loading force on the dissolution behavior and surface properties of nickel-titanium orthodontic archwires in artificial saliva. Am J Orthod Dentofac Orthop. 2011;140(2):166–76.
27. Löe H, Silness J. Periodontal disease in pregnancy. I. Prevalence and severity. Acta Odontol Scand. 1963;21:533–51.
28. Bourauel C, Fries T, Drescher D, Plietsch R. Surface roughness of orthodontic wires via atomic force microscopy, laser specular reflectance, and profilometry. Eur J Orthod. 1998;20(1):79–92.
29. Huang HH. Variation in corrosion resistance of nickel-titanium wires from different manufacturers. Angle Orthod. 2005;75(4):661–5.
30. Baričević M, Mravak-Stipetić M, Stanimirović A, Blanuša M, Kern J, Lončar B, et al. Salivary concentrations of nickel and chromium in patients with burning mouth syndrome. Acta Dermatovenerol Croat. 2011;19(1):2–5.
31. Rongo R, Ametrano G, Gloria A, Spagnuolo G, Galeotti A, Paduano S, et al. Effects of intraoral aging on surface properties of coated nickel-titanium archwires. Angle Orthod. 2014;84(4):665–72.
32. Chng CK, Foong K, Gandedkar NH, Chan YH, Chew CL. A new esthetic fiber-reinforced polymer composite resin archwire: comparative atomic force microscope (AFM) and field-emission scanning electron microscope (FESEM) study. Prog Orthod. 2014;15(1):39.
33. Jia W, Beatty MW, Reinhardt RA, Petro TM, Cohen DM, Maze CR, et al. Nickel release from orthodontic arch wires and cellular immune response to various nickel concentrations. J Biomed Mater Res. 1999;48(4):488–95.
34. Peitsch T, Klocke A, Kahl-Nieke B, Prymak O, Epple M. The release of nickel from orthodontic NiTi wires is increased by dynamic mechanical loading but not constrained by surface nitridation. J Biomed Mater Res. 2007;82(3):731–9.
35. El-Wassefy N, El-Fallal A, Taha M. Effect of different sterilization modes on the surface morphology, ion release, and bone reaction of retrieved micro-implants. Angle Orthod. 2015;85(1):39–47.
36. Kuhta M, Pavlin D, Slaj M, Varga S, Lapter-Varga M, Slaj M. Type of archwire and level of acidity: effects on the release of metal ions from orthodontic appliances. Angle Orthod. 2009;79(1):102–10.
37. Gil FJ, Espinar E, Llamas JM, Manero JM, Ginebra MP. Variation of the superelastic properties and nickel release from original and reused NiTi orthodontic archwires. J Mech Behav Biomed Mater. 2012;6:113–9.
38. Eliades T. Passive film growth on titanium alloy: physico-chemical and biologic considerations. Int J Oral Maxillofac Implants. 1997;12(5):621–7.
39. Delescluse J, Dinet Y. Nickel allergy in Europe: the new European legislation. Dermatology. 1994;189 Suppl 2:56–7.
40. Vreeburg KJ, de Groot K, von Blomberg M, Scheper RJ. Induction of immunological tolerance by oral administration of nickel and chromium. J Dent Res. 1984;63(2):124–8.
41. Setcos JC, Babaei-Mahani A, Silvio LD, Mjör IA, Wilson NH. The safety of nickel containing dental alloys. Dent Mater. 2006;22(12):1163–8.
42. Suárez C, Vilar T, Gil J, Sevilla P. In vitro evaluation of surface topographic changes and nickel release of lingual orthodontic archwires. J Mater Sci Mater Med. 2010;21(2):675–83.
43. Senkutvan RS, Jacob S, Charles A, Vadgaonkar V, Jatol-Tekade S, Gangurde P. Evaluation of nickel ion release from various orthodontic arch wires: an in vitro study. J Int Soc Prev Community Dent. 2014;4(1):12–6.

Cephalometric study to test the reliability of anteroposterior skeletal discrepancy indicators using the twin block appliance

Rahul Trivedi[1], Amit Bhattacharya[1], Falguni Mehta[1], Dolly Patel[2], Harshik Parekh[1] and Vaibhav Gandhi[1*]

Abstract

Background: The objectives of this study were to check the reliability of the five angular and two linear parameters for sagittal maxillo-mandibular discrepancy and to compare and correlate angular parameters with the ANB angle, and the linear parameter with Wits analysis.

Methods: The pre-treatment and post-functional lateral cephalograms of 25 subjects (17 males, 8 females) with class II division 1 malocclusion treated with twin block functional appliance were selected. Five angular (ANB, β angle, APDI, YEN angle, W angle) and two linear (Wits analysis, App-Bpp) parameters were traced on both sets of cephalograms. Paired Student's *t*-test, one-way ANOVA, *post hoc* test, and Karl Pearson correlation statistical analysis were performed.

Results: All the parameters considered in our study showed highly significant difference in pre-treatment and post-functional values, suggesting their reliability ($p < 0.0001$). When ANB angle was compared with the other angular parameters, a highly significant change in the mean value of the difference in pre-treatment (T1) and post-functional (T2) values was noted ($p < 0.001$). No significant change was seen when comparing the mean value of the difference in T1 and T2 between linear parameters ($p = 0.949$).

Conclusions: All the parameters used in the study can be reliably used to assess anteroposterior skeletal discrepancy. Whenever limitations of the ANB angle and Wits analysis are foreseen, the W angle and App-Bpp, respectively, can be reliably used. The YEN angle may reliably predict the post-functional change with the use of twin block appliance.

Keywords: Anteroposterior discrepancy parameters; Twin block; Lateral cephalogram; Reliability

Background

Patients seeking orthodontic treatment frequently fall in the skeletal class II category. The National Health and Nutrition Examination Survey estimated, based on overjet, that approximately 14.7% of the US population has class II malocclusion, with prevalence decreasing from 22.6% between 8 and 11 years of age, to 15.6% between 12 and 17 years of age and then to 13.4% between 18 and 50 years of age [1]. The National Center for Health Statistics reported that 20.4% of 6- to 11-year-olds have bilateral class II molar relationships, compared with 14.5% of 12- to 17-year-olds [2,3]. The prevalence of skeletal class II type of malocclusion in the Indian population is 14.6% for the age group of 10 to 13 years, 6% for the age group of 5 to 9 years, and 3.8% for the age group of 6 to 14 years [4]. Although maxillary protrusion and mandibular retrognathism are both found to be possible causative factors, McNamara reported mandibular retrognathism to be more common for skeletal class II malocclusion [5].

Evaluation of anteroposterior jaw discrepancy for diagnosis and treatment planning is one of the primary requirements in the field of orthodontics. Numerous authors have tried to assess the sagittal skeletal relationship using various landmarks, starting from Riedel (ANB angle) [6], Jacobson (Wits analysis) [7], Nanda

* Correspondence: smiledesigner1988@gmail.com
[1]Department of Orthodontics, Government Dental College and Hospital, Asarva, Ahmedabad, 380016, Gujarat, India
Full list of author information is available at the end of the article

Table 1 Short description of various parameters used in the study

Parameter	Short description
ANB	The angle formed by the intersection of the point A to N (nasion) line and the point B to N (nasion) line (Figure 1)
β angle	A perpendicular is dropped from point A to a line drawn from C (center of condyle) to point B. β angle is the angle between this perpendicular and the A-B line (Figure 2)
YEN angle	Angle between the S (sella) to M (center of the premaxilla) line and the M to D (center of the symphysis) line (Figure 3)
W angle	A perpendicular is dropped from M to the S-D line. W angle is measured between this perpendicular and the M-D line (Figure 4)
APDI	(NPg-FH plane) ± (NPg-AB) ± (FH-palatal plane) (Figure 5)
Wits appraisal	Distance between the projection of point A and point B on the occlusal plane (Figure 6)
App-Bpp	Distance between the projection of point A and point B on the palatal plane (Figure 6)

and Merrill (App-Bpp) [8], Baik and Ververidou (β angle) [9], Kim and Vietas (APDI) [10], Neela et al. (YEN angle) [11], Bhad (W angle) [12], etc. The ANB angle and Wits analysis are still one of the most commonly and reliably used parameters in assessing maxillo-mandibular relation, although there is not a single diagnostic test or cephalometric measurement that has been accepted to be used as the 'gold standard' for defining class II or class III skeletal patterns [13-16]. Accurate location of the cephalometric landmarks, growth changes, orthodontic treatment, etc. may influence the accurate assessment of the sagittal skeletal discrepancy. Limitations of these measurements add to the confusion regarding the reliability of these parameters to assess anteroposterior jaw discrepancy.

The treatment for class II malocclusion varies from skeletal growth modification to camouflage to orthognathic surgery depending upon the age of the patient. It is a well-known fact that the twin block appliance developed by Clark is an effective class II corrector in skeletal growth modification [17-19]. Although many studies have been carried out and documented showing anteroposterior skeletal assessment with twin block appliance,

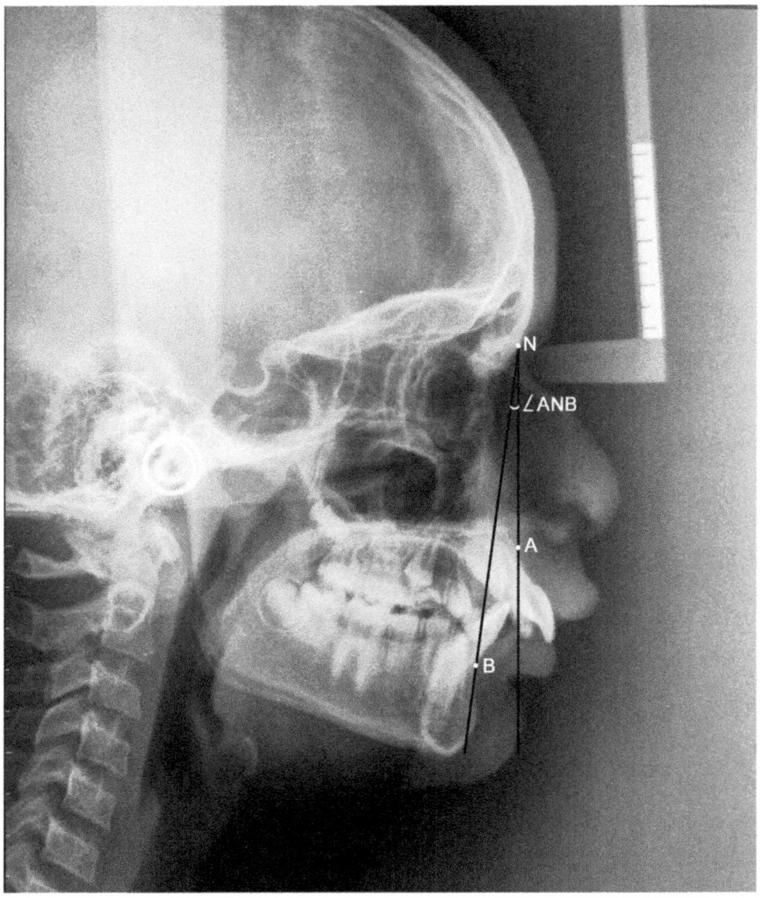

Figure 1 Angular parameter ANB.

no study has been conducted comparing and correlating all the parameters of sagittal changes using twin block. So it was considered worthwhile to do quantitative appraisal of the reliability of five angular and two linear sagittal skeletal discrepancy parameters to assess the result of using twin block appliance for correction of class II malocclusion. Taking the above stated fact into consideration, it was decided to assess the change in the maxillo-mandibular relation using five angular (ANB angle, APDI, β angle, W angle, YEN angle) and two linear (Wits analysis and App-Bpp) anteroposterior discrepancy parameters in patients who were treated with the twin block appliance.

The objectives of the study thus were as follows:

- To check the reliability of the angular and linear parameters considered in our study
- To compare and correlate the angular parameters
- To compare and correlate the linear parameters
- To evaluate which of the above parameters best predicts the sagittal correction after twin block therapy

Methods

The present cephalometric study was undertaken from the records available in the Department of Orthodontics Govt. Dental College and Hospital. Twenty-five cases (17 males, 8 females) in the age range of 11 to 14 years having CVMI in stages III and IV who fulfilled the following inclusion criteria were selected for the study:

1. Angle's class II division 1 malocclusion as evaluated from the dental study casts
2. ANB angle greater than 4° with mandibular deficiency
3. Overjet ranging from 6 to 15 mm with a mean of 10 mm
4. No prior orthodontic treatment
5. Subjects treated with only removable twin block functional appliance

All subjects were given modified twin block appliance with jack screw and labial bow incorporated in the maxillary plate. They were regularly called for follow-up and evaluated for sagittal correction. After bilateral molar class I reduction in overjet and after significant improvement in profile was achieved, post-functional records were made.

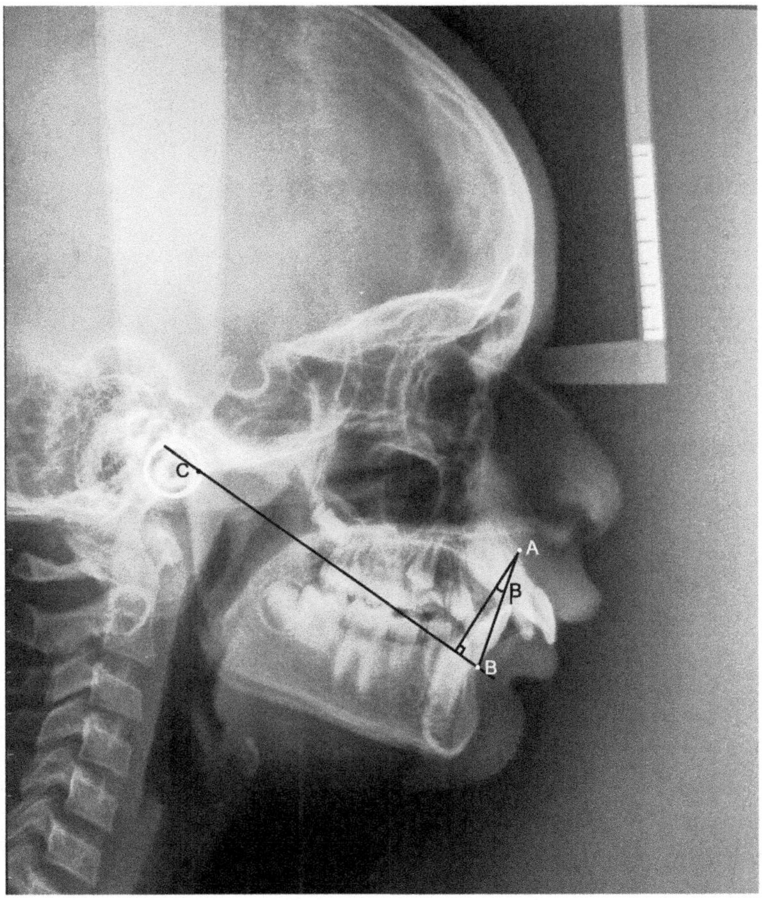

Figure 2 Angular parameter β angle.

The average treatment time of twin block functional appliance therapy was 11 months.

Pre-treatment (T1) and post-functional (T2) lateral cephalograms were obtained and traced by a single operator. Five angular and two linear parameters were taken for both sets of cephalograms and were compared and evaluated.

The angular parameters used were as follows (Table 1):

- ANB angle (Figure 1)
- β angle (Figure 2)
- YEN angle (Figure 3)
- W angle (Figure 4)
- APDI (Figure 5)

The linear parameters used were as follows (Figure 6, Table 1):

- Wits analysis
- App-Bpp

The resultant data was subjected to statistical analysis. Paired sample *t*-test was performed to evaluate the differences in the pre-treatment (T1) and post-functional (T2) values (Table 2) in the angular and linear parameters. ANOVA (Table 3) and Tukey HSD *post hoc* test (Table 4) for multiple comparisons were done to evaluate change in the mean of the difference between T1 and T2 values of the parameters. Correlations between angular parameters and linear parameters were assessed using the Karl Pearson correlation coefficient test (Table 5). The ability of a parameter to predict the probable change in the sagittal plane after treatment with the twin block appliance was evaluated using regression equations as well as the standard error of the estimate (Table 6). r, the multiple correlation coefficient, is the linear correlation between the observed and model-predicted values of the dependent variable. r^2, the coefficient of determination, is the squared value of the multiple correlation coefficient. It shows that about half the variation in time is explained by the model.

Approval for this study was obtained from the institutional review board of the Govt. Dental College and Hospital, Ahmedabad, with informed consents from the parents or guardians of all subjects.

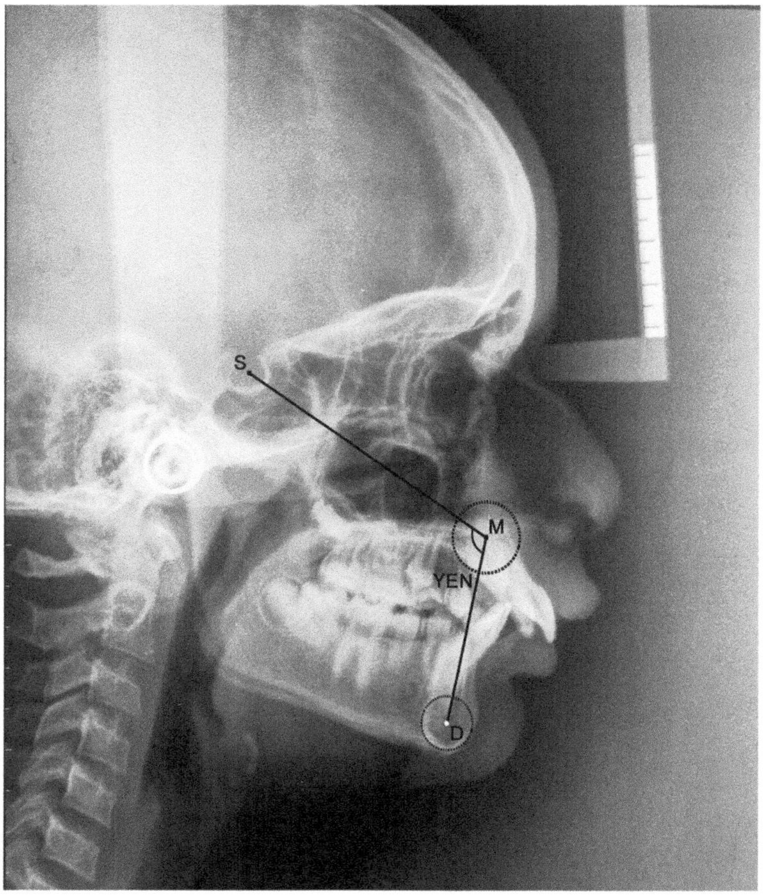

Figure 3 Angular parameter YEN angle.

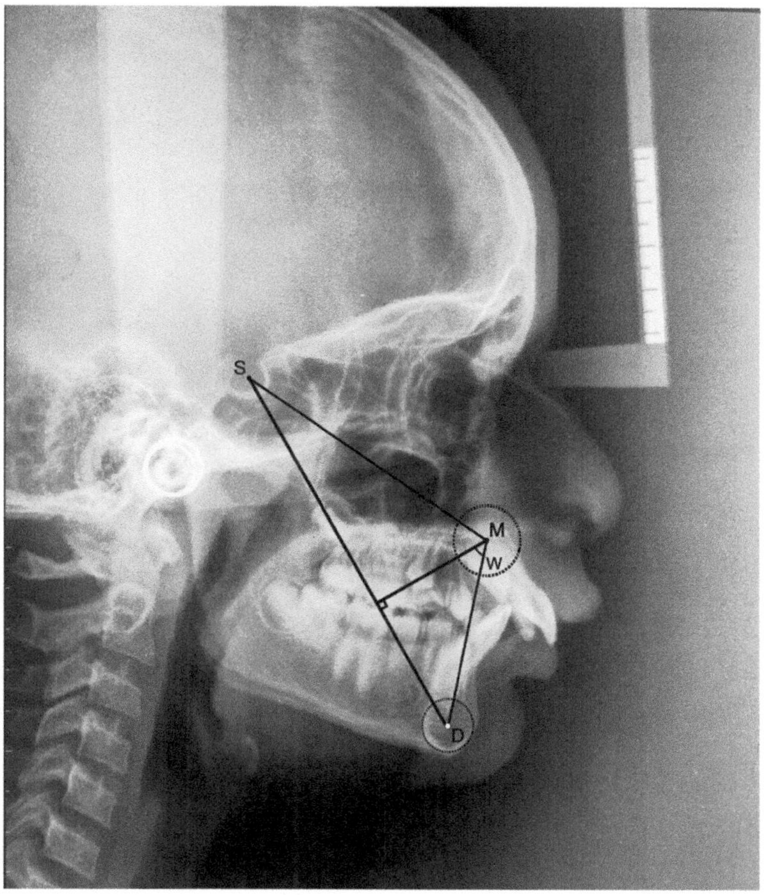

Figure 4 Angular parameter W angle.

Results and discussion

Paired sample *t*-test results showed highly significant changes between T1 and T2 for all the seven anteroposterior discrepancy parameters ($p < 0.0001$) (Table 2).

The ANOVA test showed the variation in the mean of the difference between T1 and T2 of all seven parameters to be highly significant ($p < 0.0001$) (Table 3).

Furthermore, when the ANB angle was compared with the other four angular parameters, a highly significant change in the mean of the difference between T1 and T2 values was noted (Table 4).

No significant change was seen when comparing the mean of the difference between T1 and T2 of the linear parameters ($p = 0.949$) (Table 5).

The change in the mean of the difference between T1 and T2 was highly significant for the β angle and YEN angle, β angle and W angle, and APDI and W angle ($p < 0.0001$) and were non-significant for the β angle and APDI ($p = 0.927$), and YEN angle and W angle ($p = 0.982$) (Table 4).

The Karl Pearson correlation test showed moderately negative but significant correlations for the angular parameters when they were compared to the ANB angle (Table 4). The highest correlations of all angular parameters compared with the ANB were observed for the W angle ($r = -0.613$). Moderately positive and significant correlation between App-Bpp and Wits analysis was also noted (Table 5). Strongly positive and highly significant correlations were observed only between the YEN angle and W angle ($r = 0.894$, $p < 0.0001$) (Table 5).

Regression equation analysis calculated for the YEN angle ($Y = 0.940*X + 11.697$) had the highest correlation coefficient ($r = 0.86$, $r^2 = 0.74$). The standard error of the estimate was found to be least for ANB (0.95) (Table 6).

In our study, changes in the anteroposterior plane were assessed in the same group of patients after giving them a functional appliance, thus removing the subject error. The ultimate goals of this study were to assess the reliability of five angular and two linear sagittal skeletal discrepancy parameters and to compare and correlate the angular parameters (β angle, APDI, W angle, and YEN angle) with the universally accepted ANB angle, and the linear parameter App-Bpp with Wits analysis, as indicators of successful twin block therapy in growing subjects.

The primary objective to use twin block appliance was because it is a proven potent class II corrector [17-19].

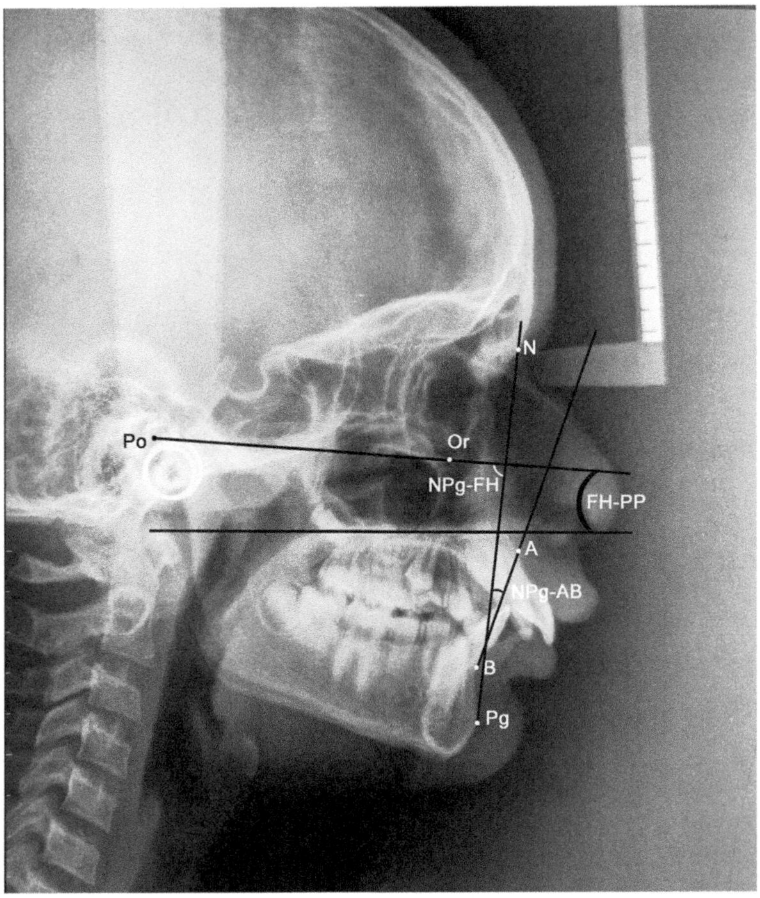

Figure 5 Angular parameter APDI.

Table 2 shows that there is a highly significant change in the pre-treatment (T1) and post-functional (T2) values of all the seven parameters considered in our study ($p = <0.0001$), suggesting that the sagittal change produced by the twin block is assessed accurately by all the seven parameters, thus confirming that any of the above parameters can be used reliably to assess antero-posterior discrepancy.

One of the oldest and widely used parameter is the ANB angle [6]; however, the stability of the nasion point is questionable as shown in growth studies by Nanda [20]. The rotation of the head sideways or upwards, rotation of the jaws either due to growth or orthodontic treatment, and rotation of the S-N plane also can affect the value of the ANB angle. Position of point A is affected by alveolar bone remodeling associated with orthodontic tooth movement of the upper incisor. Binder proposed that even the change in the vertical distance between points A and B without any change in the sagittal position may affect the ANB angle [21]. But the results of recent studies indicate that the ANB angle is still a reliable indicator to assess anteroposterior skeletal change before and after treatment, in spite of its limitation in diagnosis [22].

According to Table 3, 4, and 5, results showed that all the angular parameters vary independent of the ANB angle. Thus, it is suggested that when the abovementioned limitations of the ANB angle are anticipated, any of the other angular parameters such as the β angle (mean difference = −12.40, $r = -0.527$), APDI (mean difference = −11.60, $r = -0.420$), W angle (mean difference = −8.04, $r = -0.613$), YEN angle (mean difference = −8.64, $r = -0.445$), and especially W angle can be used to assess anteroposterior skeletal discrepancy as the limitations of the ANB angle are less likely to influence their values. Ishikawa et al. in their study found similar values for ANB and APDI [23]. Among the angular parameters considered, the W angle showed the highest correlation with the ANB angle (mean difference = −8.04, $p = < 0.0001$, $r = -0.613$).

Owing to the limitations of ANB, Jacobson came up with the Wits analysis [7]. Comparison of the linear parameters (Wits analysis and App-Bpp) from Tables 4 and 5 suggests that they do not vary independent of each other (mean difference = −0.74, $p = 0.949$, $r = 0.475$) which indicates a non-significant correlation between Wits and App-Bpp. Therefore, in cases where Wits analysis does

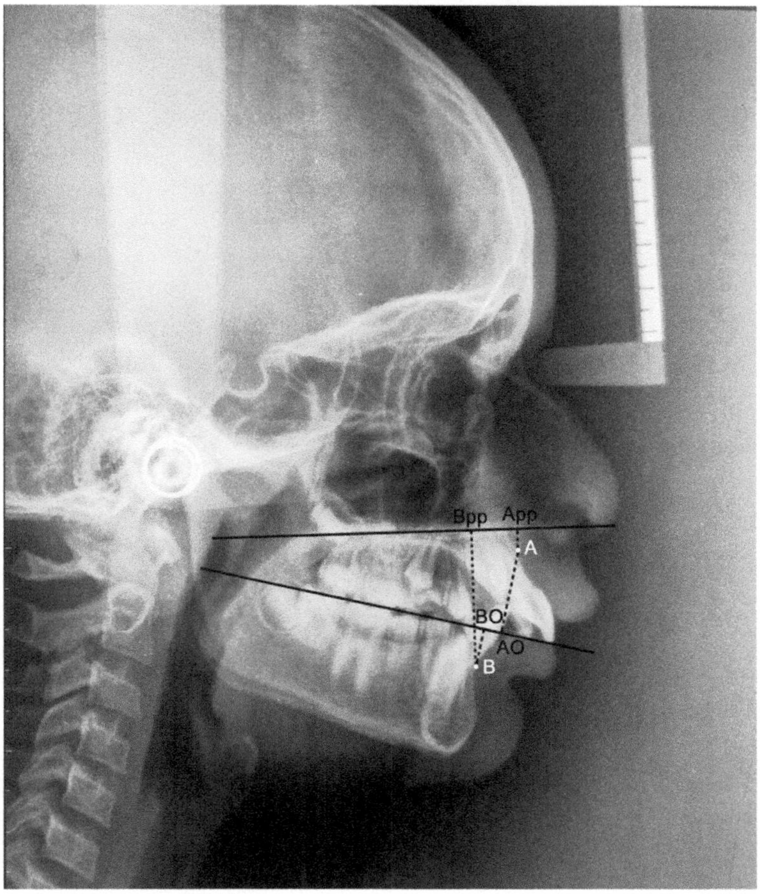

Figure 6 Linear parameters App-Bpp and Wits appraisal.

Table 2 Paired sample *t*-test comparing pre-treatment (T1) and post-functional (T2) values

	Mean	*N*	Standard deviation	Standard error of the mean	Mean difference	*p* value
ANB angle (T1)	7.36	25	1.469	0.294	−3.84	<0.0001*
ANB angle (T2)	3.52	25	1.388	0.278		
Wits appraisal (T1)	6.72	25	2.092	0.418	−5.46	<0.0001*
Wits appraisal (T2)	1.26	25	1.849	0.37		
β angle (T1)	19.12	25	3.153	0.631	8.56	<0.0001*
β angle (T2)	27.68	25	3.024	0.605		
APDI (T1)	70.2	25	3.64	0.728	7.76	<0.0001*
APDI (T2)	77.96	25	3.702	0.74		
App-Bpp (T1)	12.52	25	2.801	0.56	−4.72	<0.0001*
App-Bpp (T2)	7.8	25	2.179	0.436		
YEN angle (T1)	114.12	25	4.799	0.96	4.8	<0.0001*
YEN angle (T2)	118.92	25	5.227	1.045		
W angle (T1)	49.52	25	3.38	0.676	4.2	<0.0001*
W angle (T2)	53.72	25	3.361	0.672		

T1, pre-treatment; T2, post-functional; $*p \leq 0.05$ = significant.

Table 3 Analysis of variance test between the parameters

Parameter	N		Mean	Standard deviation	Standard error
ANB angle	25		−3.84	1.028	0.206
Wits appraisal	25		−5.46	2.291	0.458
β angle	25		8.56	3.097	0.619
APDI	25		7.76	3.767	0.753
App-Bpp	25		−4.72	2.132	0.426
YEN angle	25		4.80	2.661	0.532
W angle	25		4.20	2.102	0.420
Total	175		1.61	6.194	0.468
	Sum of squares	***Df***	**Mean square**	***F***	**Overall ANOVA *p* value**
Difference between parameters	5,569.134	6	928.189	140.853	<0.0001*
Total	6,676.214	174			

*$p \leq 0.05$ = significant.

not accurately depict the maxillo-mandibular relationship, App-Bpp also may give erroneous readings. However, since Wits analysis utilizes the occlusal plane, the value can be easily affected due to orthodontic treatment and incomplete tooth eruption. Accurate identification of the occlusal plane and its reproducibility in mixed dentition, open bite, canted occlusal plane, multiple impactions, and skeletal asymmetry subjects is difficult [24]. The palatal plane is considered to be more stable than the occlusal plane [8]. Thus, in cases where identification of anatomic landmarks required for Wits analysis is not clear, it is suggested to use App-Bpp in lieu of Wits analysis. However, when the palatal plane is severely tipped, App-Bpp may also give erroneous readings [8]. In such instances, Wits analysis can be used reliably.

According to Tables 4 and 5, it is suggested that either the YEN angle or W angle can be used to assess skeletal anteroposterior discrepancy (mean difference = −0.6, $p = 0.982$, $r = 0.894$). With reference to the YEN angle, jaw rotations due to growth and treatment can mask true skeletal dysplasia [25]. The YEN angle requires accurate tracing of the premaxilla for its assessment. The W angle also requires accurate tracing of the premaxilla and locating its center, which is difficult. Also, determining which of the jaws is prognathic or retrognathic is difficult [12]. Thus, when accurate tracing of the premaxilla for the assessment of the W angle and YEN angle is not possible, the β angle can be used as it shows least correlation with the YEN angle and W angle (Tables 4 and 5).

No significant change in the mean of the difference between T1 and T2 values of the β angle and APDI was found (mean difference = 0.8, $p = 0.927$, $r = 0.455$) (Tables 4 and 5). The β angle uses the condylion as a reference point, but its identification on a closed mouth lateral cephalogram is difficult [26-28]. Thus, APDI can be used in lieu of the β angle when locating the condylion is difficult.

Table 4 *Post hoc* tests (Tukey HSD): multiple comparisons

Parameter	Parameter	Mean difference	Standard error	*p* value
ANB angle	β angle	−12.40	0.726	<0.0001*
ANB angle	APDI	−11.60	0.726	<0.0001*
ANB angle	YEN angle	−8.64	0.726	<0.0001*
ANB angle	W angle	−8.04	0.726	<0.0001*
Wits appraisal	App-Bpp	−0.74	0.726	0.949
β angle	APDI	0.80	0.726	0.927
β angle	YEN angle	3.76	0.726	<0.0001*
β angle	W angle	4.36	0.726	<0.0001*
APDI	YEN angle	2.96	0.726	0.001
APDI	W angle	3.56	0.726	<0.0001*
YEN angle	W angle	0.60	0.726	0.982

*$p \leq 0.05$ = significant.

Table 5 A correlation matrix for the seven parameters calculated with the Karl Pearson correlation test

	ANB angle	Wits appraisal	β angle	APDI	App-Bpp	YEN angle	W angle
ANB angle	Pearson correlation (*r*)	0.563	−0.527	−0.420	0.530	−0.445	−0.613
	Significance (two-tailed) (*p*)	0.003*	0.007*	0.037*	0.006*	0.026*	0.001*
	n		25	25	25	25	25
Wits appraisal	Pearson correlation (*r*)		−0.552	−0.185	0.475	−0.217	−0.383
	Significance (two-tailed) (*p*)		0.004*	0.377	0.016*	0.297	0.059
	n			25	25	25	25
β angle	Pearson correlation (*r*)			0.455	−0.441	0.328	0.424
	Significance (two-tailed) (*p*)			0.022*	0.027*	0.110	0.035*
	n				25	25	25
APDI	Pearson correlation (*r*)				−0.552	0.593	0.591
	Significance (two-tailed) (*p*)				0.004*	0.002*	0.002*
	n					25	25
App-Bpp	Pearson correlation (*r*)					−0.548	−0.655
	Significance (two-tailed) (*p*)					0.005*	0.0004*
	n						25
YEN angle	Pearson correlation (*r*)						0.894
	Significance (two-tailed) (*p*)						<0.0001*
	n						25
W angle	Pearson correlation (*r*)						
	Significance (two-tailed) (*p*)						
	n						

*$p \leq 0.05$ = significant.

The ability of the angular and linear parameters considered in our study to predict the amount of post-functional change in the maxillo-mandibular relation was analyzed with regression equations (Table 6), and it was found that the YEN angle may reliably predict post-functional change when twin block appliance is used. Strong predictability was also found for the W angle ($r = 0.81$, $r^2 = 0.65$) and ANB angle ($r = 0.74$, $r^2 = 0.55$). Although the ANB angle showed the least error (Table 6), it has to be kept in mind that the normal range in ANB for different classes of malocclusion is also relatively small. App-Bpp showed better predictability when compared to Wits analysis (Table 6). These results are in contrast to those of Ishikawa et al. for the parameters ANB, Wits, and APDI [23].

Whenever limitations of any of the parameters used in our study are expected to cloud the clinical judgment in assessing skeletal anteroposterior relationship, use of more than one parameter in conjunction with others as described in our study is suggested.

Conclusions

Twenty-five subjects were treated with twin block appliance, and the change in their maxillo-mandibular relation was assessed with five angular and two linear parameters.

Table 6 Correlation coefficient and regression equation

Parameter	*r*	r^2	Equation	Standard error of the estimate
ANB angle	0.74	0.55	$Y = 0.702^*X - 1.645$	0.95
Wits appraisal	0.33	0.11	$Y = 0.291^*X - 0.696$	1.78
β angle	0.50	0.25	$Y = 0.478^*X + 18.549$	2.68
APDI	0.47	0.22	$Y = 0.482^*X + 44.140$	3.33
App-Bpp	0.66	0.43	$Y = 0.513^*X + 1.375$	1.67
YEN angle	0.86	0.74	$Y = 0.940^*X + 11.697$	2.70
W angle	0.81	0.65	$Y = 0.801^*X + 14.059$	2.03

r, the multiple correlation coefficient; r^2, the coefficient of determination, is the squared value of the multiple correlation coefficient.

1. All the angular and linear parameters considered in our study are reliable in assessing skeletal sagittal discrepancy.
2. Recently advocated angular parameters, especially the W angle, can be used reliably in place of the ANB angle whenever drawbacks of the ANB angle are anticipated.
3. As the palatal plane is more stable than the occlusal plane, it is suggested to use App-Bpp instead of Wits analysis.
4. The YEN angle and W angle show the highest correlation among the parameters, which suggests that either of them can be used to assess anteroposterior jaw discrepancy.
5. Then YEN angle may reliably predict the post-functional change with the use of twin block appliance.

Abbreviations

T1: Pre-treatment; T2: Post-functional.

Competing interests

The authors declare that they have no competing interests.

Authors' contributions

RT carried out the initial drafting and framing of the study and the interpretation of data. AB carried out the analysis and interpretation of data. FM has been involved in the critical revision of the manuscript for important intellectual content and agreed to be accountable for all aspects of the work in ensuring that questions related to the accuracy or integrity of any part of the work are appropriately investigated and resolved. DP has been involved in the analysis and interpretation of data and final approval of the version to be published. HP carried out the analysis and interpretation of data. VG was involved in the data collection, drafting and framing of the study, analysis and interpretation, and preparation of the manuscript. All authors read and approved the final manuscript.

Author details

[1]Department of Orthodontics, Government Dental College and Hospital, Asarva, Ahmedabad, 380016, Gujarat, India. [2]AMC Dental College, Ahmedabad, 380008, Gujarat, India.

References

1. Proffit WR. Prevalence of malocclusion and orthodontic treatment need in the United States: estimates from the NHANES III survey. Int J Adult Orthod Orthognath Surg.1998;13:97–106.s
2. Kelly JE, Sanchez M, Van Kirk LE. An assessment of the occlusion of the teeth of children: 6–11 years. Vital and Health Statistics, series 11, number 130. Washington, DC: US Public Health Service; 1977.
3. Kelly JE, Harvey CR. An assessment of the occlusion of the teeth of youths: 12–17 years. Vital and Health Statistics, series 11, number 162. Washington, DC: US Public Health Service; 1977.
4. Kharbanda OP. Orthodontics: diagnosis and management of malocclusion and dentofacial deformities. New Delhi: Elsevier; 2013. p. 459.
5. McNamara JA. Components of class II malocclusion in children 8–10 years of age. Angle Orthod. 1981;51:177–202.
6. Riedel RA. The relation of maxillary structures to cranium in malocclusion and in normal occlusion. Angle Orthod. 1952;22:142–5.
7. Jacobson A. The "Wits" analysis of jaw disharmony. Am J Orthod. 1975;67(2):125–38.
8. Nanda RS, Merrill RM. Cephalometric assessment of sagittal relationship. Am J Orthod. 1994;105(4):328–44.
9. Baik CY, Ververidou M. A new approach of assessing sagittal discrepancies: the Beta angle. Am J Orthod. 2004;126:100–5.
10. Kim YH, Vietas JJ. Anteroposterior dysplasia indicator: an adjunct to cephalometric differential diagnosis. Am J Orthod. 1978;73:619–33.
11. Neela PK, Mascarenhas R, Husain A. A new sagittal dysplasia indicator: the YEN angle. World J Orthod. 2009;10:147–51.
12. Bhad WA, Nayak S, Doshi UH. A new approach of assessing sagittal dysplasia: the W angle. Eur J Orthod 2013(1):66–70.
13. Oktay H. Comparison of ANB, WITS, AF-BF, and APDI measurements. Am J Orthod Dentofacial Orthop. 1991;99:122–8.
14. Han UK, Kim YH. Determination of class II and class III skeletal patterns: receiver operating characteristic (ROC) analysis on various cephalometric measurements. Am J Orthod Dentofacial Orthop. 1998;113:538–45.
15. Moyers RE, Bookstein FL, Guire KE. The concept of pattern in craniofacial growth. Am J Orthod. 1979;76:136–48.
16. Nanda R. Biomechanics and esthetic strategies in clinical orthodontics. St. Louis: Elsevier; 2005. p. 38–73.
17. Mills CM, Mcculloch KJ. Treatment effects of the twin block appliance: a cephalometric study. Am J Orthod. 1998;114(1):15–24.
18. Mills CM, Mcculloch KJ. Posttreatment changes after successful correction of class II malocclusions with the twin block appliance. Am J Orthod. 2000;118(1):24–33.
19. Jena AK, Duggal R. Treatment effects of twin-block and mandibular protraction appliance-IV in the correction of class II malocclusion. Angle Orthod. 2010;80(3):485–91.
20. Hussels W, Nanda RS. Analysis of factors affecting angle ANB. Am J Orthod. 1984;85(5):411–23.
21. Binder RE. The geometry of cephalometrics. J Clin Orthod 1979;13;256–263.
22. Xu TM, Ahn J, Boyd RM, Baumrind S. Sensitivity of angular cephalometric measures. J Dent Res, 1997, 76 (special issue):160
23. Ishikawa H, Nakamura S, Iwasaki H, Kitazawa S. Seven parameters describing anteroposterior jaw relationships: postpubertal prediction accuracy and interchangeability. Am J Orthod Dentofacial Orthop 2000;117(6):714–20
24. Del Santo Jr M. Influence of occlusal plane inclination on ANB and Wits assessments of anteroposterior jaw relationships. Am J Orthod. 2006;129:641–8.
25. Ghafari J, Baumrind S, Efstratiadis SS. Misinterpreting growth and treatment outcome from serial cephalographs. Clin Orthod Res. 1998;1:102–6.
26. Adenwalla ST, Kronman JH, Attarzadeh F. Porion and condyle as cephalometric landmarks: an error study. Am J Orthod. 1988;94(5):411–5.
27. Moore RN, DuBois LM, Boice PA, Igel KA. The accuracy of measuring condylion location. Am J Orthod. 1989;95(4):344–7.
28. Al-Mashhadany SM. The relation between W angle and other methods used to assess the sagittal jaw relationship. J Bagh Coll Dentistry. 2012;24(2):144–9.

Induced ankylosis of a primary molar for skeletal anchorage in the mandible as alternative to mini-implants

Matina V Angelopoulou[1*], Despina Koletsi[2], George Vadiakas[3] and Demetrios J Halazonetis[2]

Abstract

Background: Mesial protraction of mandibular posterior teeth requires increased anchorage to avoid undesired tooth movements. Orthodontic mini-implants have become a popular and successful way to increase skeletal anchorage in such cases. However, mini-implants may cause injury to adjacent teeth or anatomical structures and may lead to tissue inflammation. Induced ankylosed primary teeth have been used in the past as abutments for the protraction of the maxilla in cases of maxillary retrognathism. However, this technique has not been described in the literature for the protraction of mandibular molars. The aim of this paper is to present, through a case report, an alternative to mini-implant devices to maximize anchorage in the mandible by inducing ankylosis on a primary molar.

Findings: A 13-year-old female with class II right malocclusion, deep bite, and congenitally missing right second premolars was referred for orthodontic treatment. Treatment plan involved removal of the primary teeth and mesial protraction of the posterior. In the mandible, ankylosis was induced on the retained primary second molar by extraction, bisection, replantation of the mesial part after endodontic treatment, and bonding of a rigid splint. Ankylosis was diagnosed after 10 weeks and a closing T-loop sectional wire was inserted to move the permanent first molar mesially. At 6 months, the remaining space was closed using elastic chain on a rectangular stainless steel wire with tip-back bends, supported by class II elastics.

Conclusions: Induced ankylosis of primary teeth can be an alternative to orthodontic mini-implants in selected cases, with minimal risks and maximum biocompatibility.

Keywords: Induced ankylosis; Molar protraction; Anchorage; Congenitally missing premolars

Findings

Clinical examination

A 13-year-old Caucasian female was referred for orthodontic treatment. The patient's medical history was noncontributory. Extraoral clinical examination revealed a symmetric face, normal proportions of the upper and lower facial height, a slightly convex profile, and an acute nasolabial angle. Intraoral clinical examination showed mild generalized gingivitis with fair oral hygiene and no caries. Evaluation of the occlusion revealed a dental class II molar and canine relationship on the right side and class I molar and canine relationship on the left side, deep bite, slight malalignment of the anterior teeth, and deviation of the mandibular midline to the right by 2 mm. Both maxillary and mandibular right second primary molars were present while all other primary teeth had exfoliated (Fig. 1).

Radiographic examination revealed congenitally missing right second premolars and all third molars (Fig. 2a). Cephalometric analysis showed a skeletal class I relationship and hyperdivergent skeletal pattern (Fig. 2b, Table 1).

Treatment alternatives

Correction of the canine relationship, overbite, and midline discrepancy would be accomplished using fixed appliances. Regarding the agenesis of the second premolars, the patient was offered two choices: maintain the primary molars and prosthetically replace them when they would

* Correspondence: matinangelop@yahoo.gr
[1]Division of Pediatric Dentistry, School of Dentistry, Marquette University, 1801 W Wisconsin Ave, 53233 Milwaukee, WI, USA
Full list of author information is available at the end of the article

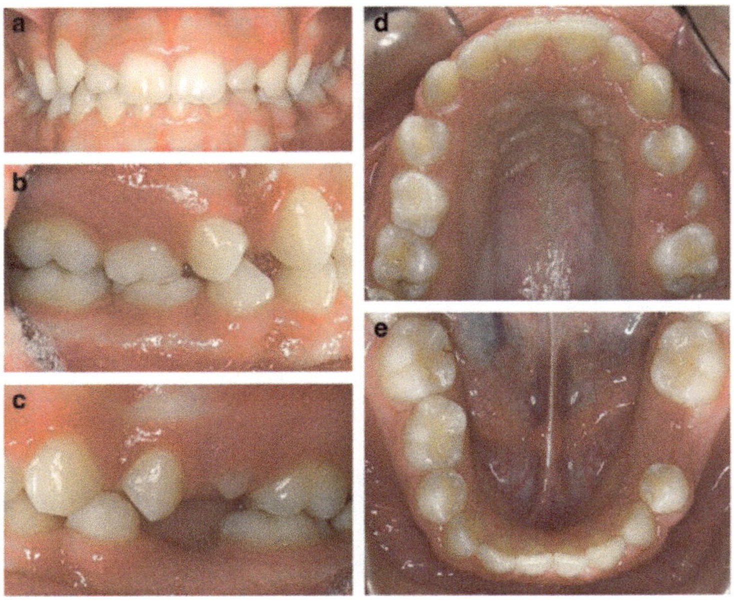

Fig. 1 Initial clinical examination of **a** frontal view, **b** right lateral view, **c** left lateral view, **d** maxillary occlusal view, and **e** mandibular occlusal view

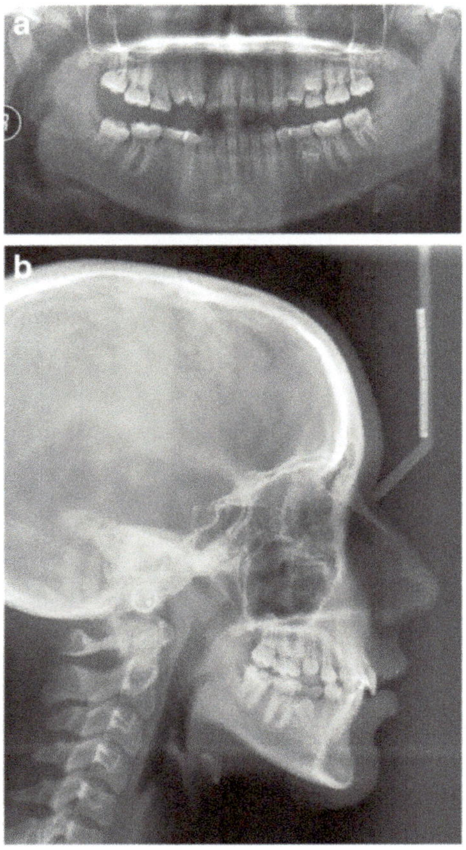

Fig. 2 a Panoramic radiograph showing congenitally missing right 2nd premolars. **b** Cephalometric radiograph at the start of treatment

eventually exfoliate, or extract them and close the space by mesial movement of the first and second permanent molars [1, 2]. The patient decided to follow the second option in order to avoid the need for implants or other prostheses in the future.

Mesial movement of molars is taxing on anchorage, especially in the mandibular arch [3–5]. Considering that the mandibular midline was already shifted to the agenesis side, skeletal anchorage was deemed an efficient option. However, instead of placing a mini-implant [3, 5, 6], we decided to use the primary molar as a biological alternative. We induced ankylosis and used the mesial root as skeletal anchorage. Induced ankylosed primary teeth have been used in the past as abutments for the

Table 1 Initial and final cephalometric measurements

	Initial	Final
SNA (°)	76.4	76.8
SNB (°)	73.3	72.7
ANB (°)	3.1	4.1
Wits (mm)	0.2	−0.4
SN to GoGn (°)	42.8	42.9
Maxillary incisor to NA (°)	19.8	13.4
Maxillary incisor to NA (mm)	4.1	−0.1
Mandibular incisor to NB (°)	25.5	27.6
Mandibular incisor to NB (mm)	4.4	3.9
Interincisal angle (°)	131.6	134.9
Mandibular incisor to GoGn (°)	89.5	92.0

protraction of the maxilla in cases of maxillary retrognathism [7–9]. However, this technique has not been described in the literature for the protraction of mandibular molars.

Treatment steps

The ankylosis technique included extraction of the primary molar under local anesthesia followed by root canal treatment of the mesial root, performed ex vivo using a zinc oxide and eugenol sealer (Fig. 3a). The crown was then restored with composite resin and a 2-mm apicoectomy and hemisectomy of the tooth was performed (Fig. 3b). To induce ankylosis, we followed the management protocol for avulsed teeth with a closed apex and extraoral dry time exceeding 60 min [10]. Periodontal ligament cells were removed from the root surface with a scaler. Sixty minutes after the extraction of the tooth, the socket was irrigated with saline solution and the mesial root was replanted with slight pressure. To stabilize the tooth and assure ankylosis, a rigid splint was applied, extending from the right canine to the right first molar, using a 0.016″ × 0.022″ stainless steel (SS) rectangular wire (Fig. 3c).

Ankylosis of the mesial root of the primary mandibular right second molar was diagnosed after 10 weeks through clinical and radiographic examination, and the splint was removed (Fig. 4). Next, a band was placed on the permanent mandibular right first molar and brackets were bonded on the primary second molar and the mandibular first premolar. A closing T-loop 0.017″ × 0.025″ TMA sectional wire was inserted between the permanent and primary molar, without any prior levelling, to move the permanent first molar mesially (Fig. 5). The T-loop was activated 9 times. At 6 months, clinical and radiographic examination revealed almost total replacement resorption of the root of the primary tooth and complete closure of the space (Fig. 6). Consequently, the bisected primary tooth was extracted and full orthodontic treatment followed. Remaining space closure was performed, during the next year, using elastic chain on a 0.017″ × 0.025″ SS wire with tip-back (Fig. 7) and support from class II elastics.

Final records show class I canine and molar relationship on both sides; full space closure of the agenesis sites, confirmed with the use of dental floss; and correction of overbite and overjet; however, a slight midline deviation remained (Figs. 8 and 9a). Cephalometric analysis showed that the mandibular incisors did not experience lingual movement as a result of molar protraction (Fig. 9b, Table 1).

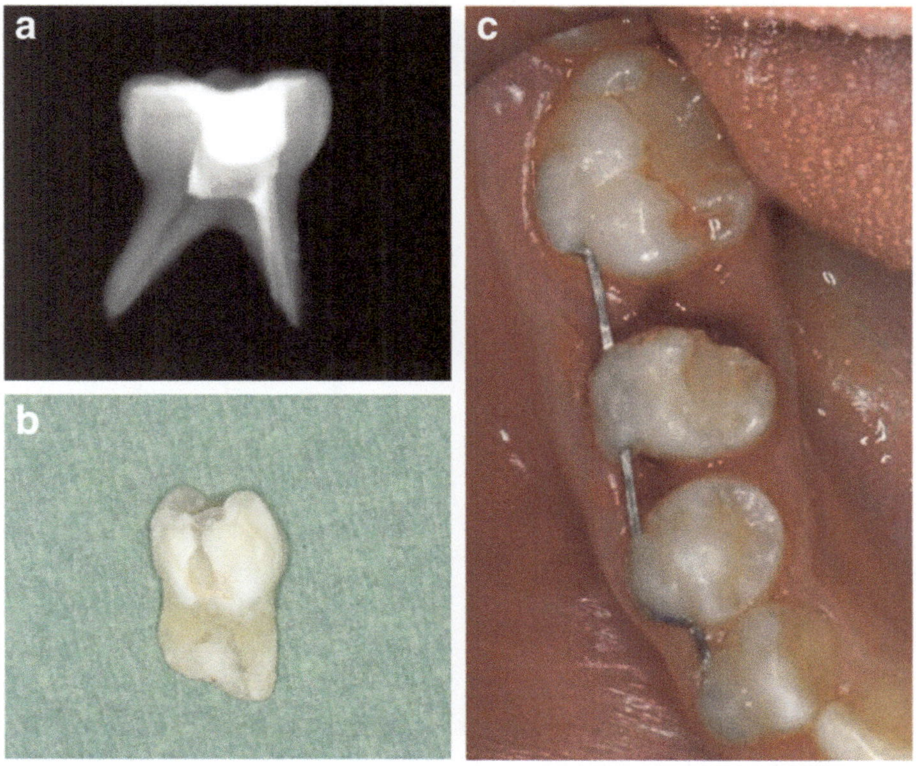

Fig. 3 Induced ankylosis technique **a** extraoral root canal treatment of the mesial root of the primary tooth, **b** hemisectomy of the primary tooth, and **c** replantation of the mesial part and splinting

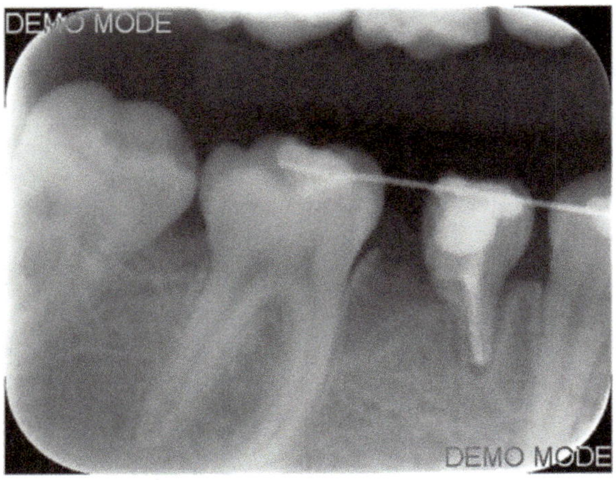

Fig. 4 Radiograph 10 weeks post replantation showing the absence of periodontal ligament and root ankylosis

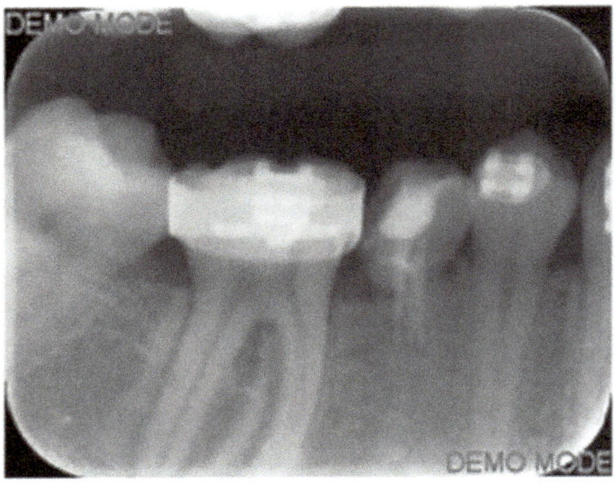

Fig. 6 Radiograph 6 months post replantation showing almost total root resorption and complete space closure between the 1st permanent molar and 2nd primary molar

Discussion

Induced ankylosed primary teeth can be used in place of temporary anchorage devices to maximize anchorage during orthodontic treatment. The technique used in the present case was based on the treatment protocol for avulsed teeth exceeding 60 min extraoral dry time, as suggested by the International Association of Dental Traumatology [11]. However, the tooth was not placed in 2 % sodium fluoride for 20 min since the goal of this step is to postpone osseous replacement of the root [10], which was not a desired outcome in this case. Also, a rigid splint was used to further assure tooth ankylosis [12]. Previous studies that have reported induced ankylosis for orthodontic protraction have used similar techniques [7–9].

Several treatment alternatives have been proposed for the management of congenital missing premolars. In cases of deep bite, spacing, and class I occlusion, the primary tooth can be kept in place until it exfoliates [2, 13]. In cases of congenitally missing premolars, the primary predecessors usually exfoliate when the patient is an adult [13, 14] and an implant can be placed, as the alveolar bone has usually been preserved [2, 15]. However, it is difficult to restore the implant since the mesiodistal dimension of the primary tooth is greater than the missing premolar and additional orthodontic treatment may be required [2, 14, 16].

An option to avoid future restorative compromise, especially when orthodontic treatment is inevitably required, is to modify the primary molar [2] by trimming it mesially and distally and restoring it as a premolar [2]. Orthodontic treatment follows and, when the primary molar exfoliates, it is replaced by an implant [2].

When the primary molar has extensive caries, restorations, or resorption, extraction is an option [1, 14]. The space can then be preserved with a space maintainer or an implant placed if the patient is an adult [2, 3, 15]. In all implant cases mentioned above, a fixed prosthesis is also an alternative [3]. It is crucial to note that when

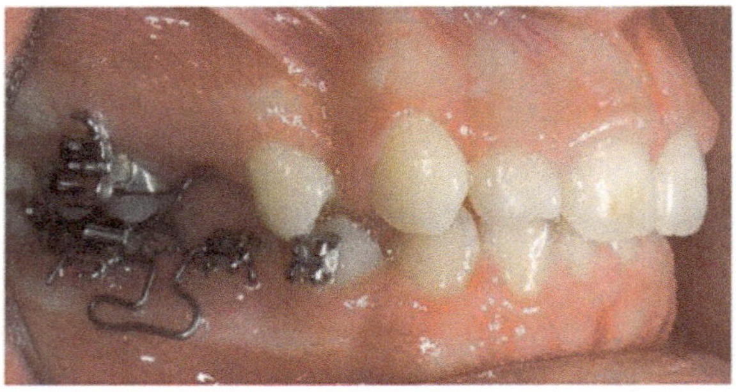

Fig. 5 Initial orthodontic space closure using a T-loop to close the space between the primary molar segment and the permanent first molar

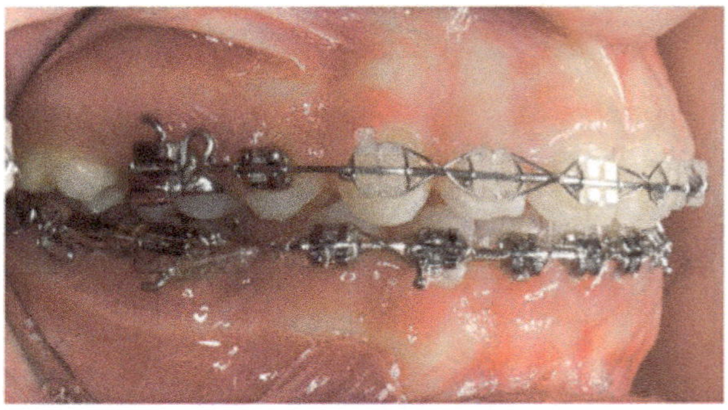

Fig. 7 Orthodontic space closure using a retraction elastic chain to close the space between the permanent first molar and the first premolar; a stop was added to the wire to maximize anchorage

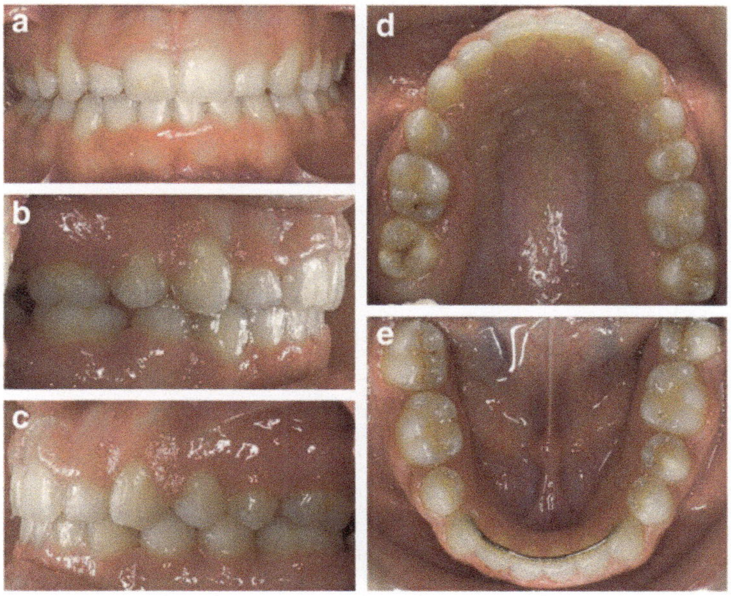

Fig. 8 Clinical examination after the completion of orthodontic treatment showing the 1st permanent molar in the position of the 2nd premolar **a** frontal view, **b** right lateral view, **c** left lateral view, **d** maxillary occlusal view, and **e** mandibular occlusal view

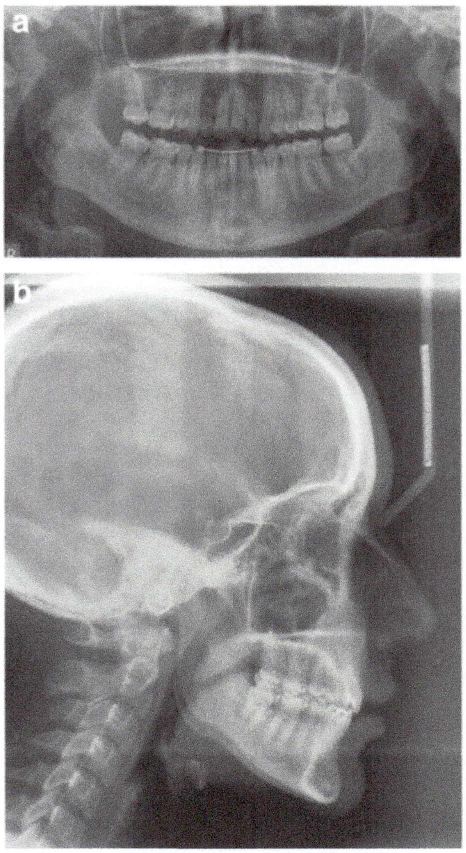

Fig. 9 **a** Panoramic radiograph at the end of orthodontic treatment showing the 1st permanent molar in the position of the 2nd premolar. **b** Final cephalometric radiograph

space is maintained for a long time, alveolar bone can become atrophic and implant placement is challenging [2, 4]. Finally, autotrasplantation of premolars or molars may also be an alternative [17].

In cases of crowding, class II malocclusion, severely damaged primary molars, or when the patient rejects the option of a prosthesis, space closure is the treatment of choice [1, 2]. When the patient is under the age of 8 years, spontaneous space closure can be achieved [18, 19]. The key point is to detect the premolar agenesis prior to root completion of the first permanent molar [18, 19]. However, even then, mild tipping of adjacent teeth can be observed [18, 19].

An alternative to space closure is the use of conventional orthodontics. In our case, this was the choice of treatment for the space closure in the maxilla, where cortical alveolar bone is less compact and thus orthodontic bodily movement is easier [20]. However, in the mandible, due to the bone's compact architecture, bodily movement is compromised leading to loss of anchorage and undesired tooth movement [3, 5, 20 21]. Lingual functional appliances [22], intermaxillary elastics [4, 16], and mandibular protraction appliances [21] have been proposed for space closure in the mandible to avoid molar tipping and anchorage loss.

Another option is controlled slicing and hemisectomy [14, 23]. Controlled slicing starts with progressive trimming of the distal surface of the primary molar which leads to hemisectomy of the tooth [14]. The hemisectomy technique is similar to the one used for induced ankylosis;

however, the primary molar is not ankylosed and cannot be used as an immovable abutment. Hemisectomy diminishes the risk of bone atrophy in the extraction site and of extreme mesial inclination of the first permanent molar [14, 23]. However, undesired movement of the anterior teeth cannot be totally prevented [23].

Recently, orthodontic mini-implants have been used successfully for space closure in mandibular molar protraction [2, 3, 6, 24]. However, they have the risk of soft tissue inflammation, damage of anatomical structures during implant placement, lack of stability, and implant fracture [25–27]. On the contrary, an induced ankylosed tooth has maximum biocompatibility leading to low inflammation risks when appropriate oral hygiene is performed. Furthermore, there is no risk to damage anatomical structures during replantation since the tooth is put in the existing socket. Finally, the root of the ankylosed tooth at the time of final extraction has almost totally been replaced by bone diminishing the risk of fracture.

The proposed technique is conservative and has advantages since (a) half of the tooth is retained, thereby retaining the alveolar process during the first phase of protraction, and (b) even if ankylosis fails to develop, other options are still open, because the tooth can be extracted and treatment can continue using other methods (e.g., mini-implant). However, this technique is indicated only for cooperative patients since procedures are time-consuming and treatment requires several visits. In addition, treatment cost can be high compared to mini-implants. Also, the ankylosed abutment cannot be placed wherever is required but where the primary tooth is located and is only partially exploited since the ankylosed root has to be extracted after 4–5 mm of protraction.

Abbreviations

TMA: Titanium molybdenum alloy; SS: Stainless steel.

Competing interests

The authors declare that they have no competing interests.

Authors' contribution

MVA performed the treatment on the primary molar to induce its ankylosis and drafted the initial manuscript. DK carried out the orthodontic treatment. GV supervised the treatment and edited the manuscript. DJH designed the treatment plan for the patient, supervised the treatment and the follow-up of the patient, and edited the manuscript. All authors read and approved the final manuscript.

Acknowledgements

The authors would like to thank Dr. Yiannis Lyros and Dr. Alina Cocos for the follow-up of the patient's orthodontic treatment. Informed consent for publication of the presented case was obtained by the parent and the child.

Author details

[1]Division of Pediatric Dentistry, School of Dentistry, Marquette University, 1801 W Wisconsin Ave, 53233 Milwaukee, WI, USA. [2]Department of Orthodontics, School of Dentistry, National and Kapodistrian University of Athens, 2 Thivon Str., 11527 Athens, Greece. [3]Department of Paediatric Dentistry, School of Dentistry, National and Kapodistrian University of Athens, 2 Thivon Str., 11527 Athens, Greece.

References

1. Santos LL. Treatment planning in the presence of congenitally absent second premolars: a review of the literature. J Clin Pediatr Dent. 2002;27(1):13–7.
2. Kokich VG, Kokich VO. Congenitally missing mandibular second premolars: clinical options. Am J Orthod Dentofacial Orthop. 2006;130(4):437–44. doi:10.1016/j.ajodo.2006.05.025.
3. Nagaraj K, Upadhyay M, Yadav S. Titanium screw anchorage for protraction of mandibular second molars into first molar extraction sites. Am J Orthod Dentofacial Orthop. 2008;134(4):583–91. doi:10.1016/j.ajodo.2006.09.055.
4. Saga AY, Maruo IT, Maruo H, Guariza Filho O, Camargo ES, Tanaka OM. Treatment of an adult with several missing teeth and atrophic old mandibular first molar extraction sites. Am J Orthod Dentofacial Orthop. 2011;140(6):869–78. doi:10.1016/j.ajodo.2010.06.027.
5. Baik UB, Chun YS, Jung MH, Sugawara J. Protraction of mandibular second and third molars into missing first molar spaces for a patient with an anterior open bite and anterior spacing. Am J Orthod Dentofacial Orthop. 2012;141(6):783–95. doi:10.1016/j.ajodo.2010.07.031.
6. Mimura H. Protraction of mandibular second and third molars assisted by partial corticision and miniscrew anchorage. Am J Orthod Dentofacial Orthop. 2013;144(2):278–89. doi:10.1016/j.ajodo.2012.08.030.
7. Kokich VG, Shapiro PA, Oswald R, Koskinen-Moffett L, Clarren SK. Ankylosed teeth as abutments for maxillary protraction: a case report. Am J Orthod. 1985;88(4):303–7.
8. Omnell ML, Sheller B. Maxillary protraction to intentionally ankylosed deciduous canines in a patient with cleft palate. Am J Orthod Dentofacial Orthop. 1994;106(2):201–5.
9. Da Silva Filho OG, Ozawa TO, Okada CH, Okada HY, Carvalho RM. Intentional ankylosis of deciduous canines to reinforce maxillary protraction. J Clin Orthod. 2003;37(6):315–20. quiz 3.
10. Andreasen FMAJ. Avulsions. In: Andreasen JOAF, Andersson L, editors. Textbook and color atlas of traumatic injuries to the teeth. 4th ed. Oxford: Blackwell; 2007. p. 444–88.
11. Andersson L, Andreasen JO, Day P, Heithersay G, Trope M, Diangelis AJ, et al. International Association of Dental Traumatology guidelines for the management of traumatic dental injuries: 2. Avulsion of permanent teeth. Dent Traumatol Off Publ Int Assoc Dent Traumatol. 2012;28(2):88–96. doi:10.1111/j.1600-9657.2012.01125.x.
12. Andreasen JO, Borum MK, Jacobsen HL, Andreasen FM. Replantation of 400 avulsed permanent incisors. 4. Factors related to periodontal ligament healing. Endod Dent Traumatol. 1995;11(2):76–89.
13. Bjerklin K, Bennett J. The long-term survival of lower second primary molars in subjects with agenesis of the premolars. Eur J Orthod. 2000;22(3):245–55.
14. Valencia R, Saadia M, Grinberg G. Controlled slicing in the management of congenitally missing second premolars. Am J Orthod Dentofacial Orthop. 2004;125(5):537–43. doi:10.1016/S0889540603010874.
15. Sabri R. Management of congenitally missing second premolars with orthodontics and single-tooth implants. Am J Orthod Dentofacial Orthop. 2004;125(5):634–42. doi:10.1016/S0889540604000022.
16. Fines CD, Rebellato J, Saiar M. Congenitally missing mandibular second premolar: treatment outcome with orthodontic space closure. Am J Orthod Dentofacial Orthop. 2003;123(6):676–82. doi:10.1016/S0889540603001628.
17. Josefsson E, Brattstrom V, Tegsjo U, Valerius-Olsson H. Treatment of lower second premolar agenesis by autotransplantation: four-year evaluation of eighty patients. Acta Odontol Scand. 1999;57(2):111–5.
18. Lindqvist B. Extraction of the deciduous second molar in hypodontia. Eur J Orthod. 1980;2(3):173–81.
19. Mamopoulou A, Hagg U, Schroder U, Hansen K. Agenesis of mandibular second premolars. Spontaneous space closure after extraction therapy: a 4-year follow-up. Eur J Orthod. 1996;18(6):589–600.
20. Roberts WE. Bone physiology, metabolism and biomechanics in orthodontic practice. In: Graber TM, Vanarsdall RLJ, editors. Orthodontics: current principles and techniques. St. Louis: Mosby; 1994. p. 193–257.
21. Coelho CM, Coelho F, White LW. Treatment of a mutilated dentition with the mandibular protraction appliance: a patient report. World J Orthod. 2009;10(4):378–82.
22. Kocadereli I, Cijger S. Congenitally missing teeth: an alternative approach for space closure. J Clin Pediatr Dent. 1993;17(4):213–6.

23. Northway W. Hemisection: one large step toward management of congenitally missing lower second premolars. Angle Orthod. 2004;74(6):792–9. doi:10.1043/0003-3219(2004)074<0792:HOLSTM>2.0.CO;2.
24. Giuliano Maino B, Pagin P, Di Blasio A. Success of miniscrews used as anchorage for orthodontic treatment: analysis of different factors. Prog Orthod. 2012;13(3):202–9. doi:10.1016/j.pio.2012.04.002.
25. Papadopoulos MA, Tarawneh F. The use of miniscrew implants for temporary skeletal anchorage in orthodontics: a comprehensive review. Oral Surg Oral Med Oral Pathol Oral Radiol Endod. 2007;103(5):e6–15. doi:10.1016/j.tripleo.2006.11.022.
26. Tsui WK, Chua HD, Cheung LK. Bone anchor systems for orthodontic application: a systematic review. Int J Oral Maxillofac Surg. 2012;41(11):1427–38. doi:10.1016/j.ijom.2012.05.011.
27. Luzi C, Verna C, Melsen B. A prospective clinical investigation of the failure rate of immediately loaded mini-implants used for orthodontic anchorage. Prog Orthod. 2007;8(1):192–201.

6

What is the best method for debonding metallic brackets from the patient's perspective?

Matheus Melo Pithon[1,2*], Daniel Santos Fonseca Figueiredo[3], Dauro Douglas Oliveira[2] and Raildo da Silva Coqueiro[2]

Abstract

Background: The aim of this clinical investigation was to compare the level of discomfort reported by patients during the removal of orthodontic metallic brackets performed with four different debonding instruments.

Methods: The sample examined in this split-mouth study comprised a total of 70 patients (840 teeth). Four different methods of bracket removal were used: lift-off debonding instrument (LODI), straight cutter plier (SC), how plier (HP), and bracket removal plier (BRP). Prior to debonding with all experimental methods, the archwire was removed. Before appliance removal, each patient was instructed about the study objectives. It was explained that at the end of debonding in each quadrant, it would be necessary to assess the discomfort of the procedure using a visual analog scale (VAS). This scale was composed of a millimeter ruler scoring from 0 to 10, in which 0 = a lot of pain, 5 = moderate pain, and 10 = painless. The level of significance was predetermined at 5 % ($p = 0.05$), and the data were analyzed using the BioEstat 5.0 software (BioEstat, Belém, Brazil).

Results: The pain scores with SC were significantly higher than in all other methods. There were no significant differences between HP and BRP pain scores, and the LODI group showed the lowest pain scores. Statistically, significant differences were observed in the ARI between the four debonding methods.

Limitations: The biggest limitation of this study is that each tooth was not assessed individually.

Conclusions: Patients reported lower levels of pain and discomfort when metallic brackets were removed with the LODI. The use of a straight cutter plier caused the highest pain and discomfort scores during debonding.

Keywords: Pain; Orthodontics brackets; Orthodontic treatment

Background

Despite all recent developments in dentistry, patient's complaints of pain or discomfort are commonly registered after different types of dental treatments and orthodontic therapy is not an exception [1, 2]. The existing literature shows that procedures such as the use of elastic separators, archwire placement and activations, as well as the application of orthopedic forces may cause pain in orthodontic patients [3–5]. It is also known that the possibility of experiencing pain or discomfort may negatively influence the willingness of patients to undergo orthodontic treatment [6–9].

Orthodontic patients may experience pain not only during the phase of active treatment but also during the removal of fixed appliances [10]. Various methods to debond metallic and ceramic brackets have been described in the literature, including the use of special debonding pliers [8], ultrasound [9, 10] or laser application [11, 12], electrothermic debonding [13–15], special instruments [8, 16], and the use of bonding materials presenting thermoexpandable microcapsules to facilitate debonding [17]. Despite the several techniques described, few authors have been concerned about understanding the discomfort the different debonding methods cause to orthodontic patients [10, 12]. Undoubtedly, the ideal debonding method should be harmless to the enamel and painless to the patients [18–20]. However, researchers have been more focused on studying pain during orthodontic treatment and the technical details of debonding rather than evaluating ways to minimize patients' discomfort during debonding [21, 22].

* Correspondence: matheuspithon@gmail.com
[1]Av. Otavio Santos, 395 sala 705, Centro Odontomédico Dr. Altamirando da Costa Lima, Vitoria da Conquista, Bahia 45020750, Brazil
[2]Southwest Bahia State University UESB, Jequié, Bahia, Brazil
Full list of author information is available at the end of the article

In an attempt to fill this gap in the literature, the aim of this clinical investigation was to compare the level of discomfort reported by patients during the removal of orthodontic metallic brackets performed with four different debonding instruments and to verify the integrity of the enamel after debonding.

Methods

Before data collection began, the project was sent for approval by the research ethics committee of Southeast Bahia State University, and it received a favorable report (number 405.944). The sample examined in this split-mouth study was collected from a single private practice and included patients who had fixed orthodontic appliances removed in both arches. The inclusion criteria were the presence of an Angle class I malocclusion and permanent teeth, except the third molars. Conversely, patients requiring extractions or presenting teeth with restorations on the buccal surface were excluded from the study. The sample comprised a total of 70 female patients (840 teeth). The mean age at the time of debonding was 31 years and 10 months, ranging from 14 years and 3 months to 45 years and 11 months. All patients or their legal guardians signed an informed consent prior to initiating their treatment.

All fixed appliances were bonded and removed by the same orthodontist, and the same brand and model of stainless steel brackets were used on all patients (Standard Edgewise 0.022 × 0.030 in.) (Morelli, Sorocaba, Brazil). Prior to bonding, the buccal surface of all teeth was pumiced with a mixture of pumice and water on slow speed, enamel was conditioned with a self-etching primer (SEP 3M/Unitek, Monrovia, CA, USA), and the same resin composite (Transbond XT 3M/Unitek, Monrovia, CA, USA) was used in all patients following the manufacturer's instructions.

Before appliance removal, each patient was instructed about the study objectives. It was explained that at the end of debonding in each quadrant, it would be necessary to assess the discomfort of the procedure using a visual analog scale (VAS). This scale was composed of a millimeter ruler scoring from 0 to 10, in which 0 = a lot of pain, 5 = moderate pain, and 10 = painless. Prior to debonding, the order and the debonding method for each quadrant were randomly selected. The teeth evaluated in this study were canine and premolars because their brackets were exactly the same.

Four different methods of bracket removal were used (Fig. 1). The first method examined was the lift-off debonding instrument (LODI) (Zatt, São Paulo, Brazil), in which a pull wire was engaged under the bracket wing producing a pulling force after a light squeeze of the handles while both plastic rests were placed on the tooth surface. The second debonding method tested was a straight cutter plier (SC) that was used to grab the bracket wings, applying pressure to the bracket base mesially and distally. The third method was the use of a how plier (HP) to press both mesial and distal wings, deforming the bracket base. The last method tested was a bracket removal plier (BRP), as shown in Fig. 1d. Prior to debonding with all experimental methods, the archwire was removed.

The amount of composite remaining on the enamel surface was examined immediately after bracket removal. The patients were instructed to rinse with a solution containing fuccina (Biodinâmica Química e Farmacêutica LTDA, Ibiporã, Brazil) for better identification of residual composite adhered to the tooth. A portable electron microscope (Vehs, Hong Kong, China) was used to evaluate the adhesive remnant index (ARI) (Fig. 2a, b) [23]. The scale had scores ranging from 0 to 3, where 0 = no adhesive remaining; 1 = less than half of adhesive remaining; 2 = more than half of adhesive remaining; and 3 = all adhesive remaining (Fig. 3). All values were assigned by a single orthodontist.

Statistical analyses

For descriptive analysis of pain scores and ARI values, mean and standard deviations were calculated. The differences registered for all debonding methods were compared with the Friedman test followed by the Wilcoxon

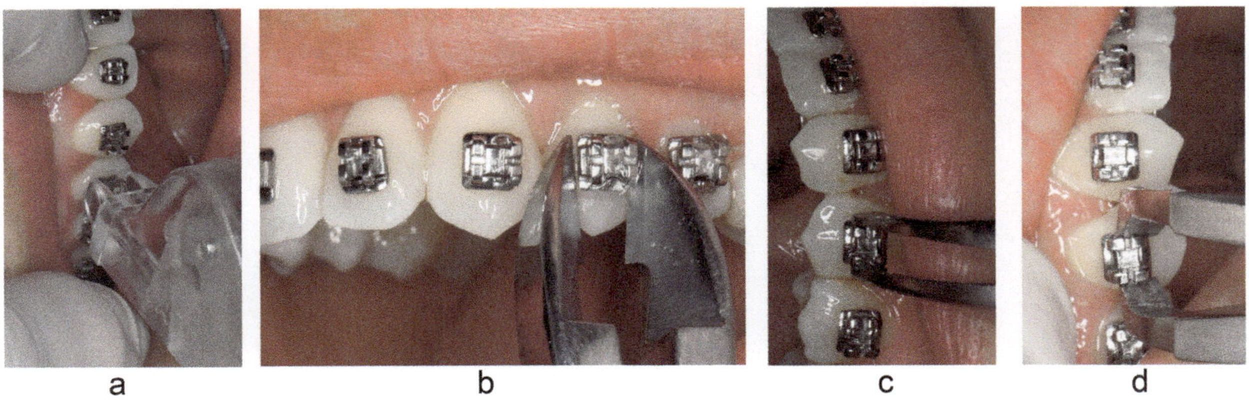

Fig. 1 Debonding methods used. **a** Lift-off debonding instrument (LODI). **b** Straight cutter (SC). **c** How plier (HP). **d** Bracket removal plier (BRP)

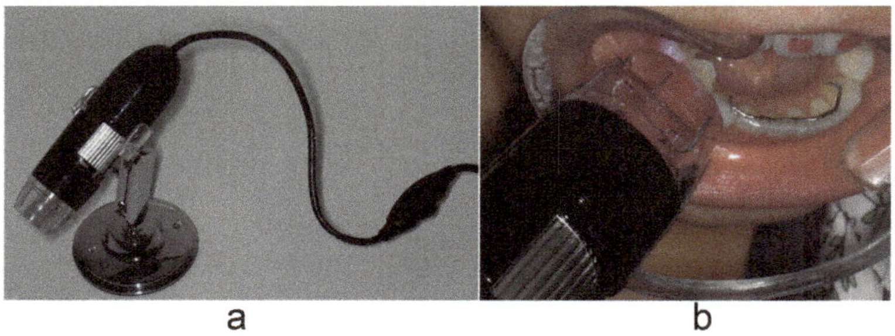

Fig. 2 **a** Portable digital microscope used to determine the ARI. **b** Microscope being used

test to compare pairs. The level of significance was predetermined at 5 % ($p = 0.05$), and the data were analyzed using the BioEstat 5.0 software (BioEstat, Belém, Brazil).

Results

Figure 4 shows the perception of discomfort reported by the participants according to the debonding method used. The Friedman test indicated that pain scores were statistically significantly different depending on the debonding method. Comparisons between pairs by the Wilcoxon test showed that pain scores with SC were significantly higher than in all other methods. There were no significant differences between HP and BRP pain scores, and the LODI group showed the lowest pain scores.

Statistically significant differences were observed in the ARI between the four debonding methods (Fig. 5). Comparisons between pairs by the Wilcoxon test showed that the methods of debonding brackets that promoted the greatest ARI were: HP > BRP > LODI > SC.

Discussion

The search for ways to reduce patient's pain and discomfort during different dental procedures has been a concern in contemporary dentistry [21, 22]. The same concern exists in orthodontics [4], however, relatively few publications on this topic have been found in the literature, especially when compared to other areas of orthodontic research [4]. For example, despite the various methods of debonding described in the literature [24–27], few have been studied in relation to pain or discomfort they may cause to the orthodontic patients. Thus, the purpose of the present paper was to evaluate four methods commonly used to debond metallic brackets, determining possible differences in patient's discomfort and their amount

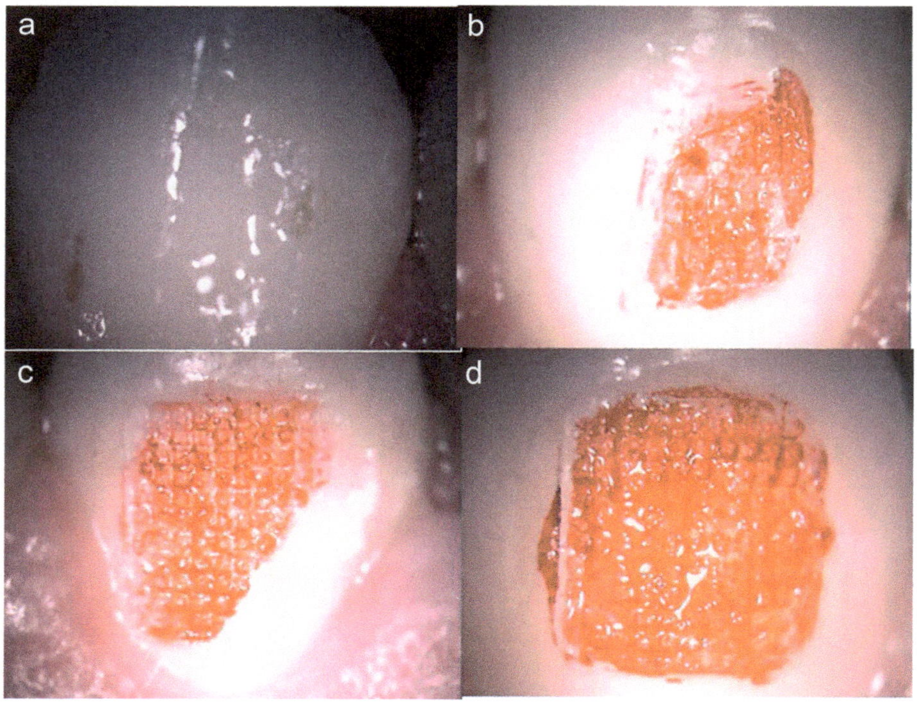

Fig. 3 Images obtained with the patient directly into portable microscope. **a** IRA = 0. **b** IRA = 1. **c** IRA = 2. **d** IRA = 3

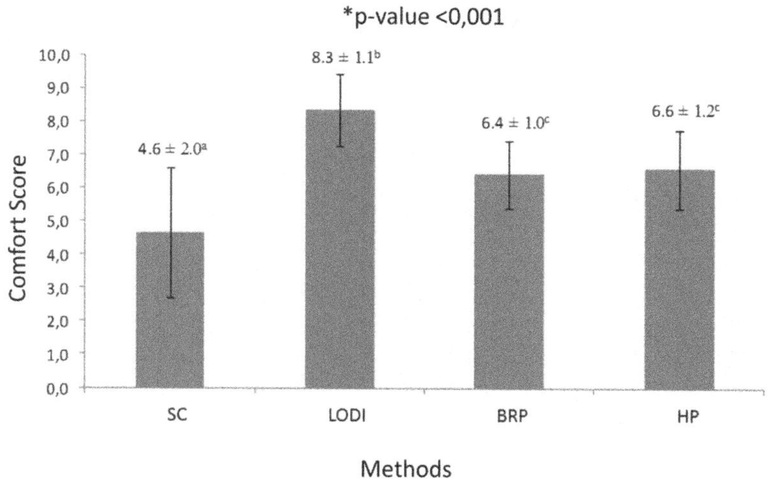

Fig. 4 Mean ± standard deviation perception of discomfort scores during bracket debonding, according to the different methods used. *Statistical difference between the methods (Friedman test). Different letters (*superscript a, b, c*) represent statistical difference (Wilcoxon test)

of adhesive remaining on the enamel surface after debonding.

The results of this study showed significant differences on the patient's discomfort between the four debonding methods. In general, the use of LODI caused lower levels of pain or discomfort to remove the brackets when compared to the other methods. Furthermore, the use of the SC was the method that presented the highest discomfort for the patients. This finding corroborates with previous clinical reports [28, 29], as well as the study of Normando et al. [12], which also compared quantitatively the discomfort caused by LODI and SC. However, that study [12] was limited to these two methods and did not evaluate other methods widely used by orthodontists, such as HP and BRP. In our study, HP and BRP showed similar scores of patient discomfort that reached intermediate levels between SC and LODI mean discomfort values.

The reasons that justify the different results found between the methods studied are unknown. However, the direction of the debonding force may influence the degree of discomfort during the removal of metallic brackets [10].

According to Williams and Bishara [10], the direction of debonding force application and the mobility of the tooth along with gender differences are seen to be factors influencing the discomfort threshold. Patients can withstand intrusive forces significantly more than forces applied in a mesial, distal, facial, lingual, or an extrusive direction [10]. Unfortunately, we have no way to standardize the direction as each instrument for removing presents a different mode of operation. However, during removal, the manufacturer's recommendations regarding the use of these instruments were followed. Therefore, the similar force systems created by the different instruments during debonding may provide an explanation for these findings. BRP, SC, and HP exert forces of similar magnitude, but in opposite direction. They cancel each other requiring greater amounts of force applied by the operator, which could lead to greater patient discomfort. Conversely, the

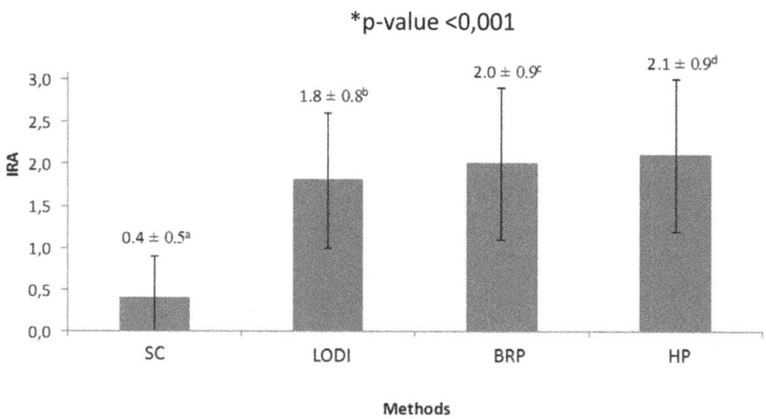

Fig. 5 Mean ± standard deviation ARI scores registered with the four debonding methods tested. *Statistical difference between the methods (Friedman test). Different letters (*superscript a, b, c*) represent statistical difference (Wilcoxon test)

LODI may require lower and more constant force levels, which may be linked to a lower score of pain or discomfort [12] Williams and Bishara [10] suggested that approximately 1000 g should be considered as an "appropriate force" limit to be directly applied to a tooth.

The discomfort felt in the premolars and canines were recorded in this study. This was an attempt to better standardize the sample. Primarily, because the brackets used for both teeth were identical. Secondly, because the type of tooth appears to influence on the threshold of pain, since the biggest complaints have been previously reported during incisor debonding [12]. This may be explained because the tactile sensory thresholds of normal people were about 1 g in the anterior portion of the dental arch and gradually increased toward the posterior segments of the arch, ranging from 5 to 10 gm [30]. Conversely, patient's gender appear to have little influence on the threshold of discomfort [10]; thus, we decided not to distinguish the groups by gender.

The four methods of debonding were also assessed for their damaging potential to the enamel surface. A crucial point for this evaluation is the line of adhesive fracture during bracket debonding. According to Artun and Bergland [23], the enamel would be protected if the adhesive line of fracture was located exclusively within the adhesive layer; thus, a thin layer of adhesive would remain attached to the enamel after debonding, covering 100 % of the bracket base's previous location, instead of having a line of fracture at the enamel-adhesive interface) [15]. Therefore, the ARI is an important indicator when assessing the integrity of the enamel surface after bracket debonding.

A portable electron microscope was used to evaluate the ARI, which due to its reduced dimension could be introduced directly into the oral cavity. After debonding and prior to microscopic evaluation, the enamel was stained with fuccina to facilitate the composite visualization and quantification.

The results of this study showed significant ARI differences among the four debonding methods tested. Despite these statistical differences, HP, LODI, and BRP showed clinically similar results, showing on average, approximately half of the enamel surface with remaining adhesive (Fig. 5). However, the ARI for SC was noticeably smaller than those registered for the other groups (Fig. 5), which seems to indicate greater potential for enamel damage. SC generates forces directly to the adhesive layer and below the bracket base, immediately transferred to the underlying enamel [28], thereby presenting higher risks to injure the enamel [14].

Therefore, when compared to the other methods tested, the use of SC seems to be far from the ideal debonding method, since it has greater potential to cause enamel damage which caused greater patient discomfort. Furthermore, if bracket rebonding is required, the use of SC may also not be considered the method of choice for removal of the brackets since another study [14, 15] reported that the majority of the brackets debonded with SC showed significant structural deformations at the base and/or at the slot. Conversely, LODI showed the highest patient acceptability. Moreover, previous reports showed that all brackets debonded with the LODI remained structurally intact afterward [14, 15], indicating that this method may also be the most recommended when bracket rebonding is necessary.

Conclusions

According to our findings, it can be concluded that:

- Patients reported lower levels of pain and discomfort when metallic brackets were removed with the lift-off debonding instrument.
- How plier and bracket removal plier generated intermediate and similar levels of patient discomfort.
- The use of a straight cutter plier caused the highest pain and discomfort scores during debonding.
- The ARI scored with all four debonding methods were not significantly different.

Competing interests
The authors declare that they have no competing interests.

Authors' contributions
MMP and DF developed the clinical session. MMP, DDO, and RSC revised the article. All authors read and approved the final manuscript.

Author details
[1]Av. Otavio Santos, 395 sala 705, Centro Odontomédico Dr. Altamirando da Costa Lima, Vitoria da Conquista, Bahia 45020750, Brazil. [2]Southwest Bahia State University UESB, Jequié, Bahia, Brazil. [3]Pontifical Catholic University of Minas Gerais, Belo Horizonte, Brazil.

References

1. d'Ornellas Pereira Jr JC, Weissheimer A, de Menezes LM, de Lima EM, Mezomo M. Change in the pulp chamber temperature with different stripping techniques. Prog Orthod. 2014;15:55.
2. Sobouti F, Rakhshan V, Chiniforush N, Khatami M. Effects of laser-assisted cosmetic smile lift gingivectomy on postoperative bleeding and pain in fixed orthodontic patients: a controlled clinical trial. Prog Orthod. 2014;15:66.
3. Loewenstein WR, Rathkamp R. A study on the pressoreceptive sensibility of the tooth. J Dent Res. 1955;34:287–94.
4. Krishnan V. Orthodontic pain: from causes to management–a review. Eur J Orthod. 2007;29:170–9.
5. Takla PM, Shivapuja PK. Pulpal response in electrothermal debonding. Am J Orthod Dentofacial Orthop. 1995;108:623–9.
6. Haynes S. Discontinuation of orthodontic treatment relative to patient age. J Dent. 1974;2:138–42.
7. Oliver RG, Knapman YM. Attitudes to orthodontic treatment. Br J Orthod. 1985;12:179–88.
8. Brown DF, Moerenhout RG. The pain experience and psychological adjustment to orthodontic treatment of preadolescents, adolescents, and adults. Am J Orthod Dentofacial Orthop. 1991;100:349–56.
9. Kluemper GT, Hiser DG, Rayens MK, Jay MJ. Efficacy of a wax containing benzocaine in the relief of oral mucosal pain caused by orthodontic appliances. Am J Orthod Dentofacial Orthop. 2002;122:359–65.

10. Williams OL, Bishara SE. Patient discomfort levels at the time of debonding: a pilot study. Am J Orthod Dentofacial Orthop. 1992;101:313–7.
11. Lee-Knight CT, Wylie SG, Major PW, Glover KE, Grace M. Mechanical and electrothermal debonding: effect on ceramic veneers and dental pulp. Am J Orthod Dentofacial Orthop. 1997;112:263–70.
12. Normando TS, Calcada FS, Ursi WJ, Normando D. Patients' report of discomfort and pain during debonding of orthodontic brackets: a comparative study of two methods. World J Orthod. 2010;11:e29–34.
13. Boyer DB, Engelhardt G, Bishara SE. Debonding orthodontic ceramic brackets by ultrasonic instrumentation. Am J Orthod Dentofacial Orthop. 1995;108:262–6.
14. Knosel M, Mattysek S, Jung K, Kubein-Meesenburg D, Sadat-Khonsari R, Ziebolz D. Suitability of orthodontic brackets for rebonding and reworking following removal by air pressure pulses and conventional debracketing techniques. Angle Orthod. 2010;80:461–7.
15. Knosel M, Mattysek S, Jung K, Sadat-Khonsari R, Kubein-Meesenburg D, Bauss O, et al. Impulse debracketing compared to conventional debonding. Angle Orthod. 2010;80:1036–44.
16. Azzeh E, Feldon PJ. Laser debonding of ceramic brackets: a comprehensive review. Am J Orthod Dentofacial Orthop. 2003;123:79–83.
17. Sheridan JJ, Brawley G, Hastings J. Electrothermal debracketing. Part I. An in vitro study. Am J Orthod. 1986;89:21–7.
18. Santos BM, Pithon MM, Ruellas AC, Sant'Anna EF. Shear bond strength of brackets bonded with hydrophilic and hydrophobic bond systems under contamination. Angle Orthod. 2010;80:963–7.
19. Pithon MM, de Oliveira Ruellas AC, Sant'Anna EF, de Oliveira MV, Alves Bernardes LA. Shear bond strength of brackets bonded to enamel with a self-etching primer. Effects of increasing storage time after activation. Angle Orthod. 2009;79:133–7.
20. Pithon MM, Oliveira MV, Ruellas AC, Bolognese AM, Romano FL. Shear bond strength of orthodontic brackets to enamel under different surface treatment conditions. J Appl Oral Sci. 2007;15:127–30.
21. Farzanegan F, Zebarjad SM, Alizadeh S, Ahrari F. Pain reduction after initial archwire placement in orthodontic patients: a randomized clinical trial. Am J Orthod Dentofacial Orthop. 2012;141:169–73.
22. Kokich VG. Do you have an evidence-based practice? Am J Orthod Dentofacial Orthop. 2013;143:1.
23. Artun J, Bergland S. Clinical trials with crystal growth conditioning as an alternative to acid-etch enamel pretreatment. Am J Orthod. 1984;85:333–40.
24. Parrish BC, Katona TR, Isikbay SC, Stewart KT, Kula KS. The effects of application time of a self-etching primer and debonding methods on bracket bond strength. Angle Orthod. 2012;82:131–6.
25. Cehreli SB, Polat-Ozsoy O, Sar C, Cubukcu HE, Cehreli ZC. A comparative study of qualitative and quantitative methods for the assessment of adhesive remnant after bracket debonding. Eur J Orthod. 2012;34:188–92.
26. Elekdag-Turk S, Isci D, Ozkalayci N, Turk T. Debonding characteristics of a polymer mesh base ceramic bracket bonded with two different conditioning methods. Eur J Orthod. 2009;31:84–9.
27. Eliades T, Gioka C, Eliades G, Makou M. Enamel surface roughness following debonding using two resin grinding methods. Eur J Orthod. 2004;26:333–8.
28. Bennett CG, Shen C, Waldron JM. The effects of debonding on the enamel surface. J Clin Orthod. 1984;18:330–4.
29. Kinch AP, Taylor H, Warltier R, Oliver RG, Newcombe RG. A clinical study of amount of adhesive remaining on enamel after debonding, comparing etch times of 15 and 60 s. Am J Orthod Dentofacial Orthop. 1989;95:415–21.
30. Manly RS, Pfaffman C, Lathrop DD, Keyser J. Oral sensory thresholds of persons with natural and artificial dentitions. J Dent Res. 1952;31:305–12.

7

The efficacy of maxillary protraction protocols with the micro-implant-assisted rapid palatal expander (MARPE) and the novel N2 mini-implant—a finite element study

Won Moon[1*], Kimberley W. Wu[1], Matthew MacGinnis[1], Jay Sung[1], Howard Chu[1], George Youssef[2] and Andre Machado[3]

Abstract

Background: Maxillary protraction with the novel N2 mini-implant- and micro-implant-assisted rapid palatal expander (MARPE) can potentially provide significant skeletal effects without surgery, even in older patients where conventional facemask therapy has limited skeletal effects. However, the skeletal effects of altering the location and direction of force from mini-implant-assisted maxillary protraction have not been extensively analyzed. In this study, the application of the novel N2 mini-implant as an orthopedic anchorage device is explored in its ability to treat patients with class III malocclusions.

Methods: A 3D cranial mesh model with associated sutures was developed from CT images and Mimics modeling software. Utilizing ANSYS simulation software, protraction forces were applied at different locations and directions to simulate conventional facemask therapy and seven maxillary protraction protocols utilizing the novel N2 mini-implant. Stress distribution and displacement were analyzed. Video animations and superimpositions were created.

Results: By changing the vector of force and location of N2 mini-implant, the maxilla was displaced differentially. Varying degrees of forward, downward, and rotational movements were observed in each case. For brachyfacial patients, anterior micro-implant-supported protraction at −45° or intermaxillary class III elastics at −45° are recommended. For dolicofacial patients, either anterior micro-implants at −15° or an intermaxillary spring at +30° is recommended. For mesofacial patients with favorable vertical maxillary position, palatal micro-implants at −30° are recommended; anterior micro-implants at −30° are preferred for shallow bites. For patients with a severe mid-facial deficiency, intermaxillary class III elastics at −30° are most effective in promoting anterior growth of the maxilla.

Conclusions: By varying the location of N2 mini-implants and vector of class III mechanics, clinicians can differentially alter the magnitude of forward, downward, and rotational movement of the maxilla. As a result, treatment protocol can be customized for each unique class III patient.

Background

Facemask has shown some effectiveness in modifying growth and eliminating surgery in select patients [1]; however, there are many limitations. Unwanted dental side effects include proclination of maxillary incisors and extrusion and mesial tipping of the maxillary molars [2–5]. In addition, the rotation of the occlusal plane with conventional facemask has been observed leading to the development of an adjustable facemask that allows altering the line of force to achieve the desired skeletal movement [6].

To overcome these limitations, some researchers propose the use of miniplates for skeletal anchorage [7, 8], which has resulted in greater skeletal effects, even in older patients. Numerous studies have shown the effectiveness of the use of miniplates placed in different locations within the maxilla in the clinical treatment of class III patients [9, 10]. While Lee et al. [10] showed that the site of miniplate placement should be specifically considered between the

* Correspondence: wmoon@dentistry.ucla.edu
[1]UCLA Section of Orthodontics, UCLA School of Dentistry, 10833 Le Conte Avenue, CHS – Box 951668, Los Angeles, CA 90095-1668, USA
Full list of author information is available at the end of the article

infrazygomatic crest and the lateral nasal walls, Kim et al. [9] showed that the placement of miniplates in the palatal area resulted in wider stress distribution and more forward displacement compared to miniplates placed at the infrazygomatic crest area and conventional tooth-borne appliances.

With the use of micro-implants, it is now possible to achieve skeletal anchorage without the surgical procedures involved with placement and removal of miniplates. While micro-implant-supported facemask has shown evidence of clinical success [11, 12], few studies have been published on this technique and few have analyzed how micro-implants can be utilized for maximal clinical effectiveness [11, 13, 14].

With the recent development of the novel N2 mini-implant (3-mm diameter, 2-mm length, tapered shape), it is believed that the short length of the implant reduces the risk of damaging anatomic structures during placement and therefore does not need to be placed interradicularly [15–17]. The aim of this study is to examine the ability of the novel micro-implant-assisted rapid palatal expander (MARPE) and N2 mini-implant to serve as an orthopedic anchorage device in creating favorable maxillary protraction protocols in lieu of the more invasive miniplates.

A finite element approach was used to simulate conventional facemask therapy, MARPE, and seven novel N2 mini-implant-supported maxillary protraction protocols to evaluate the corresponding stress patterns and skeletal changes. Our objective was to explore the ability of the novel N2 mini-implant to be used as an orthopedic anchorage and to understand how different placement locations and force directions can be used to correct different types of class III malocclusions.

Methods

The finite element method (FEM) model was generated from CT volumetric data (slice thickness of 0.300 mm) of a 42-year-old male patient of the Department of Biomedical Sciences at Ohio University, where informed consent was obtained prior to data collection. DICOM raw data was extracted from the CT and imported into Mimics 13.1 software (Materialise, Leuven, Belgium) to reconstruct a 3D model (Wu Laboratory, UCLA Bioengineering).

Utilizing Mimics, sutures 1.5–2 mm in width were manually generated (Fig. 1): mid-palatal, pterygomaxillary (2), zygomaticomaxillary (2), zygomaticotemporal (2), median nasal, and lateral nasal (2). The FEM model generated from the ANSYS software yielded 91,933 elements and 344,451 nodes. Nodes along the foramen magnum and on the center of the forehead were constrained in all degrees of freedom, with zero displacement and zero rotation.

The 3D mesh was then imported into ANSYS 12.0 (ANSYS Inc, Canonsburg, PA) FEM software program. The FEM model was defined to be linear elastic and isotropic. The bone and tooth structures in the model were assigned properties of compact bone: Poisson's ratio of $\nu = 0.3$ and a Young's modulus of $E = 1.37 \times 10^3$ (kg/mm^2) [11, 18]. Sutural elements were assigned values of connective tissue: $\nu = 0.49$ and $E = 6.8 \times 10^{-2}$ (kg/mm^2) [11, 13].

Table 1 shows different locations and directions of force application, which simulate eight clinical protocols for maxillary protraction. The location of force delineates where the elastics of the facemask appliance pull from in simulation A and the location of micro-implant placement in simulations B–H. The direction of force (denoted by the [angle]) delineates protraction in relation to the occlusal plane. Values of 1000 g per side were applied for all simulations.

Simulation A mimics conventional facemask therapy, with force applied to the buccal of the first maxillary molars, angled 30° below the occlusal plane (Fig. 2). Simulation B models a micro-implant-supported hyrax with facemask shown in Fig. 3. The forces are applied 3 mm lateral to the mid-palatal suture, at a 30° angle below the occlusal plane (Fig. 4). For simulations C, D, and E, facemask therapy directly from anterior micro-

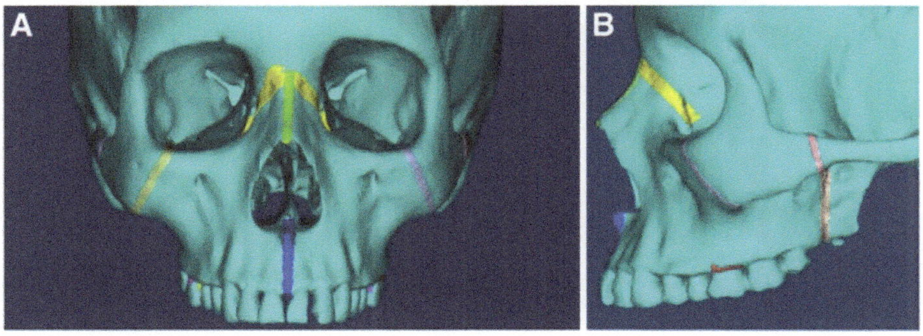

Fig. 1 3D skull with manually generated sutures. **a** Frontal view. **b** Lateral view

Table 1 Simulations of eight clinical protocols for maxillary protraction

Simulation	Clinical protocol	Location of force (bilaterally)	Direction of force (to occlusal plane)
A	FM [−30]	Buccal surface of maxillary first molars	−30
B	Pal-MI-FM [−30]	3-mm lateral of the mid-palatine suture	−30
C	Ant-MI-FM [−15]	Between roots of canine and first premolar	−15
D	Ant-MI-FM [−30]	Between roots of canine and first premolar	−30
E	Ant-MI-FM [−45]	Between roots of canine and first premolar	−45
F	Ant-MI-FM [+30]	Between roots of canine and first premolar	+30
G	Post-MI-FM [−30]	Between roots of second premolar and molar	−30
H	Post-MI-FM [−45]	Between roots of second premolar and molar	−45

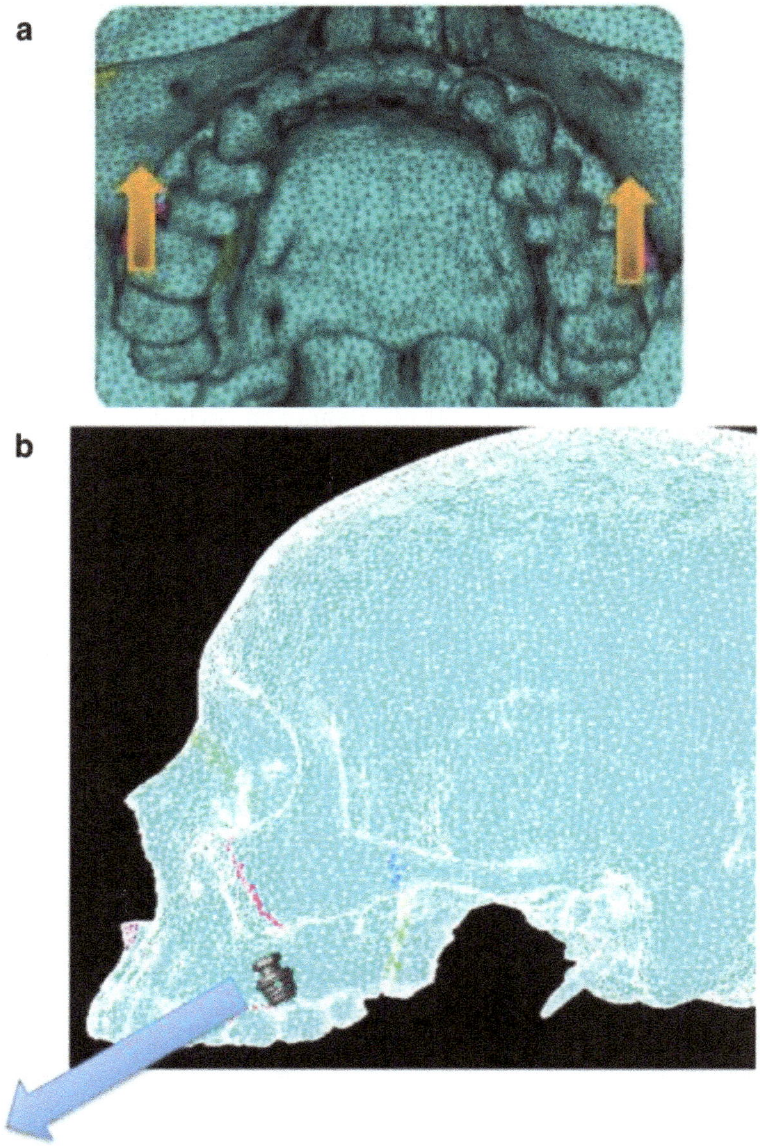

Fig. 2 **a**, **b** Location of force application for simulation A—FM [−30°]

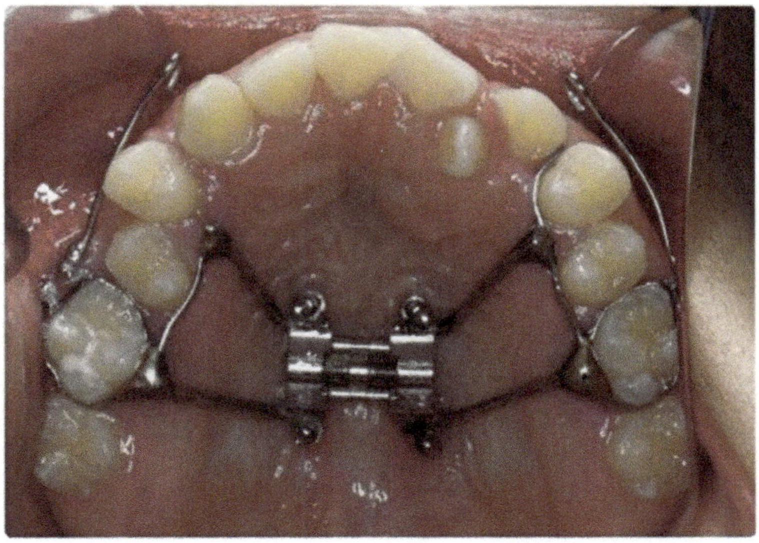

Fig. 3 Intraoral view of micro-implant-supported hyrax with facemask with Pal-MI-FM [−30°]

implants placed between the canine and first premolar roots is being modeled. The direction of force application is respectively 15°, 30°, and 45° below the occlusal plane (Fig. 5). Simulation F also has forces applied in the anterior between the canine and first premolar roots, but is directed 30° above the occlusal plane, simulating use of an intermaxillary spring pushing the maxilla forward and upward (Fig. 6). Finally, simulations G and H model the use of intermaxillary elastics from posterior maxillary micro-implants to anterior mandibular micro-implants. Point of force application is in between the roots of the second premolar and first molar, directed 30° and 45° below the occlusal plane (Fig. 7).

With ANSYS software:

1. Tensile and compressive stresses were measured separately in all simulations.
2. Video animations were developed.
3. Superimpositions were created to depict the skeletal displacement as a result of altering the location and direction of force application.

Results

First principle stress distributions depicting tensile stress are shown (Figs. 8 and 9). The color scale at the bottom of the figure shows the distribution of stress from the lowest (*blue*) to the highest (*red*).

For all simulations, there is a high concentration of tensile stress directly posterior to the location of force application. In addition, tensile stresses concentrate at the pterygoid plates in all simulations, with slightly lower levels in simulation E. Tensile stresses are also evident in the medial orbit of all simulations, with greater levels in simulations E, F, and H. Other simulations have several areas of stress concentration unique to the simulation. In simulation A, tensile stresses are also present in the maxillary buttress. In simulations E and H, tensile stresses congregate near the lateral orbit, as well as the frontal process distal to the zygoma. The most unique pattern of tensile stress involves simulation F, with additional tensile stresses involving the forehead, orbit, zygomaticomaxillary suture, frontal process of the zygoma, and extending from the pterygoid plates backward to the foramen magnum.

Third principle stresses depicting compressive stress are also shown (Fig. 10). *Dark blue areas* show areas of high compressive stress.

For all simulations, there is a high concentration of compressive stress directly anterior to the location of force application. All simulations display compressive stresses in the forehead, with significantly less in simulation F. There is also a general concentration of stresses lateral to the infraorbital foramen, although this is minimal in simulations E and H. The distribution of stresses is distinctly unique in simulation F, with areas of compressive stress involving the lateral border of the orbit, medial superior border of the orbit, maxillary buttress, zygoma, and in the frontal bone distal to the zygoma.

Animation videos and superimpositions of each simulation were created. (simulations A–H). For the superimpositions, the "before" image is shown in *blue*, while the "after" image is displayed in a *range of colors* that directly correspond to the amount of Y-displacement

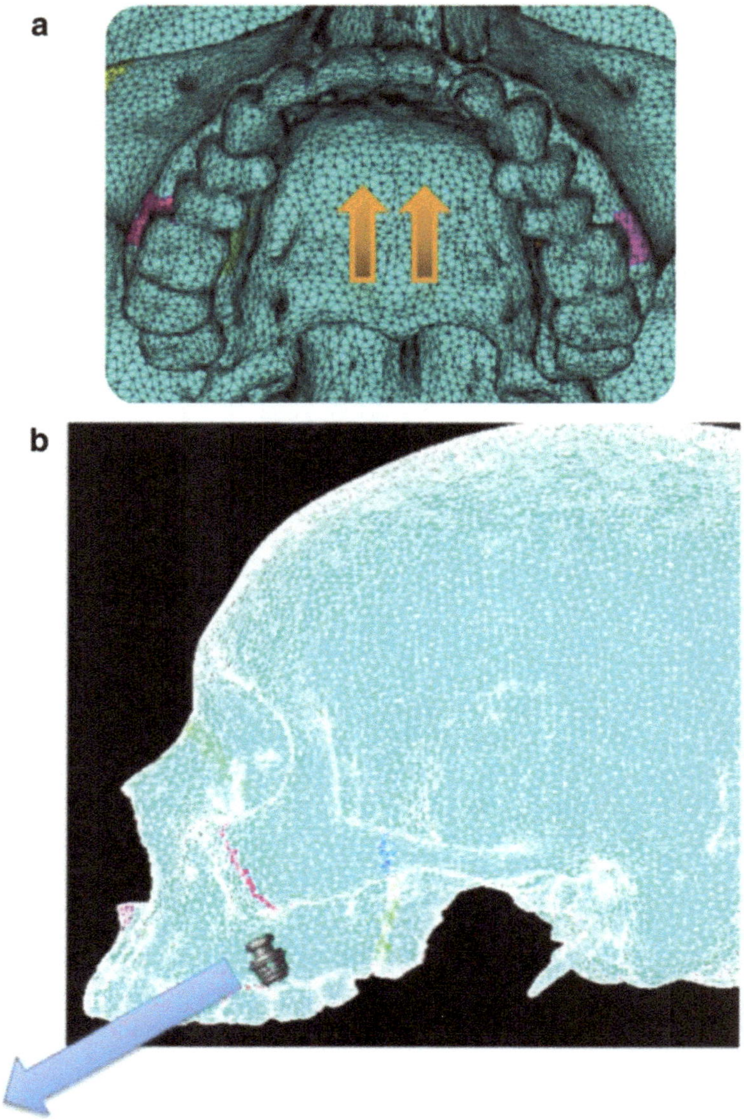

Fig. 4 a, b Location of force application for simulation B—Pal-MI-FM [−30°]

(pure protraction) following force application (Figs. 11, 12, 13, 14, 15, 16, 17, 18). As the color approaches *red* in the rainbow spectrum of colors, there is more Y-displacement of the skull model. Table 2 summarizes the significant findings from each simulation video and superimposition.

Discussion

The hypothesis being tested in this study is that different placement locations and forces applied on the novel N2 mini-implants can translate into different types of maxillary protraction. The development of different clinical protraction protocols was achieved through the various simulations.

For all simulations, 1000 g of protraction forces were applied, as studies have shown that 500–1500 g is an appropriate force load for maxillary protraction [19]. As expected, tensile stresses were visible posterior to the site and direction of force application, while compressive stresses were observed anterior. This phenomenon was observed in all simulations. This is logical, as pulling anteriorly will tend to compress the anterior and place tension on the posterior.

The video animations and superimpositions clearly portray the skeletal effects in each simulation. Because the attachment of the maxilla to the skull is complex, the center of rotation changes depending on the location and vector of force. Varying the location and direction

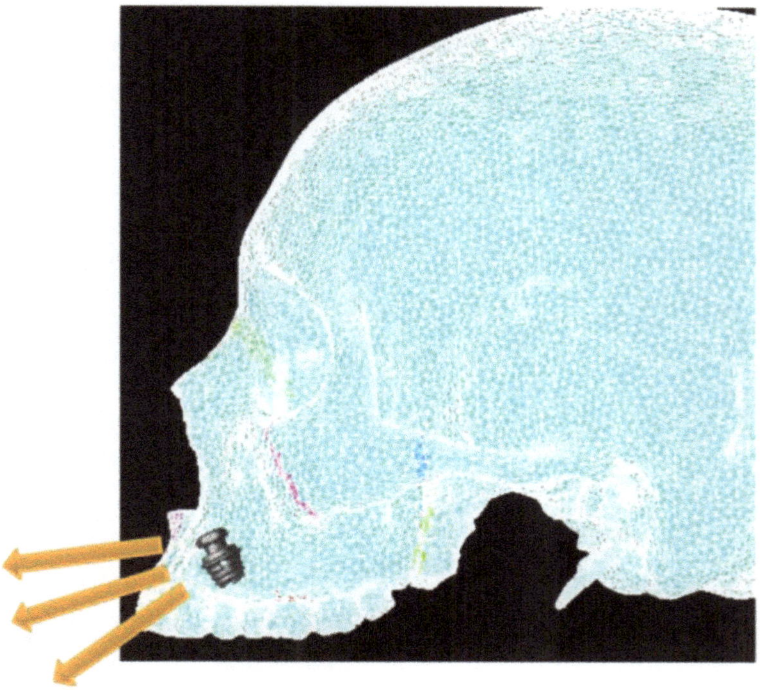

Fig. 5 Location and direction of force application for simulation C—Ant-MI-FM[−15°], simulation D—Ant-MI-FM[−30°], and simulation E—Ant-MI-FM[−45°]

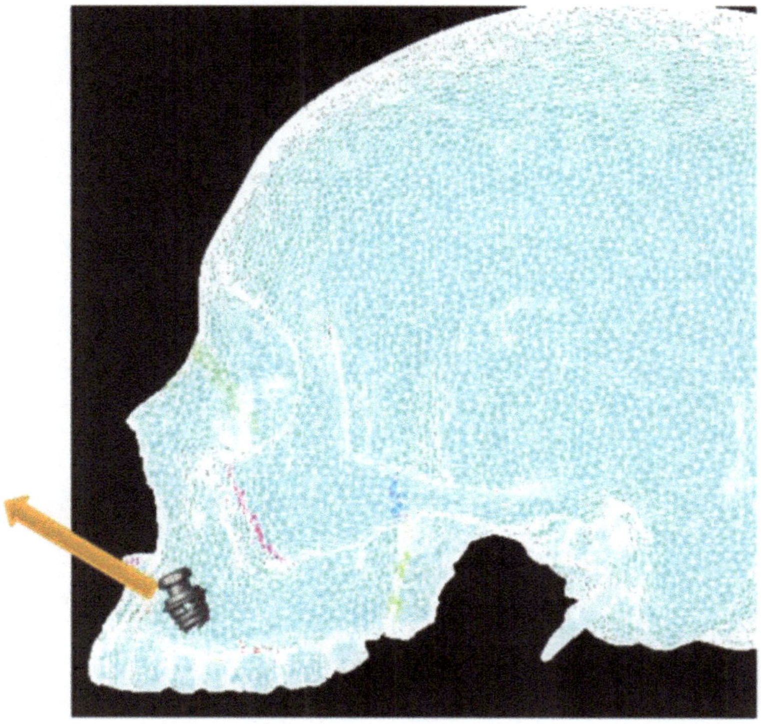

Fig. 6 Location and direction of force application for simulation F—Ant-MI-FM [+30°]

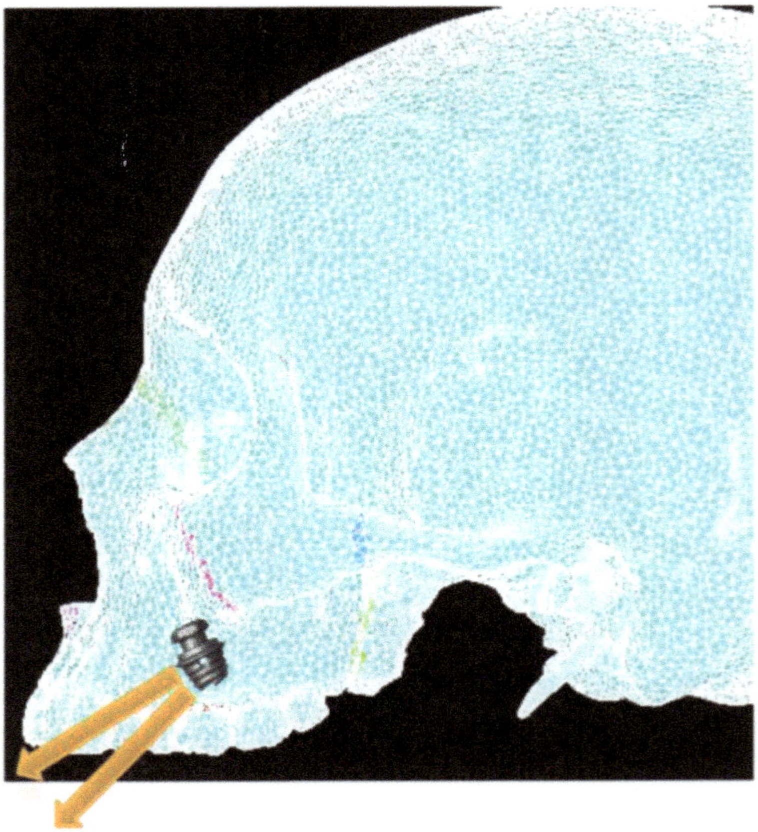

Fig. 7 Location and direction of force application for simulation G—Post-MI-FM [−30°] and simulation H—Post-MI-FM [−45°]

of force produces translation, clockwise rotation, or counter-clockwise rotation of the maxillary complex. For example, a force that is located more anteriorly in the maxilla with a strong downward vector will tend to tip the anterior segment downward. The contour plots showing first and third principle stresses also correspond with the general rotation or translation of the maxilla.

However, simulations that result in the same rotation or translation movement do not necessarily have the same anterior-posterior movement, vertical movement, and rotation. A simulation may result in upward movement of the maxilla, while another results in downward movement. In addition, the amount of forward displacement also depends on the location and direction of force. By varying the location and vector of force, the effect on sutural expansion changes. The complex anatomy of the skull and circummaxillary sutures directly influences the skeletal response from different maxillary protraction protocols. As a result, the video animations and superimpositions provide valuable additional information that can be applied to treatment of patients in the clinical setting.

Several simulations display counter-clockwise rotation of the maxilla. Conventional facemask therapy has the point of force application furthest from the maxillary fulcrum of rotation. As a result, there is significant counter-clockwise rotation. The simulation is an oversimplification, as the force is applied directly to the maxillary molars, and incorporation of periodontal ligament (PDL) into the FEM model would have revealed extrusion, buccal tipping, and mesial movement of the maxillary molars and proclination of the maxillary incisors. Also, force dissipation to the PDL results in greater dentoalveolar compensations and fewer skeletal effects. PDL could not be incorporated into the FEM model, as the element size was larger than the width of PDL. Even with PDL, the simulation will not show alveolar bone remodeling as the teeth are displaced, and the dental movement will be underestimated when using the FEM. As a result, incorporation of PDL still produces an imperfect model.

Anterior-micro-implants-facemask (Ant-MI-FM) [−15°] and Ant-MI-FM [+30°] also display counter-clockwise rotation. Ant-MI-FM [−15°] symbolizes protraction directly from anterior micro-implants while Ant-MI-FM [+30°] simulates an intermaxillary spring from mandibular posterior micro-implants to anterior maxillary micro-implants. The superimposition shows that Ant-MI-FM [−15°] impacts the maxillary complex. However, it is important to note that upward and posterior displacement will restrict

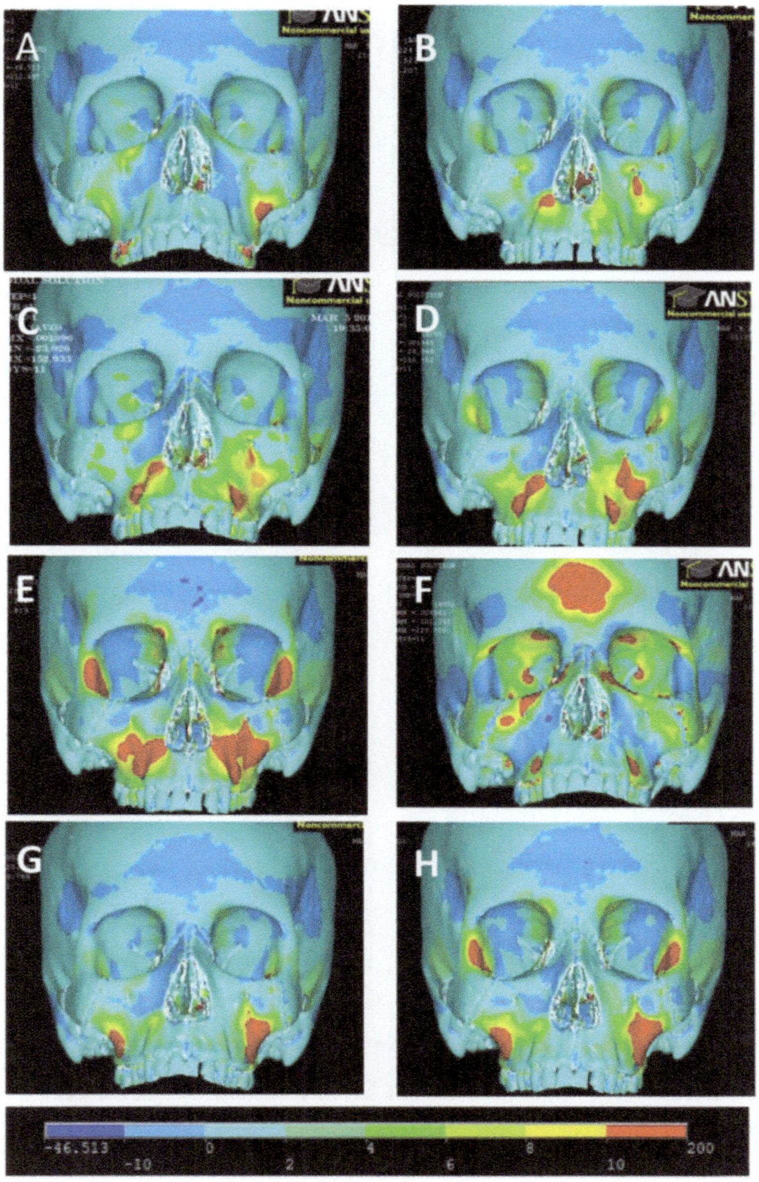

Fig. 8 Frontal view of first principle stresses. **a** FM [−30°]. **b** Pal-MI-FM [−30°]. **c** Ant-MI-FM [−15°]. **d** Ant-MI-FM [−30°]. **e** Ant-MI-FM [−45°]. **f** Ant-MI-FM [+30°]. **g** Post-MI-FM [−30°]. **h** Post-MI-FM [−45°]

maxillary growth, but will not necessarily impact it, since growth cannot be reversed or undone. Ant-MI-FM [−15°] would be beneficial in patients who display a high mandibular angle and excessive incisor show, as the force vector restricts downward displacement of the anterior maxilla. Significantly, more noticeable impaction of the maxillary complex is present in Ant-MI-FM [+30°] superimposition. This clinical protocol is unique and would be beneficial for class III malocclusions with maxillary excess displaying excessive gingiva both in the anterior and posterior regions. This protocol also results in significant protraction of the maxilla. Forward and downward displacement of the maxilla will promote sutural growth, resulting in forward and downward growth of the maxilla.

On the contrary, Ant-MI-FM [−45°] and posterior-micro-implants-facemask (Post-MI-FM) [−45°] display clockwise rotation of the maxilla. Interestingly, Ant-MI-FM [−45°], which simulates facemask protraction from anterior micro-implants, displaces the maxillary complex significantly downward and backwards, which is counterintuitive, given that the goal of maxillary protraction is to move the maxilla forward. In this case, the class III will be corrected by the clockwise rotation of the

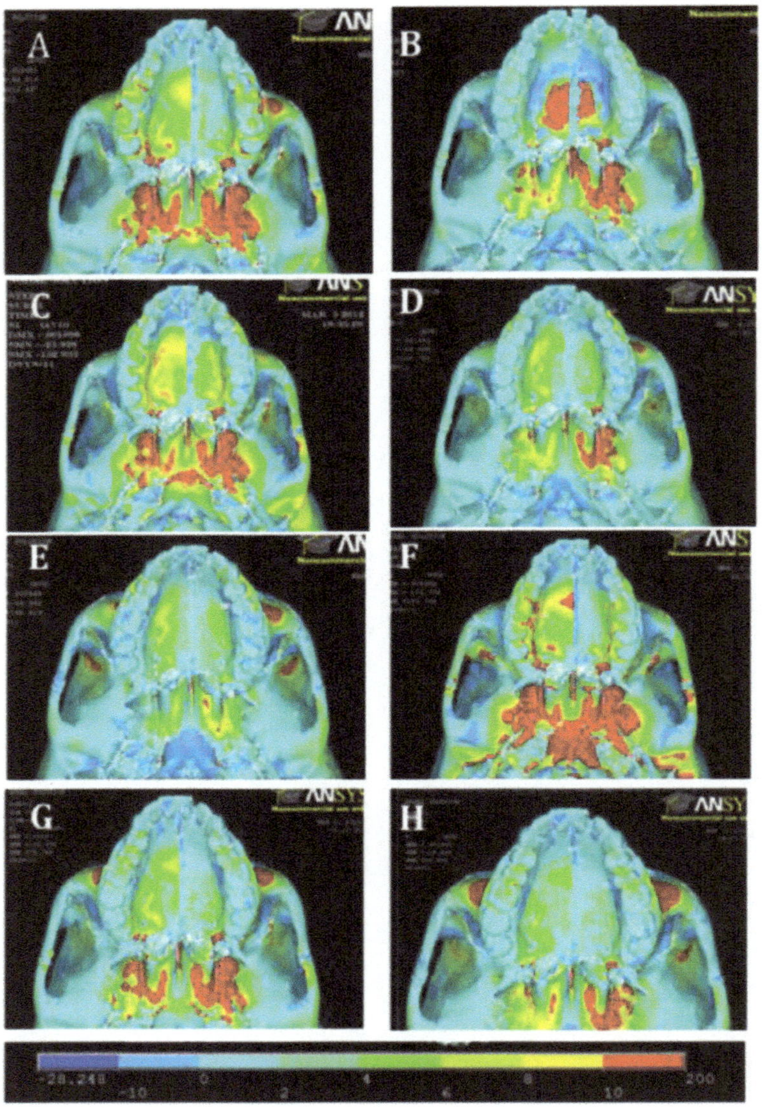

Fig. 9 Occlusal view of first principle stresses. **a** FM [−30°]. **b** Pal-MI-FM [−30°]. **c** Ant-MI-FM [−15°]. **d** Ant-MI-FM [−30°]. **e** Ant-MI-FM [−45°]. **f** Ant-MI-FM [+30°]. **g** Post-MI-FM [−30°]. **h** Post-MI-FM [−45°]

mandible, which is beneficial in select class III cases. Post-MI-FM [−45°], which simulates intermaxillary class III elastics from posterior micro-implants to anterior mandibular micro-implants, moves the maxilla downward and slightly forward. Both Ant-MI-FM [−45°] and Post-MI-FM [−45°] would be beneficial for severely brachyfacial patients with a deep bite, minimal incisal show, and reasonable maxillary A-P position.

The remaining simulations all translate the maxilla, but all in a slightly different manner. In Pal-MI-FM [−30°], the maxillary complex translates downward and forward equally, translating the whole mid-facial segment forward. The clinical effect is similar to a Le Fort III advancement. This protocol would benefit for mesocephalic class III patients with mid-facial deficiency and favorable vertical positioning of the maxilla. In face-mask therapy involving anterior micro-implants, Ant-MI-FM [−30°], the maxillary complex mainly translates downward and forward, with slight downward tipping of the anterior region. This could be useful in mesocephalic class III individuals with a shallow bite. Lastly, Post-MI-FM [−30°], simulating intermaxillary elastics to micro-implants, mainly translates the maxilla forward, with very slight upward tipping of the anterior region. Of all the simulations, Post-MI-FM [−30°] most closely resembles pure anterior protraction of the maxilla and would benefit class III patients with severe mid-facial deficiency. This suggests that a 30° vector for intermaxillary class III

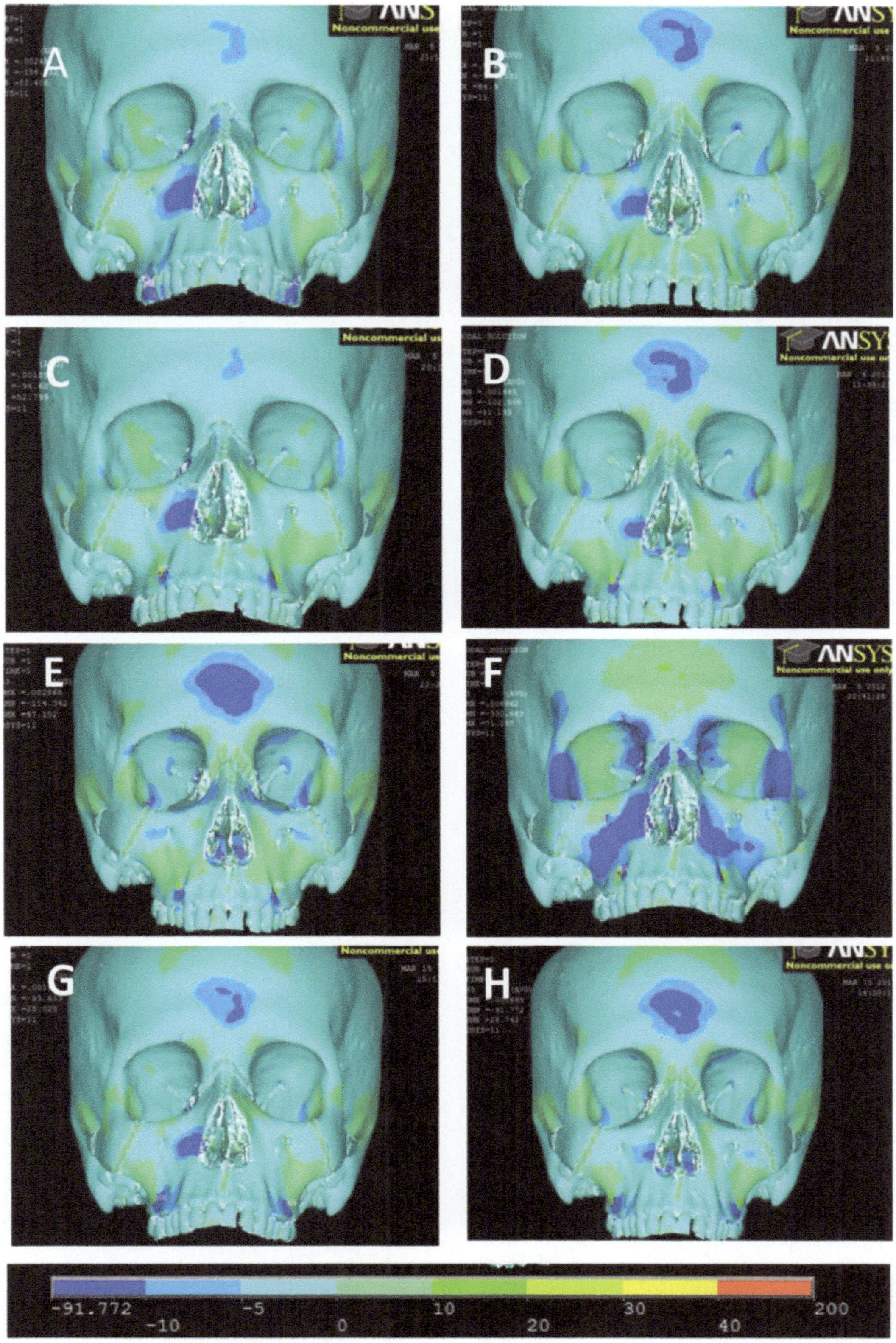

Fig. 10 Frontal view of third principle stresses. **a** FM [−30°]. **b** Pal-MI-FM [−30°]. **c** Ant-MI-FM [−15°]. **d** Ant-MI-FM [−30°]. **e** Ant-MI-FM [−45°]. **f** Ant-MI-FM [+30°]. **g** Post-MI-FM [−30°]. **h** Post-MI-FM [−45°]

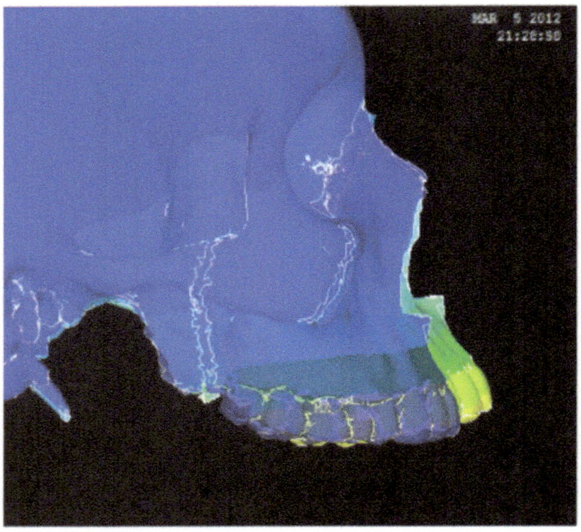

Fig. 11 Simulation A superimposition

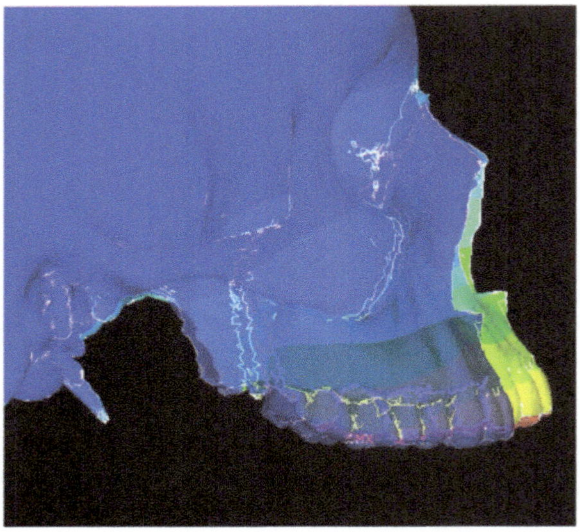

Fig. 13 Simulation C superimposition

elastics between micro-implants is most effective in promoting the anterior growth of maxilla.

The clinical application of these results is evident, given that no two patients are identical. Even though our overall goal in treating class III growing individuals may be to protract the maxilla, each patient presents with different clinical findings. Patients may be brachyfacial or dolicofacial, may present with a deep bite or open bite, may have varying severities of skeletal A-P discrepancy, and may differ in the vertical positions of the maxilla resulting in varying degrees of gingival display. As a result, the location and direction of pull from micro-implants can be altered for maximal clinical effectiveness, as each simulation resulted in a different skeletal effect.

While the study simulates the skeletal response to force application, no simulation is as reliable as real life, so there are some limitations involved with the study. First, the model utilized in this study was generated from a CT scan of a 42-year-old male patient. Even though the literature states that there are no differences in using an adult model for FEM studies [20], sutural morphology and bone anatomy may change slightly throughout growth.

The material properties of bone in this study were assumed to be linear elastic, isotropic, and time independent. This is a simplification, as real bone is more

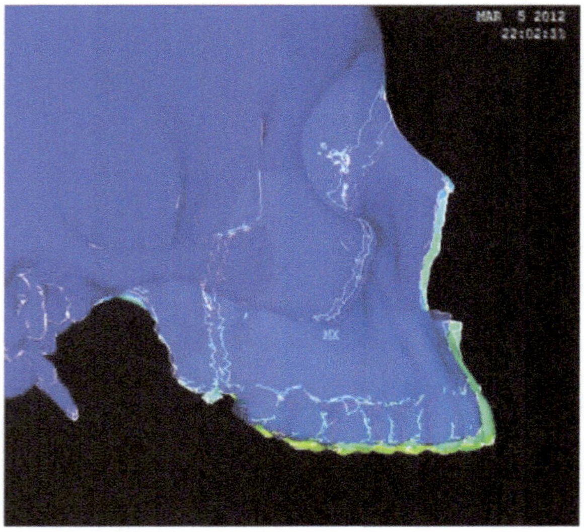

Fig. 12 Simulation B superimposition

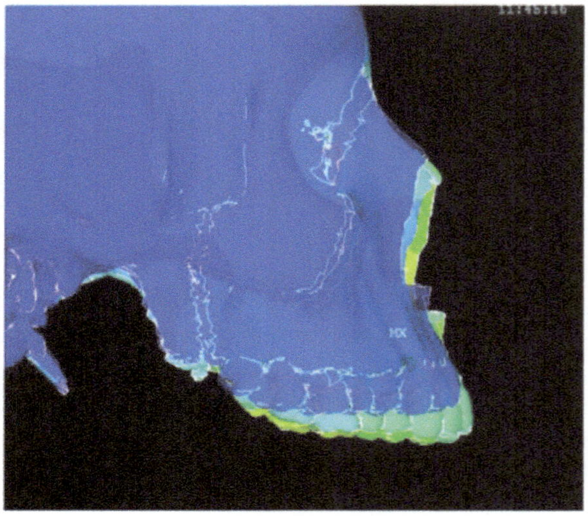

Fig. 14 Simulation D superimposition

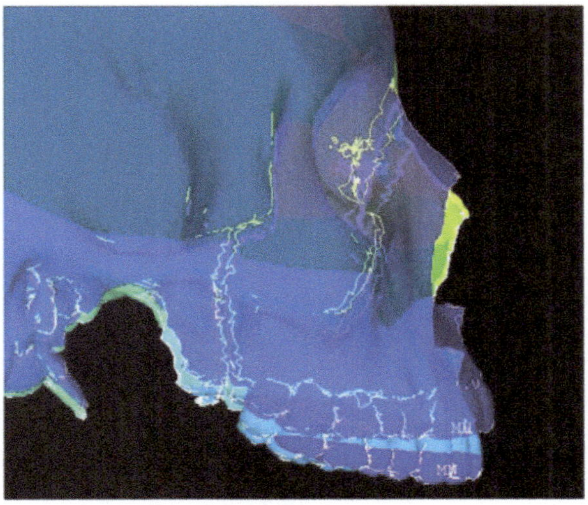

Fig. 15 Simulation E superimposition

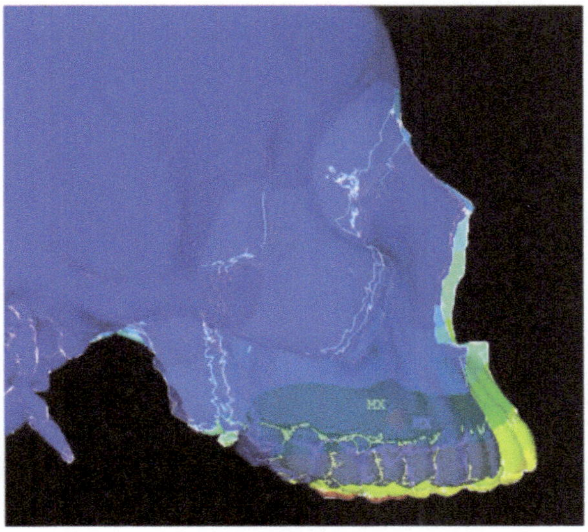

Fig. 17 Simulation G superimposition

anisotropic and time dependent. Bone growth cannot be simulated; we can only show how the internal strain can promote or restrict growth. In addition, no distinction was made between cancellous and cortical bone. The material properties of sutures, while based on several publications, are still an approximation and may not be 100% coincident with connective tissue. Suture morphology was estimated, and due to limitations in computer memory and model element size, PDL could not be accurately incorporated into the model. Logically, the PDL should absorb a proportion of the forces resulting in displacement of the teeth. In addition, FEM cannot simulate the resorption and deposition of bone that should occur in the dentoalveolar bone.

However, it may be difficult to create a perfect model with ideal properties. Anatomy and material properties change from one person to another, thus making the problem more complex.

Without PDL, soft tissues, and remodeling within the model, the teeth are essentially ankylosed within the dentoalveolar bone. While the simulation does not accurately predict the dental effects [21–23], it does, however, demonstrate the skeletal effects, which is of primary concern when it comes to growth modification procedures like maxillary protraction. This study is valid in comparing how location and vector of force alters the skeletal effects. As a result, the location and direction of

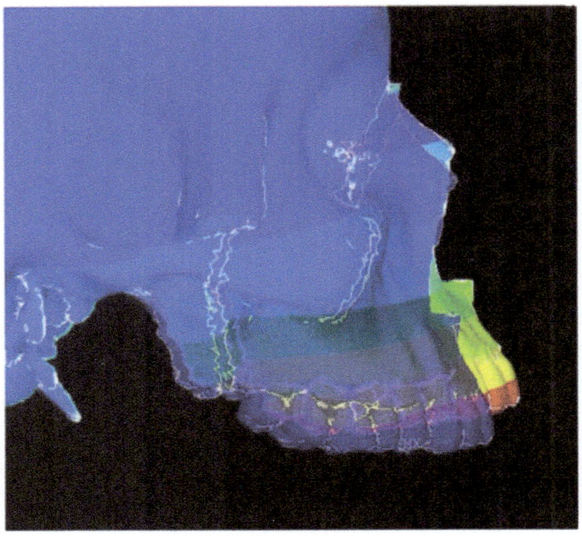

Fig. 16 Simulation F superimposition

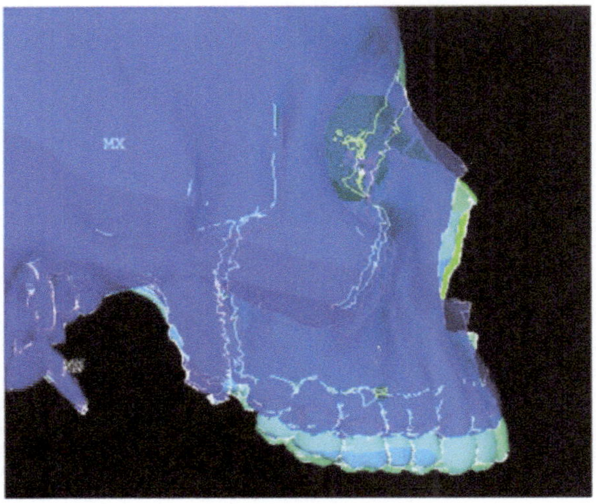

Fig. 18 Simulation H superimposition

Table 2 Skeletal effects on the maxillary complex

Simulation	Clinical protocol	Movement of maxillary complex	Details of maxillary movement
A	FM [−30]	Counter-clockwise rotation	Forward and upward movement; slight posterior downward movement
B	Pal-MI-FM [−30]	Translates forward and downward	Equal forward and downward movement
C	Ant-MI-FM [−15]	Counter-clockwise rotation	Forward and upward movement; entire maxilla moves upward
D	Ant-MI-FM [−30]	Translates; slight clockwise rotation	Forward and downward movement
E	Ant-MI-FM [−45]	Clockwise rotation	Downward and backward movement; nasal bone protracted forward
F	Ant-MI-FM [+30]	Counter-clockwise rotation	Forward and upward movement; entire maxilla moves upward
G	Post-MI-FM [−30]	Translates forward	Significant forward movement; slight downward movement
H	Post-MI-FM [−45]	Clockwise rotation	Slight forward, but mainly downward movement of maxilla

pull can be customized for treatment of different types of class III patients in the clinical setting.

Conclusions

Depending on the location and direction of force, the maxillary complex rotates clockwise, counter-clockwise, and/or translates anteriorly and vertically. By varying the location and vector of class III mechanics, orthodontists can differentially alter the magnitude of forward, downward, and rotational movement of the maxilla. As a result, we can customize the location of micro-implants and direction of force based on the patient's needs.

Competing interests

The authors declare that they have no competing interests.

Authors' contributions

WM provided the guidance and oversaw the entire investigation. KW was involved in the generation and implementation of the model. MM participated in the refinement of the model. JS was involved in the data analysis. HC was involved in running the simulations. GY was involved in writing the ANSYS simulation batch files. AM was involved in the clinical interpretation of the results.

Author details

[1]UCLA Section of Orthodontics, UCLA School of Dentistry, 10833 Le Conte Avenue, CHS – Box 951668, Los Angeles, CA 90095-1668, USA. [2]Mechanical Engineering Department, California State University, Northridge, 18111 Nordhoff Street, Northridge, CA 91330, USA. [3]Section of Orthodontics, Federal University of Bahia, Salvador, Bahia, Brazil.

References

1. Wells AP, Sarver DM, Proffit WR. Long-term efficacy of reverse pull headgear therapy. Angle Orthod. 2006;76:915–22.
2. Franchi L, Baccetti T, McNamara JA. Postpubertal assessment of treatment timing for maxillary expansion and protraction therapy followed by fixed appliances. Am J Orthod Dentofac Orthop Off Publ Am Assoc Orthod Its Const Soc Am Board Orthod. 2004;126:555–68.
3. Ngan PW, Hagg U, Yiu C, Wei SH. Treatment response and long-term dentofacial adaptations to maxillary expansion and protraction. Semin Orthod. 1997;3:255–64.
4. Sung SJ, Baik HS. Assessment of skeletal and dental changes by maxillary protraction. Am J Orthod Dentofac Orthop Off Publ Am Assoc Orthod Its Const Soc Am Board Orthod. 1998;114:492–502.
5. Yüksel S, Uçem TT, Keykubat A. Early and late facemask therapy. Eur J Orthod. 2001;23:559–68.
6. Nanda R. Protraction of maxilla in rhesus monkeys by controlled extraoral forces. Am J Orthod. 1978;74:121–41.
7. Cevidanes L, Baccetti T, Franchi L, McNamara JA, De Clerck H. Comparison of two protocols for maxillary protraction: bone anchors versus face mask with rapid maxillary expansion. Angle Orthod. 2010;80:799–806.
8. Heymann GC, Cevidanes L, Cornelis M, De Clerck HJ, Tulloch JFC. Three-dimensional analysis of maxillary protraction with intermaxillary elastics to miniplates. Am J Orthod Dentofac Orthop Off Publ Am Assoc Orthod Its Const Soc Am Board Orthod. 2010;137:274–84.
9. Kim KY, Bayome M, Park JH, Kim KB, Mo SS, Kook YA, et al. Displacement and stress distribution of the maxillofacial complex during maxillary protraction with buccal versus palatal plates: finite element analysis. Eur J Orthod. 2014. doi:10.1093/ejo/cju039.
10. Lee N-K, Baek S-H. Stress and displacement between maxillary protraction with miniplates placed at the infrazygomatic crest and the lateral nasal wall: a 3-dimensional finite element analysis. Am J Orthod Dentofac Orthop Off Publ Am Assoc Orthod Its Const Soc Am Board Orthod. 2012;141:345–51.
11. Wilmes B, Nienkemper M, Drescher D. Application and effectiveness of a mini-implant- and tooth-borne rapid palatal expansion device: the hybrid hyrax. World J Orthod. 2010;11:323–30.
12. Nienkemper M, Wilmes B, Pauls A, Drescher D. Maxillary protraction using a hybrid hyrax-facemask combination. Prog Orthod. 2013;14:5.
13. Yan X, He W, Lin T, Liu J, Bai X, Yan G, et al. Three-dimensional finite element analysis of the craniomaxillary complex during maxillary protraction with bone anchorage vs conventional dental anchorage. Am J Orthod Dentofac Orthop Off Publ Am Assoc Orthod Its Const Soc Am Board Orthod. 2013;143:197–205. doi:10.1016/j.ajodo.2012.09.019.
14. MacGinnis M, Chu H, Youssef G, Wu KW, Machado A, Moon W. The effects of micro-implant assisted rapid palatal expansion (MARPE) on the nasomaxillary complex—a finite element method (FEM) analysis. Prog Orthod. 2014;15:52. doi:10.1186/s40510-014-0052-y.
15. Hong C, Lee H, Webster R, Kwak J, Wu BM, Moon W. Stability comparison between commercially available mini-implants and a novel design: part 1. Angle Orthod. 2011;81:692–9. doi:10.2319/092410-556.1.
16. Hong C, Truong P, Song HN, Wu BM, Moon W. Mechanical stability assessment of novel orthodontic mini-implant designs: part 2. Angle Orthod. 2011;81:1001–9.
17. Song HN, Hong C, Banh R, Ohebsion T, Asatrian G, Leung HY, et al. Mechanical stability and clinical applicability assessment of novel orthodontic mini-implant design. Angle Orthod. 2013;83:832–41. doi:10.2319/111412-876.1.
18. Kircelli BH, Pektas ZO. Midfacial protraction with skeletally anchored face mask therapy: a novel approach and preliminary results. Am J Orthod Dentofac Orthop Off Publ Am Assoc Orthod Its Const Soc Am Board Orthod. 2008;133:440–9.
19. Ge YS, Liu J, Chen L, Han JL, Guo X. Dentofacial effects of two facemask therapies for maxillary protraction. Angle Orthod. 2012;82:1083–91.
20. Nakagawa M et al. Biomechanical effects of reversed headgear maxillary protraction on the craniofacial complex as determined by strain gauge measurements. Nihon Kyōsei Shika Gakkai Zasshi J Jpn Orthod Soc. 1986;45:109–18.
21. Heravi F, Salari S, Tanbakuchi B, Loh S, Amiri M. Effects of crown-root angle on stress distribution in the maxillary central incisors' PDL during application of intrusive and retraction forces: a three-dimensional finite element analysis. Prog Orthod. 2013;14:26.

22. Lombardo L, Scuzzo G, Arreghini A, Gorgun Ö, Ortan Y, Siciliani G. 3D FEM comparison of lingual and labial orthodontics in en masse retraction. Prog Orthod. 2014;15:38. doi:10.1186/s40510-014-0038-9.
23. Sardarian A, Danaei S, Shahidi S, Boushehri S, Geramy A. The effect of vertical bracket positioning on torque and the resultant stress in the periodontal ligament—a finite element study. Prog Orthod. 2014;15:50.

8

Quantitative analysis of 3-dimensional facial soft tissue photographic images: technical methods and clinical application

Vikrum Nanda[1], Boris Gutman[2], Ehab Bar[1], Suha Alghamdi[3], Sotirios Tetradis[1], Aldons J Lusis[1], Eleazar Eskin[1] and Won Moon[1*]

Abstract

Background: The recent advent of 3D photography has created the potential for comprehensive facial evaluation. However, lack of practical true 3D analysis of the information collected from 3D images has been the factor limiting widespread utilization in orthodontics. Current evaluation of 3D facial soft tissue images relies on subjective visual evaluation and 2D distances to assess facial disharmony. The objectives of this project strive to map the surface and define boundaries of 3D facial soft tissue, modify mathematical functions to average multiple 3D facial images, and mathematically average 3D facial images allowing generation of color-coded surface deviation relative to a true average.

Methods: Collaboration headed by UCLA Orthodontics with UCLA Neuroimaging was initiated to modify advanced brain mapping technology to accurately map the facial surface in 3D. 10 subjects were selected as a sample for development of the technical protocol. 3dMD photographic images were segmented, corrected using a series of topology correcting algorithms, and process to create close meshes. Shapes were mapped to a sphere using conformal and area preserving maps, and were then registered using a spherical patch mapping approach. Finally an average was created using 7-parameter procrustes alignment.

Results: Size-standardized average facial images were generated for the sample population. A single patient was then superimposed on the average and color-coded displacement maps were generated to demonstrate the clinical applicability of this protocol. Further confirmation of the methods through 3D superimposition of the initial (T0) average to the 4 week (T4) average was completed and analyzed.

Conclusions: The results of this investigation suggest that it is possible to average multiple facial images of highly variable topology. The immediate application of this research will be rapid and detailed diagnostic imaging analysis for orthodontic and surgical treatment planning. There is great potential for application to anthropometrics and genomics. This investigation resulted in establishment of a protocol for mapping the surface of the human face in three dimensions.

Background

Significance

The orthodontic profession is a specialty founded on the analysis and interpretation of geometries representing facial proportions. Dimensions and ratios are translated into representations of ideals and applied to facial aesthetics. The traditional foundation of orthodontics has relied on two-dimensional imaging to recreate the three-dimensional facial intricacies that exist in human anatomy. In the past decade, technological advancements have allowed visualization of bony anatomy and even more recently the soft tissues of the face. The orthodontic profession now has access to more information in three-dimensions than ever before [1]. It is our professional responsibility to utilize this information and apply these advancements in imaging towards patient care. There is a strong need for investigations which analyze

* Correspondence: wmoon@dentistry.ucla.edu
[1]UCLA, California, USA
Full list of author information is available at the end of the article

progress and change in three dimensions to supplement and enhance traditional treatment modalities [2].

Although frontal and lateral cephalometric radiographs, panoramic radiographs, and intraoral and extra- oral photographs are still used, more emphasis has been placed on the 3D virtual image and soft-tissue esthetics [3, 4]. The paradigm shift in treatment philosophies also means that many clinicians have started to plan from the external profile, placing importance on the soft tissues of the face largely to determine the limitations of orthodontic treatment. From the perspectives of function, stability, and esthetics, the orthodontist must plan treatment within the patient's limits of soft-tissue adaptation and contours [5].

Three-dimensional facial photographic imaging was introduced to orthodontics during the early years of the millennium. Research has demonstrated the value and increased accuracy of three-dimensional photography compared to traditional imaging modalities and has sought to develop new analyses for their application to clinical use [6, 7]. Most current methods for analysis of 3D photographic images involve simple visual evaluation or linear and angular measures between various point landmarks to evaluate facial aesthetics and proportions. The objective for this project is to develop and verify a protocol for mapping the surface of the human face in three dimensions using three-dimensional photography.

Objectives and specific aims

Facial soft tissue analysis has evolved over time, and with the latest advancements in technology, 3D photographic imaging has created the potential for comprehensive facial evaluation. However, lack of practical true 3D analysis of the information collected from 3D photographic images has been the limiting factor holding back widespread utilization in the orthodontic profession. Current evaluation of these 3D facial soft tissue images relies largely on subjective visual evaluation and 2D point-to-point distances to assess aesthetics and facial disharmony. Those that have attempted 3D averaging and analysis have failed to comprehensively and accurately describe the 3D facial surface with respect to size, color, and morphologic difference.

Ultimately, this project will contribute to the creation of a true three-dimensional craniofacial analysis and establishment of a database of 3D photographic images for generation of age, gender, and race specific normative models of the human face. Overall, this study seeks to advance 3D imaging analysis technology by aiming to:

1. Apply and modify advanced technology used in brain mapping research to accurately and efficiently map the facial surface in 3D.
2. Apply and modify existing mathematical functions to find the average of multiple facial surfaces.
3. Develop protocol for superimposing sample faces on the averaged facial model, yielding a color-coded map of surface deviation and dysmorphology.
4. Superimpose and compare the average facial models of same patients before (T1) and after (T2) a particular treatment protocol (orthognathic surgery, MARPE/SARPE, RPE, etc.)

The immediate objectives of this project strive to map the surface and define boundaries of 3D facial soft tissue, modify and apply mathematical functions to average multiple 3D facial soft tissue photographic images, and mathematically average 3D facial soft tissue images allowing generation of color-coded surface deviation relative to a true average.

Accomplishing our immediate goal would result in a protocol for mapping the surface of the human face in three dimensions using 3D photographic images. Application of this technology would allow rapid soft tissue diagnostics for treatment planning in various health care specialties (i.e. orthodontics, oral/maxillofacial and plastic surgery. As this vision is realized, the ability to analyze patients or groups of patients in three dimensions would shift the diagnostic and normative paradigms currently used in craniofacial analysis towards an ever-progressive direction.

Methods

Quantification and averaging methods

The main purpose of this project is to create an average face from a random set of faces. We are interested in finding point-to-point correspondences across a large, potentially highly variable population of human face models. Using surface mapping, this project will refine and apply tools developed in neuroimaging research to create surface-based maps of the human face. On a broad level, the project can be divided into five parts, summarized below, and described in more detail in this section:

1. Collection of sample 3D Face models
2. Surface topology correction and spherical mapping
   a. Non-manifold polygon correction
   b. Boundary closure and Smoothing
   c. Spherical Mapping
3. Shape registration
   a. Initial Spherical Matching
   b. Texture Matching
   c. Geometry Matching and Registration Model
4. Average and distance map creation
   a. Procrustes alignment/ Tensor Based Morphometry
   b. Average and distance map creation, shape statistics analysis
5. Pilot study
   a. Evaluation of individual shape morphology compared to averaged face

Collection of 3D face models

The novel nature of this investigation requires the formulation of a standard protocol for consistent image acquisition using the 3dMD facial imaging system. Our goal was to create an ideal environment and maintain consistent image acquisition for individual subjects over the duration of comprehensive treatment time. Natural head posture (NHP) was adopted for this study because it has been shown to be clinically reproducible [8–10]. IRB approval was acquired for this project.

Surface topology correction and spherical mapping

In non-technical terms, "topology" essentially refers to the number of handles, islands and boundaries of the surface. Since no well-defined correspondence between surfaces of different topologies is theoretically possible, one must perform a topological correction of each facial model before computing a dense correspondence. The simplest and most common approach is to make each surface topologically equivalent to a sphere.

Non-manifold polygon correction Removing triangles ("faces") and vertices of non-manifold nature from polygon models is a fairly common problem in 3D modeling.

Boundary closure and smoothing We propose a boundary closure and surface extrapolation procedure similar to our previous work with shape correspondence [11]. Each boundary is initially "sewn together" with a new set of triangle faces, and the surface area of the new surface patch is minimized using standard linear optimization techniques with boundary conditions [12]. The triangulation of the patch is then subdivided into more faces, and the process is repeated iteratively, until the reduction in surface area is sufficiently small. This procedure is guaranteed to produce face models of spherical topology.

Spherical mapping To enable efficient correspondence search across a dataset of faces, it is necessary to create an intermediate mapping to a common canonical space, where the final registration may be performed. A correspondence search on a sphere was performed, where all points moved around freely matching geometry appropriately, and matching extraneous tissue in some models to filler regions in others, as appropriate.

Shape registration

Several shape registration techniques exist for genus zero shapes (shapes of spherical topology), including those based on spherical parameterization. Among these

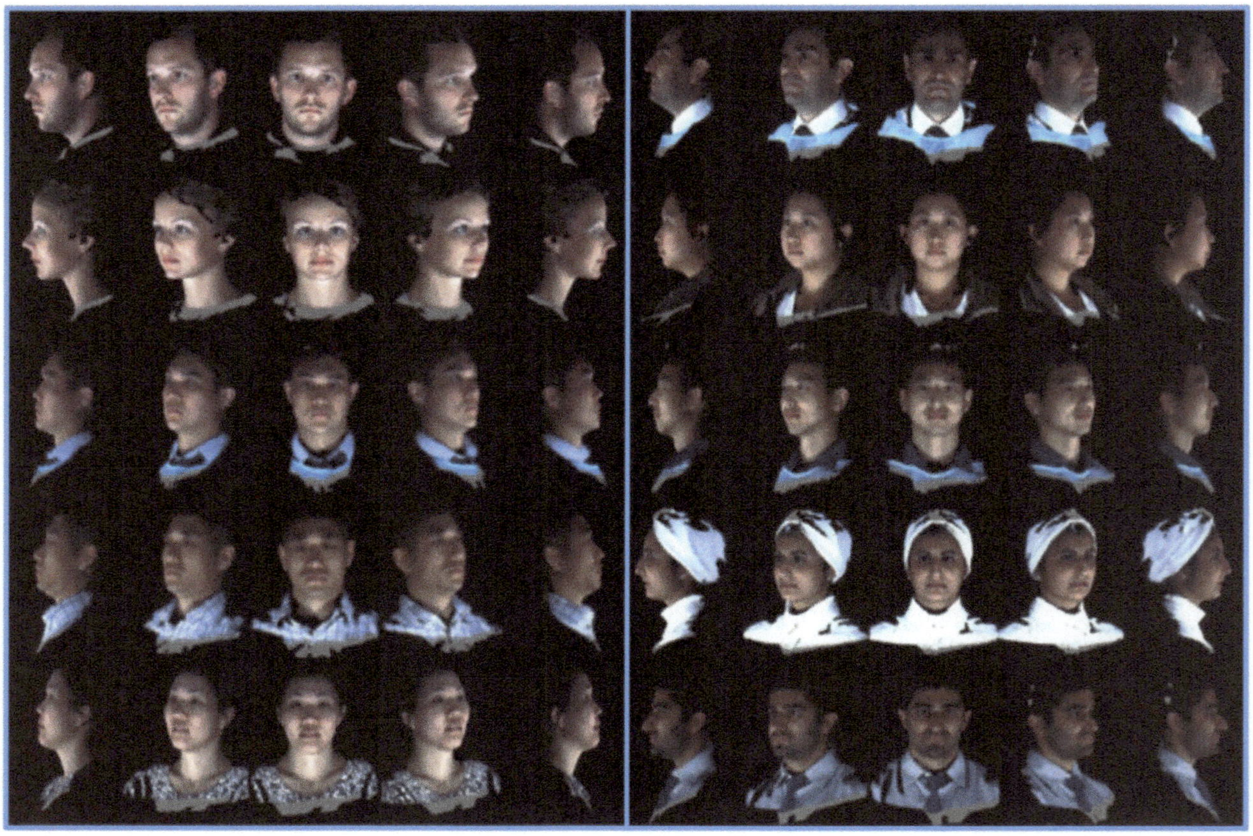

Fig. 1 10 individual 3dMD samples used to create T0 average (Frontal, ¾, Lateral Views)

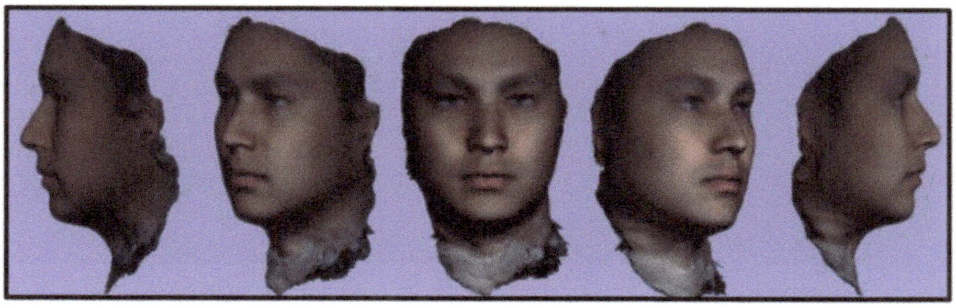

Fig. 2 T0 average of 10 samples: "The Average Face"

are the rigid spherical cross-correlation [13], spherical demons [14], Laplace-Beltrami Eigen-function registration [15], just to name a few. The unique challenge for 3D face models, not addressed by existing methods, lies in the need to combine texture information from the coloring of the face and face geometry. Our proposed method would find dense correspondence across a set of faces using both texture and geometry information, while maintaining sufficient flexibility to deal with non-face regions of the model.

Initial spherical matching To ensure a robust initial map, we used a curve-matching algorithm. A simple set of 10 curves was manually drawn on each face model using the BrainSuite 14 software, taking roughly 5 minutes per model by a trained operator. The correspondence between landmark points on the facial surface was determined automatically via the arclength map. We attain spherical displacements between corresponding curve points projected onto the sphere. This initial map suffices for further local refinement described below.

Texture matching To minimize the mismatch between texture maps, we choose to use multi-channel Mutual Information criteria, often used to match 2D and 3D medical images from different modalities [16]. This choice is motivated by the fact that facial texture correspondence is characterized by complex relationships between intensities of different color channels, without a straight-forward transfer function. For example, different individuals may have entirely different color composition of their eyes and skin.

Geometry matching and registration model In addition to texture, geometry mismatch will be simultaneously minimized following [14, 17] based on position- and orientation-invariant features such as mean and Gaussian curvature. We choose the fluid spherical registration model, which we developed recently in LONI's past study in mapping the hippocampus in Alzheimer's patients [17], because it is maximally flexible and completely agnostic with respect to the mismatch function, unlike previous methods. [13, 14] We believe that matching texture and geometry simultaneously will lead to the best most accurate mapping.

Average and distance map creation

Procrustes alignment/tensor-based morphometry To compute the average face, we must first align the shape models in their original (not parametric) space, based on the computed dense correspondence. We will use the 7-parameter Procrustes method for this [18], excluding filler patches from the mismatch cost. An alternative measure of face morphometry, called Tensor Based Morphometry, has gained popularity in recent years [19]. Unlike distance-based features above, the TBM features invariant to the position and orientation of the shapes, making accurate Procrustes alignment a non-issue.

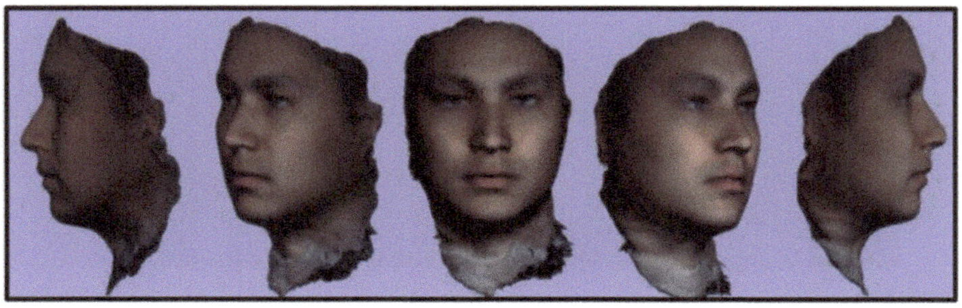

Fig. 3 T0 average of 10 samples: "The Average Face" (Repeat of Fig. 2- Here for visual purposes)

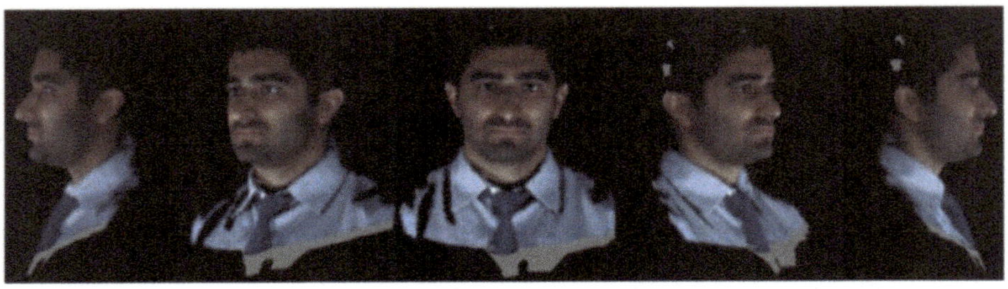

Fig. 4 T0 3dMD image of individual sample to be compared to the average T0 norm above

Distance and statistical maps Having computed the average shape, we will compute the distance from the average to each shape at each point. Distance-to-average maps are displayed as colorized surface maps. Looking to the future, given a discrete, or continuous biological variable, such as whether the subject carries a certain gene, or some clinical measure of severity of a particular deformity, it is it possible to create statistical parametric maps based on distance to the average. These typically involve parametric or non-parametric (e.g. permutation) statistical tests done at each point [20], which localize the effect of the biological variable on the face surface.

Each single 3dMD individual image consists of roughly 32,000 vertices which represent an x,y,z coordinate on a Cartesian coordinate scale. Each averaged facial image retains this 32,000 vertex mesh with each single vertex possessing a specific variance. Therefore, superimposition of two average samples essentially represents a statistical p-map representing deviation from the norm.

Proof of methods/pilot study

A critical aspect in our analysis of the human face is to demonstrate that these methods can be used to average faces with variable morphology. In order to demonstrate our proof of methods, we have subjected our pipeline to several processes to demonstrate the function, accuracy, and potential applications for our pipeline.

A) A random non-homogenous sample of 10 subjects was selected with no exclusions on gender, age, and ethnicity. These subjects' images were plugged into our averaging pipeline to create a true 3D average.

B) Furthermore, 3D distance-to-average maps displayed as colorized surface maps which will show individual deviation from our normative 10 sample average were created. This is a key feature that will allow for comparison of individual facial morphology to age, gender and race specific normative models for specific populations.

C) In order to demonstrate viability of the pipeline to average samples accurately over multiple time points, the T0 (initial) average of our 10 non-homogenous samples to their corresponding T4 (4 week) average was generated. This will illustrate the significance and accuracy of our average T0 to average T4 superimpositions and serve as a clear proof of methods.

Results

A) 3D facial photographic average

A review of 3dMD clinical records resulted in a decision to use 10 3D photographic images to demonstrate proof of methods (Fig. 1). The sample population consisted of individuals with varying demographics, including ethnicity, gender, age, and skeletal/dental type. The purpose of using such a highly diverse sample was to demonstrate the power of these methods in generating a clean average model even with a population showing high topological variability. The 10 3dMD photographic images after topological correction were loaded into the

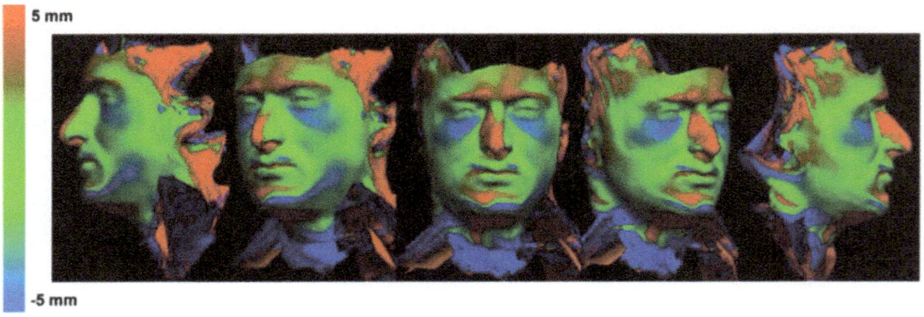

Fig. 5 T0 individual sample superimposed over our T0 10 subject average norm. Scale is -5 mm to 5 mm

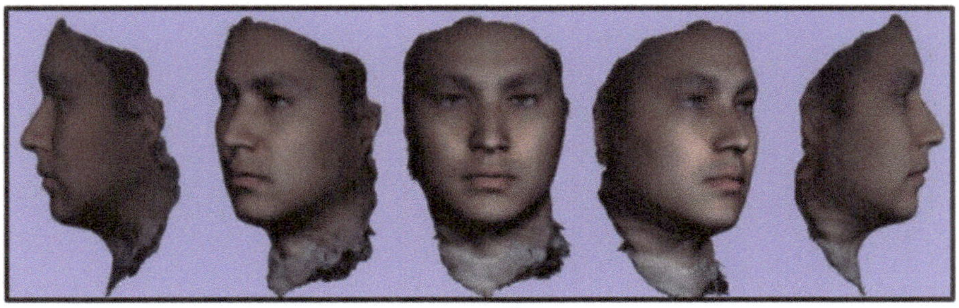

Fig. 6 T0 average of 10 samples: "The Average Face" (Repeat of Figs. 2,3)

initial software pipeline to generate the closed mesh forms of the images. These closed meshes were then traced for surface curves in areas of interest to aid in the "averaging pipeline". The result of this dual pipeline process is a clean average of 10 human three-dimensional faces after topology correction, closed mesh creation, and shape registration (Fig. 2).

B) 3D superimposition of individual sample to average

After development of an average facial normative model from the 10 image sample over two time points, our registration technique was applied to demonstrate the ability to superimpose a sample individual 3D facial image on the average model (Figs. 3, 4, 5). The orientation was maintained and registration was made possible thorugh the mesh framework, which retains point-to-point correspondence of vertices between shapes. The next step in producing clinically applicable superimpositions is to develop color-coded maps of surface deviation and dysmorphology. The color schematic that we chose to represent displacement values were as follows: Green represents no deviation from the norm; Blue represents deviation in a negative/inwards direction; Red represents deviation in a positive/outward direction. The magnitude of displacement ranged from -5 mm to 5 mm. Users have the ability to zoom in/out and

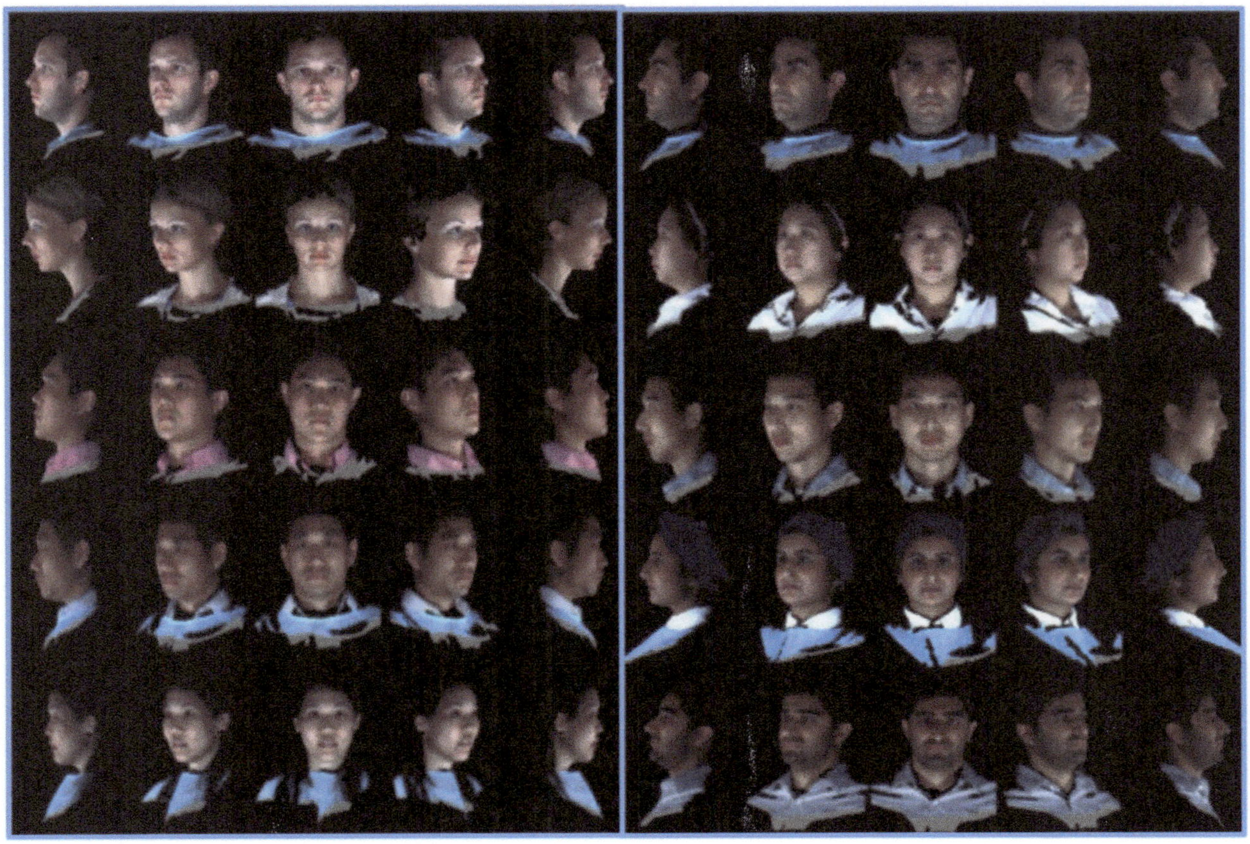

Fig. 7 10 individual 3dMD samples used to create T4 average (Frontal, ¾, Lateral Views)

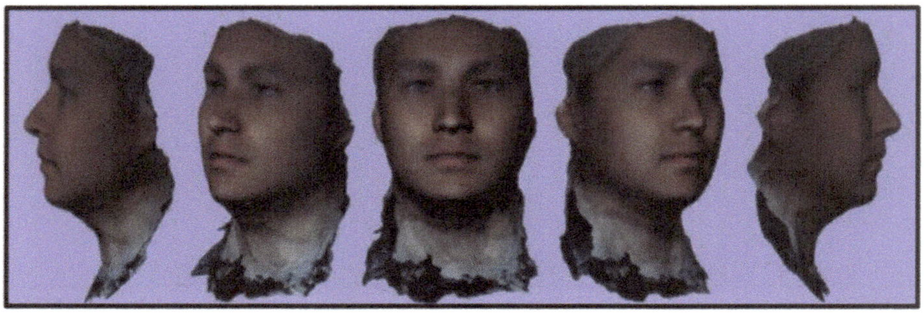

Fig. 8 T4 (4 week) average of 10 samples: "The Average Face"

manipulate the 3D superimposition to achieve any orientation desired to more appropriately view the results.

C) 3D superimposition of 10 subject average T0 to 10 subject average T4

A critical application of this averaging pipeline is to generate comparisons among groups of subjects. This goes one step beyond individual to average comparisons as seen in the previous section. Illustrating the ability to compare norm to norm over differing time points we have generated a 3D superimposition of our T0 10 subject average (Figs. 2, 3, 6) over our T4 10 subject average (Fig. 8). The scale has been adjusted for this superimposition to detect more subtle change among average to average comparison. For our purposes, the T0 average and T4 average should not vary significantly due to the fact that they were taken on subjects not undergoing any treatment modalities nor experiencing identifyable physiologic change over the 4 week test period. The scale used for the below results was -3 mm to 3 mm. An identical color schematic to the previous colorized displacement map was used here (Figs. 6, 7, 8, 9).

Discussion

A) Clinical applications

The overarching goal of this project was to successfully and accurately average the soft tissues of the human face in three dimensions. 3dMD 3D facial photographs were taken of subjects over two time points. The 3D images were piped into our developed software to process the data into a closed mesh format. The mesh geometries underlying the 3D facial photographs were topologically corrected to create a more continuous three dimensional mesh structure. Surface curves were traced using Brainsuite 14a software to identify areas of interest for the registration process. The geometries were then mapped to a sphere and aligned/registered to create an overall multi-subject average.

Creation of a true three dimensional average of the human face opens the doors to a variety of significant and novel applications. An immediate application of the basic average of a specific inclusion of samples may yield normative data for a specific demographic. This could be applied to anthropologic and genetic sciences. The ability to compare an individual to a generated average yields further potential to compare individual subjects against groups to determine detailed deviation and dysmorphology. This would prove to be invaluable in medical/dental specialties to determine appropriate treatment for correction of facial deviation from the norm.

One can imagine that comparison of norms at different time points could prove quite useful and informative when dealing with various aspects of longitudinal change. Examples include but are not limited to orthodontic

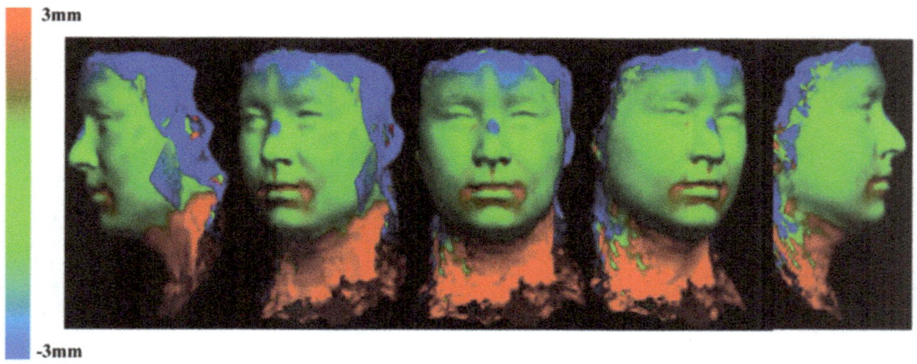

Fig. 9 T0 average to T4 average 3D superimposition

treatment, plastic/ maxillofacial surgical outcomes, longitudinal change with aging, and data collection for surgical simulations. Comparisons using this technology can be made on a macro scale involving large populations and ethnicities. Acquisition of this data poses no risk to the patient of any kind and given one 3D photographic imaging machine allows acquisition of unlimited images relying only on digital storage capacity.

The impact to orthodontics will be speedy quantitative 3D comparison of patients relative to their 3-dimensional norms in diagnostics and treatment planning. Various research opportunities will arise as a direct result of our project as 3-dimensional normative soft tissue data using our pipeline can be readily generated for ethnic, race, and gender specific populations.

The immediate objective leading to possible future publication seeks to demonstrate our project's impact to clinical orthodontics. We will follow patients over pre-treatment and post-treatment time points. We will generate a norm for the samples and create a colorized displacement map comparing the average norm pre-treatment in contrast with post-treatment. The methodologies described previously will intake individual 3-dimensional photographic patient records and output a generated average with quantifiable data allowing visualization and verification of treatment outcomes in the orthodontic profession.

B) Conclusion and future directions

As completion of this project is realized, we will set our sights towards correlation of the hard and soft tissues of the craniofacial complex. Our anticipated objectives following this project involve:

1. Overlay of facial soft tissue maintaining color and texture data on their corresponding skull CBCT data
2. Generate functions to allow comprehensive averaging of multiple skulls with their corresponding facial soft tissue
3. Create accurate methods to quantify and demonstrate differences in the craniofacial complex of an individual compared to a norm
4. Allow accurate manipulation of combined hard and soft tissue essentially creating the most accurate virtual patient known to our profession

This project will allow for the revisions of existing 2-dimensional norms which are currently being used to educate the future orthodontists of our generation.

We believe that the strength of our investigation is in the application to our profession. A software pipeline generated to create true and accurate 3D averages of facial soft tissue will attract interest from orthodontic software corporations. However, the likely impact of our methods may transcend orthodontics. Physical anthropologists and fields of surgery (such as Plastics and OMFS) would have interest in the information of norms and surface deviations of individuals which would carry applications to their respective fields.

Competing interests

The authors declare that they have no competing interests.

Authors' contributions

VN wrote the publication and coordinated the project. BG was the chief software engineer. Ehab Bar coordinated between orthodontics and software engineer. SA helped to write the publication and manually traced each facial curvature. ST, AL, EE all consulted significantly regarding appropriate imaging methodology, image. acquisition setup, etc. WM was the PI of the project, came up with the project idea and oversaw progress and obstacles. All authors read and approved the final manuscript.

Author details

[1]UCLA, California, USA. [2]USC, California, USA. [3]University of Connecticut, California, USA.

References

1. Giampietro F, Salvadori S, Nolet F, Zoia A, Davide F. Assessment of inter- and intra-operator cephalometric tracings on cone beam CT radiographs: comparison of the precision of the cone beam CT versus the latero-lateral radiograph tracing. Prog Orthod. 2014;15:1.
2. Forst D, Najjar S, Flores-Mir C, Carey J, Secanell M, Lagravere M. Comparison of in vivo 3D cone-beam computed tomography tooth volume measurement protocols. Prog Orthod. 2014;15:69.
3. Kau CH, Richmond S, Savio C, Mallorie C. Measuring adult facial morphology in three dimensions. Angle Orthodontics. 2006;76:771–6.
4. Sarver DM, Proffit WR, Ackerman J. Diagnosis and treatment planning in orthodontics. In: Vanarsdall R, Graber TM, editors. Orthodontics: current principles and techniques. St. Louis: Mosby; 2000.
5. Ackerman J, Proffit WR, Sarver DM. The emerging soft tissue paradigm in orthodontic diagnosis and treatment planning. Clin Orthod Res. 1999;2:49–52.
6. Cavalcanti MG, Rocha SS, Vannier MW. Craniofacial measurements based on 3D-CT volume rendering: implications for clinical applications. Dentomaxillofacial Radiology. 2004;33:170–6.
7. Wirthlin J, Kau C, English J, Pan F, Zhou H. Comparison of facial morphologies between adult Chinese and Houstonian Caucasian populations using three-dimensional imaging. Int J Oral Maxillofac Surg. 2013;42:1100–7.
8. Chiu CS, Clark RK. Reproducibility of Natural Head Position in Standing Subjects. J Dent. 1991;19:130–1.
9. Lundstorm A, Lundstorm F, Lebret LM, Moorrees CF. Natural Head Position and Natural Head Orientation: Basic Considerations in Cephalometric Analysis and Research. Eur J Orthodontics. 1995;17:111–20.
10. Deli R, Galantucci LM, Laino A, D'Alessio R, Di Gioia E, Savastano C. Three-dimensional methodology for photogrammetric acquisition of the soft tissues of the face: a new clinical-instrumental protocol. Prog Orthod. 2013;14:32.
11. Gutman BA, McComb R, Sung J, Moon W, Thompson P. Robust Shape Correspondence via Spherical Patch Matching for Atlases of Partical Skull Models. Mesh Processing in Medical Image Analysis. 2012;7599:89–100.
12. Saad Y. Iterative methods for sparse linear systems. Siam. 2003.
13. B. Gutman, W. Chan, P. Thompson, A. Toga. Shape Registration with Shperical Cross Correlations. Mathematical Foundations of Computational Anatomy, 2nd MICCAI Workshop on Mathematical Foundations of Computational Anatomy. 2008. pp. 56–67.
14. YEO BT, Sabuncu M, Vercauteren T, Ayache N, Fischl B, Golland P. Spherical demons:Fast diffeomorphic landmark-free surface registration. IEEE Trans Med Imaging. 2010;29(3):650–8.
15. Shi Y, Morra J, Thompson P, Toga A. Inverse-consistent surface mapping with Lapace-Beltrami eigen-features. Inf Process Med Imaging. 2009;21:476–8.

16. D'Agostino E, Maes F, Dick V, Paul S. A viscous fluid model for multimodal non-rigid image registration using mutual information. Med Image Anal. 2003;7(4):565–75.
17. Gutman B, Madsen S, Toga A, Thompson P. A family of fast Spherical registration algorithms for cortical shapes. Multimodal Brain Image Analysis. 2013.
18. Everson R. Orthogonal, but not Orthonormal Procrustes Problems. Advances in Comptutations Mathematics. 1997.
19. Wang Y, Song Y, Rajagopalan P, An T, Liu K, Chou Y. Surface-Based TBM Boosts Power to Detect Disease Effecs on the Brain: an N = 804 ADNI Study. Neuroimage. 2011;56(4):1993–2010.
20. Thompson PM, Hayashi K, De Zubicaray G, Janke A, Rose S, Semple J. Mapping Hippocampal and Ventricular Change in Alzheimer Disease. Neuroimage. 2004;22(4):1754–66.

9

Dentofacial characteristics of oral breathers in different ages: a retrospective case–control study

Rosa Carrieri Rossi[1*], Nelson José Rossi[2], Nelson José Carrieri Rossi[2], Hélio Kiitiro Yamashita[3] and Shirley Shizue Nagata Pignatari[4]

Abstract

Background: This study aimed to investigate the dental and skeletal variables associated with disturbances of craniofacial development in oral-breathing (OB) individuals and the probability that these variables are related to this condition.

Methods: This is an observational retrospective case–control study of 1596 patients divided into three groups of age n1 5–12, n2 13–18, and n3 19–57 years. Radiographic, clinical, and models data were analyzed. The control group was consisted of nasal breathing (NB) individuals. Statistical analyses of the qualitative data were performed with x^2 test to identify associations, and odds ratio (OR) tests were performed for the variables that the chi-square test (x^2) identified an association.

Results: In the descriptive analysis of the data, we observed that the class II malocclusion was the most frequent in the total sample, but when divided by age group and mode of breathing, there is a random division of these variables. In n1 group, class II, (OR = 2.02) short and retruded mandible (SM and RM) (OR = 1.65 and1.89) were associated with OB and it was considered a risk factor. In n2 group, class II (OR = 1.73), SM (OR = 1.87) and increased lower anterior height (ILAFH) (OR = 1.84) seemed to be associated and to be risk factors for OB. In the n1 group, decreased lower anterior facial height (DLAFH) and brachycephalic facial pattern (BP) seemed to be associated with NB and a protective factor against oral breathing.

Conclusions: This study showed that dental and skeletal factors are associated with OB in children, and it seems that it becomes more severe until adolescence. But adults showed no associations between OB and skeletal factors, only in dental variables, indicating that there is no cause–effect relationship between the dental and skeletal factors and OB. The treatment of nose breathing patient should be multidisciplinary, since OB remains even when dental and skeletal factors slow down.

Keywords: Mouth breathing; Oral breathing; Respiration

Background

Although the importance of nasal breathing (NB) for craniofacial growth and harmonious development is well established, a large number of studies also address oral breathing (OB) and its role in craniofacial changes [1]. The difficulty in understanding the causes and effects of respiratory patterns on craniofacial growth is a reflex of the fact that several factors acting simultaneously can influence it, and there is often inaccuracy in the diagnosis of oral and nasal breathing [2–25].

* Correspondence: rosacrossi@gmail.com
[1]Division of Pediatric Otolaryngology, Federal University of Sao Paulo-UNIFESP Brasil, Rua Botucatu 740, 4 andar, V. Clementino, São Paulo CEP:04023-062, Brazil
Full list of author information is available at the end of the article

Some authors have claimed that OB alters growth and facial development [1, 2, 4, 7, 10–13, 16, 19, 21, 22, 24, 25], but others disagree and believe that the altered growth of the dentofacial complex results from other factors that may predispose individuals to OB [2–7].

The literature has not yet clearly demonstrated the relationship between OB and the growth and development. Addressing these questions is important since patients with such respiratory disturbances more frequently exhibit chronic sleep apnea and higher mortality rates and are more likely to develop cardiovascular diseases [7].

This study aimed to investigate the dental and skeletal variables associated with disturbances of craniofacial development in oral breathing individuals and the probability that these variables are related to this condition.

Methods

This observational retrospective case–control study was approved by the Ethics Committee of the Federal University of São Paulo, protocol number 103.275. Informed consent was obtained from all patients or legal guardians.

The study population (N = 1596) was based on a consecutive sample of oral and nose breathing patients of both sexes between ages 5 and 57 years who sought orthodontic treatment in an orthodontics clinic in the city of São Paulo between the years 2006 and 2012.

The sample was consecutive and consisted of a large number of subjects in an attempt to control errors through descriptive and inferential statistical tests. The survey was conducted by the same examiner in a uniform manner to ensure consistency and quality of results [1, 2, 8–11].

Initially, the 1596 patients (N) were divided in three groups according to age range (n1, n2, n3), as previous studies:

n1- 5 to 12 years old (n = 523) child [1,6,8,10,12,20]
n2- 13 to 18 years old (n = 443) adolescent [2,4,5,7,21]
n3- 19 to 57 years old (n = 340) adult [3,22,23]

All patients had previous examinations of the same diagnostic center consisting of plaster model and side and panoramic radiographs with McNamara's cephalometric analysis [24]. Measures such as the size of the mandible (NM, RM, PM), the lower anterior facial height (NLAFH, ILAFH, DLAFH), the position of the maxilla (NMx, RMx, PMx), and mandible (NM, LM, SM), and facial pattern (NP, BP, DP) were evaluated [24, 25].

Dental characteristics were obtained by prior clinical examination and model analysis. The position of the first permanent molars followed the Angle classification [26]. Intermolar (IM) and intercanine (IC) widths (W), superior (S) and inferior (I) widths were obtained in orthodontic model with a digital caliper measuring the distance between the central fosse of molars and between the cusp tip of the canines [5, 6, 19].

The patients were divided by type of breathing presented, using the protocol described in previous studies [11]. According to their predominant breathing pattern history and the findings on clinical examination, patients were classified as either OB or NB. The OB was considered as a study group (SG) and the NB as a control group (CG).

The orthodontist performed the history and clinical examination including evaluation of lips protrusion or retrusion, and the otolaryngologist was responsible for the speech and audiologic evaluations. Patients and their guardians answered a questionnaire concerning the breathing habits, while awake, with respect to any permanency of breathing with the mouth open, oral breathing, nasal obstruction, oral malodor, hyponasal speech, and while asleep, considering snoring, sleep apnea [7], restless sleep, or hyper salivation. Most of the questions were yes or no items as the protocol [11].

Patients who reported harmful habits such as finger sucking, the use of a pacifier during sleep or during the day, patients who had been submitted to orthodontic treatment, and those whose complete record could not be verified, were excluded. The data were collected in an Excel (Microsoft, 2010) database.

Comparison of OB and NB with dental and skeletal variables was accomplished among the three age groups (n1, n2, n3).

Qualitative variables were described by means of tables showing the percentage of occurrences for each category. After the division of the groups according to exclusion criteria, each variable had different n, in the tables. Correlation analysis was made between the pattern of breathing and the following variables:

1. breathing mode and gender
2. breathing mode and Angle class
3. breathing mode and maxilla position
4. breathing mode and mandible position
5. breathing mode and mandible size
6. breathing mode and anterior-lower facial height
7. breathing mode and facial pattern

Variables OB and NB groups, separated by age (n1, n2, n3), were evaluated by the homogeneity test (chi-square-x^2). Pearson correlations were selected for a reliability of 95 % and a significance level of $p < 0.05$. Odds ratio (OR) tests were performed for the variables that the chi-square test (x^2) identified an association.

The purpose of these tests was to identify the variable associated with OB and to determine the relative influence of these variables on the risk (OR) of developing the disease. When evidence of a correlation was found, we concluded that the variable was dependent of the breathing pattern.

Quantitative variables were described using measures of central tendency (mean and median) and measures of dispersion as standard deviation (SD). The Student's t test was used to investigate the possible associations between the quantitative variables with confidence interval (CI) 95 % in each of the three groups (n1, n2, n3). Means and SD for the OB and NB, and the upper and lower intermolar and intercanine widths (IMSW, IMIW, ICSW, ICIW), were checked with the Minitab program, version 14.

For rejecting the null hypothesis we fixed the significance level of 5 %.

Results

In the descriptive analysis of the data, we observed that the class II malocclusion was the most frequent in the total sample, but when divided by age group and mode of breathing, there is a random division of these variables (Figs. 1 and 2).

Group 1 (n1 = 523) 5–12 years—Qualitative variables

For ages 5–12 years old, there was no evidence of association between gender, class III malocclusion, protruded (PMx) and retruded maxilla (RMx), protruded mandible (PM), large mandible (LM), dolichocephalic pattern (DP), increase in lower anterior face height (ILAFH), and the type of breathing.

There was a significant association between class II malocclusion, retruded mandible (RM) and short mandible (SM); there was a significantly higher percentage of oral breathing with these variables. A higher percentage of NB with normal mandible (NM) was also observed.

An association between decreased LAFH (DLAFH) and the type of breathing was observed, as was a higher percentage of OB with normal LAFH (NLAFH) and a higher percentage of NB with DLAFH. Finally, in the association between the brachycephalic facial pattern (BP) and the type of breathing, a higher percentage of OB with normocephalic pattern (NP) and a higher percentage of NB with BP were found.

We observed odds ratio (OR) between class II malocclusion (OR = 2.02; CI (95 %) = (1.32, 3.09)), RM (OR = 1.89; CI (95 %) = (0.99, 3.60)), SM (OR = 1.65; CI (95 %) = (1.06, 2.58)) with OB.

We observed DLAFH and BP with NB, and these last two presented themselves as protective factors for the development of OB (OR = 0.44; CI (95 %) = (0.26, 0.77)) and (OR = 0,43, CI (95 %) = (0.24, 0.78)), respectively.

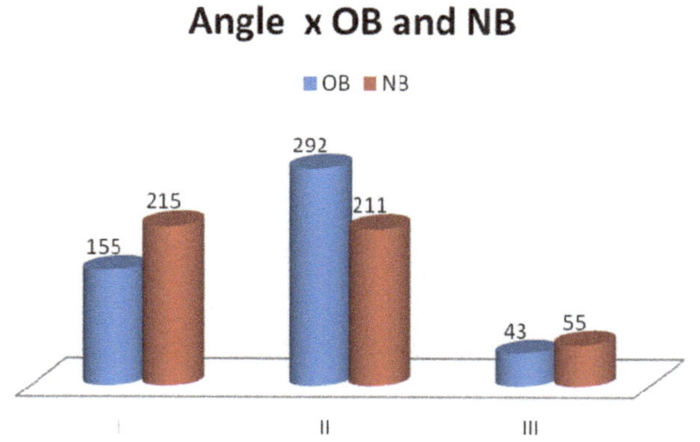

Fig. 2 Frequency of Angle classes among OB and NB. There was an homogeneous distribution of Angle malocclusion classes between OB and NB

The results of x^2 and Pearson associations, OR for qualitative variables tests, in group 1 are shown in Table 1 and Fig. 3.

Quantitative variables

There was no evidence of a difference between the mean ages of the OB and NB in group 1. No differences between the means of the upper and lower intermolars widths were detected between the OB and NB. No evidence of differences in the means of the upper and lower intercanine widths were found.

Summaries of the values of the middle range are shown in Table 2.

Group 2 (n2 = 443) 13–18 years old—qualitative variables

For the age group 13–18 years old, there is no evidence of an association between gender, class III malocclusion, PMx

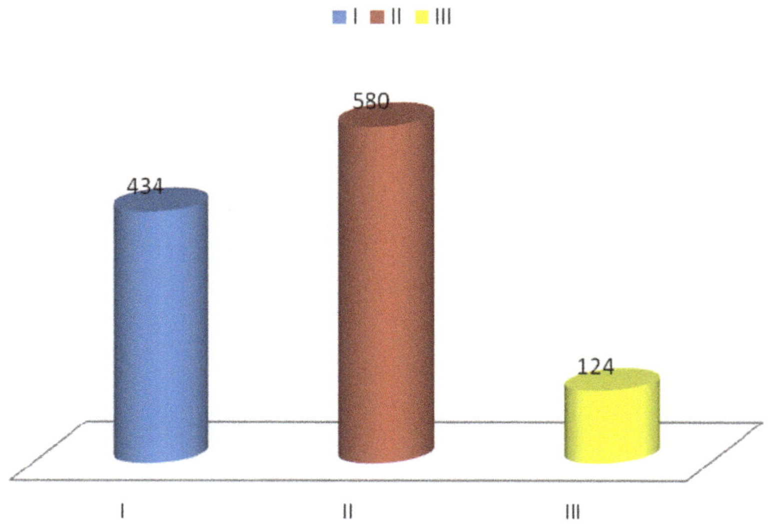

Fig. 1 Angle malocclusion in the population study. There was a greater frequency of Angle Class II in the population study

Table 1 Intra-group association tests (Pearson's x^2, odds ratio) of the qualitative variables—group n 1 (5 to 12 years of age)

Variables	OB (*n*)	OB %	NB (*n*)	NB %	Total	Pearson x^2	*p* value	DF	Lilihood x^2	OR	CI 95 %
F	152	54	130	63		2.423	1.11	1	2.43		
M	125	46	80	38							
Total	*277*		*210*		*487*						
I	67	28	73	41							
II	156	64	84	48		10.717	*0.001**	1	10672	*2.02*	*(1.32:3.09)*
III	20	8	20	11		0.057	0.811	1	0.057		
Total	*243*		*177*		*420*						
NMx	25	9	17	8							
PMx	181	66	146	71		0.263	0.608	1	0.264		
RMx	68	25	42	21		0.067	0.795	1	0.067		
Total	*274*		*205*		*479*						
NM	25	9	25	12							
PM	149	54	126	62		0.297	0.586	1	0.297		
RM	100	37	53	26		3.758	*0.053**	1	3,693		
Total	*274*		*204*		*478*						
NM	71	26	70	34							
IM	85	32	65	32		1.164	0.281	1	1.165	*1.65*	*(1.06; 2.58)*
SM	114	42	68	34		4.898	*0.027**	1	4.897		
Total	*270*		*203*		*473*						
NLAFH	70	26	41	20							
ILAFH	168	62	115	57		0.456	0.499	1	0.459	*2.31*	*(1.28; 4.15)*
DLAFH	34	12	46	23		7.926	*0.005**	1	7.957	*0.43*	*(0.24; 0.78)*
Total	*272*		*202*		*474*						
NP	65	24	33	16							
BP	56	21	64	32		8.442	*0.004**	1	1.746	*0.44*	*(1.30; 3.90)*
DP	146	55	106	52		1.746	0.186	1	1.767	*3.25*	*(0.26; 0.77)*
Total	*267*		*203*		470						

*Significant values
The values with (*) and in italics represent significant values

and RMx, PM and RM, LM, BP and DP, and the type of respiration

There is an association between class II malocclusion, SM and ILAFH, and OB. It can be seen that there is a higher percentage of OB with these variables and that there is a higher percentage of NB with class I malocclusion and of NB with NLAFH.

We calculated the OR for class II malocclusion (OR = 1.73; CI (95 %) = (1.07, 2.78), SM (OR = 1.87; CI (95 %) = (1.07, 3.24) ILAFH (OR = 1.84, CI (95 %) = (1.07, 3.17) with OB. The results of x^2 and Pearson associations, OR for qualitative variables tests, in group 2 are shown in Table 3 and Fig. 4.

Quantitative variables

There is a significant difference between the mean age of the OB and NB for the age group 13–18 years. The OB subjects are on average 0.4 years younger than NB, with the 95 % confidence level between 0.06 and 0.8 years.

There is no evidence of a difference between the average width of the maxilla and the average width of mandible, as determined by the intermolar distances and the upper and lower intercanine distances of oral and nose breathing adolescents in the 13 to 18 age group.

Summaries of the average range values are shown in Table 4.

Group 3 (n3 =312) 19–57 years old—qualitative variables

For the age group 19–57 years old, there is no evidence of an association between gender, class III malocclusion, PMx and RMx, PM and RM, LM and SM, BP and DP, and mode of breathing.

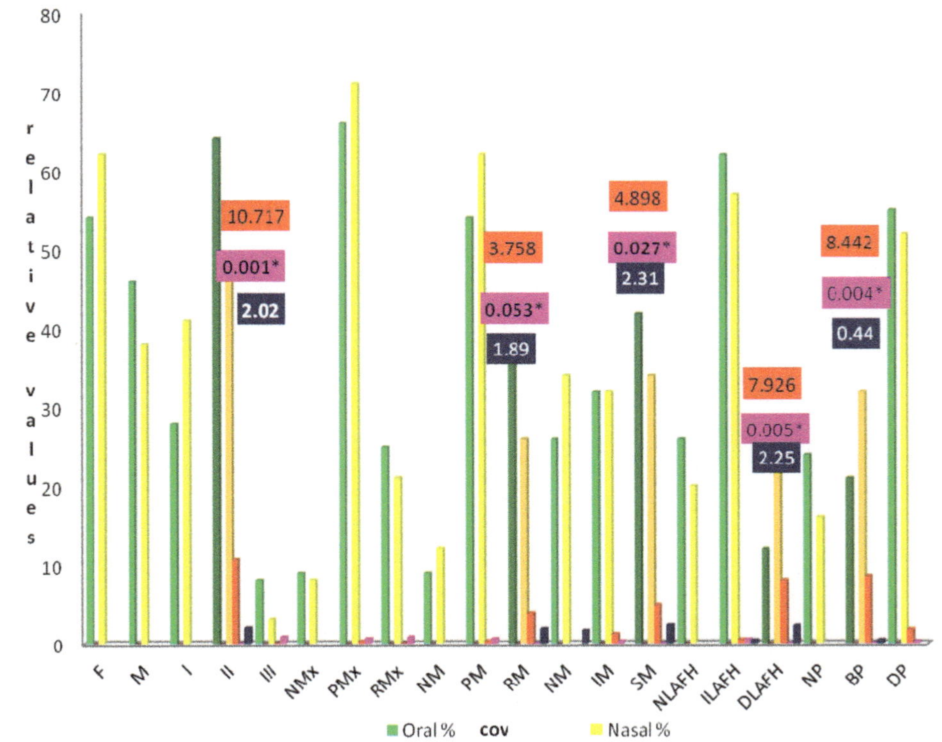

Fig. 3 Intra-groups association values (Pearson's x^2, OR) for qualitative variables, group n1 (523), 5 to 12 years of age, with OB and NB. *Significant values. The variables that showed significant associations and risk of disease were Class II, RM, SM. DLAFH and BP (protective factors)

For the age group of 19 to 57 years we found a marginally significant association between classification II malocclusion and oral breathing (OR = 1.72; CI (95 %) = (0.99, 2.98)).

The results of intra-group association tests of qualitative variables (Pearson's chi-square and odds ratio) for the age group 19–57 years with (n3 = 312) are shown in Table 5 and Fig. 5.

Quantitative values

There is a significant difference between the average width of the mandibles in OB subjects in group 3. The

Table 2 *T* tests for difference in the averages—quantitative values of n1 (5 to 12 years of age)

	(*n*)	IMSW	IMIW	ICSW	ICIW
OB	277	67	64	54	57
NB	212	49	43	47	46
Means OB	9.56	47.04	45.3	33.76	27.53
Means NB	9.79	46.54	45.3	33.34	27.06
SD OB	1.84	3.63	4.32	4.45	2.68
SD NB	1.79	3.85	4.69	3.26	2.63
OB*	0.11	0.44	0.54	0.61	0.35
NB*	0.11	0.55	0.72	0.48	0.39
Difference of means	−0.231779	0.496497	0.002362	0.423089	0.465446
CI	95 %	95 %	95 %	95 %	95 %
IC	(−0.557135; 0.093576)	(−0.905768; 1.898762)	(−1.780811; 1.785535)	(−1.106945; 1.953123)	(−0.577590; 1.508483)
T value	−1.4	0.7	0	0.55	0.89
p value	0.62	0.484	0.998	0.584	0.378
DF	459	99	85	96	97

*Significant values

Table 3 Intra-group association tests (Pearson's x^2, odds ratio) of qualitative variables for the group n3 (13 to 18 years of age)

Variables	OBI(n)	OBI % NB (n)	NB %	Total	Pearson X	*p*-value DF	Lilihood x	*p*-value	DF OD	IC 95 %	DF	OR	IC 95 %
F	91	54	104	56									
M	76	46	82	44		0.072	0.788	1	0.072	0.7888	1		
Total	**167**		**186**		**353**								
I	52	39	85	50									
II	73	54	69	40		5.102	**0.024***	1	5.121	**0.024***	1	1.73	**(1.07; 2.78)**
III	10	7	17	10		0.008	0.928	1	0.008	0.928	1		
Total	**135**		**171**		**306**								
NMx	21	13	15	8									
PMx	113	69	127	70		1.586	0.208	1	1.59	0.207	1		
RMx	29	18	40	22		2.521	0.112	1	2.528	0.112	1		
Total	**163**		**182**		**345**								
NM	17	10	23	13									
PM	83	51	103	56		0.06	0.806	1	0.06	0.806	1		
RM	64	39	57	31		1.299	0.254	1	1.302	0.254	1		
Total	**164**		**183**		**347**								
NM	45	28	63	35									
IM	60	37	73	41		0.288	0.592	1	0.288	0.591	1		
SM	56	35	42	24		4.924	*0.026**	1	4.943	*0.026**	1	1.87	(1.07; 3.24)
Total	**161**		**178**		**339**								
NLAFH	27	17	47	27									
ILAFH	109	68	103	58		4.902	*0.027**	1	4.957	*0.026**	1	1.84	(1.07; 3.17)
DLAFH	25	15	26	15									
Total	**161**		**176**		**337**								
NP	29	18	35	19									
BP	42	26	55	31		0.063	0.801	1	0.063	0.801	1		
DP	90	56	89	50		0.465	0.495	1	0.466	0.495	1		
Total	**161**		**179**										

*Significant p values <0.05

OB have mandibles that are on average 2.4 mm wider than NB, with a 95 % confidence level (0.4 and 4.5 mm). Summaries of the values of the middle range are shown in Table 6.

Discussion

We assessed skeletal and dental changes in a large group of patients, to minimize the probable random errors. Statistical tests helped to widespread the results and confirmed the associations (x^2) and disease risk (OR).

OB is a result of the influence of genetic and environmental factors [4, 13]. Some authors claim that diseases such as allergies [17], chronic colds, habits [22, 27], head position [12], or shape of the upper airway [2, 7] may lead to nasal obstruction and consequent OB [1, 8, 12, 13, 16, 28]. However, the relative influence of these factors in the genesis of OB remains unclear [2, 5–7, 10, 11, 14, 20, 21]. Studies indicate that factors that cause OB do not cause malocclusion [20] or modify facial patterns [2, 5].

Most studies included children and adolescents, because more significant changes occur in these groups [1–10, 12, 16–19, 21–23, 27–29] and the changes become less apparent in adulthood [15]. Dentition and aging affect the initiation and persistence of craniofacial changes [8, 15, 18]. Alterations in early age do not persist into adulthood [17, 20]. The influence of OB on craniofacial development becomes evident from the ages of 8 to 10 years [18].

Class II malocclusion remained present in all patients with OB, as disease risk. This condition improved in adult patients in our study (n3), with only a marginal association with class II and OB [17, 20]. It seems reasonable to suggest that early treatment of that condition may be beneficial, especially in young individuals. Treatment should be multidisciplinary [14].

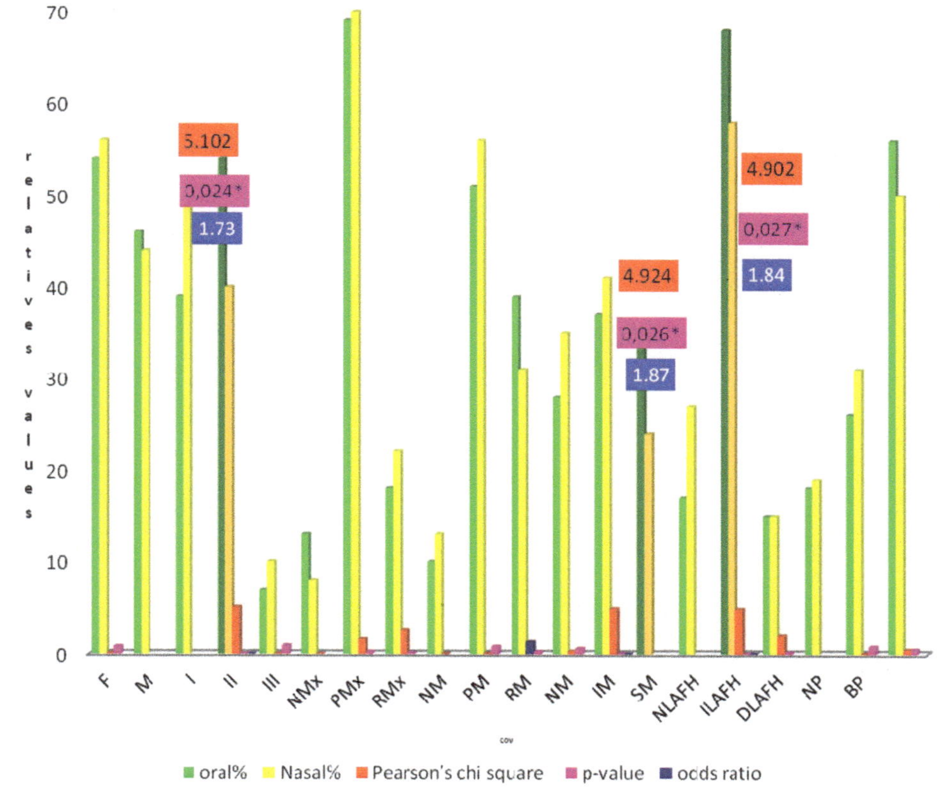

Fig. 4 Intra-groups association values (Pearson's x^2 odds ratio) for qualitative variables, n2 (924), 13 to 18 years of age, with oral and nasal breathing. *Significant values. The variables that showed significant associations and the risk of disease were Class II, SM and ILAFH

Table 4 *T* tests for difference in the averages—quantitative values for group n2 (13 to 18 years of age)

	(*n*)	IMSW	IMIW	ICSW	ICIW
OB	167	46	42	42	45
NB	186	49	46	45	45
Means OB	14.83	47.39	45.55	34.61	27.3
Means NB	15.25	47.02	46.1	34.5	27.81
SD OB	1.76	3.2	3.57	3.22	2.8
SD NB	1.7	3.32	4.22	3.16	2.9
OB*	0.14	0.47	0.55	0.5	0.31
NB*	0.12	0.47	0.62	0.47	0.43
Dif of means	−0.426341	0.370896	−0.550207	0.111905	−0.777778
CI	95 %	95 %	95 %	95 %	95 %
IC	(−0.789891; −0.062791)	(−0.958786; 1.700578)	(−2.203110; 1.102696)	(−1.250651; 1.474461)	(−1.837129; 0.281573)
T value	−2.31	0.55	−0.66	0.16	1.46
p value	*0.022**	0.581	0.51	0.871	0.148
DF	343	92	85	84	79

*Significant values

Table 5 Intra-group association tests (Pearson's x^2, odds ratio) of qualitative variables—group n3 (19 to 57 years of age)

Variables	OB (*n*)	OB %	NB (*n*)	NB %	Total	Pearson x^2	*p* value	DF	Lilihood x^2	OR	CI 95 %
F	95	47	110	53		1.012	0,314	1	1.012		
M	56	53	51	47							
Total	*151*		*161*		*312*						
I	36	32	57	43							
II	63	56	58	43		3.773	*0.052**	1	3.792	*1.72*	*(0.99; 2.98)*
III	14	12	19	14		0.14	0.708	1	0.14		
Total	*113*		*134*		*247*						
NMx	15	10	8	5							
PMx	107	73	122	80		2.862	0.091	1	2.894		
RMx	25	17	22	15		0.912	0.34	1	0.923		
Total	*147*		*152*		*299*						
NM	21	14	16	10							
PM	81	55	90	59		1.073	0.3	1	1.075		
RM	46	31	47	31		0.564	0.453	1	0.565		
Total	*148*		*153*		*301*						
NM	42	30	39	26							
IM	57	40	61	41		0.242	0.623	1	0.242		
SM	43	30	48	33		0.363	0.547	1	0.363		
Total	*142*		*148*		*290*						
NLAFH	26	18	34	23							
ILAFH	100	71	94	63		1.237	0.266	1	1.24		
DLAFH	15	11	21	14		0.026	0.873	1	0.026		
Total	*141*		*149*		*290*						
NP	22	16	26	18							
BP	43	31	50	34		0.002	0.964	1	0.002		
DP	74	53	70	48		0.444	0.505	1	0.445		
Total	*139*		*146*		285						

*Significant values

In our groups, we observed a higher proportion of subjects class II. Initially, we made the separation of groups by age and by mode of breathing, so the occlusal and skeletal variables were divided into groups, regardless of their initial ratio.

We obtained different results for each age group. In group n1, most children BP and with DLAFH, breathe through the nose and were class I, and these characteristics were shown to be protective factors found in the OR [18]. In group n2, we found that the oral breathers tended to be younger than nasal breathers. We did not identify sexual dimorphism in any group [18], although some studies claim a slight prevalence of OB in females [5, 13]. There were fewer changes in group n3 that exhibited only significant associations with dental changes as class II malocclusion and mandibular width suggesting an increased tendency to posterior cross bite, agreeing with many studies [2, 5, 10, 15–17, 19, 20] and disagreeing with others [1, 3]. Most patients reported "crooked teeth" as the main complain, and the information of OB and NB was obtained following the protocol [1, 2, 6, 8–11, 13, 19, 28].

Some authors postulate that facial, skeletal [1, 7, 8, 10, 13, 15, 17, 20, 28], and dental [1, 7, 8, 15, 17, 20, 22, 28] changes result from the influence of oral breathing [1, 7, 13, 29]. We confirmed this statement: In group 1, we found evidence of associations of SM and RM and OB in agreement with several studies [8, 10, 13, 15, 28], and a DLAFH and BP with NB, which appeared to be protective for disease, in disagreement with some studies [8, 10, 13, 15, 28]. In group n2 we found a clear association of SM and ILAFH agreeing with previous publications [2, 10, 16]. In group 3, we found a marginally significant association between class II malocclusion and OB, confirming the literature [8, 15, 18].

The condition of exclusive oral breathing is rare; alternation between OB and NB is much more common. The boundary between the air passages for OB and NB is small,

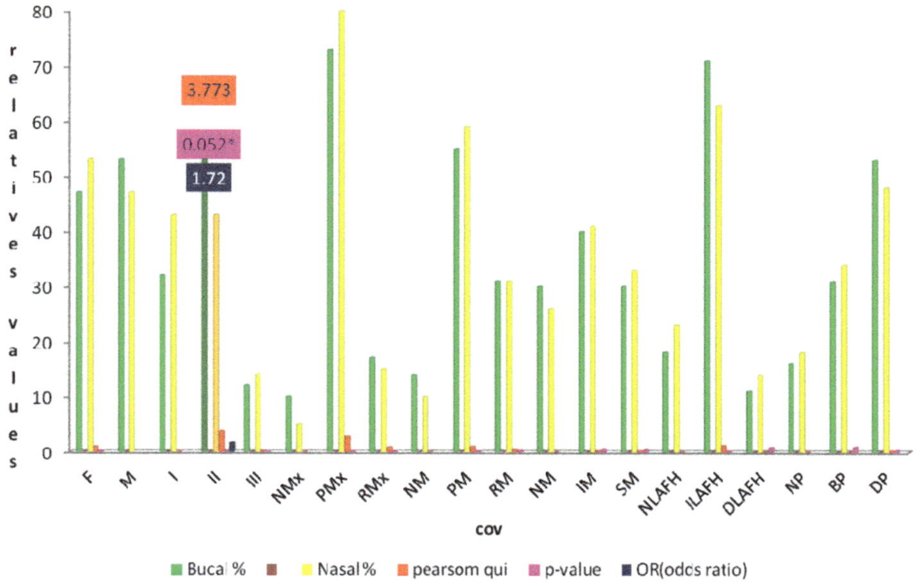

Fig. 5 Intra-groups association values, (Pearson's x^2, OR, for qualitative variables n3 (19 to 57 years of age), with OB and NB. *Significant values. The variable that showed significant associations and the risk of disease was the Angle Class II

and sometimes, even though the nasal air passages are of normal size, nasal breathing is replaced by oral [3, 16].

We could not obtain concordances in the literature for the diagnosis of OB. Few studies evaluated OB using calibrated instruments, but they are not gold standards. Even as the assessments may have been made at a time when the breathing mode was alternating [3, 12, 16, 23].

Most of the literature uses subjective information obtained through questionnaires, where the patient states his mode of breathing, and some clinical trials are not carefully constructed and do not lead to results that generate confidence [1, 2, 8–11, 13, 19, 20, 28]. Our diagnosis of OB and NB was based on clinical examination and a questionnaire [11].

Conclusions

This study showed that dental and skeletal factors are associated with OB in children, and it seems that it becomes more severe until adolescence. But adults showed no associations between OB and skeletal factors, only in dental variables, indicating that there is no cause–effect relationship between the dental and skeletal factors and

Table 6 *T* test for differences of averages- Quantitative values for group n3 (19 to 57 years of age)

	(*n*)	IMSW	IMIW	ICSW	ICIW
OB	151	41	36	43	43
NB	161	43	39	37	37
Means OB	26.17	47.93	47.07	35.01	28.37
Means NB	27.95	46.7	44.65	34.86	27.64
SD OB	6.71	4.01	4.09	4.57	3.03
SD NB	7.35	4.29	4.74	3.61	2.91
OB*	0.55	0.63	0.68	0.7	0.46
NB*	0.58	0.65	0.66	0.79	0.48
Dif of means	−1.77813	1.22915	2.4156	0.146763	0.736958
CI	95 %	95 %	95 %	95 %	95 %
IC	(−3.34477; −0.21148)	(−0.57221; 3.03052)	(0.38313; 4.44807)	(−1.675761; 1.969287)	(−0.587233; 2.061149)
T value	−2.23	1.36	2.37	0.16	1.11
p value	*0.026**	0.178	*0.021**	0.873	0.271
DF	309	81	72	77	77

*Significant
There was a significant difference between the OB and NB: OB are younger, and the inferior molar widths are larger than the superior molar widths

OB. The treatment of nose breathing patient should be multidisciplinary, since OB remains even when dental and skeletal factors slow down.

Abbreviations

BP: brachycephalic facial pattern; CG: control group; CI: confidence interval; DLAFH: decreased lower anterior facial height; DP: dolichocephalic pattern; IC: intercanine; ICIW: intercanine width inf; ICSW: intercanine width sup; ILAFH: increased lower anterior facial height; IMIW: intermolar width inf; IMSW: intermolar width sup; LM: large mandible; NB: nasal breathing; NLAFH: normal lower anterior facial height; NM: normal mandible; NP: normocephalic pattern; OB: oral breathing; OR: odds ratio; OSA: sleep apnea; PM: protruded mandible; PMx: protruded maxilla; RM: retruded mandible; RMx: retruded maxilla; SD: standard deviations; SG: study group; SM: short mandible.

Competing interests

The authors declare that they have no competing interests.

Authors' contributions

RRC participated in all phases of the study. RNJ and RNC participated in data collection. YHK collaborated with images evaluation and measurements. PSSn coordinated the study and collaborated with writing and reviewing of the text. All authors read and approved the final manuscript.

Acknowledgements

This clinical study was conducted at the Federal University of Sao Paulo (UNIFESP), and it is part of the thesis for obtaining the title of Doctor DDs, Ms, Rosa Carrieri Rossi. There was no previous publication of this research. The Institutional Ethics Committee (UNIFESP) approved the study project (1739/11 02/12/2011).

Financial support

The research was financially supported by Fundação Capes Ministério de Educação-Brasil CAPES Foundation—MEC Brasil. The authors, the educational institutions and the agency responsible for Research, have no conflict of interest.

Author details

[1]Division of Pediatric Otolaryngology, Federal University of Sao Paulo-UNIFESP Brasil, Rua Botucatu 740, 4 andar, V. Clementino, São Paulo CEP:04023-062, Brazil. [2]Educational Association of Brazil- FUNORTE/SOEBRAS, Rua Tijuco Preto 1694, Sao Paulo, Tatuapé CEP:03316-000, Brazil. [3]Department of Diagnostic Imaging, Division of Otolaryngology and Head and Neck Imaging, Federal University of Sao Paulo- UNIFESP, Rua Botucatu 740, 4 andar, V. Clementino, São Paulo CEP:04023-062, Brazil. [4]Department of Otolaryngology and Head and Neck Surgery, Division of Pediatric Otolaryngology, Federal University of Sao Paulo- UNIFESP, Rua Botucatu 740, 4 andar, V. Clementino, São Paulo CEP:04023-062, Brazil.

References

1. Kluemper GT, Vig PS, Vig KW. Nasorespiratory characteristics and craniofacial morphology. The European Journal of Orthodontics. 1995;17(6):491–5.
2. Bianchini AP, Guedes ZC, Vieira MM. A study on the relationship between mouth breathing and facial morphological pattern. Braz J Otorhinolaryngol. 2007;73(4):500–5.
3. Warren DW, Hairfield WM, Seaton D, Morr KE, Smith LR. The relationship between nasal airway size and nasal-oral breathing. Am J Orthod Dentofacial Orthop. 1988;93(4):289–93.
4. Retamoso LB, Knop LAH, Guariza Filho O, Tanaka OM. Facial and dental alterations according to the breathing pattern. J Appl Oral Sci. 2011;19(2):175–81.
5. Coelho ARDP, Tanaka O, Ribeiro JS, Machado MAN, Camargo ES. Transverse craniofacial dimensions in Angle Class II, Division 1 malocclusion according to breathing mode Braz. Oral Res. 2010;24(1):70–5.
6. de OLIVEIRA JML, Carvalho ES, Dutra ALT, Bezerra ACB, de TOLEDO OA. Transverse measurements of the jaws of patients with a predominance of nose and mouth breathing in children between 6 and 14 years of age. RGO. 2012;60(1):61–9.
7. Ucar FI, Uysal T. Comparision of orofacial airway dimensions in subject with different breathing pattern. Progress in Orthod. 2012;13(3):210–7.
8. Harari D, Redlich M, Miri S, Hamud T, Gross M. The effect of mouth breathing versus OB on dentofacial and craniofacial development in orthodontic patients. Laryngoscope. 2010;120(10):2089–93.
9. Bakor SF, Enlow DH, Pontes P, De Biase NG. Craniofacial growth variations in nasal-breathing, oral-breathing, and tracheotomized children. Am J Orthod Dentofacial Orthop. 2011;140(4):486–92.
10. Malhotra S, Pandey RK, Nagar A, Agarwal SP, Gupta VK. The effect of mouth breathing on dentofacial morphology of growing child. J Indian Soc Pedod Prev Dent. 2012;30:27–31.
11. Wieler WJ, Barros AM, Barros LA, Camargo ES, Ignácio SA, Maruo H. A combined protocol to aid diagnosis of breathing mode. Rev Clin Pesq Odontol. 2007;3(2):101–14.
12. Solow B, Siersbæk-Nielsen S, Greve E. Airway adequacy, head posture, and craniofacial morphology. Am J Orthod. 1984;86(3):214–23.
13. Padzys GS, Tankosic C, Trabalon M, Martrette JM. Craniofacial development and physiological state after early oral breathing in rats. Eur J Oral Sci. 2012;120(1):21–8.
14. Harvold EP, Tomer BS, Vargervik K, Chierici G. Primate experiments on oral respiration. Am J Orthod. 1981;79(4):359–72.
15. Souki BQ, Pimenta GB, Souki MQ, Franco LP, Becker HM, Pinto JA. Prevalence of malocclusion among mouth breathing children: do expectations meet reality? Int J Pediatr Otorhinolaryngol. 2009;73:767–73.
16. Zicari AM, Albani F, Ntrekou P, Rugiano A, Duse M, Mattei A, et al. Oral breathing and dental malocclusions. European journal of paediatric dentistry: official journal of European Academy of Paediatric Dentistry. 2009;10(2):59–64.
17. Bresolin D, Shapiro PA, Shapiro GG, Chapko MK, Dassel S. Mouth breathing in allergic children: its relationship to dentofacial development. Am J Orthod. 1983;83(4):334–40.
18. Muñoz ICL, Orta PB. Comparison of cephalometric patterns in mouth breathing and nose breathing children. Int J Pediatr Otorhinolaryngol. 2014;78(7):1167–72.
19. Mattar SEM, Matsumoto MAN, Valera FCP, Anselmo-Lima WT, Faria G. The effect of adenoidectomy or adenotonsillectomy on occlusal features in mouth-breathing. Pediatr Dent. 2012;34(5):108–12.
20. Souk BQ, Petrus B, Lopes TBJ, Pereira LP, Franco HMG, Becker DO. Mouth breathing children and cephalometric pattern: does the stage of dental development matter? Int J Pediatr Otorhinolaryngol. 2012;76:837–8.
21. Young T, Larel F, Hyon K. Nasal obstruction as a risk factor for sleep-disordered breathing. J Allergy Clin Immunol. 1997;99(2):s757–62.
22. Vig PS, Sarver DM, Hall DJ, Warren DW. Quantitative evaluation of nasal airflow in relation to facial morphology. Am J Orthod. 1981;79(3):263–72.
23. Fujimoto S, Yamaguchi K, Gunjigake K. Clinical estimation of mouth breathing. Am J Orthod Dentofacial Orthop. 2009;136(5):e630–1.
24. Namara Jr M. A method for cephalometric evaluation. Am J Orthod. 1984;86(5):449–69.
25. Durão AR, Pittayapat P, Rockenbach MI, Olszewski R, Ferreira AP, Jacobs R. Validity of 2D lateral cephalometry in orthodontics: a systematic review. Progress in Orthod. 2013;14:31.
26. Angle EH. Classification of malocclusion. Dental Cosmos 1899: 248–264.
27. MCNAMARA JA. Influence of respiratory pattern on craniofacial growth. Angle Orthod. 1981;51(4):269–300.
28. Trask GM, Shapiro GG, Shapiro PA. The effects of perennial allergic rhinitis on dental and skeletal development: a comparison of sibling pairs. Am J Orthod Dentofacial Orthop. 1987;92(4):286–93.
29. Souki BQ, Lopes PB, Veloso NC, Avelino RA, Pereira TB, Souza PE, et al. Facial soft tissues of mouth-breathing children: do expectations meet reality? Int J Pediatr Otorhinolaryngol. 2014;78(7):1074–9.

10

Comparison between rapid and mixed maxillary expansion through an assessment of arch changes on dental casts

Vincenzo Grassia[1], Fabrizia d'Apuzzo[1], Abdolreza Jamilian[2], Felice Femiano[1], Lorenzo Favero[3] and Letizia Perillo[4*]

Abstract

Background: Aim of this retrospective observational study was to compare upper and lower dental changes in patients treated with Rapid Maxillary Expansion (RME) and Mixed Maxillary Expansion (MME), assessed by dental cast analysis.

Methods: Treatment groups consisted of 42 patients: the RME group (n = 21) consisted of 13 female and 8 male subjects with the mean age of 8.8 years ± 1.37 at T0 and 9.6 years ± 1.45 at T1; the MME group (n = 21) consisted of 12 female and 9 male patients with a mean age of 8.9 years ± 2.34 at T0 and 10.5 years ± 2.08 at T1. The upper and lower arch analysis was performed on four dental bilateral landmarks, on upper and lower casts; also upper and lower arch depths were measured. The groups were compared using independent sample t-test to estimate dental changes in upper and lower arches.

Results: Before expansion treatment (T0), the groups were similar for all examined variables ($p>0.05$). In both RME and MME group, significant increments in all the variables for maxillary and mandibular arch widths were observed after treatment. No significant differences in maxillary and mandibular arch depths were observed at the end of treatment in both groups. An evaluation of the changes after RME and MME (T1) showed statistically significant differences in mandibular arch depth ($p<0.001$) and maxillary intercanine widths ($p<0.05$). Differences in maxillary arch depth and arch width measurements were not significant.

Conclusions: RME and MME can be considered two effective treatment options to improve transverse arch dimensions and gain space in the dental arches. A greater lower arch expansion was observed in the MME group, which might be attributed to the "lip bumper effects" observed in the MME protocol.

Background

Dento-skeletal maxillary constriction can be treated by opening the mid-palatal suture, and widening the roof of the mouth and floor of the nose [1–5].

Skeletal expansion allows the correction of a posterior crossbite, when present [6–10]. In addition, a space gain is achieved in the arch, and the underlying permanent tooth buds are buccally repositioned [11–14].

Maxillary expansion can be performed with different methods: rapid maxillary expansion (RME) [15–17], semi-rapid maxillary expansion (SRME) [18], slow maxillary expansion (SME) [19–21] and mixed maxillary expansion (MME) [22–24]. Each treatment protocol is based on a different rationale, but all produce both skeletal and dental changes.

MME separates the two maxillary halves at the first appointment, by applying all the expansion forces to maxillary bones, thereby increasing skeletal effects and reducing unwanted dental side movements. In a previous study comparing MME-induced dento-skeletal changes on postero–anterior cephalograms in pre-pubertal patients with those in an untreated control group [22], MME was found to be an effective treatment option for improving dento-skeletal transverse dimensions and correcting posterior crossbite. These positive outcomes were associated with major skeletal and minor dental changes. A further research comparing the arch changes on dental

* Correspondence: letizia.perillo@unina2.it
[4]Multidisciplinary Department of medical-Surgery and Dental Specialties, Second University of Naples; Post-Graduate Orthodontics Programme and Operative Unit, Via Luigi De Crecchio 6, 80138 Napoli, Italy
Full list of author information is available at the end of the article

casts, using the same sample and treatment procedures, confirmed the validity of MME as a useful alternative protocol for improving transverse arch dimensions and correcting posterior crossbite, as well as for gaining arch space to relieve mild-to-moderate tooth-size/arch discrepancies [23]. A third paper compared the dento-skeletal changes on postero–anterior cephalograms in two groups of pre-pubertal patients treated with MME or RME [24, 25]. Both expansion procedures proved effective in increasing skeletal transverse dimensions by opening the mid-palatal suture in growing patients. However, MME had significantly fewer dental side effects than RME. To complete this latter research, in the light that one of the outcomes of expansion is often to increase arch widths and achieve space gain [26–31], it could be useful to investigate whether differences in arch changes were present.

Thus, the aim of this study was therefore to compare the changes in arch widths on dental casts in two groups of pre-pubertal patients treated with MME or RME.

Methods

Appropriate ethical approval was secured by the Health Research Ethics Board of the Second University of Naples (No.429), in July 22, 2014.

Consecutive records of patients treated with maxillary expansion at the Orthodontic Unit of the Second University of Naples, Italy, and in a private practice (LP) from October 2010 to March 2012 were examined. The parents of all children involved in the study gave informed consent. Inclusion criteria of this retrospective study were unilateral or bilateral posterior crossbite and/or variable degree of crowding, mixed dentition with fully erupted upper permanent molars, Cervical Vertebral Maturation Stage (CVMS) 1 or 2, treatment performed with RME or MME, dental casts, high quality latero–lateral, postero–anterior and occlusal radiographs at pre-expansion (T0) and post-expansion (T1). Exclusion criteria were cranio-facial anomalies or syndromes, periodontal diseases, dental trauma or anomalies and previous orthodontic treatment.

Forty-two patients met the inclusion criteria. Of these, 21 were treated with RME and 21 with MME using a palatal Hyrax-type expander (Fig. 1) applied in mixed dentition and bonded to the first upper molars and either first deciduous molars or first bicuspids.

Activation

In both groups, activation started immediately after the appliance was fitted, and ended when overcorrection was achieved with the palatal cusps of the upper molars riding up on the buccal cusps of the lower molars. The activation schedule of both protocols is reported in Table 1.

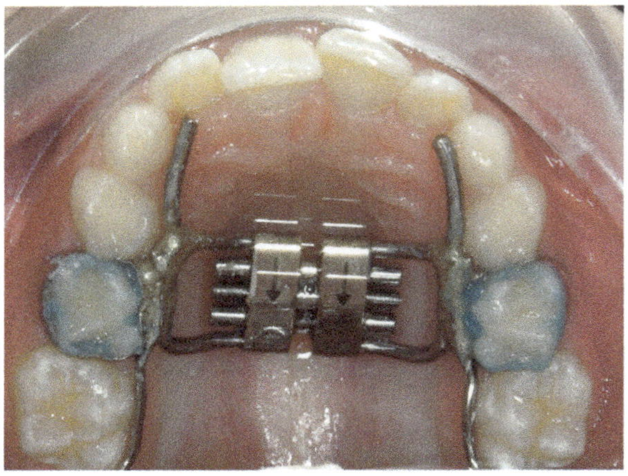

Fig. 1 Palatal Hyrax-type expander

RME group activation

In the RME group, the operator began activation at the chairside with two turns of the expansion screw (0.25 mm per turn). Parents were then instructed to continue activation at home with two turns per day.

During the expansion phase, which lasted from 1 to 3 weeks depending on the degree of maxillary constriction and/or crowding, patients were monitored once a week.

MME group activation

In the MME group, the protocol comprised two phases: an initial, very rapid opening of the device followed by a second, slower activation. The first phase, started at the chair side, included three steps with four, two and one turn (0.25 mm per turn), respectively. The three steps were carried out at the same appointment until the suture was opened.

The second expansion phase then began and parents were instructed to continue activation at home with one turn every 3 days.

During the expansion phase, which lasted from 4 to 6 months depending on the degree of maxillary constriction and/or of crowding, patients were monitored once every 2 weeks.

Clinical procedure for MME

After the first step, the patient usually experiences tenderness of the bonded teeth, which disappears in 20 to 30 min. After the second step, tenderness lasting 10–15 min then shifts to the palatal incisor area and, finally, following the third step, to the suture area. A decrease in tenderness of the bonded teeth and/or tenderness in the sutural area may indicate that the maxillary halves have been separated. However, a successful separation can only be confirmed by occlusal radiograph, before and after maxillary expansion. In the event of increased palatal suture resistance, a fourth step with two additional turns

Table 1 Characteristics of RME and MME sample groups

	Expansion				Retention	Total treatment duration
	Phase	Turns	Duration	Controls		
RME group	One: rapid	2/day	1–3 weeks	4/months	8 months ± 2	1.2 year ± 0.3
MME group	First: very rapid	4–2–1/day	1 h	2/months	8 months ± 2	1.3 year ± 0.2
	Second: slow	2/week	4–6 months			

may be performed. In this case, tenderness in the temporo- and fronto-zygomatic areas may be experienced. The number of steps and associated turns therefore depends on suture intercuspidation.

Retention phase

After the expansion phase, the Hyrax device was removed in both groups in order to stabilize the screw with acrylic. The device was then re-cemented so that it could be used as a retainer. The retention phase lasted on average 8 months. The retention schedule of both protocols is shown in Table 1.

Data collection

Digital occlusal photographs were taken of all maxillary and mandibular casts according to a standard technique and imported into Adobe Photoshop, version 5.0 (Adobe Systems, San Jose, CA). Each photograph was saved with a 5-mm grid and then imported into Scion Image (Scion, Frederick, MD; a version of the Macintosh program, NIH Image, from the National Institutes of Health). Each point in Scion was recorded to an x, y coordinate system and imported into a Microsoft Excel program to orient the coordinates and align the maxillary and mandibular casts. The dental casts were measured at T0 and T1 for each patient.

Landmark identification

Landmarks were identified on the distal, facial, mesial and lingual surfaces of each tooth from the right first permanent molar to the left first permanent molar in the same arch (Fig. 2). These points were selected in accordance with guidelines reported in literature to determine the geometric centre of each tooth, known as the tooth centroid. This point provides a more accurate measurement of arch width as it removes the effect of tooth rotation.

Landmarks were not recorded if the teeth were in the process of exfoliation, ectopically erupted or in the process of eruption if the height of the four outer surfaces (distal, facial, mesial and lingual) were visible.

Measurements

For each dental arch, at T0 and T1, four transversal linear measurements (arch widths) connecting the centroid of a tooth (Fig. 3) and its antimere, and one sagittal measurement (arch depth) were analysed.

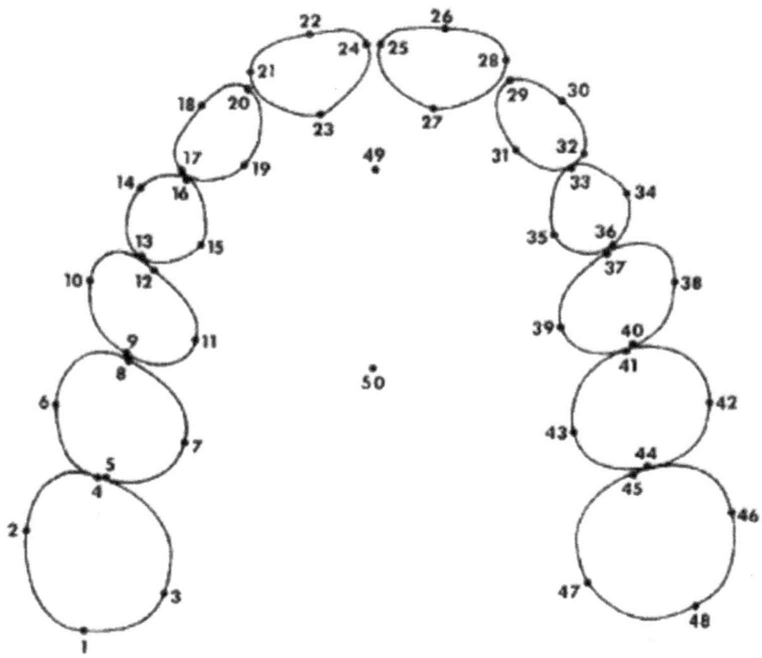

Fig. 2 Location of landmarks on maxillary dental casts. Similar dental landmarks were located on the mandibular dental arch

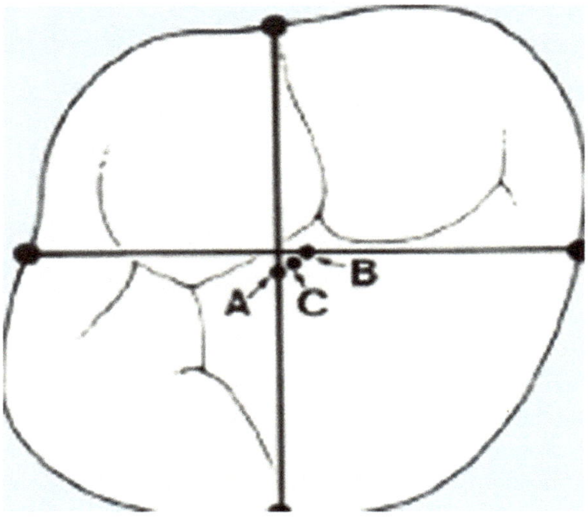

Fig. 3 Location of the centroid of each posterior tooth. (A) Midpoint of a line connecting mesial and distal landmarks. (B) Midpoint between buccal and lingual landmarks. (C) Centroid located midway between points A and B

For each tooth, the midpoint of a line connecting mesial and distal landmarks was determined, and another midpoint was constructed midway between the buccal and lingual landmarks of the tooth; the centroid is located midway between the midpoints. In the majority of teeth studied, the centroid and the midpoint between the approximal midpoints coincided or were very close to each other.

Arch width was measured between the following teeth on both arches: primary/permanent canines, first primary molars/first premolars, second primary molars/second premolars, and first permanent molars.

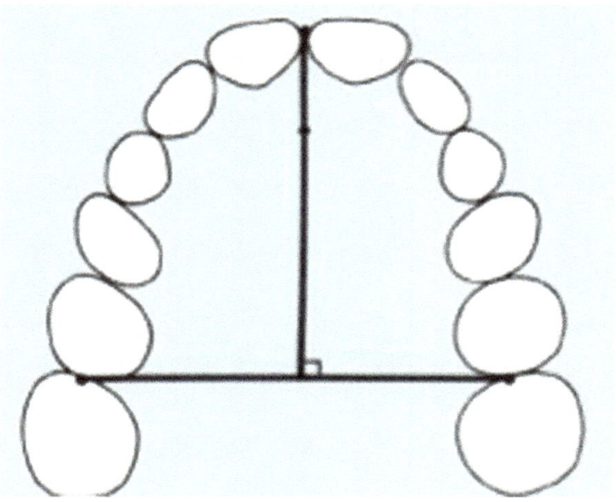

Fig. 4 Arch depth measured as distance from a point midway between facial surfaces of central incisors to a line tangent to mesial surfaces of first permanent molars

Arch depth was determined by measuring the length of a perpendicular line constructed from the contact point between mesial contact points of central incisors to a line connecting points between second premolars and first molars (Fig. 4).

Error method

All measurements were carried out by the same operator. A combined error of the landmark location and tracing was determined. The method error was calculated from the double determinations of 12 randomly selected dental casts, re-measured after an interval of 1 week, using Dahlberg's formula. The mean value of the method error was 0.5 ± 0.2 mm, within acceptable limits for the analysis of serial dental casts.

Statistical analysis

Descriptive statistics were performed on dental cast measurements at T0 and T1 for RME and MME groups.

Statistical comparisons were performed on:

- starting forms: RME group vs. MME group at T0
- treatment effects: RME group T1–T0
- treatment effects: MME group T1–T0
- final forms: RME group vs. MME group at T1.

All data were tested as for the normality; therefore, a parametric test was applied for the comparisons of the groups. Comparison of continuous variables between groups was made through unpaired *t*-tests, while changes within groups were tested through paired *t*-tests. The level of statistical significance set at $p < .05$ for all statistical tests. The statistical Package for the Social Sciences (version 22; SPSS, Chicago, III) was used for data analysis.

Results

The main characteristics of the samples are summarized in Table 2.

RME and MME groups were matched for number, sex, chronological age and CVMS. The RME group ($n = 21$) consisted of 13 girls and 8 boys with a mean age of 8.8 years ± 1.37 at T0 and 9.6 years ± 1.45 at T1. The MME group ($n = 21$) consisted of 12 girls and 9 boys with a mean age of 8.9 years ± 2.34 at T0 and 10.5 years ± 2.08 at T1. The CVMS ranged from 1 to 2 at T0 and from 2 to 3 at T1. The mean value of the method error was 0.5 ± 0.2 mm, within acceptable limits for the analysis of serial dental casts.

Descriptive statistics for values and changes of the dental measurements with comparisons are reported in Table 3.

1. *Comparison of starting forms: RME group vs. MME group at T0*

Table 2 Characteristics of RME and MME sample groups

		Male	Female	Mean age ± SD (year/month)		CVM stage	
				T0	T1	T0	T1
RME group	21	8	13	8.8 ± 1.37	9.6 ± 1.45	CS1–CS2	CS2–CS3
MME group	21	9	12	8.9 ± 2.39	10.5 ± 2.08	CS1–CS2	CS2–CS3

Before expansion treatment (T0), the groups were similar for all width and depth measurements for maxillary and mandibular arch examined ($p > 0.05$).

2. *Treatment effects: RME group T1–T0*
   In the RME group, significant increments in all the variables for maxillary and mandibular arch widths were observed after treatment. Maxillary intermolar, inter second premolar, inter first premolar and intercanine widths changed considerably ($p < 0.001$), while increases in mandibular intermolar and inter second premolar were slightly greater ($p < 0.05$). No significant differences in maxillary and mandibular arch depths were observed at the end of treatment.
3. *Treatment effects: MME group T1–T0*
   In the MME group, significant increases in all the variables for maxillary and mandibular arch widths were observed after treatment. Maxillary intermolar, inter second premolar, inter first premolar and intercanine widths changed considerably ($p < 0.001$), while increases in mandibular intermolar, inter second premolar, inter first premolar ($p < 0.01$) and intercanine widths ($p < 0.05$) were slightly greater. No significant differences in maxillary and mandibular arch depths were observed at the end of treatment.
4. *Comparison of final forms: RME group vs. MME group at T1*
   An evaluation of the changes after RME and MME (T1) showed statistically significant differences in mandibular arch depth ($p < 0.001$) and maxillary intercanine widths ($p < 0.05$). Differences in maxillary arch depth and arch width measurements were not significant.

Discussion

The purpose of this retrospective study was to compare the changes in arch widths and depths on dental casts in two groups of pre-pubertal patients treated with MME or RME.

The method error was low, indicating the high reliability of procedures and measurements.

At baseline (T0), all the parameters were similar in the RME and MME groups ($p > 0.05$) and were thus comparable. All the upper measurements confirmed constriction of the dental arch associated with unilateral or bilateral posterior crossbite. In contrast, the lower values showed no abnormalities in arch widths, as reported in

Table 3 Dental cast analysis in RME and MME groups

	Initial					Change after treatment				Final				
	RME group		MME group			RME group		MME group		RME group		MME group		
	T0		T0			T1–T0		T1–T0		T1		T1		
Cast measure (mm)	Mean	SD	Mean	SD	*p* value	Mean	*p* value	Mean	*p* value	Mean	SD	Mean	SD	*p* value
Maxillary arch width														
Intermolar	43.2	1.576	41.62	3.72	ns	8.8	***	8.7	***	52	2.40	50.31	5.30	ns
Inter second premolar	38.39	1.784	36.93	2.78	ns	7.28	***	6.9	***	45.67	2.15	43.83	4.52	ns
Inter first premolar	33.9	1.698	32.66	2.23	ns	6.82	***	7.33	***	40.72	2.47	40	4.40	ns
Intercanine	29.32	2.135	28.62	2.26	ns	4.3	***	3.70	***	33.62	1.55	32.33	2.12	*
Mandibular arch width														
Intermolar	41.37	2.139	41.2	2.57	ns	1.5	*	2.09	**	42.87	2.35	43.29	2.62	ns
Inter second premolar	36.02	1.874	35.27	2.61	ns	1.17	*	2.36	**	37.2	1.69	37.63	2.79	ns
Inter first premolar	30.55	2.356	29.88	1.85	ns	0.8	ns	1.91	**	31.35	1.38	31.79	2.44	ns
Intercanine	24.9	1.382	24.45	1.50	ns	0.85	ns	1.13	*	25.75	1.58	25.59	1.68	ns
Maxillary arch depth	28.61	1.909	27.5	1.98	ns	−0.59	ns	−0.16	ns	28.02	2.80	27.34	2.18	ns
Mandibular arch depth	25.17	1.599	23.59	1.86	ns	0.3	ns	−0.59	ns	25.47	1.59	23	2.37	***

ns not significant
*$p < 0.05$; **$p < 0.01$; ***$p < 0.001$;

our previous study comparing the MME sample with an untreated control group [11].

After treatment, significant increases in upper and lower arch widths were observed in both the RME and MME group.

Changes in the upper arch intermolar, inter second premolar, inter first premolar and intercanine widths were significant ($p < 0.001$) in both groups.

Lower arch changes were significant for intermolar and inter second premolar in both the MME ($p < 0.01$) and RME ($p < 0.05$) group, whereas increases in inter first premolar ($p < 0.01$) and intercanine widths ($p < 0.05$) were significant only in the MME group. Conversely, no significant differences in upper and lower arch depth between the groups were noted.

Therefore, both procedures were found to be useful for increasing upper arch widths and gaining space to resolve unilateral or bilateral posterior crossbite and/or mild-to-moderate upper crowding.

However, as previously reported, the expansion obtained with MME presents minor dental side effects [22–24]. We may thus speculate that, although comparable at T1 in both groups, the increase in transverse diameters in the upper arch following MME is due to skeletal basal expansion rather than dental tipping. Upper arch changes obtained with MME are therefore subject to less relapse and consequently more stable.

A larger increase in lower widths was found in the MME group. This could be explained by a greater "lip bumper effect" observed after MME [23, 32]. When the upper widths increased slowly during the second step of activation, the cheeks were distanced from the buccal surfaces of mandibular teeth, causing the lower teeth to upright. Uprighting was greater in the molar than in the canine area as a consequence of greater posterior upper arch changes.

At T1, the two groups overlapped for all measurement increases, except for upper intercanine width ($p < 0.05$) and mandibular arch depth ($p < 0.001$). The difference in upper intercanine width is likely a result of the greater anterior opening of the mid-palatal suture, a consequence of increased skeletal expansion obtained by MME, as shown in our previous studies [22–24].

Interestingly, a statistically significant difference in mandibular arch depth between the two groups was observed. The loss in mandibular depth in the MME group might be related to the greater increase in transversal lower arch dimensions compared to the RME group. This study had some limitations. The first is due to the observational design although randomized controlled trials (RCTs) in orthodontic research are still very rare. Second, the small size of the sample can be explained with the very restrictive inclusion criteria. Third, the error method was low, but it does not mean high reliability, so the validity may be not high.

Our future goals are to compare the results obtained with MME and RME through the analysis of the cone beam for skeletal pattern and 3D model analysis for dental arches changes.

Conclusions

RME and MME can be considered two effective treatment options to improve transverse arch dimensions and gain space in the dental arches. Few statistically significant differences in measurements of dental changes were found. RME and MME were both effective in increasing dental transverse dimensions by opening the mid-palatal suture in growing patients. A greater lower arch expansion was observed in the MME group, which might be attributed to the "lip bumper effects" observed in the MME protocol.

Competing interests

The authors declare that they have no competing interests.

Authors' contributions

VG and Fd'A performed the clinical assessments. AJ did the statistical analysis. FF and LF carried out the x-ray examinations. LP conceived the protocol and revised the manuscript. All authors read and approved the final manuscript.

Author details

[1]Multidisciplinary Department of Medical-Surgical and Dental Specialties, Second University of Naples, Via Luigi De Crecchio 6, 80138 Napoli, Italy. [2]Department of Orthodontics, Dental Branch, Craniomaxillofacial Center Islamic Azad University, No.2713, Vali Asr St, Tehran, Iran. [3]Department of Neurosciences, University of Padua, Via Giustiniani 2, 35128 Padova, Italy. [4]Multidisciplinary Department of medical-Surgery and Dental Specialties, Second University of Naples; Post-Graduate Orthodontics Programme and Operative Unit, Via Luigi De Crecchio 6, 80138 Napoli, Italy.

References

1. Gracco A, Malaguti A, Lombardo L, Mazzoli A, Raffaelie R. Palatal volume following rapid maxillary expansion in mixed dentition. Angle Orthod. 2010;80:153–9.
2. Lagravère MO, Major PW, Flores-Mir C. Long-term dental arch changes after rapid maxillary expansion treatment: a systematic review. Angle Orthod. 2005;75:155–61.
3. Perillo L, Femminella B, Farronato D, Baccetti T, Contardo L, Perinetti G. Do malocclusion and temporomandibular disorders correlate with body posture? J Oral Rehabil. 2011;38:242–52.
4. Da Silva Filho OG, Montes LA, Torelly LF. Rapid maxillary expansion in the deciduous and mixed dentition evaluated through posteroanterior cephalometric analysis. Am J Orthod Dentofacial Orthop. 1995;1(07):268–75.
5. Cameron CG, Franchi L, Baccetti T, McNamara Jr JA. Long-term effects of rapid maxillary expansion: a posteroanterior cephalometric evaluation. Am J Orthod Dentofacial Orthop. 2002;121:129–35.
6. Sandikçioğlu M, Hazar S. Skeletal and dental changes after maxillary expansion in the mixed dentition. Am J Orthod Dentofacial Orthop. 1997;111:321–7.
7. Hesse KL, Artun J, Joondeph DR, Kennedy DB. Changes in condylar position and occlusion associated with maxillary expansion for correction of functional unilateral posterior crossbite. Am J Orthod Dentofacial Orthop. 1997;111:410–8.

8. Erdinç AE, Ugur T, Erbay E. A comparison of different treatment techniques for posterior crossbite in the mixed dentition. Am J Orthod Dentofacial Orthop. 2002;116:287–300.
9. Baccetti T, Franchi L, Cameron CG, McNamara Jr JA. Treatment timing for rapid maxillary expansion. Angle Orthod. 2001;71:343–50.
10. Martina R, Cioffi I, Farella M, Leone P, Manzo P, Matarese G, et al. Transverse changes determined by rapid and slow maxillary expansion–a low-dose CT-based randomized controlled trial. Orthod Craniofac Res. 2012;15:159–68.
11. Adkins MD, Nanda RS, Currier GF. Arch perimeter changes on rapid palatal expansion. Am J Orthod Dentaf Orthop. 1990;9:194–9.
12. Lagravere MO, Major PW, Flores-Mir C. Long-term skeletal changes with rapid maxillary expansion: a systematic review. Angle Orthod. 2005;75:1046–52.
13. Lagravere MO, Heo G, Major PW. Meta-analysis of immediate changes with rapid maxillary expansion treatment. J Am Dent Assoc. 2006;137:44–53.
14. Sandstrom RA, Klapper L, Papaconstantinou S. Expansion of the lower arch concurrent with rapid maxillary expansion. Am J Orthod Dentofacial Orthop. 1988;94:296–302.
15. Cross DL, McDonald JP. Effect of rapid maxillary expansion on skeletal, dental, and nasal structures: a postero-anterior cephalometric study. Eur J Orthod. 2000;22:519–28.
16. Haas AJ. Rapid expansion of the maxillary dental arch and nasal cavity by opening the midpalatal suture. Angle Orthod. 1961;31:73–90.
17. Haas AJ. Long-term posttreatment evaluation of rapid palatal expansion. Angle Orthod. 1980;50:189–217.
18. Işeri H, Ozsoy S. Semirapid maxillary expansion-a study of long-term transverse effects in older adolescents and adults. Angle Orthod. 2004;74:71–8.
19. Defraia E, Marinelli A, Baroni G, Tollaro I. Dentoskeletal effects of a removable appliance for expansion of the maxillary arch: a postero-anterior cephalometric study. Eur J Orthod. 2008;30:57–60.
20. Skieller V. Expansion of the midpalatal suture by removable plates, analysed by the implant method. Trans Eur Orthod Soc. 1964;40:143–58.
21. Lione R, Franchi L, Cozza P. Does rapid maxillary expansion induce adverse effects in growing subjects? Angle Orthod. 2012;83:172–82.
22. Grassia V, D'Apuzzo F, Ferrulli VE, Matarese G, Femiano F, Perillo L. Dento-skeletal effects of mixed palatal expansion evaluated by postero-anterior cephalometric analysis. Eur J Paediatr Dent. 2014;15(1):59–62.
23. Grassia V, d'Apuzzo F, DiStasio D, Jamilian A, Lucchese A, Perillo L. Upper and lower arch changes after Mixed Palatal Expansion protocol. Eur J Paediatr Dent. 2014;15(4):375–80.
24. Perillo L, De Rosa A, Iaselli F, d'Apuzzo F, Grassia V, Cappabianca S. Comparison between rapid and mixed maxillary expansion through an assessment of dento-skeletal effects on posteroanterior cephalometry. Prog Orthod. 2014;1815:46.
25. Akkaya S, Lorenzon S, Uçem TT. Comparison of dental arch and arch perimeter changes between bonded rapid and slow maxillary expansion procedures. Eur J Orthod. 1998;20:255–61.
26. Braun S, Bottrel JA, Lee KG, Lunazzi JJ, Legan HL. The biomechanics of rapid maxillary sutural expansion. Am J Orthod Dentofacial Orthop. 2000;118:257–61.
27. Asanza S, Cisneros GJ, Nieberg LG. Comparison of Hyrax and bonded expansion appliances. Angle Orthod. 1997;67:15–22.
28. Mew J. Relapse following maxillary expansion. A study of twenty-five consecutive cases. Am J Orthod. 1983;83:56–61.
29. Vardimon AD, Graber TM, Voss LR, Lenke J. Determinants controlling iatrogenic external root resorption and repair during and after palatal expansion. Angle Orthod. 1991;61:113–24.
30. Perillo L, Castaldo MI, Cannavale R, Longobardi A, Grassia V, Rullo R, et al. Evaluation of long-term effects in patients treated with Fränkel-2 appliance. Eur J Paediatr Dent. 2011;12:261–6.
31. Paolantonio M, D'Ercole S, Pilloni A, D'Archivio D, Lisanti L, Graziani F, et al. Clinical, microbiologic, and biochemical effects of subgingival administration of a Xanthan-based chlorhexidine gel in the treatment of periodontitis: a randomized multicenter trial. J Periodontol. 2009;80(9):1479–92.
32. Fastuca R, Zecca PA, Caprioglio A. Role of mandibular displacement and airway size in improving breathing after rapid maxillary expansion. Prog Orthod. 2014;15(1):40.

11

In vitro study of the potential protection of sound enamel against demineralization

Mona A Montasser[1*], Noha A El-Wassefy[2] and Mahasen Taha[1]

Abstract

Background: The objective of this study was to study the potential protection effect of different treatments against sound enamel demineralization around orthodontic brackets.

Methods: This is an in vitro randomized controlled study; artificial enamel demineralization of human premolars was created and compared with reference to control. The three materials used for enamel treatment were resin infiltrate (ICON), fluoridated varnish (Clinpro), and the self-etch primer system (Transbond Plus Self-Etch Primer). Fifty premolars divided equally into five groups were included in the study for quantitative surface micro-hardness assessment using a micro-hardness tester (MHT). Qualitative assessment of the enamel demineralization with a polarized light microscope (PLM) was also used. Enamel was demineralized by subjecting the specimens to cycling between artificial saliva solution and a demineralizing solution for 21 days.

Results: The mean Vickers hardness in kgf/mm^2 was as follows: intact enamel = 352.5 ± 13.8, demineralized enamel = 301.6 ± 34.0, enamel treated with Clinpro = 333.6 ± 18.0, enamel treated with SEP = 370.7 ± 38.8, and enamel treated with ICON = 380.5 ± 53.8.

Conclusions: ICON, Clinpro, and Transbond Plus Self-Etch Primer (TPSEP) increased enamel resistance to demineralization. Attempting to protect the enamel around the orthodontic brackets could be done by applying a preventive material before bonding, if not compromising the bond strength, the orthodontic brackets.

Keywords: Enamel; Demineralization; Protective methods

Background

Demineralization and appearance of white spot lesions around brackets and bands have become a major concern during orthodontic treatment especially with the potential of these lesions to develop into caries when oral hygiene maintenance is compromised. During orthodontic treatment, an acidic environment develops at the periphery of the orthodontic brackets and bands due to accumulation of bacterial plaque. Enamel demineralization has been repeatedly reported [1–3], and efforts continue to develop ways to prevent development of white spot lesions that are not only unaesthetic but also remineralize poorly increasing the risk of developing carious lesions [4, 5]. Increasing the resistance of the enamel in these areas would control development of white spot lesions.

* Correspondence: mmontasser11@yahoo.com
[1]Orthodontic Department, Faculty of Dentistry 35516, Mansoura University, Mansoura, Egypt
Full list of author information is available at the end of the article

Multiple preventive agents had been tested over years to evaluate their effectiveness in prevention and treatment of white spot lesions associated with orthodontic treatment [6–11]. It was assumed that the most efficient method of delivering preventive agents during orthodontic treatment would be one independent of patient compliance and specific to those areas most susceptible to demineralization [12]. These included adhesives and cements containing fluoride (F), casein phosphopeptide-amorphous calcium phosphate (CPP-ACP), or amorphous calcium phosphate (ACP); fluoride applications; and sealants. Fluoride has been proven to be effective in fighting demineralization [13, 14] that Rølla et al. [13] considered it the only factor that explains the caries reduction in recent years with a synergistic effect from the improved oral hygiene. Fluoride has been found to be effective in reducing the development of white spot lesions associated with fixed orthodontic treatment [15, 16]. Therefore, incorporating preventive agents in orthodontic bonding composite was considered a potential method to reduce white spot lesions during orthodontic treatment even with the general agreement that it is not simple to predict what might occur when the bonding adhesive is used in the demanding environment of the oral cavity [17–19]. Clinpro, a fluoridated varnish, has been introduced to the market and supposed to be most beneficial in a neutral pH environment. Sealants were suggested as protective enamel agents that do not require patient co-operation, but sealants on areas adjacent to brackets are subject to physical challenges as tooth brushing and acid attacks that limit their effect [20, 21]. Recently, resin infiltrants were found to decrease the dissolution of enamel and so limit the appearance of white spot lesions. In an in vitro study to compare a conventional adhesive, a caries infiltrant (ICON), and a combination of both in resisting demineralization, it was found that in both sound enamel and artificial caries lesions, the application of the caries infiltrant was effective in protecting the enamel against dissolution [22].

Systematic reviews of previous studies found a lack of reliable evidence on a protocol or a method to protect the enamel against development of white spot lesions during orthodontic treatment or to remineralize post-orthodontic white spot lesions [23, 24]. The objective of this study was to study the potential protection of different treatments against sound enamel demineralization around orthodontic brackets.

Methods

This is an in vitro randomized controlled study; artificial enamel demineralization of human premolars was created and compared with reference to control. Quantitative surface micro-hardness assessment of the specimens was done with a digital display Vickers micro-hardness tester (MHT) (Model HVS-50, Laizhou Huayin Testing Instrument Co., Ltd., China). The study also used a qualitative polarized light microscope (PLM) (Olympus dual stage polarized light microscope, Model BH-2, Dualmont Corporation, Minneapolis, MN).

The materials used in this study together with the study design are given in Table 1. The three materials used for enamel treatment were Clinpro (3M Unitek, Monrovia, CA, USA), a fluoridated varnish containing 5 % sodium fluoride; ICON (DMG, Hamburg, Germany), a resin infiltrant; and Transbond Plus Self-Etch Primer (TPSEP) (3M Unitek, Monrovia, CA, USA). All materials were used according to the manufacturers' instructions.

The software EpiCalc 2000 version 1.02 (Brixton Books, Brixton, UK) indicated 10 specimens for each group to be a reliable sample size at power 80 % and confidence interval 95 %. For micro-hardness testing, 50 specimens were prepared and then randomly assigned to 5 groups of 10. A similar sample was prepared for the PLM part of the study. Specimens' preparation included separation of the crown from the root, removing any calculus or debris, and polishing with non-fluoride prophylaxis. The crown was then sectioned mesio-distally with a diamond separating disc leaving only a thin layer of the underlying dentin. For PLM examination, 140- to 160-μm-thick sections were prepared from each tooth segment.

To create artificial carious lesions of the enamel, artificial saliva solution [19] was prepared consisting of 20 mmol/L $NaHCO_3$, 3 mmol/L NaH_2PO_4, and 1 mmol/L $CaCl_2$ at neutral pH. Alongside, a demineralizing solution consisting of 2.2 mmol/L Ca^{2+}, 2.2 mmol/L $PO4^{3-}$, and 50 mmol/L acetic acid at pH 4.4 was prepared. Deionized water was used in the preparation of the two solutions. Solutions were measured using a pH/mV meter (Accumet Portable, Fisher Scientific, Pittsburgh, PA) and calcium electrode (Thermo Electron Co., Beverly, MA). The specimens were placed in the prepared artificial saliva solution for 12 h before subjecting them to the demineralizing solution. The specimens were subjected to cycling between the artificial saliva and the demineralizing solutions for 21 days [25].

Surface micro-hardness of the specimens was determined using MHT with a Vickers diamond indenter and a ×20 objective lens. A load of 200 g was applied to the surface of the specimens for 10 s. Three indentations equally placed over a circle and each no closer than 0.5 mm to the adjacent indentations were made on the surface of each specimen. The diagonals' length of the indentations was measured by a built-in scaled microscope, and Vickers values were converted into micro-hardness values. Micro-hardness was obtained using the following equation: $HV = 1.854\ P/d^{2}$, where HV is Vickers

Table 1 Study groups and examination methods

Group	Description	Treatment duration	Examination method	
1	Enamel, no demineralization, no treatment (control)	21 days	MHT	PLM
2	Enamel, demineralization, no treatment (control)			
3	Enamel, demineralization, ICON treatment			
4	Enamel, demineralization, Clinpro treatment			
5	Enamel, demineralization, SEP treatment			

hardness in kgf/mm^2, P is the load in kgf, and d is the length of the diagonals in mm. For the qualitative part of the current study, the prepared specimens were analyzed with the PLM. Each specimen was wetted with deionized water and then was oriented longitudinally on a glass cover slide and mounted, and the stage rotated to allow maximum illumination. The area of demineralization was centered in the field of view and photographed under maximum illumination at ×10 magnification.

Statistical analysis of the results of micro-hardness testing included one-way ANOVA followed by least significant difference (LSD) post-hoc analysis for comparisons between groups.

Results

Descriptive statistics of the enamel hardness of each group are presented in Table 2 and Fig. 1. The demineralized untreated enamel group followed by the Clinpro group showed the lowest hardness values of the enamel surface. The ICON group, the SEP group, and the intact undemineralized enamel group showed the highest hardness values of the enamel surface in descending order.

The one-way ANOVA (Table 2) indicated a significant difference in the enamel hardness between groups ($P = 0.009$). There was no significant difference between the intact enamel and the demineralized enamel groups ($P = 0.09$), the Clinpro group ($P = 0.52$), the SEP group ($P = 0.19$), and the ICON group ($P = 0.10$). However, there was a significant difference between the demineralized enamel group and both the SEP group ($P = 0.004$) and the ICON group ($P = 0.001$).

On the other hand, there was no significant difference between the two treated groups: Clinpro group and SEP group ($P = 0.05$), and Clinpro group and ICON group ($P = 0.24$). The SEP group and ICON group were not significantly different ($P = 0.71$).

A representative photomicrograph for each of the five groups from polarized light microscopy is shown in Fig. 2. The photomicrographs showed that all the three groups of ICON, Clinpro, and SEP were less affected by the demineralization, with smaller lesions and a bright color.

Table 2 Descriptive statistics of the enamel hardness

Group	*N*	Mean (kgf/mm^2)	SD	Minimum	Maximum
1	10	352.5	±13.8	334.8	370.0
2	10	301.6	±34.0	227.3	341.3
3	10	380.5	±53.8	309.4	679.4
4	10	333.6	±18.0	314.3	373.4
5	10	370.7	±38.8	304.1	660.1

$F = 3.42$; $P = 0.009$. Significance at $P \leq 0.05$

Discussion

Micro-hardness is a linear function of the local calcium content [26] that can be used not only as a comparative measure of hardness but also as a direct measure of mineral gain or loss as a consequence of demineralization and remineralization [27, 28]. The method was proved as valid and useful for assessment of the changes in enamel surface demineralization [29, 30].

In the current study, the mean enamel hardness of the control group was 352.5 ± 13.8 kgf/mm^2, while that of the demineralized enamel was 301 ± 34.0 Kgf/mm^2. Applying the fluoridated varnish Clinpro to the enamel surface before demineralization helped to preserve the enamel hardness to some extent as the enamel hardness in this group remained less than that in the control group; the mean enamel hardness in this group was 333.6 ± 18.0 kgf/mm^2. Clinpro™ is a white varnish with tri-calcium phosphate (TCP) ingredient to deliver fluoride, phosphate, and calcium. According to the manufacturer, a protective barrier is created around this ingredient during manufacturing, and as the varnish flows on the teeth, it comes into contact with saliva, breaking down the protective barrier and so makes calcium, phosphate, and fluoride ions available to the teeth to decrease the demineralization. Although enamel treated with Clinpro™ was not as hard as the intact untreated enamel, the change might be clinically significant taking into consideration the long duration of orthodontic treatment that on average ranges from 2 to 3 years. Multiple applications of Clinpro over the period of orthodontic treatment may be recommended for further enhancing its protective effect.

The increased surface hardness of the enamel in the ICON group (380.5 ± 53.8 kgf/mm^2) could be interpreted in light of the mode of action of this material. The low-viscosity light-cured resin material infiltrates the etched enamel surface creating a barrier on the enamel surface, and it is this superficial layer that increases the enamel surface hardness and subsequently increases the resistance to surface demineralization and the development of white spot lesions. Earlier studies as the study of Yetkiner et al. [31] found that the use of low-viscosity caries infiltrant ICON increased sound enamel resistance to demineralization. The mean enamel hardness in group 5 in which the specimens were treated with TPSEP and then subjected to the same protocol of demineralization used in the other groups was 370.7 ± 38.8 kgf/mm^2. This group, therefore, presented the second highest mean enamel hardness in the current study. TPSEP is a F-releasing self-etch primer, and it acts as other self-etch primers through three mechanisms to stop the etching process and complete the priming: (1) the acid groups attached to the etching monomers are neutralized by forming a complex with

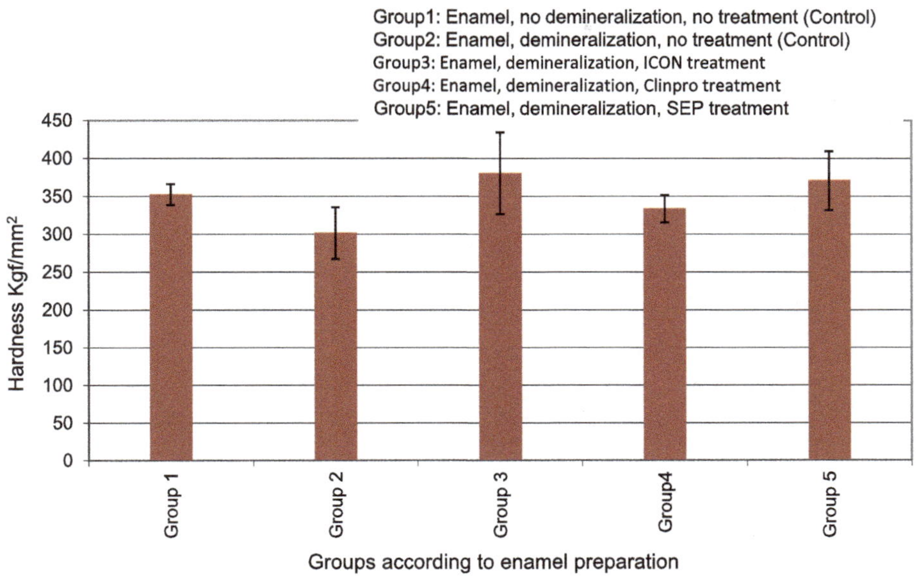

Fig. 1 Mean ± SD of the enamel hardness (kgf/mm^2) of the five tested groups

the calcium from the hydroxyapatite; (2) the viscosity increases with the air drying, slowing the transport of acid groups to the enamel interface; and (3) the primer polymerizes and the transport of acid groups to the interface stops [32]. The results of the current study suggest that it is not only the effect of the F that increased the enamel hardness but the polymerized surface layer also contributed to this effect. Both group 3 (ICON) and group 5 (SEP) showed increased enamel hardness compared to group 2 (demineralized enamel) and even to group 1 (untreated enamel); this could be contributed by the polymerized surface layer.

On the other hand, the polarized light microscope, with its unique ability to deliver information about the submicroscopic structure of the material under examination utilizing polarized light to form highly magnified images, could qualitatively show the areas of mineral loss and mineral gain represented by areas with different porosities and birefringence [33, 34]. The results of the PLM photomicrographs, as shown in Fig. 2, supported the micro-hardness results; the three groups of ICON, Clinpro, and SEP showed better resistance to enamel demineralization. The photomicrographs showed smaller lesions in the three groups where the enamel was treated with ICON, Clinpro, and SEP compared to the demineralized untreated enamel.

Attempting to protect the enamel around orthodontic brackets could be done through different techniques that each could be effective. This could be by applying a preventive material before bonding the orthodontic brackets or around the brackets after bonding. Regarding the three materials used in the current study, the use of self-etch

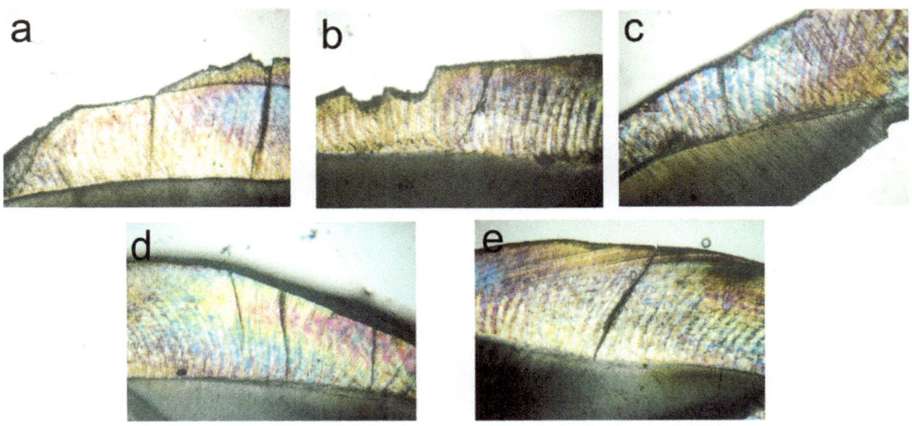

Fig. 2 Showing polarized light microscope micrograph at ×10 magnification. **a** Intact enamel. **b** Demineralized enamel. **c** Enamel treated with ICON. **d** Enamel treated with Clinpro. **e** Enamel treated with SEP

primers for orthodontic bracket bonding is well documented and has proven not to compromise bond strength [35–37]. A previous study which tested the effect of using ICON and Clinpro before bonding orthodontic brackets with self-etch primer and conventional adhesive systems on the shear bond strength found no significant effect [38].

However, although the observed increase in the enamel hardness would logically suggest more resistance to demineralization, it is not possible to simply expect a solution to the problem of developing white spot lesions during orthodontic treatment with the use of these materials. A systematic review of in vivo studies on the caries-inhibiting effect of preventive measures during orthodontic treatment with fixed appliances considered the effect significant if only it was over 50 % [24].

Conclusions

ICON, Clinpro, and TPSEP increased enamel resistance to demineralization. Attempting to protect the enamel around the orthodontic brackets could be done by applying a preventive material before bonding, if not compromising the bond strength, the orthodontic brackets.

Competing interests

The authors declare that they have no competing interests.

Authors' contributions

MM formulated the idea and the design of the study, participated in preparing the samples and did the writing of the manuscript. NA participated in preparing the samples and, did the statistics and the MH and PLM testing. MT participated in designing the study, selecting the material, preparing the samples, and interpreting the results. All authors read and approved the final manuscript.

Author details

[1]Orthodontic Department, Faculty of Dentistry 35516, Mansoura University, Mansoura, Egypt. [2]Dental Biomaterials Department, Faculty of Dentistry 35516, Mansoura University, Mansoura, Egypt.

References

1. Gorelick L, Geiger AM, Gwinnett AJ. Incidence of white spot formation after bonding and banding. Am J Orthod. 1982;81:93–8.
2. O'Reilly MM, Featherstone JD. Demineralization and remineralization around orthodontic appliances: an in vivo study. Am J Orthod Dentofacial Orthop. 1987;92:33–40.
3. Mitchell L. Decalcification during orthodontic treatment with fixed appliances—an overview. Br J Orthod. 1992;19:199–205.
4. Årtun J, Thylstrup A. A 3-year clinical and SEM study of surface changes of carious enamel lesions after inactivation. Am J Orthod. 1989;95:327–33.
5. Øgaard B. Prevalence of white spot lesions in 19-year olds: a study on untreated and orthodontically treated persons 5 years after treatment. Am J Orthod. 1989;96:423–7.
6. Pol TR, Naik CR, Gupta R, Pol A, Sanghvi S. Incorporation of casein phosphopeptide-amorphous calcium phosphate into glass-ionomer cement for orthodontic band cementation—an in vitro study. Int J Stomatol Res. 2013;2:5–10.
7. Tüfekçi E, Pennella DR, Mitchell JC, Best AM, Lindauer SJ. Efficacy of a fluoride-releasing orthodontic primer in reducing demineralization around brackets: an in-vivo study. Am J Orthod Dentofacial Orthop. 2014;146:207–14.
8. Yap J, Walsh LJ, Naser-Ud Din S, Ngo H, Manton DJ. Evaluation of a novel approach in the prevention of white spot lesions around orthodontic brackets. Aust Dent J. 2014;59:70–80.
9. Benson PE, Parkin N, Dyer F, Millett DT, Furness S, Germain P. Fluorides for the prevention of early tooth decay (demineralised white lesions) during fixed brace treatment. Cochrane Database Syst Rev. 2013 Dec12;12:CD003809.
10. Ballard RW, Hagan JL, Phaup AN, Sarkar N, Townsend JA, Armbruster PC. Evaluation of 3 commercially available materials for resolution of white spot lesions. Am J Orthod Dentofacial Orthop. 2013;143(4 Suppl):S78–84.
11. Zanarini M, Pazzi E, Bonetti S, Ruggeri O, Alessandri Bonetti G, Prati C. In vitro evaluation of the effects of a fluoride-releasing composite on enamel demineralization around brackets. Prog Orthod. 2012;13:10–6.
12. Gwinnett JA, Ceen F. Plaque distribution on bonded brackets. Am J Orthod. 1979;75:667–77.
13. Rølla G, Ogaard B, Cruz Rde A. Clinical effect and mechanism of cariostatic action of fluoride-containing toothpastes: a review. Int Dent J. 1991;41:171–4.
14. Featherstone JD, Glena R, Shariati M, Shields CP. Dependence of in vitro demineralization of apatite and remineralization of dental enamel on fluoride concentration. J Dent Res. 1990;69:620–5. discussion 634–636.
15. Lodaya SD, Keluskar KM, Naik V. Evaluation of demineralization adjacent to orthodontic bracket and bond strength using fluoride-releasing and conventional bonding agents. Indian J Dent Res. 2011;22:44–9.
16. Chow CK, Wu CD, Evans CA. In vitro properties of orthodontic adhesives with fluoride or amorphous calcium phosphate. Int Dent. 2011;2011:ID 583521.
17. Lee SY, Greener EH, Menis DL. Detection of leached moieties from dental composites in fluids simulating food and saliva. Dent Mater. 1995;11:348–53.
18. Söderholm K, Mukherjee R, Longmate J. Filler leachability of composites stored in distilled water or artificial saliva. J Dent Res. 1996;75:1692–9.
19. Miller JR. Commentary basic concepts concerning bracket failure research. Angle Orthod. 1997;67:167–8.
20. Gorton J, Featherstone JDB. Demineralization and remineralization around orthodontic brackets. Am J Orthod Dentofac Orthop. 2003;123:10–40.
21. Paschos E, Kleinschrodt T, Clementino-Luedemann T, Huth KC, Hickel R, Kunzelmann KH, et al. Effect of different bonding agents on prevention of enamel demineralization around orthodontic brackets. Am J Orthod Dentofac Orthop. 2009;135:603–12.
22. Schmidlin PR, Sener B, Attin T, Wiegand A. Protection of sound enamel and artificial enamel lesions against demineralization: caries infiltrant versus adhesive. J Dent. 2012;40:851–6.
23. Chen H, Liu X, Dai J, Jiang Z, Guo T, Ding Y. Effect of remineralizing agents on white spot lesions after orthodontic treatment: a systematic review. Am J Orthod Dentofacial Orthop. 2013;143:376–82.
24. Derks A, Katsaros C, Frencken JE, van't Hof MA, Kuijpers-Jagtman AM. Caries-inhibiting effect of preventive measures during orthodontic treatment with fixed appliances. A systematic review. Caries Res. 2004;38:413–20.
25. Uysal T, Amasyali M, Koyuturk AE, Sagdic D. Efficiency of amorphous calcium phosphate-containing orthodontic composite and resin modified glass ionomer on demineralization evaluated by a new laser fluorescence device. Eur J Dent. 2009;3:127–34.
26. Davideson CL, Hoeksra IJ, Arends J. Microhardness of sound, decalcified and etched tooth enamel related to calcium content. Caries Res. 1974;8:135–44.
27. Featherstone JDB, Rodgers BE, Smith MW. Physicochemical requirements for rapid remineralization of early carious lesions. Caries Res. 1981;15:221–35.
28. Featerstone JDB, Cutress TW, Rodgers BE, Dennison PJ. Remineralization of early carious lesion in vivo by a self-administered mouthrinse or paste. Caries Res. 1982;16:235–42.
29. Featherstone JD, Ten Cate JM, Shariati M, Arends J. Comparison of artificial caries-like lesions by quantitative microradiography and microhardness profiles. Caries Res. 1983;17:385–91.
30. White DJ, Featherstone JD. A longitudinal microhardness analysis of fluoride dentifrice effects on lesion progression in vitro. Caries Res. 1987;21:502–12.
31. Yetkiner E, Ozcan M, Wegehaupt FJ, Attin R, Attin T. Caries infiltrant combined with conventional adhesives for sealing sound enamel in vitro. Angle Orthod. 2013;83:858–63.
32. Vicente A, Bravo L, Romero M, Ortiz AJ, Canteras M. Shear bond strength of orthodontic brackets bonded with self-etching primers. Am J Dent. 2005;18:256–60.

33. Silverstone LM. Structure of carious enamel including the early lesion. Orl Sic Rev. 1973;3:100–60.
34. Theuns HM, Arends J, Groeneveld A. Polarizing microscopy and microradiography of sound enamel. J Biol buccal. 1980;8:229–38.
35. Rajagopal R, Padmanabhan S, Gnanamani J. A comparison of shear bond strength and debonding characteristics of conventional, moisture insensitive, and self-etching primers in vitro. Angle Orthod. 2004;74:264–8.
36. Arnold RW, Combe EC, Warford JH. Bonding of stainless steel brackets to enamel with a new self-etching primer. Am J Orthod Dentofac Orthop. 2002;122:274–6.
37. Nikaido T, Nakajima M, Higashi T, Kanemura N, Pereira P, Tagami J. Shear bond strength of a single-step bonding system to enamel and dentin. Dent Mater. 1997;16:40–7.
38. Montasser MA, Taha M. Effect of enamel protective agents on the shear bond strength of orthodontic brackets. Prog Orthod. 2014;18:15-34.

12

Synergistic effect of wire bending and salivary pH on surface properties and mechanical properties of orthodontic stainless steel archwires

Marieke G. Hobbelink[1,2], Yan He[1,3*], Jia Xu[1], Huixu Xie[1], Richard Stoll[1] and Qingsong Ye[1*]

Abstract

Background: The aim of this study was to investigate the corrosive behaviour of stainless steel archwires in a more clinically relevant way by bending and exposing to various pH.

Methods: One hundred and twenty pieces of rectangular stainless steel wires (0.43 × 0.64 mm) were randomly assigned into four groups. In each group, there were 15 pieces of bent wires and 15 straight ones. Prior to measurements of the wires, as individual experimental groups (group 1, 2, and 3), the wires were exposed to artificial saliva for 4 weeks at pH 5.6, 6.6, and 7.6, respectively. A control group of wires (group 4) remained in air for the same period of time before sent for measurements. Surface roughness (Ra-value) was measured by a profilometer. Young's modulus and maximum force were determined by a four-point flexural test apparatus. Scanning electron microscopy was used to observe the surface morphology of straight wire. Differences between groups were examined using a two-way analysis of variance (ANOVA).

Results: Mean surface roughness values, flexural Young's moduli, and maximum force values of bent wires are significantly different from those of the straight wires, which was the main effect of wire bending, ignoring the influence of pH. A significant effect was found between Ra-values regarding the main effect of pH, ignoring the influence of shape. There was a significant interaction effect of bending and pH on flexural Young's moduli of stainless steel archwires, while pH did not show much impact on the maximum force values of those stainless steel wires. Bigger surface irregularities were seen on SEM images of straight wires immersed in artificial saliva at pH 5.6 compared to artificial saliva at other pH values. Surface depth (Rz) was more sensitive than Ra in revealing surface roughness, both measured from 3D reconstructed SEM images. Ra showed a comparable result of surface roughness to Ra-value measured by the profilometer.

Conclusions: Bending has a significant influence on surface roughness and mechanical properties of rectangular SS archwires. pH plays a synergistic effect on the change of mechanical properties of stainless steel (SS) wires along with wire bending.

Keywords: Stainless steel archwire, Surface roughness, Young's modulus, Maximum force, Salivary pH, Corrosion

* Correspondence: Helen-1101@hotmail.com; qingsongye@hotmail.com
[1]Orthodontic Department, College of Medicine and Dentistry, James Cook University, Cairns, Australia
Full list of author information is available at the end of the article

Background

Stainless steel (SS) has been introduced around 1930 as an alloy for the fabrication of orthodontic archwires and is still a broadly used appliance in orthodontic practice [1]. Stainless steel is a convenient material to act as a spring because it is, among other materials, a ductile material and it is able to maintain its shape after bending. This behaviour of a SS alloy can be explained by consideration of its mechanical properties. Examination of mechanical properties is the key to understand the clinical application of a material since mechanical properties determine the behaviour of the wire in generating forces and thus influence tooth movement.

An important parameter is the flexural Young's modulus (Fig. 1). It represents the flexibility of an archwire and can be calculated as the slope of a force-deflection curve. Researchers have been reporting a flexural Young's modulus of ~120–217 GPa [2] for as-received stainless steel archwires. Another important parameter is the maximum force. This is defined as the maximum amount of force the wire can withstand before it starts to fail [3].

Mechanical properties of stainless steel orthodontic archwires can be influenced by a variety of causes, for example, corrosion [4, 5]. Electrolytic corrosion of orthodontic appliances in the mouth regularly occurs due to the wet oral environment [6]. The pH value of saliva in the oral environment has a significant effect on the corrosion rate [7]. The resting pH of human saliva ranges from 5.6 to 7.6, which can be caused by dietary habits [8] and internal stimuli like vomitingor by diseases [9, 10].

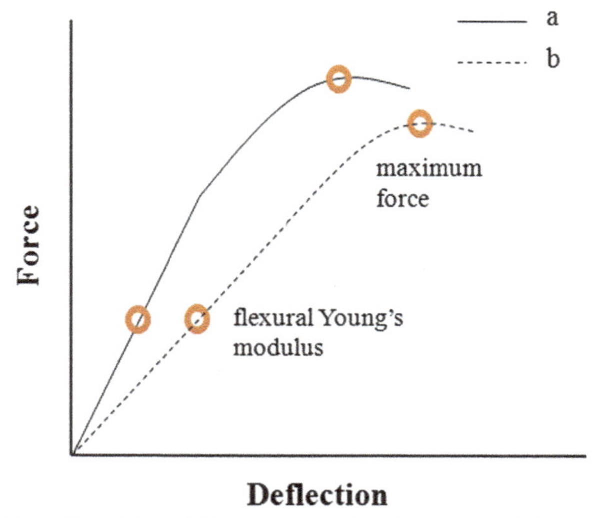

Fig. 1 Typical force-deflection curves of an elastic material. The flexural Young's modulus and maximum force value are indicated as *brown circles*. The flexural Young's modulus is calculated as the slope of the linear portion of the curve by taking into account the dimensions of the wire. The maximum force is the maximum amount of force a material can withstand before it starts to fail. Curve *a* represents a stiffer material than curve *b*

Corrosive damage to archwires can result in deterioration of its mechanical properties. Limited studies have been performed to investigate the influence of corrosion on mechanical properties of stainless steel archwires [4, 5, 11]. The corrosion phenomenon may not only influence the mechanical properties of the orthodontic archwires but also affect surface properties, such as the surface roughness and surface texture [7, 12].

A variety of experiments have measured the surface roughness of as-received stainless steel archwires [10], resulting in a description of the surface of SS archwires as smooth, compared to titanium archwires [13, 14]. Regarding corrosion resistance, literature describes that SS archwires corroded more than titanium archwires [7, 15]. Surface roughness and texture increase with the increase of incubation time in acid solutions [13] and the decrease of pH [7].

Surface texture can be observed by a scanning electron microscope (SEM). SEM images of as-received SS archwires showed an inhomogeneous surface with different surface irregularities [2, 16], scratches, and pits [17]. SEM images of in vitro corroded SS archwires show pitting corrosion, localized corrosion, and scratches [13]. An increase in variety, type, and number of surface irregularities were observed due to wear and friction of archwires from in vivo studies [16, 18].

The corrosion phenomenon influences the mechanical properties and surface properties of stainless steel orthodontic archwires [19]. Such degradation processes can have serious clinical implications resulting in weakening the efficacy of the force delivering system. It also increases the potential for failure [15]. Previous experimental set-ups had been performed to investigate the influence of corrosion on the mechanical properties and surface properties of SS archwires [13]. However, those studies investigated straight archwire pieces only. In orthodontic clinic, archwire bending is an integral part of orthodontic treatment. Straight archwires are hardly used in a patient's mouth. Bending causes stress in the material, which alters the wire properties and its behaviour upon challenges, e.g., corrosion.

So, the aim of this study was to investigate the corrosive behaviour of bent SS archwires in a more clinically relevant manner comparing the bent with the as-received straight wires in a clinically relevant pH solution.

Methods

Wire preparation

Rectangular stainless steel orthodontic archwires, 0.43 × 0.64 mm (3M Unitek, USA), were cut into pieces with a distal-end cutter (Hu-Friedy, USA) for further sample preparation. A curved shape was bent following the Ovoid Arch Form OrthoForm™ III (3M Unitek, USA) with an Adams Plier (678-320-U5 Hu-Friedy, USA). The length of the pieces was measured with an electronic digital calliper to ±0.1 mm accuracy. The total sample size of 120 pieces, 60 pieces per wire shape type, was determined by a multiple comparisons Power Analysis (Tukey-Kramer) test. These archwires were randomly divided into four groups, three experimental groups and one control group. Each group contained 30 pieces of wires, including 15 bent wires and 15 straight wires (24 mm). Additionally, one short straight wire (10 mm) was included for each group to study surface characteristics under a scanning electron microscope.

Immersing experiment

A total of 1 L of artificial saliva was prepared (0.400 g/L NaCl, 0.400 g/L KCl, 0.795 g/L $CaCl_2$, 0.010 g/L Na_2S9H_2O, 1.000 g/L CH_4N_2O, 0.789 g/L KH_2PO_4) and divided into three portions equally, which were calibrated to pH 5.6, 6.6, and 7.6, respectively. Experimental groups were marked as groups 1, 2, and 3 in the same order as pH values. The wires were immersed in 20 mL artificial saliva and placed in the incubator (SANYO Electric Biomedical Co., Japan) at 37 °C for 4 weeks. The solution was refreshed every week to ensure a constant pH. The wires of group 4 were exposed to air at room temperature, served as the control group.

Surface roughness test

Surface roughness test was carried out by a calibrated contact profilometer (RTD-200 Portable Surface Roughness tester, New Star, Australia). Mean surface roughness values (Ra-values, μm) are defined as the arithmetic mean of the absolute departures of the roughness profile from the mean line. The software of profilometer was set at a Gauss roughness filter type with a cut-off length of 0.25 mm and an assessment length of 0.75 mm. The measurement was performed by a diamond point ($\phi = 5$ μm) moving along the wire with a traversing speed of 0.135 mm/s at a pressing force of 4 mN. Prior to surface roughness test, the wires were taken out of the immersion solution and air-dried on a paper towel. Each wire was measured at three different positions. To ensure the reliability of measurements, these positions were indicated by lines as shown in Fig. 2a. The mean of three Ra-values per wire was used for statistical analysis.

Four-point flexural test

In this research, the flexural test was performed by a Z2.5 ZwickiLine Universal Testing Machine (Zwick/Roell, Germany) with a customized four-point appliance (Fig. 2b), which consists of two loading pins and two supporting pins. A 500-N maximal force, 2-mV/V

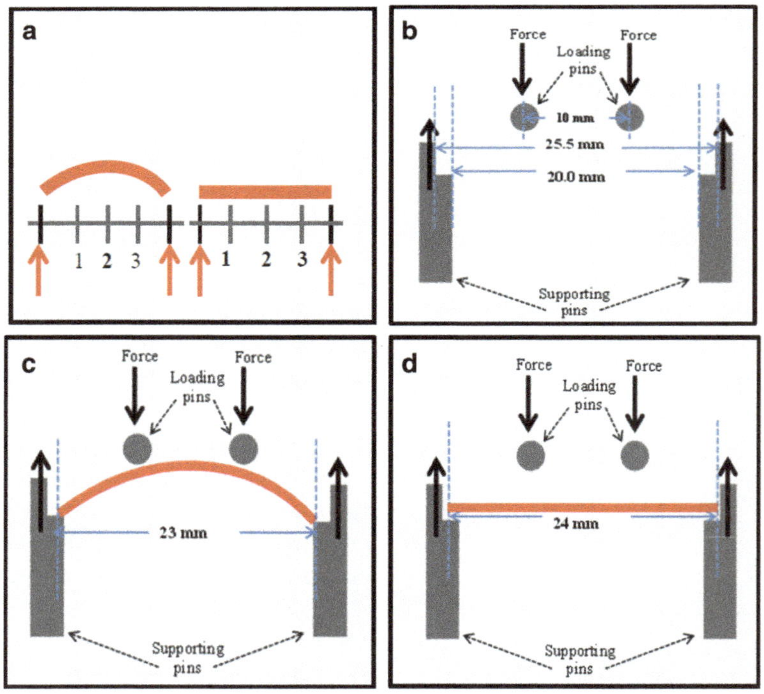

Fig. 2 Schematics of measurements of surface roughness and mechanical properties. **a** Schematic of surface roughness of bent and straight wires measurement by a profilometer. Wire placed in-between two outer lines, indicated by *red arrows*. Bent wires were measured at around position *2* and straight wires were measured at positions *1*, *2*, and *3*. **b** Schematic drawing of the four-point flexural test apparatus for measurements of flexural Young's modulus and maximum force of bent and straight wires. The distance between the supporting pins ranges from 20 to 25.5 mm (support span), and the distance between the loading pins is 10 mm (load span). Both loading pins move downward to produce force on the wires. **c–d** Bent and straight wire placed in-between the supporting pins, where the 0.43-mm side of wires are resting upon

sensitivity load cell (XforceP, Zwick/Roell, Germany), containing two loading pins, was installed in the machine with a crosshead speed of 1 mm/min. The load span, distance between both loading pins, was set at 10 mm. Loading pins deformed the wire at a speed of 1 mm/min until a threshold of 25 N was reached (Fig. 2). The load-deflection data obtained from the test were plotted as force-deflection curves, and the flexural Young's modulus was calculated by the computer software testXpert II (Zwick/Roell, Germany) (Fig. 3).

Scanning electron microscopy

The surface of 10-mm straight wires was observed by SEM apparatus (G2 Pro, Phenom-World BV, The Netherlands) on its 0.43-mm side with a ×2000 magnification. Three places on each sample were randomly chosen for image scanning. The SEM software (Phenom Pro Suite, Phenom-World BV, The Netherlands) was used to quantity the surface morphology by reconstructing a 3D surface, from which mean surface roughness values (Ra) and mean surface depth values (Rz) were calculated. Three different regions of each image were selected for 3D reconstruction and calculation. Ra is the arithmetic mean of the absolute departures of the roughness profile from the mean line. Rz is the roughness depth, calculated as the sum of the height of the highest profile peak from the mean line and the depth of the deepest profile valley from the mean line.

Statistical analyses

All data were analysed by SPSS 22 (IBM® SPSS®, USA). A two-way analysis of variance (ANOVA) test was carried out for surface roughness (Ra-values), flexural Young's moduli, and maximum force values, followed by post hoc multiple comparison tests. A significance level of $p = 0.05$ was used.

Results

Surface roughness

The Ra-value of the bent wires was significantly higher than that of the straight wires in all three pH groups ($p < 0.000$), where the straight wires in the control group had the lowest Ra-value $(8.2 \pm 0.9) \times 10^{-2}$ μm and the bent wire had the roughest surface $(24.1 \pm 4.5) \times 10^{-2}$ μm after being immersed in artificial saliva of pH 5.6 for 4 weeks (Table 1). Surface roughness from different pH groups showed highly varied Ra-values in both the bent and straight wires ($p < 0.000$) (Fig. 4).

Compared to the wires in control group, the surface roughness of the bent and straight wires immersed in pH 5.6 and 7.6 were significantly rougher ($p < 0.000$) (Table 1). The surface roughness of both wires at pH 5.6 was also significantly different from that of the wires at pH 6.6 and 7.6 ($p < 0.05$) (Table 1). There is no difference in surface roughness of wires between the control and pH 6.6 groups ($p = 0.740$). A bigger distribution of data for the immersion groups than for the control group was observed, where higher SD were noted for immersion groups than for control groups. Similarly, higher SD values were noted on bent wires than on straight wires (Table 1).

Flexural young's modulus

The flexural Young's modulus of SS wires had been distinctively reduced after bending ($p < 0.000$). In the control group, Young's modulus was 496 ± 18.62 GPa measured in the straight wires and 345 ± 85.90 GPa in the bent wires (Table 1). This discrepancy between the bent and straight wires was not diminished by immersion in artificial saliva

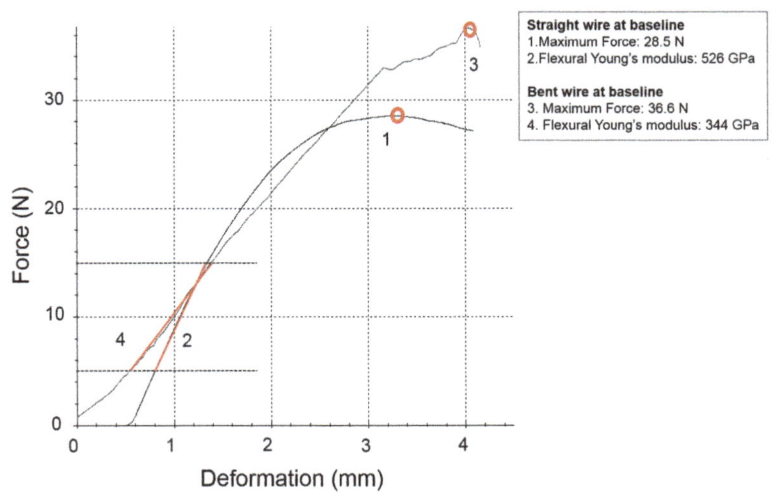

Fig. 3 Force-deflection curves of two SS wires obtained by four-point flexural testing. The flexural Young's moduli were the slope of the section on the curve indicated by a *red line* and the maximum force values are *circled* in *red*. Their corresponding values are given in the legend

Table 1 Surface roughness, Young's modulus, and maximum force of bent/straight wires before and after immersion

Groups		Surface roughness ×10^{-2} (μm)			Mean flexural young's modulus (GPa)	Mean Maximum force (N)
		Ra-value	Ra	Rz		
1 (pH 5.6)	Bent	24.1 ± 4.5	30.2 ± 5.7	117.3 ± 43.4	295 ± 46.98	32.5 ± 3.24
	Straight	11.1 ± 2.5			505 ± 38.34	27.9 ± 1.07
2 (pH 6.6)	Bent	18.3 ± 3.8	11.5 ± 1.5	81.2 ± 4.8	300 ± 46.72	31.4 ± 5.86
	Straight	9.4 ± 2.9			502 ± 52.48	27.6 ± 1.40
3 (pH 7.6)	Bent	20.5 ± 4.2	14.0 ± 0.9	78.8 ± 8.5	242 ± 35.07	29.2 ± 7.43
	Straight	10.1 ± 2.4			485 ± 92.66	27.2 ± 3.00
4 (Control)	Bent	17.9 ± 2.2	4.4 ± 0.6	28.4 ± 6.8	345 ± 85.90	32.5 ± 3.72
	Straight	8.2 ± 0.9			496 ± 18.62	28.4 ± 0.42

Mean roughness (Ra-value), mean flexural Young's modulus, and mean maximum force of bent/straight wires as well as mean roughness (Ra and Rz) of straight wires before (control group 4) and after immersion in artificial saliva at pH 5.6, 6.6, and 7.6 (experiment groups 1, 2, and 3). Data are shown as mean ± SD

of various pH. On the contrary, the discrepancy was enlarged as pH increased, which was mainly contributed by the decrease of Young's moduli of bent wires because Young's moduli of straight wires were hardly influenced by pH ($p = 0.772$) (Fig. 4). The lowest Young's modulus measured in this study was 242 ± 35.07 GPa, marked by the bent wires immersed in pH 7.6 (Table 1).

Maximum force values

The maximum force of the bent wires was significantly higher than that of the straight wires throughout the experiment groups and control group ($p < 0.00$). After wire bending, the maximum force increased from 28.4 ± 0.42 N to 32.5 ± 3.224 N ($p < 0.05$). After immersion in artificial saliva for 4 weeks, there was a mild decrease in maximum force of the straight wires as pH increased, whereas a dramatic drop in maximum force in bent wires was noticed (Fig. 4). Yet pH did not make significant influence on SS wires regarding the maximum force values in either the bent or straight wires ($p = 0.127$).

Scanning electron microscopy

Scratches along the axial of wires were observed in all SEM images, which are typical defects of SS surface indicated by white arrows. The SEM image of SS wire from the control group showed a relatively smooth

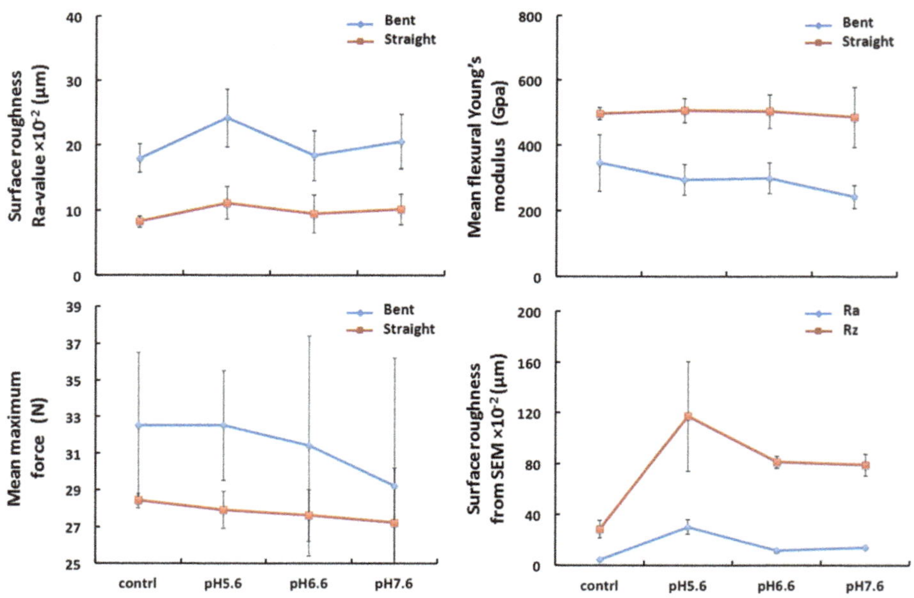

Fig. 4 Comparison of surface roughness, Young's modulus, and maximum force of bent and straight wires. Surface roughness (Ra-value, μm) of bent and straight SS archwires was measured by a profilometer; flexural Young's modulus (GPa) and maximum force (N) of bent and straight SS archwires were measured by a four-point bending test; surface roughness (Ra and Rz,μm) of straight SS wires were measured via 3D reconstruction of SEM images. All measured wires were exposed to air or immersed in artificial saliva at pH 5.6, 6.6, and 7.6 for 4 weeks according to protocol

surface except for the typical striations and flaws existing on the wires from the experimental groups as well (Fig. 5a). The surface roughness of the wire from the control group had a mean Ra of 4.4×10^{-2} μm and Rz of 28.4×10^{-2} μm, which were the lowest values compared to the rest ($p < 0.05$) (Table 1).

Figure 5b depicts the surface of SS wire immersed in artificial saliva at pH 5.6 for 4 weeks. An increased corrosion pattern was observed compared to other pH groups. Irregularities on the surface were broader and the roughness peaks were bigger (green arrow). Scratch lines are more pronounced on the sample wire from this pH group than in the other pH groups (white arrow). These observations were in line with the measurements made upon SEM images, mean Ra and Rz were 30.2×10^{-2} μm and 177.3×10^{-2} μm, respectively, where the parameters from pH 5.6 group were higher than those from other pH groups ($p < 0.05$) (Table 1).

Figure 5c and d show the surface of SS wire immersed in artificial saliva at pH 6.6 and 7.6. These surfaces revealed more irregularities than the wire surface from the control group and those irregularities were smaller than those observed in Fig. 5b. In Fig. 5d, pores (green arrow) are seen in higher frequency than in the other pH groups. But they were smaller in diameter and depth than the surface irregularities in Fig. 5b. This was in accordance with a mean Rz of 78.8×10^{-2} μm and Ra of 14.0×10^{-2} μm (Table 1).

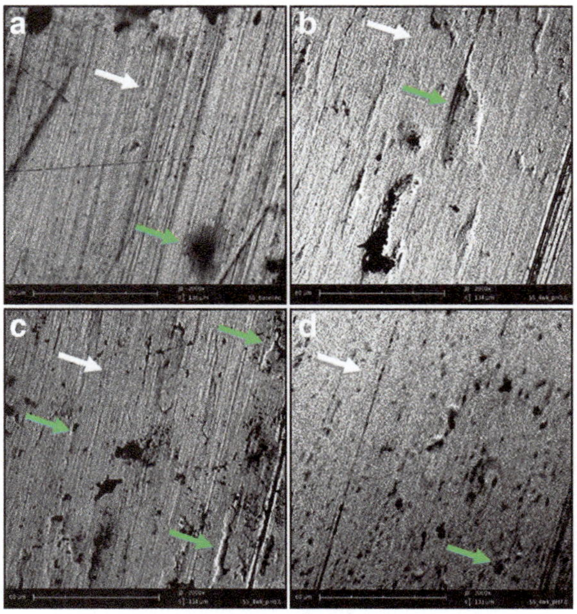

Fig. 5 SEM images of straight rectangular SS wires at ×2000 magnification (**a–d**). Representative SEM images of SS wire of control group, pH 5.6, 6.6, and 7.6, respectively. *White arrows* indicate typical manufacturing striations; *green arrows* indicate specific surface irregularities

Although Rz was more sensitive than Ra in revealing surface roughness, both parameters showed that SS wires had the most rough surface after bending and immersion at pH 5.6 ($p < 0.05$) (Table 1). The influence of pH on surface roughness quantified by 3D construction of SEM images was consistent with the surface roughness measured by profilometer, which was much more obvious than observation done via a profilometer (Fig. 5). Especially, the Ra derived from SEM images was comparable to the measurements done by profilometer except that it was $(11.1 \pm 2.5) \times 10^{-2}$ μm as measured by profilometer and $(30.2 \pm 5.7) \times 10^{-2}$ μm by 3D reconstruction of SEM images (Table 1).

Discussion

Surface properties

Determining the surface roughness of stainless steel wires is a fundamental concern in corrosion resistance of a wire for orthodontic clinic. Straight archwires are hardly used in a patient's mouth, and wire bending is an integral part of the orthodontic treatment. Even though the preformed SS archwires are popularly used nowadays, the chairside wire bending is inevitable due to the variations in the malocclusions of individual patient. In this research it is determined that bent SS wires have a highly significantly rougher surface than straight SS wires, ignoring pH. These divergences in surface roughness between bent and straight wires could be caused by the use of pliers when bending the wires, which could easily cause damages to the protective oxide layer.

In this research, Ra-values revealed that bent wires immersed in pH 5.6 and 7.6 solutions have a significantly rougher surface than bent wires at baseline. The increase of surface roughness by decreasing the pH is in agreement with results of other study. However, the surface of SS wires has also been roughened by artificial saliva at pH 7.6 according to our experiment. So far, no researchers had investigated the influence of basic saliva on SS archwires. This phenomenon of basic solution corroding SS wire was minute on straight wires and was amplified on bent wires, which has been echoed by images and measurements of SEM. Hence, it is recommendable that more research should be done regarding immersion in artificial saliva at basic pH because of its clinical relevance that the pH of resting saliva ranges from pH 5.6 to 7.6 [9, 10]. On the other hand, pH 6.6 seemed to be an optimal pH for SS archwire to perform and thus this might be our goal to balance oral pH especially during orthodontic treatment.

Mechanical properties

Mechanical properties of SS wires are key to understand the wire application clinically since it determines the force generated for tooth movement. It has been reported that a flexural Young's modulus of ~133–184 GPa for as-received SS archwires was measured by a three-point flexural test [13], while 468–526 GPa of Young's modulus on SS wires was measured in this study by a four-point bending test, which was about threefold of the former. The explanation for the differences could be the support span. A support span of 20 mm was used in this research (Fig. 5), while other researchers used a lower support span of 14 and 9 mm [14, 20]. Alteration of the support span alters the load-deflection rate, even as alteration of the wire diameter [21]. Another explanation might be that smaller cross section increases the wire stiffness [2]. In other research, the wires were tested on their 0.64-mm side, whereas they were tested on their 0.43-mm side in this research [13].

In our study, we found that wire bending played an essential role on the mechanical properties of SS wires. It lowered Young's modulus, and this influence was enhanced by the increase of pH. A higher flexural Young's modulus indicates a stiffer wire with a greater resistance to deformation. Wire bending was originally introduced to elongate the length of a wire and thus to increase the flexibility and to lower Young's modulus in order to deliver a moderate and persistent optimal force for tooth movement. As our finding pointed out that bending discounts the flexibility and Young's modulus of the material, it might have been the effective elongation that guarantees a desired result on this bending of wires.

Regarding the influence of corrosion on mechanical properties of bent and straight SS archwires, it is revealed that bent wires became vulnerable to pH and the mechanical properties were altered.

Conclusions

Bending has a significant influence on surface roughness and mechanical properties of rectangular SS archwires. pH plays a synergistic effect on the change of mechanical properties of SS wires along with wire bending.

The clinical implications of this study are as follows: (1) salivary pH tests for patient with fixed orthodontic appliance should be recommended and (2) bending on SS archwires should be done carefully for patients with imbalanced salivary pH (especially for basic pH) due to the synergistic effect.

Competing interests

The authors declare that they have no competing interests.

Authors' contributions

QY and MGH conceived of the study; MGH and YH participated in its design; MGH, QY, JX, and RS helped to carry out the experiments in the laboratory; YH and HX were involved in the data analysis and further literature searching; and MGH, YH, and QY drafted the manuscript. All authors read and approved the final manuscript.

Author details

[1]Orthodontic Department, College of Medicine and Dentistry, James Cook University, Cairns, Australia. [2]School of Dentistry, University Medical Centre Groningen, Groningen, The Netherlands. [3]School and Hospital of Stomatology, Wenzhou Medical University, Wenzhou, China.

References

1. Sankar SG, Shetty V, Karanth H. A comparative study of physical and mechanical properties of the different grades of Australian stainless steel wires. Trends Biomater Artif Organs. 2011;25:67–74.
2. Verstrynge A, Van Humbeeck J, Willems G. *In-vitro* evaluation of the material characteristics of stainless steel and beta-titanium orthodontic wires. Am J Orthod Dentofacial Orthop. 2006;130:460–70.
3. Nucera R, Giudice AL, Matarese G, Artemisia A, Bramanti E, Crupi P, et al. Analysis of the characteristics of slot design affecting resistance to sliding during active archwire configurations. Prog Orthod. 2013;14:35.
4. Walker MP, Ries D, Kula K, Ellis M, Fricke B. Mechanical properties and surface characterization of beta titanium and stainless steel orthodontic wire following topical fluoride treatment. Angle Orthod. 2007;77:342–8.
5. Srivastava K, Chandra PK, Kamat N. Effect of fluoride mouth rinses on various orthodontic archwire alloys tested by modified bending test: An *in vitro* study. Indian J Dent Res. 2012;23:433.
6. Kim H, Johnson JW. Corrosion of stainless steel, nickel-titanium, coated nickel-titanium, and titanium orthodontic wires. Angle Orthod. 1999;69:39–44.
7. Huang HH. Corrosion resistance of stressed NiTi and stainless steel orthodontic wires in acid artificial saliva. J Biomed Mater Res A. 2003;66:829–39.
8. Duffó GS, Farina SB. Corrosion behaviour of a dental alloy in some beverages and drinks. Mater Chem Phys. 2009;115:235–8.
9. Vasudevan DM, Sreekumari S, Vaidyanathan K. Textbook of biochemistry for dental students: JP Medical Ltd. 2011.
10. Bourne M. Food texture and viscosity: concept and measurement: Academic press. 2002.
11. Lombardo L, Ortan YÖ, Gorgun Ö, Panza C, Scuzzo G, Siciliani G. Changes in the oral environment after placement of lingual and labial orthodontic appliances. Prog Orthod. 2013;14:1-8.
12. Saranya R, Rajendran S, Krishnaveni A, Pandiarajan M, Nagalakshmi R. Corrosion resistance of metals and alloys in artificial saliva-an overview. Eur Chem Bull. 2013;2:163–70.
13. Juvvadi SR, Kailasam V, Padmanabhan S, Chitharanjan AB. Physical, mechanical, and flexural properties of 3 orthodontic wires: an *in-vitro* study. Am J Orthod Dentofacial Orthop. 2010;138:623–30.
14. Krishnan V, Kumar KJ. Mechanical properties and surface characteristics of three archwire alloys. Angle Orthod. 2004;74:825–31.
15. Konda P, Kamble R, Kumar A. An evaluation and comparison of surface corrosion of orthodontic archwires using scanning electron microscope: an *in vitro* study. J Indian Orthod Soc. 2013;47:16–20.
16. Daems J, Celis J-P, Willems G. Morphological characterization of as-received and *in vivo* orthodontic stainless steel archwires. Eur J Orthod. 2009;31:260–5.
17. Kao C-T, Huang T-H. Variations in surface characteristics and corrosion behaviour of metal brackets and wires in different electrolyte solutions. Eur J Orthod. 2010;32:555–60.
18. Edie JW, Andreasen GF, Zaytoun MP. Surface corrosion of nitinol and stainless steel under clinical conditions. Angle Orthod. 1981;51:319–24.
19. Raucci G, Elyasi M, Pachêco-Pereira C, Grassia V, d'Apuzzo F, Flores-Mir C, et al. Predictors of long-term stability of maxillary dental arch dimensions in patients treated with a transpalatal arch followed by fixed appliances. Prog Orthod. 2015;16:1-6.
20. Rucker BK, Kusy RP. Elastic properties of alternative versus single-stranded leveling archwires. Am J Orthod Dentofacial Orthop. 2002;122:528–41.
21. Nanda R. Biomechanics and esthetic strategies in clinical orthodontics: Elsevier Health Sciences. 2005.

13

Comparison of the effects of preemptive acetaminophen, ibuprofen, and meloxicam on pain after separator placement: a randomized clinical trial

Hooman Zarif Najafi[1], Morteza Oshagh[2], Parisa Salehi[1], Neda Babanouri[1*] and Sepideh Torkan[3]

Abstract

Background: This study aims to evaluate and compare the effect of pre-procedural administration of acetaminophen, ibuprofen, and meloxicam in reducing pain after separator placement.

Methods: Three hundred twenty-one patients who needed orthodontic treatment and aged above 15 were randomly assigned to one of the three study groups: group A: 650 mg acetaminophen, group B: 400 mg ibuprofen, and group C: 7.5 mg meloxicam. All subjects received a single dose of medication 1 h prior to separator placement. Using visual analog scale, patients recorded their pain perception during rest, fitting posterior teeth together, and chewing at time intervals of immediately, 2, 6, 24, and 48 h after separator placement.

Results: There was no significant difference between acetaminophen, ibuprofen, and meloxicam in post-separator placement pain control when administered 1 h before the procedure. In all the groups, at rest, pain level elevated after separator placement and reached its peak at 24 h and then subsided until 48 h. But during chewing and fitting of the posterior teeth, some of the groups reached a peak in pain at 48 h. No significant difference was found in pain experience between males and females.

Conclusions: Meloxicam can be used as an effective analgesic in orthodontic pain control considering it has less gastric side effects compared to the conventional nonsteroidal anti-inflammatory drugs.

Trial registration: Iranian Registry of Clinical Trials, IRCT2015041821828N1

Keywords: Orthodontic pain; Non-selective NSAIDs; Meloxicam

Background

Pain is an unpleasant sensation caused by some tissue changes. These tissue changes in orthodontic treatment are caused by the compression of periodontal ligament and alteration of blood flow to the tooth, resulting in releasing chemical mediators like prostaglandins [1, 2]. About 95 % of the patients undergoing orthodontic therapy report varying degrees of pain and discomfort during some stages of treatment such as separator or arch wire placement [3, 4]. It has also been reported that pain is the foremost reason for patient aversion and discontinuing treatment [5, 6]. It has been claimed that degree of pain experienced by patient varies based on gender, age, patient anxiety level, and emotional stress [1, 4, 7, 8].

Despite the concerns stated by the orthodontists and patients, no standard of care has still been defined to control pain caused by orthodontic appliances [9, 10]. Several methods have been proposed such as administration of analgesics, introducing vibratory stimulation, chewing on a bite wafer, and most recently, the use of low-level laser therapy [11–22].

Analgesics are the most common treatment modality used to control the pain associated with orthodontic treatment [15]. Several studies evaluated the effect of pre- and postoperative use of various medications including aspirin, acetaminophen, ibuprofen, piroxicam,

* Correspondence: nedababanouri@yahoo.com
[1]Orthodontic Research Center, Orthodontics Department, School of Dentistry, Shiraz University of Medical Sciences, Shiraz, Iran
Full list of author information is available at the end of the article

etc. on the orthodontic-induced pain [11–18, 20, 23]. Acetaminophen is an over-the-counter medication with antipyretic and analgesic effects via central inhibition of the third isoform of cyclooxygenase enzyme (COX_3), which is mostly found in the cerebral cortex and heart [13, 24]. The conventional nonsteroidal anti-inflammatory drugs (NSAIDs) like ibuprofen, piroxicam, aspirin and naproxen sodium block the production of prostaglandins through inhibiting the other isoforms of cyclooxygenase (COX) enzyme [24].These medications are called non-selective COX inhibitors, since they block both COX_1 and COX_2 isoforms [24]. Inhibition of COX_1 is responsible for the adverse effects of NSAIDs such as gastric ulceration and bleeding disorders [25]. Many studies have been conducted to evaluate the effects of this family of NSAIDs on the pain relief during orthodontics treatment [11–18]. Bird et al. reported that there was no difference between the single preemptive use of acetaminophen and ibuprofen in pain control after separator placement whereas Bradley et al. showed that ibuprofen was more effective than acetaminophen [13, 14].

Another class of NSAIDs that has been recently introduced is selective COX_2 inhibitors (coxibs) like celecoxib, valdecoxib, and lumiracoxib [26]. They retain the benefits of anti-inflammatory action with minimum side effects like gastric irritation and platelet functional alteration, and also, they have longer dose interval [25–28]. Young et al. showed that pre- and postoperative use of valdecoxib compared to placebo can effectively decrease pain after archwire placement, while Bruno et al. found no significant difference in post-separator pain between placebo and lumiracoxib [29, 30].

Meloxicam is one of most popular relatively selective COX_2 inhibitors used in the treatment of acute and chronic inflammatory painful disorders like rheumatoid arthritis, dental pain, and postoperative pain [31–33]. It is now clear that meloxicam has a lower gastric effect compared to other NSAIDs [31]. Efficacy of this drug in controlling post-endodontic pain and pain after third molar removal and oral surgery has been investigated previously [27, 32, 33].

Recently, there have been some concerns regarding the increased risk of cardiovascular and renal events associated with administration of selective COX_2 inhibitors such as valdecoxib, rofecoxib, and lumiracoxib [9, 30]. COX_2 inhibitors decrease the production of vascular prostaglandin I_2 (PGI_2) which is a vasodilator and anti-aggregator mediator [34]. In addition, COX_2 inhibitors do not inhibit thromboxane A_2 (TxA_2) production, one of COX_1 products from arachidonic acid in platelets which causes irreversible platelet aggregation, vasoconstriction, and smooth muscle proliferation [34]. However, available data and systematic reviews suggest that meloxicam has more desirable cardiovascular and renal safety profile than other COX_2 inhibitors like celecoxib and rofecoxib [35].

Considering that only few studies have evaluated the effect of selective COX inhibitors on orthodontic pain control and no studies have evaluated the effect of meloxicam as a relatively selective COX_2 inhibitor in orthodontic pain control and given the adverse effects of conventional NSAIDs, the authors of this study designed this double-blinded parallel arm randomized clinical trial study to compare the effect of preemptive administration of meloxicam with acetaminophen and ibuprofen on the experienced pain following orthodontic separator placement.

Methods

The sample size was determined to be 70 in each group based on the mean pain scores recorded in the similar study (acetaminophen (31.6 ± 18.8) and ibuprofen (22.8 ± 17.7)) at $\alpha = 0.05$ and power = 80 % [13]. One hundred seven patients were recruited in this study to account for the potential patient dropouts during the course of the study. Three hundred twenty-one patients who needed fixed orthodontic therapy and were referred to the Orthodontic Clinic of Dental School at Shiraz University of Medical Sciences, Iran, were selected for this prospective double-blind randomized clinical trial investigation. This study was approved by the ethical committee of Shiraz University of Medical Sciences. All participants had the following criteria:

1. Need separator placement to begin orthodontic treatment in the maxillary arch
2. Aged 15 years or older
3. Were informed and signed the written informed consent
4. Not currently using antibiotics, analgesics, anti-inflammatory, anti-coagulative, diuretics, oral anti diabetics, lithium, cyclosporine, and methotrexate
5. No need for antibiotic prophylaxis
6. No chronic systemic disease or clotting disorders
7. Not reporting contraindication for NSAIDs
8. Not pregnant or nursing

The block randomization method was used with block length 9, and number of repetition for each group $m = 3$, to allocate subjects in each group. This method was used separately for each sex group to provide groups with equal numbers of male and female. The patients were divided to three equal groups which were consisted of 78 women and 29 men: group A (650 mg acetaminophen), group B (400 mg ibuprofen) and group C (7.5 mg meloxicam (7.5 mg; BohringerIngelheim Pharms, Germany)). In each group, all tablets were covered by identical gelatin cover, so the investigators, the patients, and the statistician were all blind to the treatment groups. All patients were given only one tablet, 1 h before separator placement (Alastiks S-2separator modules; lot number A2508, 3M UnitekMonorvia, Calif) .The time and the quadrant in which the separators were placed were recorded.

A visual analog scale (VAS) was used to determine the level of pain and discomfort at the following intervals: immediately after separator placement (T_0), 2 h post-treatment (T_1), 6 h post-treatment (T_2), 24 h post-treatment (T_3), and 48 h after separator placement (T_4). Each patient received a booklet consisted of five series of VAS. The VAS format was a 10 cm line from 0 indicating no pain to 10 indicating the worst pain a patient has ever experienced. Patients were instructed to mark the degree of the pain with a short vertical line on the VAS during three oral situations including rest, fitting posterior teeth, and chewing, and return the questionnaire in the next visit (a week later). While fitting the posterior teeth, the patients were instructed to bring the teeth together with a light force and not to eat anything in the process. For the chewing function, the subjects were instructed to chew on a slice of granny smith apple and mark the level of the subsequent pain on the VAS. The patients were asked to not use other analgesics during the period of the study, and in case they did so, they would be excluded from the investigation. Before this study, a pilot study was carried out with 20 patients who needed to have separators placed prior to orthodontic treatment. The patients did not take any medications before the treatment. They were asked to record their pain score according to the instructions, and their functions were evaluated via the questionnaire. This pilot study was just performed to ensure the ease of comprehending the instructions by the participants, and none of the subjects were included in the main study.

Statistical analysis

Statistical analysis was done using the Statistical Package for Social Sciences (Version 15.0, SPSS Inc., Chicago, Illinois, USA). Descriptive analysis was performed for pain scores in three treatment groups for all different time intervals, at rest, fitting the posterior teeth, and chewing. The normal distribution of the data was tested with Kolmogorov Smirnov normality test, before application of parametric tests. Differences in the mean pain score between experimental groups were evaluated by analysis of variance (ANOVA) and Tukey test. Repeated measure ANOVA and paired *t* test was conducted to determine the difference in the pain scores at each time interval. The level of significance for all tests in our study was set at $p < 0.05$.

Results

Eighty patients (25 %) were dropped out of the study, of whom 18 patients used other analgesics during the time of study, 46 patients did not complete the questionnaires correctly, and 16 did not return the questionnaires. The final sample consisted of 60 men (25 %) and 181 women (75 %), of whom 57 women and 19 men were in the acetaminophen group, 55 women and 21 men in the ibuprofen group, and 68 women and 21 men in the meloxicam group (Fig. 1). No statistical difference was found between the three study groups in terms of age; the mean age of the acetaminophen group was 21.7 ± 3.5 and a mean age of 22.1 ± 3.2 and 21.2 ± 3.8 were recorded for the ibuprofen and the meloxicam groups, respectively. Table 1 outlines the descriptive information and ANOVA results for the three groups.

Although, there was no statistically significant difference in the pain perception scores between the three treatment groups (Table 1), patients consistently experienced more pain on T_0 and T_1 in the meloxicam group and on T_3 and T_4 in the ibuprofen group. Additionally, when considering the peak pain scores, the highest values were in the ibuprofen group during the rest, and two masticatory functions and the lowest ones were seen in the meloxicam group during rest and fitting posterior teeth. In the chewing function, the difference between the mean pain score of the three groups tended to be significant 48 h after separator placement ($P = 0.095$). Tukey test showed the difference was between the ibuprofen and the acetaminophen groups ($P = 0.091$). Although, in all study groups and at all time intervals, subjects experienced more pain when chewing compared to at rest and while fitting posterior teeth, but the difference was not significant. Our results also showed that gender had no significant effect on pain perception scores in any treatment groups and for any time intervals.

Significant differences were found in pain perception scores at different times ($P = 0.001$), although the trend was almost similar in all groups and for all masticatory functions (Figs. 2, 3, and 4). The changes in pain perception with the time are presented individually for each medication.

1. *Acetaminophen.* Generally, pain increased immediately following separator placement and reached a peak at 24 h and then subsided until 48 h. There was no significant change in the level of pain perceived at rest over time. The results of the paired *t* test showed significant difference between T0 and T1 ($P = 0.025$), T1 and T2 ($P = 0.005$), and T2 and T3 ($P = 0.001$) while fitting posterior teeth and between T0 and T1 ($P = 0.031$), T1 and T2 ($P = 0.003$), T2 and T3 ($P = 0.001$) and T3 and T4 ($P = 0.011$) in chewing function.
2. *Ibuprofen.* Subjects experienced significant increase in the level of pain from 2 h after separator placement until 24 h at rest (T_1–T_2 ($P = 0.038$),

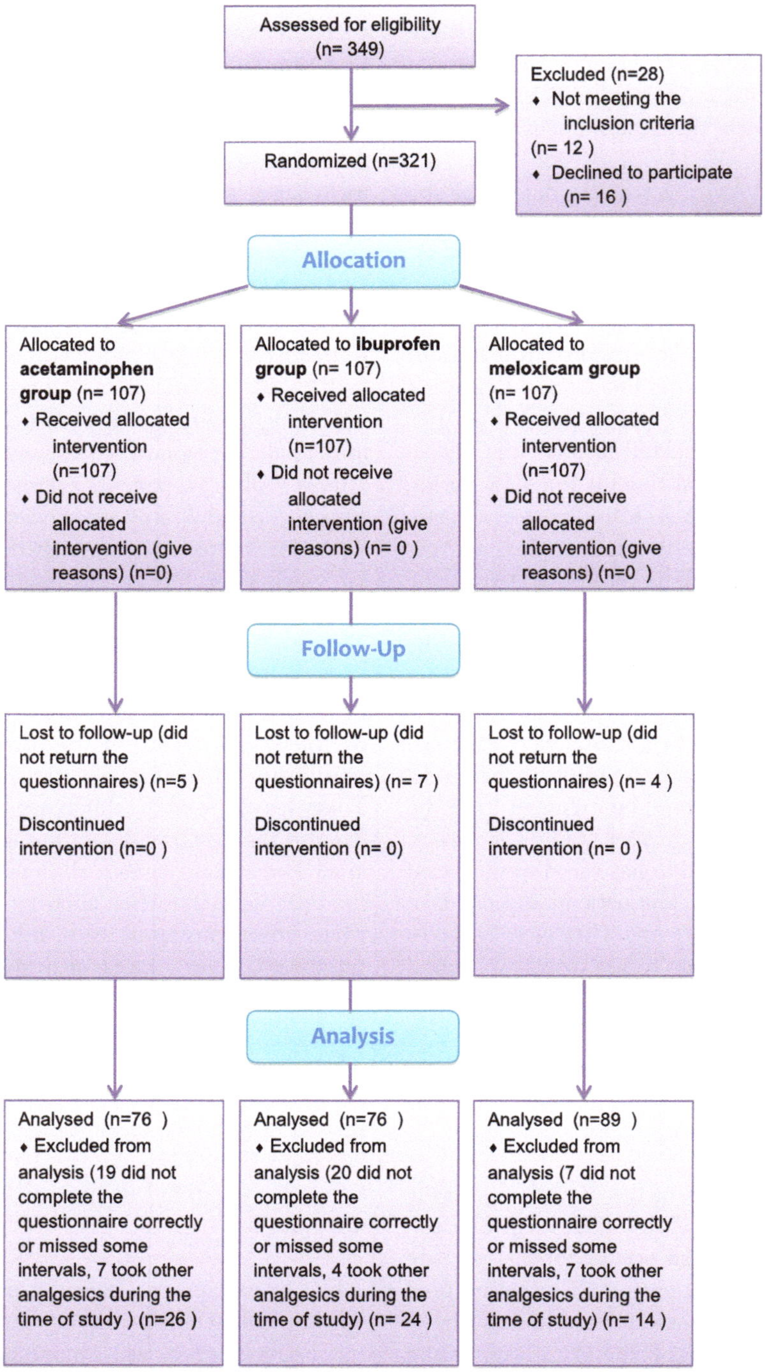

Fig. 1 CONSORT flow diagram

T_2–T_3 ($P = 0.001$)). During the two other functions, patients experienced increased level of pain until its peak at 48 h. The paired *t* test showed significant increase between T_2–T_3 ($P = 0.001$) and T_3–T_4 ($P = 0.001$).

3. *Meloxicam.* The mean pain score increased immediately after separator placement and reached the peak at 24 h at rest. There was a significant increased only between T_1 and T_2 ($P = 0.001$); however, the difference between T_2 and T_3 ($P = 0.061$) tended to be significant during this function. During the fitting of posterior teeth, the mean pain score increased immediately after separator placement until the peak at 24 h (T_0–T_1 ($P = 0.011$), T_1–T_2 ($P = 0.001$), T_2–T_3 ($P = 0.002$)). In the chewing function, pain increased immediately after

Table 1 Descriptive information and ANOVA results of three treatment groups

Function	Group	T0	T1	T2	T3	T4
Rest	Acetaminophen	0.58 ± 0.97	0.78 ± 1.26	1.08 ± 1.50	1.48 ± 1.91	1.20 ± 2.01
	Ibuprofen	0.54 ± 1.05	0.69 ± 1.30	0.95 ± 1.66	1.78 ± 2.43	1.71 ± 2.24
	Meloxicam	0.66 ± 0.93	0.80 ± 1.16	1.13 ± 1.58	1.42 ± 1.98	1.33 ± 1.84
	P value[a]	0.739	0.844	0.758	0.532	0.276
Fitting posterior teeth	Acetaminophen	0.84 ± 1.24	1.13 ± 1.26	1.65 ± 1.69	2.65 ± 2.68	2.10 ± 2.68
	Ibuprofen	0.69 ± 1.10	1.06 ± 1.84	1.48 ± 2.04	2.89 ± 3.00	3.02 ± 2.86
	Meloxicam	0.99 ± 1.28	1.27 ± 1.52	1.73 ± 2.06	2.44 ± 2.48	2.35 ± 2.54
	P value[a]	0.281	0.675	0.694	0.566	0.095
Chewing	Acetaminophen	1.01 ± 1.46	1.36 ± 1.56	1.96 ± 1.84	3.08 ± 2.97	2.79 ± 3.17
	Ibuprofen	0.98 ± 1.52	1.37 ± 2.15	1.89 ± 2.42	3.63 ± 3.24	3.75 ± 3.29
	Meloxicam	1.22 ± 1.65	1.50 ± 1.86	2.01 ± 2.14	3.05 ± 2.81	3.16 ± 3.10
	P value[a]	0.560	0.871	0.939	0.397	0.177

T0 (immediately after separator placement), T1 (2 h), T2 (6 h), T3 (24 h), T4 (48 h)
[a]ANOVA results

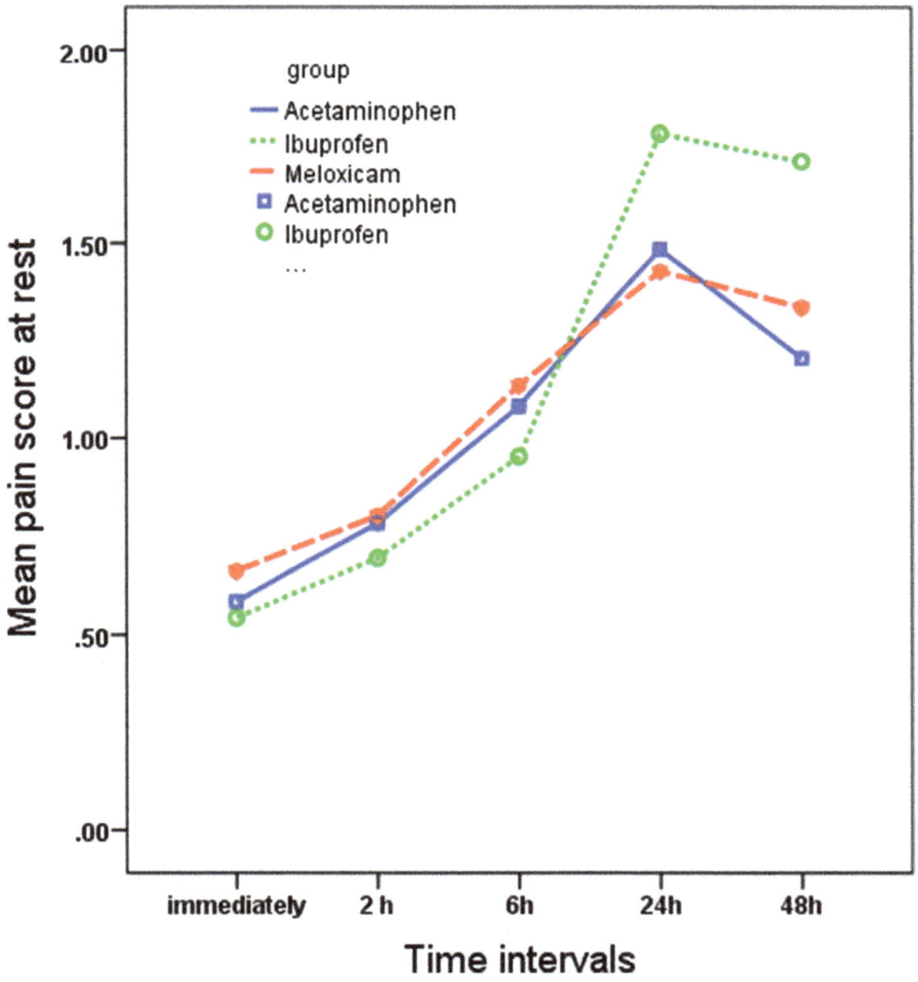

Fig. 2 Comparison of the mean pain scores on VAS among the three study groups over the time in the rest position

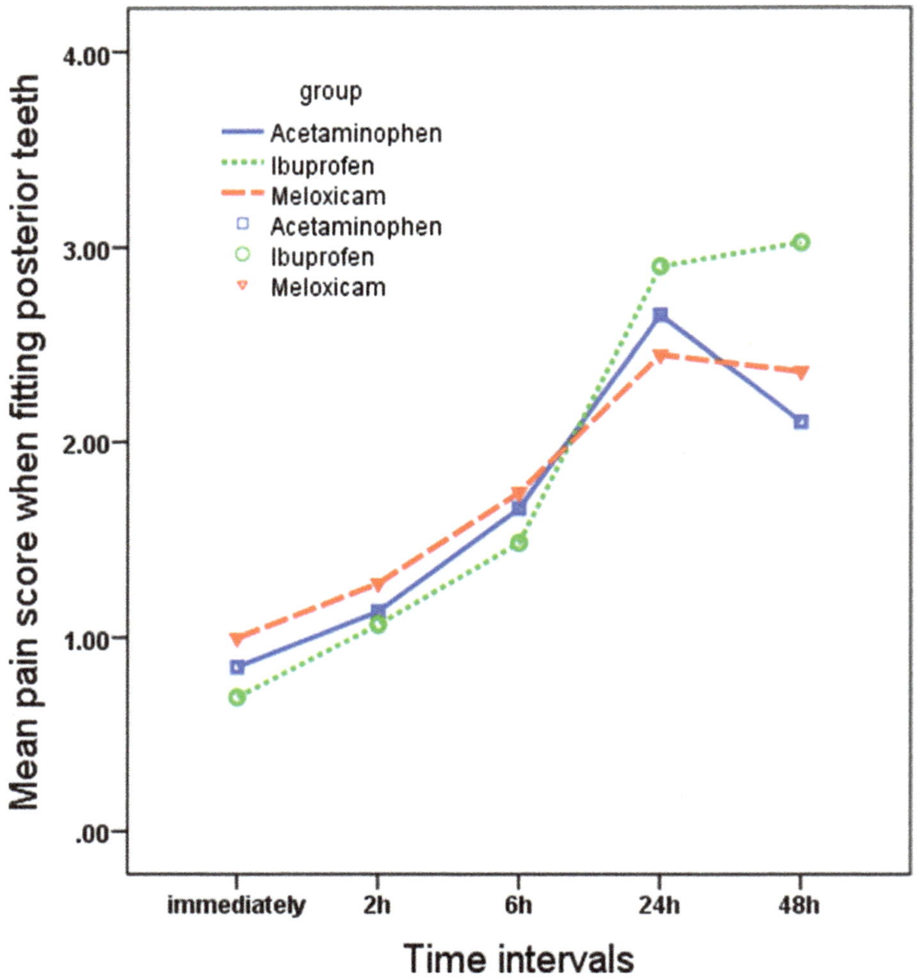

Fig. 3 Comparison of the mean pain scores on VAS among the three study groups over the time when fitting posterior teeth

separator was placed until 48 h. Significant differences were found between $T_0–T_1$ ($P = 0.024$), $T_1–T_2$ ($P = 0.001$), and $T_2–T_3$ ($P = 0.002$)].

Discussion

In this study, the effect of preemptive administration of acetaminophen, ibuprofen, and meloxicam in controlling post-separator pain was evaluated and compared using visual analog scale (VAS). VAS is generally accepted as a reliable and valid instrument for measuring acute and chronic pain, and is more sensitive for measuring positive responses to treatment compared to verbal descriptors [14, 36]. Our results indicated that there was no significant difference among three analgesics when administered 1 h prior to separator placement. Generally, pain increased immediately after separators were placed and in most cases reached a peak at 24 h. This result is in accordance to what has been reported in most of the previous studies [9, 11, 12, 21].However, slight increase in pain was observed after 24 h in meloxicam group in chewing function and in ibuprofen group when fitting posterior teeth. These results are comparable to those of Law et al. and Farzanegan et al. for 400 mg ibuprofen [12, 21]. Law et al. showed no alleviation in pain after 24 h "when fitting front teeth together," and Farzanegan reported no reduction in pain levels after 24 h "when chewing" [12, 21]. It may be attributed to the blood level of medication not reaching its optimum to reduce pain efficiently in this interval.

Similar to other studies evaluating orthodontic pain level, the greatest reported pain occurred on chewing rather than at fitting posterior teeth or at rest [9, 11, 12, 21, 29]. It is not surprising because the orthodontic pain is the result of compression, inflammation, and edema in the periodontal ligament, and there is greater compression during function in the periodontal ligament (PDL) [21, 29].

Our results showed no difference between acetaminophen and ibuprofen when administered 1 h before the procedure. These findings are similar to those of Bird et al. that used single pretreatment dose of ibuprofen

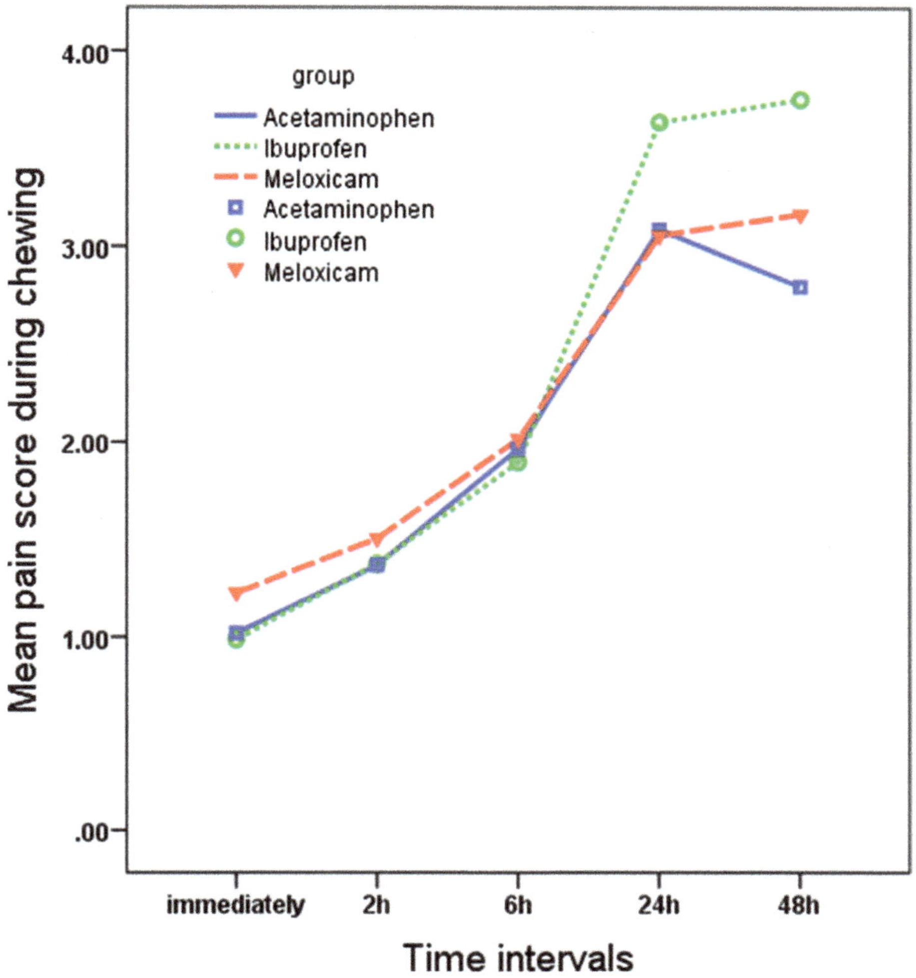

Fig. 4 Comparison of the mean pain scores on VAS among the three study groups over the time in chewing function

(400 mg) and acetaminophen (650 mg) 1 h prior to separator placement [14]. However, Patel et al. and Bradley et al. reported that ibuprofen was more effective than acetaminophen in post-separator pain control [13, 17]. It may be attributed to the administration of the follow-up doses of medication in the two latter studies. Patel et al. administered 400 mg ibuprofen or 650 mg acetaminophen 1 h before and 3 and 7 h after separator placement [17]. Bradley et al. used 400 mg ibuprofen or 1 g acetaminophen 1 h before and 6 h post-treatment [13].

Bird et al. observed a decrease in pain 2 to 3 h after separators were placed in ibuprofen (400 mg) and acetaminophen (650 mg) group when used 1 h prior to the treatment [14]. Although this trend was not found in our study, but during all the masticatory functions in the ibuprofen group and at rest in the meloxicam group, there was no significant increase in the mean pain scores until 2 h. A possible explanation could be that Bird's study was performed on a different age range (9 to 19 years) compared to our study (≥15 years) and thus might have required lower doses of medication to reach its optimum efficacy.

Our results showed no significant difference between preoperative administration of meloxicam and the two other medications in post-separator placement pain control. To the best of our knowledge, no other studies have assessed the effectiveness of meloxicam in orthodontic pain reduction, so there is no previous report for comparison. Young et al. conducted a study on valdecoxib (a selective COX_2 inhibitor) and showed that preemptive administration of the medication followed by five postoperative doses could effectively control post archwire placement pain [29]. It should be noted that valdecoxib has been removed from US and European markets because of the increased risk of cardiovascular events and skin reactions [29]. Bruno et al. showed that a single preoperative dose of lumiracoxib did not significantly reduced post-separator pain [30]. Nekoofar et al. proposed that there was no significant difference between meloxicam (15 mg), piroxicam (20 mg), and placebo in reducing postoperative endodontic pain when administered after treatment [27]. Aoki et al. reported that premedication with 10 mg meloxicam could reduce postsurgical pain in patients after lower third molar extraction [33]. Calvo et al. reported that pain levels after lower third molar extraction not requiring osteotomy can be successfully controlled by a single dose regimen of 7.5 mg meloxicam once daily [32].

This is clearly shown that pain during orthodontic treatment is related to inflammatory responses in the PDL [1].Orthodontic forces produce ischemia and inflammation in compressed areas that lead to the release of high levels of mediators such as prostaglandin in the PDL [1, 2]. COX_2 is the main isoenzyme in the production of pro-inflammatory prostaglandin and also plays an important role in centrally generated hypersensitivity process [28, 33].

Meloxicam is a relatively COX_2 inhibitor with more inhibitory effects on COX_2 than COX_1. Via this inhibitory effect on COX_2, it could be effective in orthodontic pain control. In addition, as it was already mentioned, COX_1 inhibition is responsible for the adverse gastric effects of non-selective NSAIDs [25]. It has been shown that meloxicam doses ≤15 mg decreased the incidence of gastrointestinal side effects such as perforation, ulceration, and bleeding than non-selective NSAIDs [37]. As mentioned before, there has been an increased concern regarding the risk of cardiovascular thrombotic event associated with the administration of selective NSAIDs [9, 30]. However, it seems that meloxicam is relatively safer compared to other medications of this class of NSAIDs; specifically in lower doses such as what was used in the current study (a single 7.5 mg), the risk of cardiovascular events may be very low [33, 35].

Prostaglandins play an important role in stress-related bone remodeling [38], and the potential effects of NSAIDs on the rate of orthodontic tooth movement have been considered. Acetaminophen, an NSAID from para-aminophenol family, differs from the majority of selective and non-selective NSAIDs; it does not inhibit or slightly inhibits the formation of prostaglandins and thus does not affect orthodontic tooth movement [39, 40]. It has been shown that meloxicam does not affect orthodontic tooth movement after 2 weeks of administration via drinking water in Wistar rats and seems to be safer than other selective NSAIDs [39]. There is no clear evidence on long-term effects of meloxicam on the rate of orthodontic tooth movement, and it could be an area of interest for future studies. In the absence of comprehensive study, it needs to be prescribed with caution.

In contrast to the generally accepted concept that females have greater perception of pain and lower pain threshold than males, we found no significant difference in pain experience between males and females [2, 4]. This finding is similar to several other studies that have investigated orthodontic pain [16–18, 41].

At the end, it should be noted that the pain is a subjective sensation which can be influenced significantly by factors such as cultural background, previous traumatic experience, sex, age, and psychological factors [1, 4, 7, 8, 17, 42]. We expected that the large sample volume used in the present study could offset the effects of these variables on our results.

In the present study, we compared the effect of a single preemptive dose of meloxicam with ibuprofen and acetaminophen in the control of the separator orthodontic pain. It can be suggested that a comparison between the pre- and post-administration of meloxicam and conventional analgesics be carried out in future studies, but the effect of long-term use of this drug on the rate of orthodontic tooth movement should be noted.

Conclusions

Our findings suggest preoperative administration of meloxicam (7.5 mg) was as effective as acetaminophen (650 mg) and ibuprofen (400 mg) to control the post-separator pain. However, acetaminophen can be considered as the treatment of choice due to the fact that it does not cause gastrointestinal (GI) ulcers and does not affect the rate of tooth movement. Considering the low GI toxicity, meloxicam can be recommended as a good alternative for those patients who cannot take other NSAIDs or acetaminophen.

Competing interests

The authors declare that they have no competing interests.

Authors' contributions

HZN designed and conducted the study and participated in the drafting the manuscript. MO participated in the conducting the study. PS participated in the conducting the study. NB gathered and analyzed the data and drafted the manuscript. ST participated in the drafting the manuscript and English editing. All authors read and approved the final version of the manuscript.

Acknowledgements

The authors thank the Vice-Chancellery of Shiraz University of Medical Science for supporting this research (2186). The authors also thank Dr. Salehi from Dental Research Development Center, for the statistical analysis.

Funding

This work was supported by the Vice-Chancellery of Shiraz University of Medical Science (2168).

Author details

[1]Orthodontic Research Center, Orthodontics Department, School of Dentistry, Shiraz University of Medical Sciences, Shiraz, Iran. [2]Private Practice, Tehran, Iran. [3]Orthodontics Department, University of Washington, Seattle, WA, USA.

References

1. Krishnan V. Orthodontic pain: from cause to management—a review. Eur J Orthod. 2007;29:170–79.
2. Furstman L, Bernik S. Clinical considerations of the periodontium. Am J Orthod. 1972;61:138–55.

3. Lew KK. Attitudes and perceptions of adults towards orthodontic treatment in an Asian community. Community Dent Oral Epidemiol. 1993;21:31–5.
4. Scheuer PA, Firestone AR, Burgin WB. Perception of pain as a result of orthodontic treatment with fixed appliances. Eur J Orthod. 1996;18:349–57.
5. Oliver RG, Knapman YM. Attitudes to orthodontic treatment. Br J Orthod. 1985;12:179–88.
6. Fujiyama K, Honjo T, Suzuki M, Matsuoka S, Deguchi T. Analysis of pain level in cases treated with Invisalign aligner: comparison with fixed edgewise appliance therapy. Prog Orthod. 2014;15:64.
7. Ngan P, Kess B, Wilson S. Perception of discomfort by patients undergoing orthodontic treatment. Am J Orthod Dentofacial Orthop. 1989;96:47–53.
8. Brown DF, Moerenhout RG. The pain experience and psychological adjustment to orthodontic treatment of preadolescents, adolescents, and adults. Am J Orthod Dentofacial Orthop. 1991;100:394–56.
9. Bernhardt MK, Southard KA, Batterson KD, Logan HL, Baker KA, Jakobsen JR. The effect of preemptive and/or postoperative ibuprofen therapy for orthodontic pain. Am J Orthod Dentofacial Orthop. 2001;120:20–7.
10. Berguis M, Berggren U, Kiliaridis S. Experience of pain during an orthodontic procedure. Eur J Oral Sci. 2002;110:92–8.
11. Ngan P, Wilson S, Shanfeld J, Amini H. The effect of ibuprofen on the level of discomfort in patient undergoing orthodontic treatment. Am J Orthod Dentofacial Orthop. 1994;106:88–95.
12. Steen Law SL, Southard KA, Law AS, Logan HL, Jakobsen JR. An evaluation of preoperative ibuprofen for treatment of pain associated with orthodontic separator placement. Am J Orthod Dentofacial Orthop. 2000;118:629–35.
13. Bradley R, Ellis P, Thomas P, Bellis H, Ireland A, Sandy J. A randomized clinical trial comparing the efficacy of ibuprofen and paracetamol in the control of orthodontic pain. Am J Orthod Deantofacial Orthop. 2007;132:511–7.
14. Bird S, Williams K, Kula K. Preoperative acetaminophen vs ibuprofen for control of pain after orthodontic separator placement. Am J Ortho Dentofacial Orthop. 2007;132:504–10.
15. Xiaoting L, Tin T, Yangxi C. Intervention for pain during fixed orthodontic appliance therapy—a systematic review. Angle Orthod. 2010;80:925–32.
16. Kohli SS, Kohli VS. Effectiveness of piroxicam and ibuprofen premedication on orthodontic patients' pain experiences—a randomized control trial. Angle Orthod. 2011;81:1097–102.
17. Patel S, McGorray SP, Yezierski R, Fillingim R, Logan H, Wheeler T. Effects of analgesics on orthodontic pain. Am J Orthod Dentofacial Orthop. 2011;139:e53–8.
18. Minor V, Marris CK, McGorray SP, Yezierski R, Fillingim R, Logan H, et al. Effects of preoperative ibuprofen after separator placement. Am J Orthod Dentofacial Orthop. 2009;136:510–7.
19. Marie SS, Powers M, Sheridan JJ. Vibratory stimulation as a method of reducing pain after orthodontic appliance adjustment. J Clin Orthod. 2003;37:205–8.
20. Proffit WR, Fields HW. Biologic basis of orthodontic therapy. In: Proffit WR, Fields HW, editors. Contemporary orthodontics. 3rd ed. St Louis: Mosby; 2000.
21. Farzanegan F, Zebarjad SM, Alizadeh S, Ahrari F. Pain reduction after initial archwire placement in orthodontic patients. Am J Orthod Dentofacial Orthop. 2012;141:169–73.
22. Ren C, McGrath C, Yang Y. The effectiveness of low-level diode laser therapy on orthodontic pain management: a systematic review and meta-analysis. Lasers Med Sci 2015; in press.
23. Sudhakar V, Vindohini TS, Moham AM, Srinivasan B, Rajkumar BK. The efficacy of different pre- and post-operative analgesics in the management of pain after orthodontic separator placement: a randomized clinical trial. J Pharm Bioallied Sci. 2014;6 Suppl S1:80–4.
24. Dionne RA, Berthold CW. Therapeutic uses of non-steroidal anti-inflammatory drugs in dentistry. Crit Rev Oral Biol Med. 2001;12:315–30.
25. Jackson LM, Hawkey CJ. COX-2 selective nonsteroidal anti-inflammatory drugs, do they really offer any advantages? Drugs. 2000;59:1207–16.
26. Fitz Gerald GA, Patrono C. Thecoxibs, selective inhibitors of cyclo-oxygenase-2. N Engl J Med. 2001;345:433–42.
27. Nekoofar MH, Sadeghipanah M, Dehpuor AR. Evaluation of meloxicam (a Cox-2 inhibitor) for management of postoperative endodontic pain: a double-blind placebo-controlled study. J Endod. 2003;29:634–37.
28. Lee Y, Rodriguez C, Dionne RA. The role of COX-2 in acute pain and the use of selective COX-2 inhibitors for acute pain relief. Curr Pharm Des. 2005;11:1737–55.
29. Young AN, Taylor RW, Taylor SE, Linnebur SA, Buschang PH. Evaluation of preemptive valdecoxibthrapy on initial archwire placement discomfort in adults. Angle Orthod. 2006;76:251–59.
30. Bruno MB, Bruno MA, Krymchantowski AV, da Motta AF, Mucha JN. A double-blind, randomized clinical trial assessing the effects of a single dose of preemptive anti-inflammatory treatment in orthodontic pain. Prog Orthod. 2011;12:2–7.
31. Euller-Ziegler L, Velicitat P, Bluhmki E, Türcy D, Scheuerer S, Combe B. Meloxicam: a review of its pharmacokinetics; efficacy and tolerability following intramascular administration. Inflamm Res. 2001;50:S5–9.
32. Calvo AM, Sakai VT, Giglio FPM, Modensa KCS, Colombini BL, Benetello V, et al. Analgesic and anti-inflammatory dose-response relationship of 7.5 and 15 mg meloxicam after lower third molar removal: a double blind, randomized, crossover study. Int J Oral MaxillofacSurg. 2007;36:26–31.
33. Aoki A, Yamaguchi H, Naito H, Shiiki K, Izawa K, Ota Y, et al. Premedication with cyclooxygenase-2 inhibitor meloxicam reduced postoperative pain in patients after oral surgery. Int J Oral Maxillofac Surg. 2006;35:613–17.
34. Weir MR, Sperling RS, Reicin A, Gertz BJ. Selective COX-2 inhibition and cardiovascular effects: a review of the rofecoxib development. Am Heart J. 2003;146:591–604.
35. Asghar W, Jamali F. The effect of COX-2 selective meloxicam on myocardial, vascular and renal risks: a systemic review. Inflammopharmacology. 2015;23:1–16.
36. Bijur PE, Silver W, Gallagher EJ. Reliability of the visual analog scale for measurement of acute pain. Acad Emerg Med. 2001;8:1153–7.
37. Fleischmann R, Iqbal I, Slobodin G. Meloxicam. Expert Opin Pharmacother. 2002;3:1–12.
38. Nimeri G, Kau CH H, Abou-Kheir NS, Corona R. Acceleration of tooth movement during orthodontic treatment—a frontier in orthodontics. Prog Orthod. 2013;14:42.
39. Gonzales C, Hotokezaka H, Matsuo KI, Shibazaki T, Yozgatian JH, Darendeliler MA, et al. Effect of steroidal and nonsteroidal drugs on tooth movement and root resorption in the rat molar. Angle Orthod. 2009;79:715–26.
40. Shetty N, Patil AK, Ganeshkar SV, Hegde S. Comparison of the effects of ibuprofen and acetaminophen on PGE_2 levels in the GCF during orthodontic tooth movement: a human study. Prog Orthod. 2013;14:6.
41. Abdelrahman RS, Al-Nimiri KS, Al Maaitah EF. Pain experience during initial alignment with three types of nickel-titanium archwires: a prospective clinical trial. Angle Orthod 2015; in press.
42. Sergl HG, Klages U, Zentner A. Pain and discomfort during orthodontic treatment: causative factors and effects on compliance. Am J Orthod Dentofacial Orthop. 1998;114:684–91.

14

Effect of single-dose low-level helium-neon laser irradiation on orthodontic pain: a split-mouth single-blind placebo-controlled randomized clinical trial

Farhad Sobouti[1], Maziar Khatami[2], Nasim Chiniforush[3], Vahid Rakhshan[4,5] and Mahsa Shariati[6*]

Abstract

Background: Pain is the most common complication of orthodontic treatment. Low-level laser therapy (LLLT) has been suggested as a new analgesic treatment free of the adverse effects of analgesic medications. However, it is not studied thoroughly, and the available studies are quite controversial. Moreover, helium neon (He-Ne) laser has not been assessed before.

Methods: This split-mouth placebo-controlled randomized clinical trial was performed on 16 male and 14 female orthodontic patients requiring bilateral upper canine retraction. The study was performed at a private clinic in Sari, Iran, in 2014. It was single blind: patients, orthodontist, and personnel were blinded of the allocations, but the laser operator (periodontist) was not blinded. Once canine retractor was activated, a randomly selected maxillary quarter received a single dose of He-Ne laser irradiation (632.8 nm, 10 mw, 6 j/cm^2 density). The other quarter served as the placebo side, treated by the same device but powered off. In the first, second, fourth, and seventh days, blinded patients rated their pain sensed on each side at home using visual analog scale (VAS) questionnaires. There was no harm identified during or after the study. Pain changes were analyzed using two- and one-way repeated-measures ANOVA, Bonferroni, and *t*-test ($\alpha = 0.01$, $\beta > 0.99$). This trial was not registered. It was self-funded by the authors.

Results: Sixteen males and 11 females remained in the study (aged 12–21). Average pain scores sensed in all 4 intervals on control and laser sides were 4.06 ± 2.85 and 2.35 ± 1.77, respectively (*t*-test $P < 0.0001$). One-way ANOVA showed significant pain declines over time, in each group ($P < 0.0001$). Two-way ANOVA showed significant effects for LLLT ($P < 0.0001$) and time ($P = <0.0001$).

Conclusions: Single-dose He-Ne laser therapy might reduce orthodontic pain caused by retracting maxillary canines.

Keywords: Low-level laser therapy (LLLT); Helium-neon (He-Ne) laser; Orthodontic pain; Canine retraction; Placebo; Visual analog scale (VAS); Laser irradiation

* Correspondence: mahsa.shariati@gmail.com
[6]Craniomaxillofacial Surgery Research Center, Shariati Hospital, Tehran University of Medical Sciences, Postal Code: 14174North Kargar Ave., 16 Azar ST, Tehran, Iran
Full list of author information is available at the end of the article

Background

The most common sequela of orthodontic treatment and one of its most significant problems is pain and discomfort [1–8]. Its intensity might be comparable with the highest ranked general pains such as wasp sting or spraining one's ankle [1]. About 90 % of orthodontic patients find that orthodontic treatment is painful [9, 10]. Therefore, it is a critical deterrent to orthodontic treatment and a common cause of treatment discontinuation [1, 5–9, 11–14]. Despite its substantial clinical value, orthodontic pain is broadly neglected and underestimated [1, 7, 9, 14].

Various methods have been proposed to relieve orthodontic pain. According to recent reviews, the most effective approach is the administration of non-steroidal anti-inflammatory drugs (NSAID) [7, 11, 15]. However, besides their adverse effects, these analgesics might disrupt the osteoclastic mechanisms responsible for tooth movement by inhibiting prostaglandins and thus reduce the efficacy of orthodontic treatment [7, 11, 15]. Moreover, over-the-counter NSAID doses might inhibit tooth movement while might not necessarily relieve pain [9, 16]. Other methods for pain control include vibratory stimulation, transcutaneous electrical nerve stimulation, and chewing gum or plastic wafers [7, 11, 15]. However, the clinical application of such alternatives has been limited due to scant evidence, unclear influence, and poor tolerance [15]. Moreover, masticating firm objects might cause pain and discomfort [16].

Owing to unique advantages in bio-stimulation, pain relief, therapeutic effects, and lack of adverse effects, low-level laser therapy (LLLT) has attracted increasing attention in recent years [7, 11, 15]. This method might be relatively safer than some traditional approaches [11]. The efficacy of LLLT in reducing orthodontic pain has been studied recently [17–23]. Three systematic reviews/meta-analyses have been published in 2013 [24], 2014 [25], and 2015 [15], summarizing the emerging literature. Each of them independently concluded that the evidence is still lacking and further randomized clinical trials are necessary. This was mainly because of the rather small number of studies, controversial results, and methodological issues in almost all of them [15].

An issue with the methods was that most studies evaluated pain invoked by local separator placement [15], which cannot simulate common orthodontic pain caused by real tooth movements. A few studies have induced a generalized orthodontic pain by activating archwires [18, 26]; nevertheless, this method disallows effective split-mouth designs with proper contrasts between the left/right sides of the mouth.

Evaluating subjective phenomena like pain is a challenge, since it varies considerably between patients and even between different times in a single patient [15]. The best approach for dealing with such situations is conducting a split-mouth design which eliminates both interindividual and intra-individual confounders and thus allows deriving stronger conclusions based on smaller samples [15]. A way to assess localized pain (which is more reliable) in a split-mouth setup is to evaluate the pain caused by canine retraction. However, due to the design difficulties, only three studies have evaluated the pain of canine retraction [27–29], on 12 [29], 20 [27], and 30 patients [28].

Furthermore, all previous studies have evaluated aluminum-gallium lasers. There is no study on helium-neon (He-Ne) lasers. Therefore, we aimed to conduct this split-mouth clinical trial on the analgesic effect of a single-dose He-Ne laser irradiation on pain caused by canine retraction. The null hypotheses were the absence of any differences between the pains felt at laser or placebo sides as well as the absence of any changes in pain levels over time.

Methods

This single-blind split-mouth placebo-controlled randomized clinical trial was performed (in 2014, Sari, Iran) on 60 bilateral maxillary canines retracted in 30 orthodontic patients (16 males, 14 females).

Ethical considerations and potential harms

The ethics were approved by the university's research committee, in accordance with the Helsinki declaration. This trial was not registered. Subjects or their parents were thoroughly briefed written and orally. Subjects could leave the study at their wish in any stage. They signed written consent forms.

The patients and the operator wore protective goggles. No harms were identified during the study, except for those being a routine part of the process of canine retraction (pain and discomfort).

Screening for potential subjects

The patients were selected from attendees to a private orthodontic clinic in Sari, during 2013. The subjects were sequentially acquired until reaching the predetermined sample size.

Eligibility criteria and sample

The inclusion criteria comprised the subjects' willingness to participate, the indication for bilateral canine retraction (through the extraction of maxillary first premolars), the absence of any systemic diseases or mental disorders (e.g., anxiety disorders etc.), any history of medication intake as of 4 days before the treatment, any local or systemic condition affecting or inducing pain, as well as no history of previous orthodontic treatment of any kind. Patients were excluded if they did not return the completed questionnaires, used any analgesics during the trial period, were not available at the scheduled phone call, and if the treatment was interrupted [23, 30–32].

Randomization

In this split-mouth design, each patient had a treatment side (real laser therapy) and a placebo side (simulated laser therapy) simultaneously. These sides were randomly pre-assigned in each patient, based on a random number table, by a periodontist who was the only person knowing the allocations (and did all the laser irradiations).

Blinding

The patients, orthodontist, and personnel were blinded of the allocations. The results were coded. During the irradiation, personnel would leave the room, so only the periodontist would know the allocations (hence, single blind). Patients were not told of the experimental side. The placebo was the simulation of irradiation with the same duration but with the device turned off. Therefore, patients could not distinguish the placebo/experimental sides. Since the data were coded, the statistician did not know the grouping as well.

Uniform treatment protocols

Orthodontic treatment plan included extraction of upper premolars for crowding correction or treatment of maxillary dental protrusion. Patients were treated using metal pre-adjusted brackets of slot 0.022 in. (MBT 3 M, Unitek, Monrovia, CA). After banding and bracket bonding, the stages of aligning and leveling were started. According to common treatment sequence, this treatment stage was done by nickel titanium archwires (Ormco, CA, USA) with diameters of 0.014, 0.016, and 0.018 in.

After finishing the aligning and leveling stages, canine retraction began using 0.018-in-stainless steel wires containing offset for canines, molar toe in and tip back in the mesial side of first molars. For more anchorage preservation, second molars were banded and engaged in wires in both sides. A closed power chain (3 M Unitek, USA) was used to apply forces of 150–175 g. Both sides were treated in the same session and immediately after each other. The side to begin the canine retraction with (left or right) was selected randomly as stated above. This randomization was absolutely independent of the randomization of the laser treatment side (left/right) and its order (being performed first or second). The force was standardized between both sides and among all patients, using a force gauge. All the canine retraction (and laser irradiation) procedures were performed at evening sessions (between 17 and 20 o'clock).

Laser irradiation

All the experiments were performed in a single location and in the evening. In the experimental side, laser irradiation was conducted as follows: A single dose of laser emission was applied immediately after the initiation of force exertion. The used laser was He-Ne of red color (632.8 nm) emitted at a 10-mW power and an energy density of 6 J/cm^2. The tip diameter was 5 mm. From the tooth CEJ to the end of the root apex, irradiation was separately done from the buccal and palatal. During the irradiation, the tip was directed perpendicular to the long axis of the tooth. Since the thickness of alveolar bone is greater over the apical part of the root, the duration of irradiation was decided to be as twice longer in the apical one half of the root, compared to its coronal half. Therefore, radical apical and coronal halves were irradiated for 40 and 80 s, respectively (on each of buccal or lingual sides). The phototherapy of each root section (buccal/lingual in combination with coronal/apical) was performed by a slow up-and-down movement of the device tip in a gentle touch with soft tissue, within the predetermined duration. The amount of laser irradiated at each point was standardized by the constant speed of the device tip being moved on the desired root section/side.

In the placebo side, the phototherapy was simulated [pretended] in terms of timing and every procedural detail with the same equipment, however, turned off. The patient was unaware of the placebo and experimental sides as well as the order of performing laser/placebo treatments.

Pain measurement

In each patient, the pain was assessed on each side of the mouth using a visual analog scale (VAS). The patients were thoroughly instructed regarding filling VAS for left and right sides. A written instruction was as well given to them. The evaluations were done at home, on the first, second, fourth, and seventh days after imposing the force. Patients were called on their landline and/or mobile phones after 24, 48, 96, and 168 h after the treatment. On the phone, they were reminded of filling their VAS questionnaires.

The VAS was converted to 10 distances of equal length, between the 11 scores of 0–10. The score zero meant the absence of any pain/discomfort. The score 10 meant any pain considered intolerable by the patient OR causing the patient to seek emergency visits OR waking them from sleep [30].

Statistical analysis

Descriptive statistics for pain levels, as the outcome, were calculated. The sample size was predetermined based on a pilot study of 17 patients, to obtain powers

Table 1 Descriptive statistics for pain values

Day	Treatment	N	Mean	SD	CV	Min	Q1	Med	Q3	Max	95 % CI	
1	Placebo	27	6.63	1.94	29.3	2.0	5.0	7.0	8.0	10.0	5.86	7.40
	Laser	27	4.59	1.39	30.4	2.0	4.0	5.0	5.0	7.0	4.04	5.14
2	Placebo	27	5.22	0.93	17.9	3.0	5.0	5.0	6.0	7.0	4.85	5.59
	Laser	27	3.74	1.26	33.6	1.0	3.0	4.0	5.0	6.0	3.24	4.24
4	Placebo	27	2.81	0.96	34.2	1.0	2.0	3.0	4.0	5.0	2.43	3.20
	Laser	27	1.89	0.89	47.2	0.0	2.0	2.0	2.0	3.0	1.54	2.24
7	Placebo	27	1.59	0.93	58.4	0.0	1.0	2.0	2.0	3.0	1.22	1.96
	Laser	27	1.19	0.83	70.3	0.0	1.0	1.0	2.0	3.0	0.86	1.52

SD standard deviation, *CV* coefficient of variation (%), *Min* minimum, *Q1* 25th percentile, *Med* median, *Q3* 75th percentile, *Max* maximum, *CI* confidence interval for the mean

greater than 90 %. It sufficed to provide post hoc test powers greater than 99 % ($n = 216$ measurements, $\alpha = 0.01$, mean difference = 1.213 ± 1.326). The difference between the control and experimental groups was assessed using a paired *t*-test of the SPSS program (v 20.0, IBM, USA). Repeated-measures one- and two-way analyses of variance (ANOVA) and a Bonferroni post hoc test were used to assess the effects of treatment and time on pain. The level of significance was set at 0.01.

Results

More than 80 patients were assessed until 30 patients were enrolled. The excluded patients did not meet the inclusion criteria. Of the 30 included patients, 3 girls were dropped out of the study because of consuming analgesics or failure to answer the phone and fill the questionnaire on time. The remaining volunteers (16 males and 11 females) aged 12–21 years (mean = 15.3).

Differences between pain sensed on placebo and laser sides

The average pain scores sensed in all 4 intervals on control and laser sides were 4.06 ± 2.85 and 2.35 ± 1.77, respectively. The paired *t*-test showed a significant difference between the pain level senses on each side ($P < 0.0001$). The paired *t*-test also detected significant differences between the treatment/placebo groups, at each of time intervals (Tables 1 and 2).

Pain changes over time

- *Control group*
  The one-way repeated-measures ANOVA showed a significant overall time-dependent decline in pain perceived in the placebo side ($P < 0.0001$). The Bonferroni test showed significant differences between each of the intervals (all *P* values ≤0.001).
- *Experimental group*
  The time-dependent pain decrease was significant in the laser side as well (ANOVA $P < 0.0001$). All pairwise comparisons were significant (all Bonferroni *P* values ≤0.005).

Effect of treatment and time on pain

According to the two-way repeated-measures ANOVA, the effect of treatment ($P < 0.0001$) and time ($P < 0.0001$) were significant. The interaction of the variables "time and treatment" was not significant ($P = 0.022$). According to the Bonferroni post hoc test, all pairwise comparisons were significant (all *P* values <0.001, Fig. 1, Table 1).

Discussion

Pain is a part of all orthodontic treatments [1, 3, 9, 14, 33], although its intensity, prevalence, and duration are disputed [1–7, 9–14, 16, 33–37]. About 90 % of patients experience pain during fixed orthodontic treatment [1–7, 11, 14]. In this study, all patients firstly felt pain in the first 24 h, which although decreased significantly, did not completely eliminate within 1 week. This was in line with earlier studies [1–3, 5, 6, 9, 16], most of which asserting that the pain peaks within the first 24 h and lasts for a short period [2, 5, 11–14, 33–35], while some others state that it might last for a rather long duration [6, 16]. Although not completely understood, orthodontic pain is mainly attributed to the compression of

Table 2 Pairwise comparisons between laser and placebo-matched sides presented as mean pain difference in 27 patients (control pain minus experimental pain)

Day	Groups	N	Mean	SD	95 % CI		P
1	Control–laser	27	2.04	1.60	1.40	2.67	<0.0001
2	Control–laser	27	1.48	1.31	0.96	2.00	<0.0001
4	Control–laser	27	0.93	0.92	0.56	1.29	<0.0001
7	Control–laser	27	0.41	0.75	0.11	0.70	0.0088

SD standard deviation, *CI* confidence interval for the pain difference

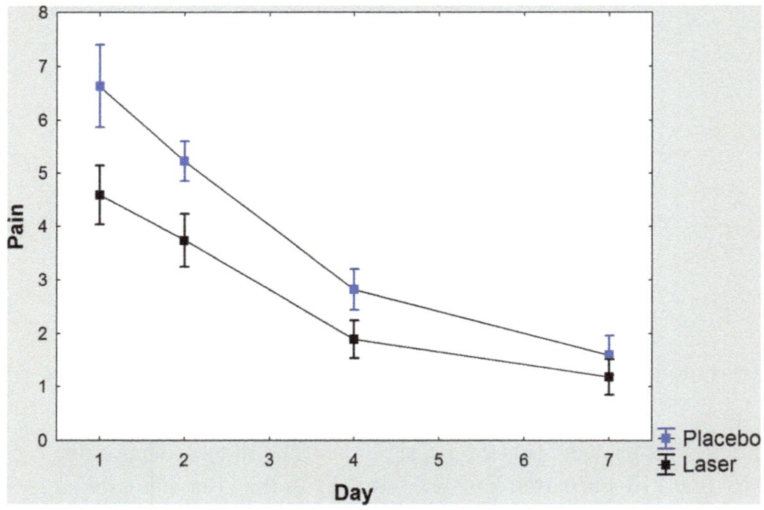

Fig. 1 Pain levels on each side and at each evaluated day. *Error bars* represent 95 % confidence intervals

periodontal ligament under orthodontic forces [2, 7, 12, 14]. The immediate response to orthodontic forces characterizes by ischemia and PDL compression. After a few hours of prostaglandin release, the sensitivity of the pain receptors to noxious chemicals (e.g., histamine, bradykinin, acetylcholine, etc.) increases, marking the PDL hyperalgesia phase. This mechanism together with other phenomena (such as osteoclastic activity, neurogenic inflammation, and vasodilatation in the PDL) might cause pain [2, 3, 5, 7, 12, 14, 16, 35]. Different methods proposed to reduce orthodontic pain are NSAID consumption, chewing plastic wafers or gum, vibratory and transcutaneous electrical stimulation, and a diet of softer foods [7, 11, 15, 16]. It seems that fixed appliances might cause higher levels of pressure, tension, pain, and sensitivity of the teeth compared to removable appliances [13, 38]. However, the differences between the levels of pain treated with various fixed appliances such as with self-ligation, lingual, or conventional brackets were mostly not significant [33, 38, 39]. Recently, Invisalign approach has been suggested as a less painful method, although it has its own limitations [38].

Low-level laser therapy can be performed by He-Ne lasers. Irradiation with He-Ne laser at 632.8-nm wavelength and energy of 7.5 J/cm^2 might reduce inflammation and accelerate the healing [40]. In this study, a single dose of He-Ne laser was shown effective in reducing the orthodontic pain sensed after beginning of tooth movement. There was no previous study on this particular type of laser, and all studies focused on laser wavelengths longer than ours. Therefore, we are limited to compare these results with other laser types. In this study, laser treatment contributed to about 12.1 % pain reduction in the laser side compared with the matched placebo side (1.21 out of 10 points). Our result was within the range reported in split-mouth studies [19, 26, 41] while it was smaller than the differences observed in parallel designs [18, 21, 42]. Of the few split-mouth studies conducted in this regard, only two found a significant difference. In one of them, laser irradiation accounted for 36.7 % pain reduction (3.67 out of 10) [26], while in the other one, laser reduced orthodontic pain for a statistically significant main score of 6.4 % (0.64 score out of 10) favoring laser irradiation [19]. The other two split-mouth designs failed to find a significant difference with very small differences (0.6 % in favor of the placebo side [41] and 2.4 % in favor of laser [17]). On the other hand, all parallel designs showed significant differences between the laser and placebo groups, with differences ranging from 19.6 to 52.5 % all favoring laser groups [18, 21, 42–44]. The differences can be attributable to the highly different methodologies including the orthodontic technique applied, laser dosimetry and parameters, the number of laser irradiation sessions, the laser types used, sample sizes, age ranges, gender compositions, analgesic consumption, and many other factors [15]. Mechanisms responsible for the pain-reducing effect of LLLT are unclear [15]. Perhaps, because of having anti-inflammatory and neural regenerative properties—as a probable result of photobioactive reaction which stimulates cell differentiation and proliferation—low-level laser therapy might be useful for pain control [20, 42–46]. Also, it might improve blood supply and enhance tissue recovery [42, 47]. Other factors contributing to the analgesic effect of LLLT might be the reactivation of enzymes targeted at pain-inductive factors, inhibiting nerve depolarization (C fibers in particular), ATP production, and prostaglandin reduction [15, 48].

Also, LLLT might alter nerve conduction by influencing the synthesis, release, and metabolism of encephalin and endorphins and many other neurochemicals [15, 49].

Limitations and strengths

This study was limited by some factors. Pain is subjective, and numerous factors (such as sex, age, genetics, pain threshold, stress, emotional state, response to analgesics, sociocultural differences, past pain experiences, and the magnitude of the force applied) can affect it [1, 2, 4, 5, 7, 9, 11, 14–16, 30, 46, 32]. On the other hand, the sample size was based on a pilot study and the post hoc power was very high because of the specific design of the study, excluding the abovementioned confounding variables [30, 50]. Moreover, VAS is understandable by patients and is reliable, sensitive, and reproducible [5, 11, 12, 14, 16, 46]. Still, standardizing the intolerable pain was virtually impossible, as patients might have different levels of tolerance to pain. However, this could favor the generalizability since it was similar to what happens in a clinical condition, as what is relevant to patient is not a pain which can necessarily keep them awake at night (as might be incorrectly considered as a standardized response), but a pain which can render that specific patient seek emergency treatment.

Some studies did not exclude patients taking analgesics and only monitored the number of analgesics taken [19]. However, taking analgesics could disrupt the reliability and validity of the responses [30, 32]. Therefore, this and some other studies [21, 23] excluded such patients. Since there was no bias in delivering proper treatment towards the excluded patients and patients had voluntarily participated, they were unlikely secretly taking painkillers while falsely reporting the opposite. Therefore, the pain-related side effects might not be biased. It was possible that excluding patients consuming analgesics might skew the sample to more cooperating and psychologically prepared patients (and perhaps also to those with lower pains) [30]. However, including patients taking analgesics would not help in improving the generalizability, since they would as well perceive lower pains and skew the results [30]. Finally, the inclusion of both genders and a rather broad range of ages favored the generalizability, as pain perception might differ between ages [7, 16] and between genders [1, 3, 7]. The role of age in pain is debated, since the methodologies differ [3], and the correlation between pain threshold and age might be non-linear [7, 16]. There might be a linear negative correlation between general pain and age until the age 25 years [14, 16]. Nevertheless, in orthodontics, the relationship is not necessarily linear, and the most sensitive age might be between 13 and 16 years old [7, 14]. Some studies have observed more intense pains in older subjects [3, 14, 36] while some others have found no correlations between pain and age [12, 16, 33]. Besides sample and methodological differences, this again might be caused by a non-linear correlation pattern, with adolescence or another age range having lower pain thresholds compared to ages younger or older than it [7, 16]. With this in mind, enrolling subjects from different ages seem advantageous over pooling a narrow age range, since results of a study on pain in children might not be necessarily generalizable to pain perceived by adults and vice versa. Since, in this split-mouth design each subject was matched with himself/herself, such variations in patients' demographics less likely confound the results, since the laser (treatment) sides were perfectly matched with their counterpart placebo quarters, in terms of age, gender, genetics, etc.

Conclusions

Single-dose low-level laser therapy might reduce orthodontic pain caused by retracting maxillary canines. Regardless of the presence or absence of laser therapy, orthodontic pain might considerably decrease after a week, although not completely eliminated in this period.

Competing interests
The authors declare that they have no competing interests.

Authors' contributions
FS conceived and designed the study, selected the patients, performed the orthodontic treatments, interpreted the findings, and drafted the methods. NC searched the literature, designed the study, interpreted the findings, and drafted the methods. MK designed the study, selected the patients, performed the laser irradiation, interpreted the findings, and drafted the methods. VR searched the literature, specified and performed the analyses, interpreted the findings, and drafted the article. MS searched the literature and interpreted the findings. All authors read and approved the final manuscript.

Author details
[1]Department of Orthodontics, Dental Faculty, Mazandaran University of Medical Sciences, Sari, Iran. [2]Department of Periodontics, Dental Faculty, Mazandaran University of Medical Sciences, Sari, Iran. [3]Laser Research Center of Dentistry, Dental Research Institute, Tehran University of Medical Sciences, Tehran, Iran. [4]Iranian Tissue Bank and Research Center, Tehran University of Medical Sciences, Tehran, Iran. [5]Department of Dental Anatomy and Morphology, Dental Branch, Islamic Azad University, Tehran, Iran. [6]Craniomaxillofacial Surgery Research Center, Shariati Hospital, Tehran University of Medical Sciences, Postal Code: 14174North Kargar Ave., 16 Azar ST, Tehran, Iran.

References
1. Bergius M, Berggren U, Kiliaridis S. Experience of pain during an orthodontic procedure. Eur J Oral Sci. 2002;110:92–8.
2. Tecco S, D'Attilio M, Tete S, Festa F. Prevalence and type of pain during conventional and self-ligating orthodontic treatment. Eur J Orthod. 2009;31:380–4.
3. Scheurer PA, Firestone AR, Bürgin WB. Perception of pain as a result of orthodontic treatment with fixed appliances. Eur J Orthod. 1996;18:349–57.
4. Firestone AR, Scheurer PA, Bürgin WB. Patients' anticipation of pain and pain-related side effects, and their perception of pain as a result of orthodontic treatment with fixed appliances. Eur J Orthod. 1999;21:387–96.

5. Erdinc AM, Dincer B. Perception of pain during orthodontic treatment with fixed appliances. Eur J Orthod. 2004;26:79–85.
6. Miyawaki S, Yasuhara M, Koh Y. Discomfort caused by bonded lingual orthodontic appliances in adult patients as examined by retrospective questionnaire. Am J Orthod Dentofacial Orthop. 1999;115:83–8.
7. Krishnan V. Orthodontic pain: from causes to management—a review. Eur J Orthod. 2007;29:170–9.
8. Sandhu SS, Sandhu J. Orthodontic pain-an interaction between age and sex in early and middle adolescence. Angle Orthod. 2013;83:966–72.
9. Krukemeyer AM, Arruda AO, Inglehart MR. Pain and orthodontic treatment. Angle Orthod. 2009;79:1175–81.
10. Lew KK. Attitudes and perceptions of adults towards orthodontic treatment in an Asian community. Community Dent Oral Epidemiol. 1993;21:31–5.
11. Xiaoting L, Yin T, Yangxi C. Interventions for pain during fixed orthodontic appliance therapy. A systematic review. Angle Orthod. 2010;80:925–32.
12. Scott P, Sherriff M, Dibiase AT, Cobourne MT. Perception of discomfort during initial orthodontic tooth alignment using a self-ligating or conventional bracket system: a randomized clinical trial. Eur J Orthod. 2008;30:227–32.
13. Sergl HG, Klages U, Zentner A. Pain and discomfort during orthodontic treatment: causative factors and effects on compliance. Am J Orthod Dentofacial Orthop. 1998;114:684–91.
14. Bergius M, Kiliaridis S, Berggren U. Pain in orthodontics. A review and discussion of the literature. J Orofac Orthop. 2000;61:125–37.
15. Ren C, McGrath C, Yang Y. The effectiveness of low-level diode laser therapy on orthodontic pain management: a systematic review and meta-analysis. Lasers Med Sci. 2015;30:1881–93.
16. Rakhshan H, Rakhshan V. Pain and discomfort perceived during the initial stage of active fixed orthodontic treatment. Saudi Dent J. 2015;27:81–7.
17. Eslamian L, Borzabadi-Farahani A, Hassanzadeh-Azhiri A, Badiee MR, Fekrazad R. The effect of 810-nm low-level laser therapy on pain caused by orthodontic elastomeric separators. Lasers Med Sci. 2014;29:559–64.
18. Tortamano A, Lenzi DC, Haddad ACSS, Bottino MC, Dominguez GC, Vigorito JW. Low-level laser therapy for pain caused by placement of the first orthodontic archwire: a randomized clinical trial. Am J Orthod Dentofacial Orthop. 2009;136:662–7.
19. Artes-Ribas M, Arnabat-Dominguez J, Puigdollers A. Analgesic effect of a low-level laser therapy (830 nm) in early orthodontic treatment. Lasers Med Sci. 2013;28:335–41.
20. Turhani D, Scheriau M, Kapral D, Benesch T, Jonke E, Bantleon HP. Pain relief by single low-level laser irradiation in orthodontic patients undergoing fixed appliance therapy. Am J Orthod Dentofacial Orthop. 2006;130:371–7.
21. Nobrega C, da Silva EM, de Macedo CR. Low-level laser therapy for treatment of pain associated with orthodontic elastomeric separator placement: a placebo-controlled randomized double-blind clinical trial. Photomed Laser Surg. 2013;31:10–6.
22. Marini I, Bartolucci ML, Bortolotti F, Innocenti G, Gatto MR, Alessandri BG. The effect of diode superpulsed low-level laser therapy on experimental orthodontic pain caused by elastomeric separators: a randomized controlled clinical trial. Lasers Med Sci. 2015;30:35–41.
23. Abtahi SM, Mousavi SA, Shafaee H, Tanbakuchi B. Effect of low-level laser therapy on dental pain induced by separator force in orthodontic treatment. Dent Res J (Isfahan). 2013;10:647–51.
24. He WL, Li CJ, Liu ZP, Sun JF, Hu ZA, Yin X, et al. Efficacy of low-level laser therapy in the management of orthodontic pain: a systematic review and meta-analysis. Lasers Med Sci. 2013;28:1581–9.
25. Li FJ, Zhang JY, Zeng XT, Guo Y. Low-level laser therapy for orthodontic pain: a systematic review. Lasers Med Sci. 2014;30:1789–803.
26. Dominguez A, Velasquez SA. Effect of low-level laser therapy on pain following activation of orthodontic final archwires: a randomized controlled clinical trial. Photomed Laser Surg. 2013;31:36–40.
27. Heravi F, Moradi A, Ahrari F. The effect of low level laser therapy on the rate of tooth movement and pain perception during canine retraction. Oral Health Dent Manag. 2014;13:183–8.
28. Doshi-Mehta G, Bhad-Patil WA. Efficacy of low-intensity laser therapy in reducing treatment time and orthodontic pain: a clinical investigation. Am J Orthod Dentofacial Orthop. 2012;141:289–97.
29. Angelieri F, Sousa MVS, Kanashiro LK, Siqueira DF, Maltagliati LÁ. Effects of low intensity laser on pain sensitivity during orthodontic movement. Dental Press J Orthod. 2011;16:95–102.
30. Haraji A, Rakhshan V. Chlorhexidine gel and less difficult surgeries might reduce postoperative pain, controlling for dry socket, infection, and analgesic consumption: a split-mouth controlled randomized clinical trial. J Oral Rehab. 2015;42:209–19.
31. Amini F, Harandi S, Mollaei M, Rakhshan V. Effects of fixed orthodontic treatment using conventional versus metal-injection molding brackets on salivary nickel and chromium levels: a double-blind randomized clinical trial. Eur J Orthod. 2015. [Epub ahead of print].
32. Haraji A, Rakhshan V, Khamverdi N, Khanzadeh-Alishahi H. Effects of intra-alveolar placement of 0.2 % chlorhexidine bioadhesive gel on dry socket incidence and postsurgical pain: a double-blind split-mouth randomized controlled clinical trial. J Orofac Pain. 2013;27:256–62.
33. Ngan P, Kess B, Wilson S. Perception of discomfort by patients undergoing orthodontic treatment. Am J Orthod Dentofacial Orthop. 1989;96:47–53.
34. Jones M, Chan C. The pain and discomfort experienced during orthodontic treatment: a randomized controlled clinical trial of two initial aligning arch wires. Am J Orthod Dentofacial Orthop. 1992;102:373–81.
35. Fujita K. New orthodontic treatment with lingual bracket mushroom arch wire appliance. Am J Orthod. 1979;76:657–75.
36. Jones ML. An investigation into the initial discomfort caused by placement of an archwire. Eur J Orthod. 1984;6:48–54.
37. Jones ML, Richmond S. Initial tooth movement: force application and pain—a relationship? Am J Orthod. 1985;88:111–6.
38. Fujiyama K, Honjo T, Suzuki M, Matsuoka S, Deguchi T. Analysis of pain level in cases treated with Invisalign aligner: comparison with fixed edgewise appliance therapy. Prog Orthod. 2014;15:64.
39. Wu AKY, McGrath C, Wong RWK, Wiechmann D, Rabie ABM. A comparison of pain experienced by patients treated with labial and lingual orthodontic appliances. Eur J Orthod. 2010;32:403–7.
40. Fahimipour F, Mahdian M, Houshmand B, Asnaashari M, Sadrabadi AN, Farashah SE, et al. The effect of He-Ne and Ga-Al-As laser light on the healing of hard palate mucosa of mice. Lasers Med Sci. 2013;28:93–100.
41. Bicakci AA, Kocoglu-Altan B, Toker H, Mutaf I, Sumer Z. Efficiency of low-level laser therapy in reducing pain induced by orthodontic forces. Photomed Laser Surg. 2012;30:460–5.
42. Kim WT, Bayome M, Park JB, Park JH, Baek SH, Kook YA. Effect of frequent laser irradiation on orthodontic pain. A single-blind randomized clinical trial. Angle Orthod. 2013;83:611–6.
43. Harazaki M, Takahashi H, Ito A, Isshiki Y. Soft laser irradiation induced pain reduction in orthodontic treatment. Bull Tokyo Dent Coll. 1998;39:95–101.
44. Harazaki M, Isshiki Y. Soft laser irradiation effects on pain reduction in orthodontic treatment. Bull Tokyo Dent Coll. 1997;38:291–5.
45. Verschueren RC, Koudstaal J, Oldhoff J. The carbon dioxide laser; some possibilities in surgery. Acta Chir Belg. 1975;74:197–204.
46. Sobouti F, Rakhshan V, Chiniforush N, Khatami M. Effects of laser-assisted cosmetic smile lift gingivectomy on postoperative bleeding and pain in fixed orthodontic patients: a controlled clinical trial. Prog Orthod. 2014;15:66.
47. Abi-Ramia LB, Stuani AS, Stuani AS, Stuani MB, Mendes AM. Effects of low-level laser therapy and orthodontic tooth movement on dental pulps in rats. Angle Orthod. 2010;80:116–22.
48. Mizutani K, Musya Y, Wakae K, Kobayashi T, Tobe M, Taira K, et al. A clinical study on serum prostaglandin E2 with low-level laser therapy. Photomed Laser Surg. 2004;22:537–9.
49. Sun G, Tuner J. Low-level laser therapy in dentistry. Dent Clin North Am. 2004;48:1061–76. viii.
50. Kazemi M, Geramipanah F, Negahdari R, Rakhshan V. Active tactile sensibility of single-tooth implants versus natural dentition: a split-mouth double-blind randomized clinical trial. Clin Implant Dent Relat Res. 2014;16:947–55.

15

Facial asymmetry assessment in adults using three-dimensional surface imaging

Arti Patel[1], Syed Mohammed Shamsul Islam[1*], Kevin Murray[2] and Mithran S. Goonewardene[1]

Abstract

Background: The use of three-dimensional (3D) surface imaging is becoming more popular and accepted in the fields of Medicine and Dentistry. The present study aims to develop a technique to automatically localise and quantify soft-tissue asymmetry in adults using 3D facial scans. This may be applied as a diagnostic tool to monitor growth and dynamic changes and to evaluate treatment outcomes.

Methods: 3D facial surface data were captured from 55 adults comprising 28 symmetrical faces and 27 asymmetrical faces using a 3dMDface system. A landmark-independent method, which compared the original and the mirrored 3D facial data, was developed to quantify the asymmetry. A Weibull distribution-based probabilistic model was generated from the root-mean-square (RMS) error data for the symmetrical group to designate a level of asymmetry which represented a normal range.

Results: Statistically significant ($p < 0.0001$) differences in the RMS error values were found when comparing symmetrical with asymmetrical groups and a similarly significant difference was identified between the lower and the upper face of the asymmetrical group.

Conclusions: The proposed 3D imaging-based method of identifying and quantifying facial soft-tissue asymmetry was fast and effective. The Weibull distribution-based comparison of a person's asymmetry with respect to a large sample of symmetrical faces may also be used to evaluate growth, soft-tissue compensations and surgical outcomes.

Keywords: Facial aesthetics; Facial soft-tissue asymmetry; 3D surface imaging; Landmark-independent analysis; RMS distance measure; Weibull distribution

Background

Symmetry is a common occurrence in nature. It is defined as "equality or correspondence in the form of parts distributed around a centre or an axis, at the two extremes or poles, or in opposite sides of the body" [1]. Although a mild degree of asymmetry is common in the face of normal human individuals [2–7], orthodontists and surgeons often encounter patients with severe asymmetries. Facial symmetry is historically associated with attractiveness [8–11], and a severe asymmetry may have a psychosocial impact [12]. Severe asymmetries combined with other skeletal deformities may require surgical intervention [13]. Therefore, accurate localisation and quantification of the extent of facial asymmetry are crucial in order to facilitate orthodontic diagnosis and establish treatment goals.

According to Proffit and Severt [14], the prevalence of asymmetry is dependent on the type of presenting malocclusion. Asymmetry was found to be present in 28 % of class II subjects, and a prevalence of 40 % was noted in others (class III patients, patients with a long face and class I). However, the most severe asymmetries are usually associated with craniofacial syndromes such as hemifacial microsomia, clefting anomalies and craniosynostoses [15, 16]. Skeletal asymmetries not linked to craniofacial syndromes are considered related to asymmetrical skeletal development of individual craniofacial structures. This may include asymmetry in the position of the glenoid fossa or asymmetrical development of the mandible. Trauma and infection in the condylar region may also result in the development of asymmetry and perhaps ankylosis of the temporomandibular joint leading to a

* Correspondence: syed.islam@uwa.edu.au
[1]Department of Orthodontics, School of Dentistry, The University of Western Australia, 35, Stirling Hwy, Crawley, Western Australia 6009, Australia
Full list of author information is available at the end of the article

secondary functional impairment. This may have a profound impact on future growth [17].

The surface of the face is the most visible area that clinicians and lay people appreciate and often forms the basis of aesthetic judgments. Since there is greater emphasis placed on the soft tissues, it is important to have reliable data on the external soft-tissue integument and its balance with the underlying hard-tissue skeleton.

Currently, there are several available methods for capturing and quantifying craniofacial surface morphology. These include direct anthropometry and digital photography as well as newer three-dimensional (3D) surface imaging systems. 3D imaging-based methods of measuring facial asymmetry have become popular and have created a virtual reality paradigm. In addition, 3D image analysis methods have greatly assisted in reducing the magnification errors produced from geometric distortions that commonly affect conventional 2D-acquisition methods. The use of 2D projections, which aim to quantify 3D asymmetric objects, introduces inaccuracies [18] because reference points are imprecise. In a recent report which assessed ten human skulls, de Moraes et al. found poor reproducibility of reference points in digital 2D images and the true physical measurements (kappa = 0.609) and an almost perfect agreement (kappa = 0.92) when 3D data were analysed [19]. Cheung et al. and Tai et al. [20, 21] also reported similar and supportive results. From an anthropometric perspective, 3D surface capture has many additional advantages over traditional methods. Craniofacial angles, surface areas and volumes may be quantified along with linear distances. The extraction of X, Y and Z coordinate data, as well as the generation of a permanent archival record of a subject's face, has been made possible [18, 20–22].

Previous reports have indicated that asymmetry largely exists in the lower third of the face [14, 23–25]. However, most studies have focused on hard-tissue asymmetry. Further information related to the dominance of soft-tissue asymmetry in the facial thirds is needed, particularly since it has been demonstrated that the nasal region is more critically evaluated as an observer's focus is initially directed to the central region of the face [26].

In addition to a pretreatment morphological assessment and quantification of soft tissue, 3D soft-tissue scanning may be useful for assessing the impact of treatment in the management of asymmetry by appropriately developed superimposition techniques [27]. Furthermore, it may be possible and advantageous to monitor growth or treatment-induced changes in three dimensions.

The aim of the present study was to devise a relatively quick, simple and landmark-independent 3D imaging-based technique that might potentially be valuable as a diagnostic tool for orthognathic and cosmetic surgical planning for patients with soft-tissue asymmetry. Moreover, it was expected that the technique would establish a threshold, above and below which asymmetry might be identified in a region-specific analysis.

Methods

Ethics approval to conduct this study was obtained from the Human Research Ethics Committee of The University of Western Australia. All assessments were performed in accordance with the guidelines of the National Health and Medical Research Council of Australia.

The study was a retrospective evaluation of two groups of male and female subjects, 20 years of age and older who were treated in the Dental School Clinic and a Private Orthodontic Practice in Perth, Western Australia. The first group was comprised of 27 patients who presented for the management of an obvious facial asymmetry. The second group was formed with 28 subjects with no apparent facial asymmetry. Appropriate group allocation was confirmed by three different orthodontists on separate occasions based on the comprehensive evaluation of the facial radiographs and photographs collected as part of the subjects' treatment records. The subjects in the first group were a combination of different angle classifications (classes I, II or III), and all of these patients required combined orthognathic surgery to correct their asymmetry. The subjects in the second group were all angle class I subjects. Patients who presented with a craniofacial deformity or syndrome were not included in any of the groups.

The method of the facial asymmetry analysis is illustrated in Fig. 1. Initially, each subject was scanned using a 3dMDface scanning system (3dMD Inc., Atlanta, GA, USA). The scanner incorporated a multi-camera configuration mounted on a wall. Three cameras were arranged on each side of the subject who was seated on an adjustable chair and asked to adopt a natural head posture by looking at a specific point marked on an opposing wall. Natural head posture was adopted for this study as it has been shown to be clinically reproducible [28-30]. The subjects were also required to keep their jaws in a relaxed state just before the images were taken. If the subject moved during scanning, the procedure was repeated.

The 3dMDface scanning system scanned a subject's head and neck area (a 180° facial image from ear to ear) in 1.5 ms at the highest resolution available (1236 × 1624 pixels). The two acquired stereo camera viewpoints (captured by the cameras located on two sides) were combined using a stereophotogrammetry technique which produced a single 3D image.

The scanned images were refined on a personal standard desktop computer using the 3dMDpatient software (3dMD Inc., Atlanta, GA). The software provided automatic tools

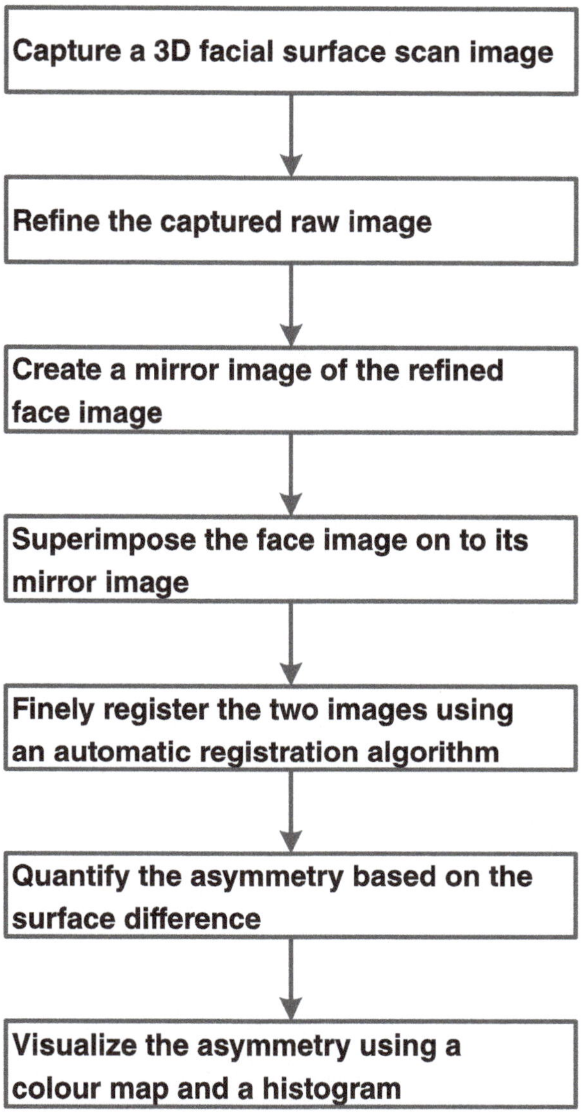

Fig. 1 Basic block diagram of the proposed approach for facial asymmetry analysis

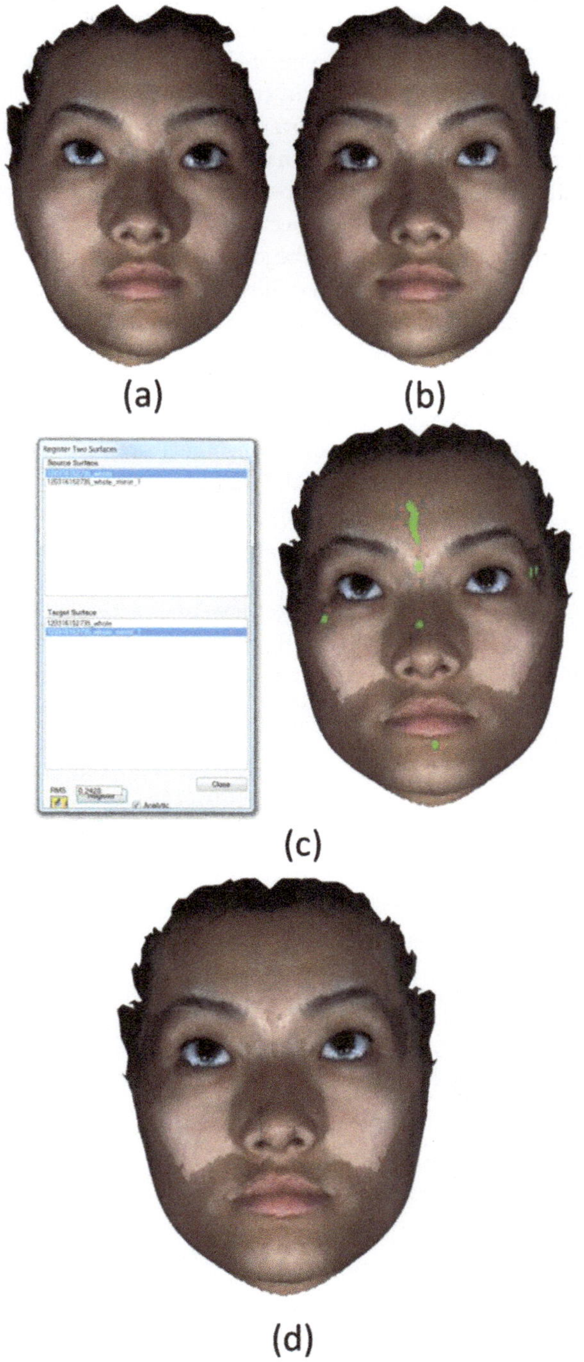

Fig. 2 Image registration process. **a** Original image. **b** Mirror image of **a** constructed along an arbitrary plane. **c** Initial registration based on some selected regions (shown with *green colour*). **d** The fine registration of the two images using that Levenberg-Marquardt algorithm

for removing 'defects' such as spikes or holes in the point cloud generated by the scanner. A cylindrical area of the face extending from ear to ear was cropped to eliminate the shoulders and neck.

The quantification of facial asymmetry was performed on each patient's 3D data using the 3dMDvultus software (3dMD Inc., Atlanta, GA) by superimposing an image onto its mirror image, similar to the approach described by Nonda et al. [27]. The mirror image was created, in accordance with Cevidanes et al. [31] by reflecting along an arbitrary plane outside of the face (Fig. 2). Subsequently, the original and the mirror images were aligned with respect to surface features of the forehead, over the root of the nose and zygoma. Following manual registration, an automatic fine registration was performed using the Levenberg-Marquardt algorithm [32] carried out to an error level below 0.5.

The distances between the data points of the two registered surfaces were colour-coded for the purpose of asymmetry visualisation. Every data point of the original surface image was assigned a colour based on its distance from the corresponding data point in the mirrored surface image. A histogram (colour-coded scale), corresponding to the distances, was also generated as illustrated in Fig. 3. Colours at the positive end of the histogram depicted regions which had outward movement or convexity with respect to the reference (original) surface. Colours at the negative end represented regions which had inward movement or concavity with respect to the reference surface. Colours at the middle of the histogram highlighted regions which had almost no differences between the two superimposed surfaces. The parameters noted in the histogram were defined as follows:

- *N*—number of data points in the selected region
- RMS (root-mean-square)—the square root of the mean of the squares of the discrete values
- Min (minimum)—the smallest area of deviation between the two selected surfaces displayed in millimetres
- Max (maximum)—he largest area of deviation between the two selected surfaces displayed in millimetres
- Std dev—the standard deviation of the negative and positive values over the selected region

Minimum and maximum measurements are found to be greatly influenced by the boarder of the images (especially the hairline) and by the changes near the eyes (due to blinking) or mouth (due to lip posture) which may result in arbitrary minimum and maximum measurements. Therefore, these two measurements are discarded in the analysis.

The middle and lower facial thirds were separated by horizontal lines running through the outer canthus of the eye to the outer commissure of the lips (upper third) and below the outer commissure of the lips (lower third) as illustrated in Fig. 4. This separation was performed after the registration of the original and mirror whole face images. Colour maps were also generated for the lower and middle third of the faces to visualise the asymmetry in those regions.

Statistical analysis

A linear mixed model approach was used to determine the impact of the fixed factors of location (whole, mid or lower face) and symmetry (asymmetrical or symmetrical subjects), on the response variables of the RMS, minimum, maximum and mean. A variance stabilising log transformation was used for the RMS. Additionally, given the skewed nature of the whole-face RMS measurements, a two-parameter Weibull distribution was fitted to the data on the 28 symmetrical subjects, using methods of maximum likelihood to estimate the parameters from the data.

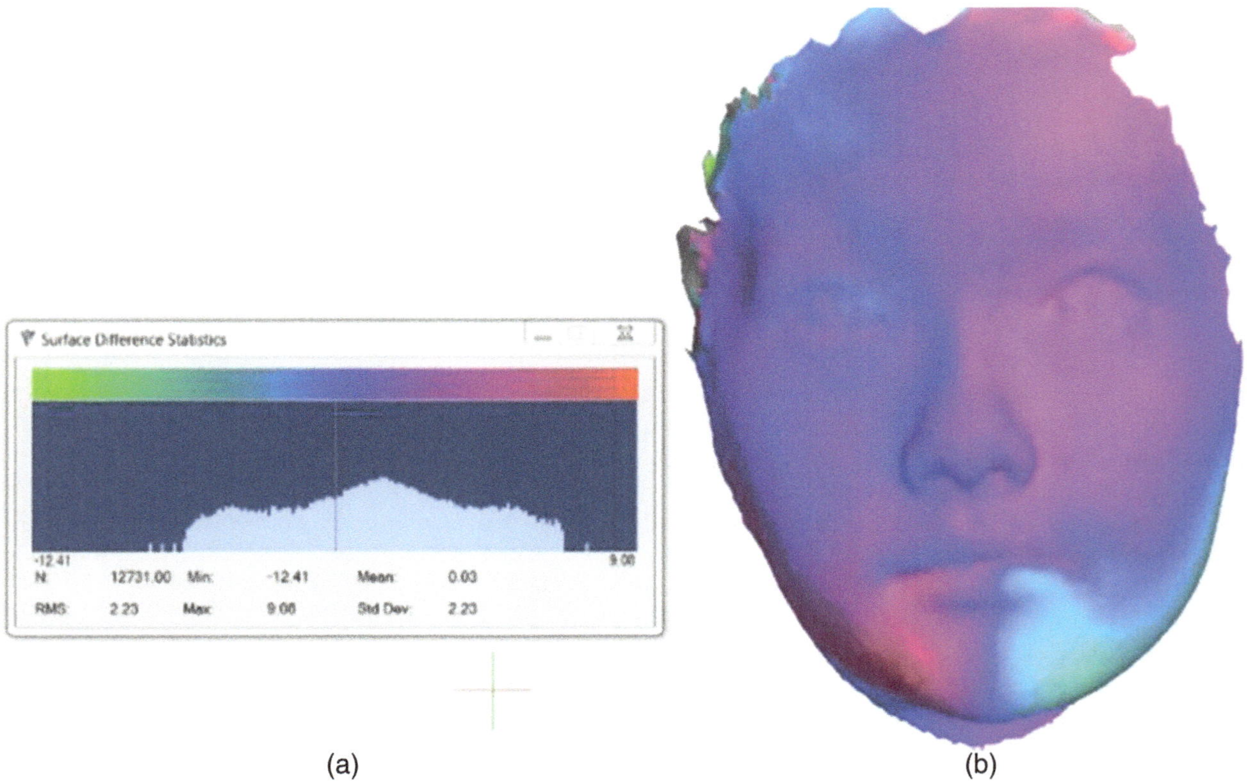

Fig. 3 Quantification and visualisation of facial asymmetry. **a** Statistics of the difference of two registered facial surfaces (original and mirror). **b** Registered face images with *colour map*

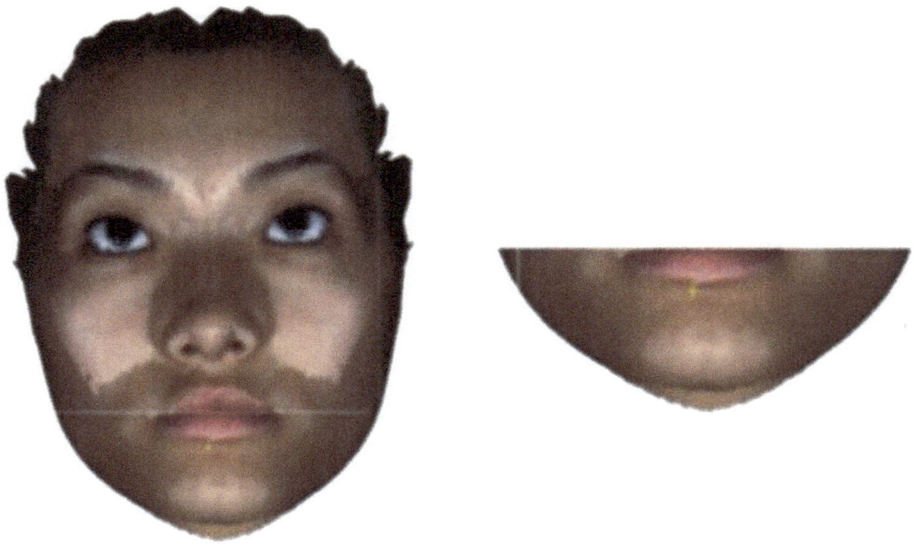

(a) (b)

Fig. 4 Segmentation of the lower third of the face. **a** *Line* along which the lower face was segmented. **b** Lower face after segmentation

To investigate the intra-observer reliability, the 3D data of five randomly selected subjects were analysed for a second time 2 weeks later and intraclass correlation coefficients (ICC) were estimated. The interpretation of the ICCs was based on a sliding scale characterised by Landis and Koch [33], indicating values <0 as no agreement, 0–20 as slight, 21–40 as fair, 41–60 as moderate, 61–80 as substantial and 81–100 as almost perfect agreement. All statistical analyses were performed using R environment for statistical computing [34].

Results

The Intraclass Correlation Coefficients (ICC) were calculated by face type (asymmetrical or symmetrical), location (upper or lower face) and type of measurement (RMS error, mean, minimum, and maximum). Apart from a couple of measures, the ICCs were generally high.

Table 1 shows the summary statistics for the different measurements of the upper, lower and whole face in the 27 asymmetrical and 28 symmetrical subjects, whilst Table 2 and Fig. 5 provide comparisons of upper/lower face and asymmetry/symmetry combinations separately for each of the measurements (RMS error and mean value). On average, the RMS error was higher in the asymmetrical groups compared with the symmetrical groups when considering all three locations (lower, upper and whole faces) separately (3.33, 2.39 and 2.85 versus 1.37, 1.23 and 1.52, respectively). Upon comparison of the lower face in the asymmetrical subjects against the lower face in the symmetrical subjects, the difference in the RMS error values was statistically significant ($p < 0.0001$). Similarly, a statistically significant difference in the RMS error values ($p < 0.0001$) can be seen in comparison of the lower face and upper face in the asymmetrical subjects and the upper face in the asymmetrical subjects against the upper face in the symmetrical subjects ($p < 0.0001$). No statistically significant differences ($p = 0.2505$) were observed when comparing the lower and upper face in the symmetrical subjects.

Table 1 Summary statistics for different measurements on the upper, lower and whole faces in the 27 asymmetrical and 28 symmetrical subjects

Measurements		Asymmetrical			Symmetrical			Total
		Lower	Upper	Whole	Lower	Upper	Whole	
RMS	Average	3.33	2.39	2.85	1.37	1.23	1.52	2.10
	Std dev	1.82	1.88	1.54	0.52	0.42	0.39	1.48
Mean	Average	0.04	0.07	0.06	−0.07	−0.02	−0.00	0.01
	Std dev	0.43	0.25	0.30	0.29	0.14	0.19	0.28

On average, the mean value measurements were higher in the asymmetrical groups compared with the symmetrical groups at the three locations (lower, upper and whole faces) separately (0.04, 0.07 and 0.06 versus −0.07, −0.02 and −0.00, respectively). Although the summary statistics indicated variation in the asymmetrical and symmetrical subjects in the mean value measurements, the comparative data indicated no statistically significant differences between all combinations in facial symmetry (asymmetrical versus symmetrical) and location (upper and lower faces).

Figure 6 illustrates a two-parameter (shape and scale) *Weibull distribution* fitted to the RMS error data for the whole face in the 28 symmetrical subjects. The Weibull curve is superimposed over the histogram and thus

Table 2 Statistical differences in different measurements upon comparison of the upper and lower faces in the asymmetrical and symmetrical subjects

Pairwise comparison	Measurements	Estimated value	Std err	*T* value	*p* value
Lower asymmetrical vs. lower symmetrical	RMS	0.8033	0.1273	6.31	<0.0001*
	Mean	0.1097	0.07940	1.38	0.1711
Lower asymmetrical vs. upper asymmetrical	RMS	0.3563	0.08098	4.40	<0.0001*
	Mean	−0.02630	0.05130	−0.51	0.6104
Lower symmetrical vs. upper symmetrical	RMS	0.09239	0.07952	1.16	0.2505
	Mean	−0.04893	0.05038	−0.97	0.3358
Upper asymmetrical vs. upper symmetrical	RMS	0.5394	0.1273	4.24	<0.0001*
	Mean	0.08704	0.07940	1.10	0.2763

*Statistically significant differences

provides a percentile measurement for any given individual. Therefore, this curve can be used to predict the severity of asymmetry in a given subject. For example, as illustrated in Fig. 7, an asymmetrical subject with an observed RMS measurement of 2.6 (the square of which is 6.76) falls in the 99.8th percentile (represented by the red dotted line). This percentile value indicates 99.8 % of the symmetrical patients (according to this group) would have a value less than the observed RMS measurement value for this patient. Since a large RMS value is proportional to the level of asymmetry, the extreme RMS value potentially indicates that this particular patient is unlikely to be from the symmetrical distribution.

Discussion

The development and advancement of technology has improved diagnosis and treatment planning for significant dentofacial deformities [35]. Peck et al. [36] demonstrated that the extent of skeletal asymmetry was confounded by significant deviations in overlying soft-tissue dimensions. Therefore, correction of the skeletal and dental asymmetry may not result in a symmetrical aesthetic soft-tissue form.

Historically, a 2D analysis of asymmetry with facial photographs has complemented a clinical examination using linear and planar differences between each side of the face which are prone to measurement error [19]. With the advancement of 3D technology, cost effective, fast, reliable, accurate and noninvasive methods have been developed to provide 3D scanning of facial soft tissues. Since the 3D facial analysis methods described in the present study are independent of the 3D image capturing system, any 3D facial scanner may be used for acquiring 3D facial surface data.

In the present study, the quantitative analysis of facial asymmetry was performed by measuring the distances between the original and mirror images of a subject. It was observed that the RMS errors between the two sides of the face were higher for asymmetrical compared with symmetrical faces regardless of the location (upper and lower) (Table 1 and Fig. 5). This implied that an asymmetrical face, on average, has a wider range of points (minimum to maximum) in comparison with symmetrical faces.

The statistical differences in the RMS error measurements (Table 2) indicated highly significant differences

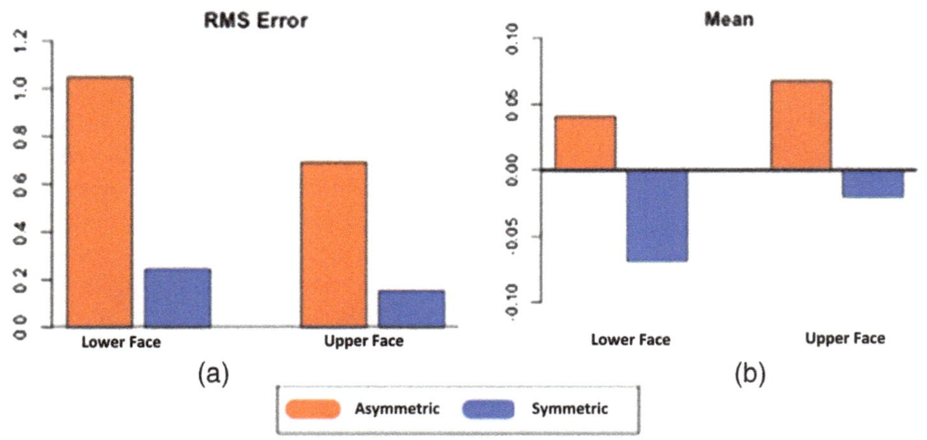

Fig. 5 The changes in the upper and lower faces of asymmetrical and symmetrical subjects measured in **a** RMS **b** mean values

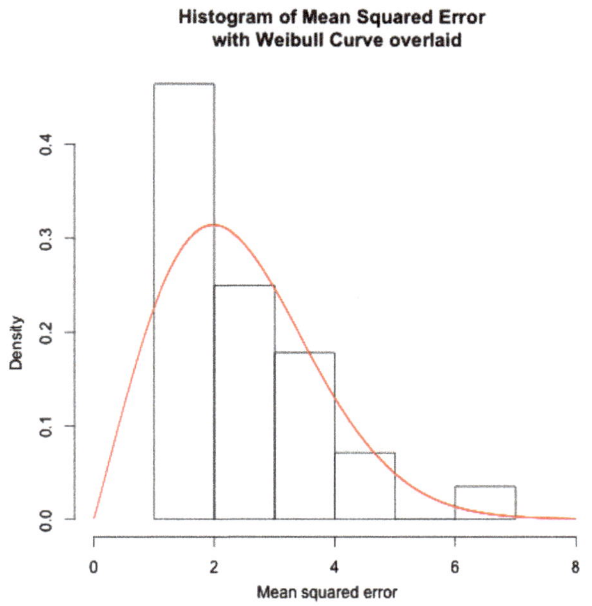

Fig. 6 A Weibull graph created from a histogram of the whole face in the symmetrical subject group

for the upper and lower faces independently between the asymmetrical and symmetrical subjects. A statistically significant difference in the RMS values in the upper and lower face in the asymmetrical subjects was observed. This finding matches those of previous studies which indicated facial asymmetry predominated in the lower third of the face [3, 23–25]. However, similar to Djordjevic et al. [37], no statistically significant difference was identified in symmetrical subjects.

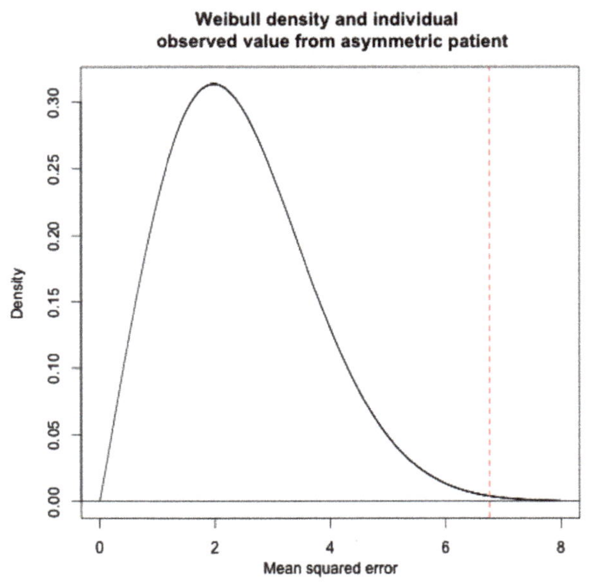

Fig. 7 An illustration of an example on how to utilise the Weibull distribution graph created from a dataset of symmetrical subjects. The *dotted line* illustrates a patient that lies in the 99.8th percentile

The mean value analysis calculated the mean of the number of data points in a selected region. The mean value measurements were higher in the asymmetrical groups compared with the symmetrical groups at the three locations (lower, upper and whole faces) separately (Table 1 and Fig. 5). A comparison of the mean difference data (Table 2) indicated no statistically significant effects for all combinations in facial asymmetry (asymmetrical versus symmetrical) and location (upper versus lower face). This may be explained by a subject who is asymmetrical would be expected to have a wide spread in minimum and maximum values, and hence, the mean value could potentially be zero. In addition, it would be expected that a smaller spread in the minimum and maximum values would occur in symmetrical subjects and hence, still result in a mean value of zero.

One of the strengths of the present study is that a face was only compared with its mirror image which avoided the problem of assessing faces of different sizes. Using an arbitrary plane outside of the face eliminated the problem of identifying a midsagittal plane which is difficult to define, especially in patients with asymmetry [38]. Moreover, the colour maps (Fig. 3) obtained by the superimposition (best fit registration) of the original and mirror facial images provided a detailed quantitative assessment of asymmetry using all of the available facial points instead of a limited number of facial landmarks. This also prevented inaccuracies associated with individual landmark identification. The number of registered points relied on the size of the superimposed area and the proportion of asymmetrical facial regions. Therefore, two surfaces were first registered based on the entire face and then segmented into lower and middle thirds for a more in-depth assessment of asymmetry of specific regions.

It is important to select the most appropriate reference region when manually superimposing the 3D images. The ideal reference region should be a stable area such as the forehead [39] which is unlikely to be affected by surgical intervention. Some rotational errors were encountered during forehead registration as the forehead is relatively flat and lacks unique 3D shape features. Therefore, similar to Jayaratne et al. [40], surfaces over the root of the nose and zygoma were chosen. The relatively thin and immobile nature of the overlying soft tissues in these regions helped eliminate some of the spatial image malalignments. Guest et al. [41] evaluated four methods of superimposition in two surgical patients. All methods were found to produce errors in the calculation of final surface changes. However, the registration algorithm chosen in the present study produced promising and realistic results because no assumptions were made about the direction of displacement between surfaces.

The Weibull distribution-based probabilistic model illustrated in Figs. 6 and 7 was generated from a data set of 28 symmetrical subjects. Therefore, it may be too simplistic to make a clinical recommendation regarding the use of this curve. However, as this curve represents the quantification of symmetry distribution, it may be a useful diagnostic tool in identifying asymmetries not immediately recognised by the naked eye. It may also enable the clinician or researcher to monitor the progress of diagnosed asymmetries, if they are progressive. The probabilistic model may be useful in the identification of significant deviation beyond a particular threshold. An individual can have their RMS value converted to a corresponding percentile from the Weibull curve, to represent the level of deviation from symmetry, thus potentially providing a reference to evaluate treatment outcomes when asymmetries have been addressed.

Apart from the smaller dataset, the present study has the following limitations. The methodology in selecting an external reference plane and mirror imaging was not fully automated; therefore, minor individual technique differences may account for user-related error. It would also be interesting to prepare subset dependent on class of malocclusion to determine if there are class-based associations with distribution and magnitude of facial asymmetry. Unfortunately this was not possible with the database currently available but would be considered with subsequent follow-up studies.

Conclusions

This study presents a method to automatically localise and quantify soft-tissue asymmetry in adults from their 3D facial scans. The method is relatively fast, simple and landmark independent and is a valuable diagnostic and treatment planning tool for orthognathic and cosmetic surgery patients with soft-tissue asymmetry. Our method can enhance clinician-patient communication by identifying areas of deformity, the level of asymmetry and relative relationships between different components of the face and presenting these interactively on a screen in front of the patient. The results of this study suggest that the use of RMS error measurements is predictable and useful as an indication of facial soft-tissue asymmetry. By utilising a Weibull curve in this study, we have identified a prospective means to assess quantitative comparisons of growth, tissue compensation, and surgery outcomes. However, to make better use of the distribution, this probabilistic model needs to be generated from a larger dataset which presents an opportunity for future research.

Competing interests

The authors declare that they have no competing interests.

Authors' contributions

MG and SI designed the research protocol, AP carried out the measurements, AP and SI drafted the manuscript, KM carried out the data processing and statistical analysis, MG and SI supervised the research. All authors read and approved the final manuscript.

Acknowledgments

This research is sponsored by the Australian Society of Orthodontists Foundation for Research and Education (ASOFRE) Special Donation grants (PG51311900 and PG51312000) and, by The University of Western Australia under Research Development Award grant (PG12104373).

Author details

[1]Department of Orthodontics, School of Dentistry, The University of Western Australia, 35, Stirling Hwy, Crawley, Western Australia 6009, Australia. [2]School of Mathematics and Statistics, The University of Western Australia, 35, Stirling Hwy, Crawley, Western Australia 6009, Australia.

References

1. Stedman T. Stedman's medical dictionary. Baltimore: The Williams and Wilkins Company; 1966.
2. Lu KH. Harmonic analysis of the human face. Biometrics. 1965;21:491–505.
3. Pirttiniemi P, Kantomaa T, Lahtela P. Relationship between craniofacial and condyle path asymmetry in unilateral cross-bite patients. Eur J Orthod. 1990;12(4):408–13.
4. Vig PS, Hewitt AB. Asymmetry of human facial skeleton. Angle Orthod. 1975;45(2):125–9.
5. Kowner R. Facial asymmetry and attractiveness judgment in developmental perspective. J Exp Psychol Hum Percept Perform. 1996;22(3):662–75.
6. Langlois JH, Roggman LA. Attractive faces are only average. Psychol Sci. 1990;1(2):115–21.
7. Langlois JH, Roggman LA, Musselman L. What is average and what is not average about attractive faces. Psychol Sci. 1994;5(4):214–20.
8. Grammer K, Thornhill R. Human (Homo sapiens) facial attractiveness and sexual selection: the role of symmetry and averageness. J Comp Psychol. 1994;108(3):233–42.
9. Jones D, Hill K. Criteria of facial attractiveness in five populations. Human Nature-an Interdisciplinary Biosocial Perspective. 1993;4(3):271–96.
10. Rhodes G, Proffitt W, Grady J, Sumich A. Facial symmetry and the perception of beauty. Psychon Bull Rev. 1998;5(4):659–69.
11. Sforza C, Laino A, D'Alessio R, Grandi G, Dellavia C, Tartaglia G, et al. Three dimensional facial morphometry of attractive Italian women. Prog Orthod. 2007;8:282–93.
12. Shaw WC, Rees G, Dawe M, Charles CR. The influence of dentofacial appearance on the social attractiveness of young adults. Am J Orthod. 1985;87(1):21–6.
13. Eubanks RJ. Surgical correction of masseter muscle hypertrophy associated with unilateral prognathism: report of case. J Oral Surg (Chic). 1957;15(1):66–9.
14. Proffit W, Severt T. The prevalence of facial asymmetry in the dentofacial deformities population at the University of North Carolina. Int J Adult Orthodon Orthognath Surg. 1997;12:171–5.
15. Kronmiller JE. Development of asymmetries. Semin Orthod. 1998;4(3):134–7.
16. Sanders DA, Chandhoke TK, Uribe FA, Rigali PH, Nanda R. Quantification of skeletal asymmetries in normal adolescents: cone-beam computed tomography analysis. Prog Orthod. 2014;15(1):26.
17. Erickson GE, Waite DE. Mandibular asymmetry. J Am Dent Assoc. 1974;89(6):1369–73.
18. Hajeer MY, Millett DT, Ayoub AF, Siebert JP. Applications of 3D imaging in orthodontics: part I. J Orthod. 2004;31(1):62–70.
19. de Moraes ME, Hollender LG, Chen CS, Moraes LC, Balducci I. Evaluating craniofacial asymmetry with digital cephalometric images and cone-beam computed tomography. Am J Orthod Dentofacial Orthop. 2011;139:e523–31.
20. Cheung G, Goonewardene MS, Islam SMS, Murray K. The validity of transverse intermaxillary analysis on traditional PAC compared to cone-beam computed tomography. Aust Orthod J. 2013;29(1):116–25.
21. Tai B, Goonewardene M, Koong B, Murray K, Islam SMS. The reliability of using posteroanterior cephalometry and cone-beam CT to determine transverse dimensions in clinical practice. Aust Orthod J. 2005;30(2):132–42.

22. Weinberg SM, Kolar JC. Three-dimensional surface imaging: limitations and considerations from the anthropometric perspective. J Craniofac Surg. 2005;16(5):847–51.
23. Chew MT. Spectrum and management of dentofacial deformities in a multiethnic Asian population. Angle Orthod. 2006;76(5):806–9.
24. Maeda M, Katsumata A, Ariji Y, Muramatsu A, Yoshida K, Goto S, et al. 3D-CT evaluation of facial asymmetry in patients with maxillofacial deformities. Oral Surg Oral Med Oral Pathol Oral Radiol Endod. 2006;102(3):382–90.
25. You KH, Lee KJ, Lee SH, Baik HS. Three-dimensional computed tomography analysis of mandibular morphology in patients with facial asymmetry and mandibular prognathism. Am J Orthod Dentofacial Orthop. 2010;138(5):540. e1-8; discussion 540–1.
26. Meyer-Marcotty P, Alpers GW, Gerdes ABM, Stellzig-Eisenhauer A. Impact of facial asymmetry in visual perception: a 3-dimensional data analysis. Am J Orthod Dentofacial Orthop. 2010;137(2):168. e1-168.e8.
27. Nanda V, Gutman B, Bar E, Alghamdi S, Tetradis S, Lusis AJ, et al. Quantitative analysis of 3-dimensional facial soft tissue photographic images: technical methods and clinical application. Prog Orthod. 2015;16:21.
28. Chiu CS, Clark RK. Reproducibility of natural head position in standing subjects. J Dent. 1991;19:130–1.
29. Lundstorm A, Lundstorm F, Lebret LM, Moorrees CF. Natural head position and natural head orientation: basic considerations in cephalometric analysis and research. Eur J Orthodontics. 1995;17:111–20.
30. Deli R, Galantucci LM, Laino A, D'Alessio R, Di Gioia E, Savastano C. Three-dimensional methodology for photogrammetric acquisition of the soft tissues of the face: a new clinical-instrumental protocol. Prog Orthod. 2013;14:32.
31. Cevidanes LH, Alhadidi A, Paniagua B, Styner M, Ludlow J, Mol A, et al. Three-dimensional quantification of mandibular asymmetry through cone-beam computerized tomography. Oral Surg Oral Med Oral Pathol Oral Radiol Endod. 2011;111(6):757–70.
32. Gavin H. The Levenberg-Marquardt method for nonlinear least squares curve-fitting Problems. Duke University: Department of Civil and Environmental Engineering; 2011.
33. Landis JR, Koch GG. The measurement of observer agreement for categorical data. Biometrics. 1977;33(1):159–74.
34. The R Core Team. R: a language and environment for statistical computing. Vienna, Austria: R Foundation for Statistical Computing; 2013. http://www.R-project.org/
35. Fuhrmann R, Feifel H, Schnappauf A, Diedrich P. Integration of three-dimensional cephalometry and 3D-skull models in combined orthodontic/surgical treatment planning. J Orofac Orthop. 1996;57(1):32–45.
36. Peck S, Peck L, Kataja M. Skeletal asymmetry in esthetically pleasing faces. Angle Orthod. 1991;Spr;61(1):43–8.
37. Djordjevic J, Toma AMT, Zhurov AI, Richmond S. Three-dimensional quantification of facial symmetry in adolescents using laser surface scanning. Eur J Orthod. 2014;36(2):125–32.
38. Ferrario VF, Sforza C, Poggio CE, Tartaglia G. Distance from symmetry: a three-dimensional evaluation of facial asymmetry. J Oral Maxillofac Surg. 1994;52(11):1126–32.
39. Miller L, Morris DO, Berry E. Visualizing three-dimensional facial soft-tissue changes following orthognathic surgery. European J Orthodontics. 2007;29(1):14–20.
40. Jayaratne YS, Zwahlen RA, Lo J, Cheung LK. Three-dimensional color maps: a novel tool for assessing craniofacial changes. Surg Innov. 2010;17(3):198–205.
41. Guest E, Berry E, Morris D. Novel methods for quantifying soft-tissue changes after orthognathic surgery. Int J Oral Maxillofac Surg. 2001;30(6):484–9.

16

Missing upper incisors: a retrospective study of orthodontic space closure versus implant

Abdolreza Jamilian[1*], Letizia Perillo[2] and Marco Rosa[3]

Abstract

Background: The aim of this retrospective study was to compare the esthetic, periodontal, and functional outcomes of orthodontic space closure versus implant substitution in patients with missing maxillary incisors 5 years after completion of treatment.

Methods: The study group consisted of ten patients treated with orthodontic space closure (six males, four females, mean age 19 ± 2.1 years at the completion of treatment) and ten patients treated with implant insertion (five males, five females, mean age 20 ± 1.4 years at the time of implant insertion). Tooth mobility, plaque index, probing depth, infraocclusion, open gingival embrasure (black triangle), and temporomandibular joint function were recorded at the 5.6 years follow-up. Self-perceived dental esthetic appearance was also evaluated through a visual analog scale (VAS) questionnaire. *T*-test was used to evaluate the data.

Results: All patients were equally satisfied with the appearance of their teeth 5.6 ± 0.4 years after the completion of treatment. No statistically significant differences were found in relation to the VAS scores of the subjects ($P < 0.857$). No significant differences were found in tooth mobility, plaque index ($P < 0.632$), and the prevalence of signs and symptoms of temporomandibular disorders. However, significant infraocclusion was noticed in all implant patients ($P < 0.001$). Probing depth was also significantly higher in implant patients ($P < 0.001$).

Conclusions: Orthodontic space closure and implant of missing maxillary incisors produced similar, well-accepted esthetic results. None of the treatments impaired temporomandibular joint function. Nevertheless, infraocclusion was evident in implant patients. Space closure patients also showed better periodontal health in comparison with implant patients.

Keywords: Implant; Orthodontic space closure; Missing maxillary incisor; Infraocclusion; Periodontal health

Background

The absence of upper incisors is a serious problem and often needs a challenging treatment. The treatment alternatives of missing upper incisors include orthodontic space closure, resin-bonded bridgework, osseointegrated implants, removable partial dentures, and autotransplantation of developing premolars [1-7]. Although each of these methods is a viable treatment option, implant insertion and space closure are more popular among clinicians.

Implant substitution is considered an optimal solution considering the possibility of obtaining an ideal occlusion and the indisputable advantage of avoiding any damage to the adjacent teeth [1,8]. Orthodontic space closure, by mesial movement of the adjacent teeth, also provides satisfactory esthetic and functional long-term results [9,5,10]. One of the major advantages of space closure is that treatment is finished immediately after orthodontics and, in the case of adolescents, there is no necessity of waiting years until the 'end of growth' to replace the missing tooth. Moreover, the result is natural and all the changes in the long term will also be natural, unlike what could happen in the presence of a foreign body.

The aim of this study was to examine and compare, 5 years post treatment, the esthetic outcomes, function, and periodontal health in two groups of subjects with one or two missing maxillary incisors and

* Correspondence: info@jamilian.net
[1]Department of Orthodontics, Dental Branch, Craniomaxillofacial Center Islamic Azad University, No 2713, Vali Asr St., Tehran 1966843133, Iran
Full list of author information is available at the end of the article

Table 1 Distribution of age, sex, and left or right missing teeth in the OSC and implant groups

Treatment group		OSC group	Implant group	Significance
Age at the time of treatment completion		19 ± 2.1	20 ± 1.4	NS
Gender	Male	6	5	NS
	Female	4	5	NS
Lateral incisor	Left	3	1	NS
	Right	4	3	NS
Central incisor	Left	4	4	NS
	Right	6	6	NS
Treatment time (months)		29 ± 7	18 ± 4	$P < 0.001$

OSC, orthodontic space closure; NS, not significant.

treated either with implant substitution or orthodontic space closure.

Methods

This retrospective observational study was carried out in accordance with the ethical standards set forth in the 1964 Declaration of Helsinki. Informed written consent was obtained from each patient and a parent or guardian.

Twenty-six patients with missing maxillary incisors, who were treated by one orthodontist between 2004 and 2006 in two centers, were all invited to a follow-up examination. One of the patients was omitted from the study because she could have only been treated by means of implant insertion. Five of the patients refused to attend. Out of the 20 remaining patients, 10 were treated by implant insertion and 10 by orthodontic space closure.

The selection criteria included patients who had the following:

- Congenital absence of the maxillary central and/or lateral incisor.
- Patients treated with orthodontic space closure and/or implant.

Table 2 Clinical records of periodontal states

Index	Assessment method
Tooth mobility	Mobility more than 1 mm was recorded
Probing depth	Pockets exceeding 3 mm were recorded
Infraocclusion	Infraocclusion exceeding 1 mm was recorded
TMD	Tooth clenching, grinding, and TMJ sounds were recorded

TMD, temporomandibular joint dysfunction; TMJ, temporomandibular joint.

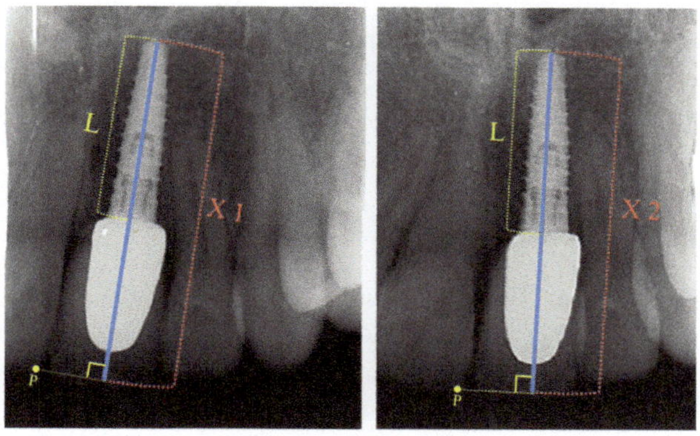

Figure 1 Method of measuring infraocclusion.

- Patients who could have been treated by either space closure or implant insertion.
- Patients not treated with autotransplantation or crown bridge.
- No periodontal breakdown or history of periodontal disease.

The implant group (IG) consisted of ten patients (five males, five females, mean age 20 ± 1.4 years at the time of implant insertion). All the implants were of the same type and were inserted by the same surgeon. Fourteen teeth including four lateral and ten central maxillary incisors were totally missing in the implant group. The average treatment time of these patients was 18 ± 4 months. The orthodontic space closure (OSC) group consisted of ten patients (six males, four females, mean age 19 ± 2.1 years at the completion of treatment). Seventeen teeth including

Table 3 Questionnaire for assessing TMD

Severity of occurrence	0	1	2	3
1. Do you have difficulty in opening your mouth?				
2. Do you have difficulty in moving or using your jaw?				
3. Do you have tenderness or muscular pain when chewing?				
4. Do you have frequent headaches?				
5. Do you have neck aches or shoulder pain?				
6. Do you have pain in or about the ears?				
7. Are you aware of noises in the jaw joints?				
8. Do you consider your bite "normal"?				
9. Do you use only one side of your mouth when chewing?				
10. Do you have morning facial pain?				

Table 4 Comparison of parameters between implant and space closure groups

Recorded scores	Tooth mobility (number of teeth)	Probing depth (number of teeth)	Infraocclusion (number of teeth)	Plaque index (mean ± SD)	TMD (mean ± SD)
Implant group	1	12	14	3.1 ± 1.2	1.3 ± 1.1
OSC group	0	3	0	2.9 ± 1.1	1.5 ± 1.03
P value	NS	0.001*	0.001*	0.632	0.605

*Level of significance set at $P < 0.05$. TMD, temporomandibular joint dysfunction; SD, standard deviation; OSC, orthodontic space closure.

seven lateral and ten central maxillary incisors were totally missing in the OSC group. The average treatment time of these patients was 29 ± 7 months (Table 1). For retention, upper and lower Hawley retainers were worn by all the patients for 1 year.

The follow-up records were taken 5 years or more after the completion of treatment (mean interval was 5.6 ± 0.4 years).

Tooth mobility (TM) [11], plaque index (PI) [12,13], probing depth (PD), infraocclusion (I), open gingival embrasure (black triangle) [14], and temporomandibular joint dysfunction (TMD) of the patients were recorded at the follow-up examinations (Table 2).

Probing depth was recorded at four sites for each upper central and lateral incisor with a periodontal probe. Identical intra-oral radiographs, taken with the 'parallel technique', were used for assessment of infraocclusion. Evaluation of the image distortion was done by measuring the length of the implant (L) as it appears on the radiography and comparing it to the real length of the implant (Figure 1). In order to evaluate infraocclusion, a reference point (p) was selected on the intersection between the incisal and mesial borders of the tooth adjacent to the implant. Afterwards, a line was drawn from this point perpendicular to the longitudinal axis of the implant creating the projection of p. The distance between the projection of p and the apex of the implant was measured, and the difference between this distance after the completion of treatment and follow-up examination was recorded as infraocclusion ($X2 - X1$) (Figure 1). The distance of the alveolar crest to the contact point of the teeth was used to evaluate the presence of an open embrasure (black triangle). A distance of more than 5 mm was considered as black triangle [14].

The prevalence of signs and symptoms of TMD was assessed by means of an anamnestic questionnaire [15] (Table 3). A score '0' indicated the absence of symptoms, whereas '1' was given for a report of an occasional occurrence. Grade 2 indicated the presence of symptoms, and a score of '3' was used to indicate severe pain or bilateral symptoms. The sum of the scores was used to classify the sample into four categories: (1) from 0 to 3, TMD free; (2) from 4 to 8, mild TMD; (3) from 9 to 14, moderate TMD; and (4) from 15 to 23, severe TMD. Plaque was measured by the plaque index developed by Quigley and Hein [12] and modified by Turesky et al. [13]. The scoring system is as follows: 0 = no plaque, 1 = separate flecks of plaque at the cervical margin of the tooth, 2 = a thin continuous band of plaque at the cervical margin, 3 = a band of plaque wider than 1 mm but covering less than one third of the crown, 4 = plaque covering at least one third but less than two thirds of the crown, 5 = plaque covering two thirds or more of the crown. None of the patients had systemic diseases or long-term pharmacological treatment until the end of follow-up studies.

Patient satisfaction was assessed using the visual analog scale (VAS) [16,17]. The subjects were asked to record their happiness with their dental and facial appearance on a 10-cm VAS having phrases 'very dissatisfied' (score 0) on the left end and 'very satisfied' (score 10) on the right end.

Each patient was examined by two examiners in two sessions with an interval of 1 week. The inter-examiner agreement was calculated through kappa analysis. A kappa value of 0.96 showed perfect agreement. *T*-test was used to evaluate the data of the study.

Results

Tables 4 and 5 show the results 5.6 ± 0.4 years after treatment. Increased mobility was noticed in only one implant, but no tooth mobility was present in any of the OSC patients. More than 3 mm increase of probing depth was found in 12 implants, while it increased more than 3 mm in only 3 teeth in the OSC group ($P < 0.001$). The vertical step measured on radiographs of implant patients varied between 1.2 and 1.6 mm, which showed that all implant-supported teeth had increased infraocclusion of more than 1 mm, while none of the OSC patients showed infraocclusion ($P < 0.001$) (Figure 1). Black triangle was seen in one of the implant patients and three of the OSC patients.

Table 5 Patient satisfaction assessed by visual analog scale (VAS) after 5 years since the completion of treatment

	Implant group Mean ± SD	OSC group Mean ± SD	*P* value
VAS scores	8.7 ± 1.3	8.8 ± 1.2	0.857

OSC, orthodontic space closure; SD, standard deviation.

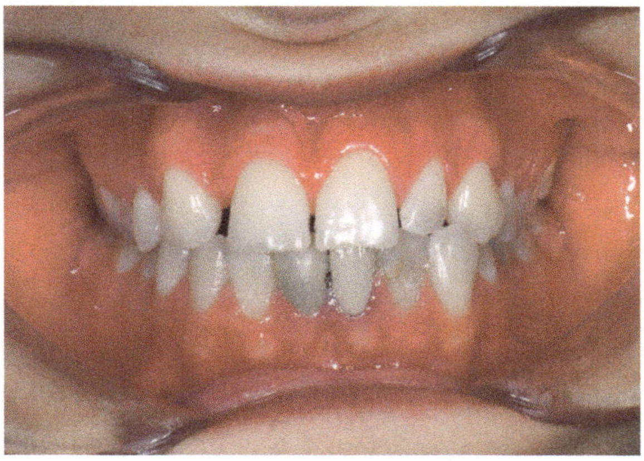

Figure 2 A patient with a missing maxillary lateral incisor.

No signs and symptoms of temporomandibular joint dysfunction including history of headache, locking, difficulty in opening/closing mouth, and tooth clenching were noticed in any of the patients, and *T*-test showed that there were no statistically significant differences between the two groups ($P < 0.605$). Five years after the completion of treatment, the plaque indexes of the implant and OSC patients were 3.1 ± 1.2 and 2.9 ± 1.1, respectively ($P < 0.632$) (Table 4).

VAS scores of 8.7 ± 1.3 and 8.8 ± 1.2 were recorded for the implant and OSC patients, subjectively. The scores which ranged from 7 to 10 showed that both groups were almost equally satisfied with the appearance of their teeth after 5 years. *T*-test did not show any statistically significant difference between the two groups (Table 5).

Figures 2 and 3 show a patient with a missing upper lateral incisor, and Figures 4 and 5 show the same patient 5 years after implant insertion. Figures 6 and 7 show a patient with missing maxillary lateral incisors treated by orthodontic space closure, and Figures 8 and 9 show the same patient 5 years after the completion of treatment.

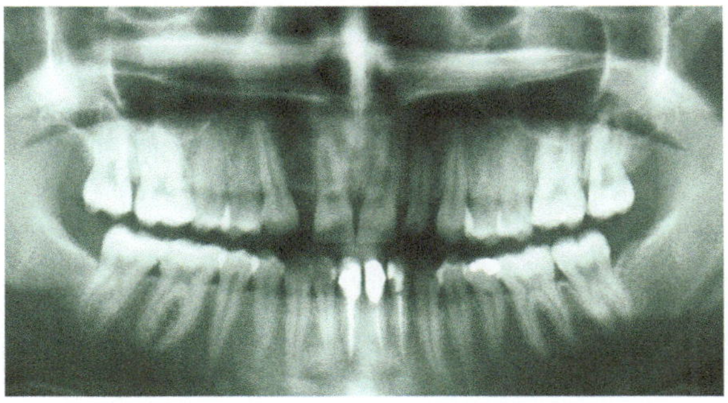

Figure 3 Panoramic radiograph of the same patient with a missing maxillary lateral incisor.

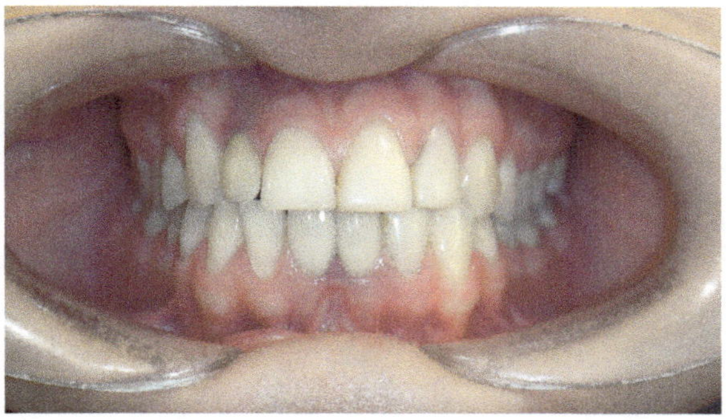

Figure 4 The same patient 5 years after implant insertion.

Discussion

The present retrospective study shows that both treatment modalities resulted in satisfactory and well-accepted esthetic outcomes after 5 years. However, infraocclusion and increased probing depth were seen in the implant patients.

These findings correspond to the findings of Bernard et al. [18], Kuijpers et al. [19], and Jemt et al. [20] who reported that even if the implant is inserted after 19 years of age, the adjacent teeth and surrounding alveolar bone may continue to develop vertically and may continue to erupt resulting in infraocclusion of the implant restoration, i.e., a discrepancy between the gingival margin of the implant restoration and the gingival margin of the adjacent natural teeth may appear in a few years after treatment, and the implant becomes submerged. In cases where the upper and lower incisors are not in contact, the resulted extrusion might be 0/2 to 0/3 mm per year. Implants behave like ankylosed teeth, and their position cannot change in contrast to their neighboring natural teeth; therefore, even small tooth movements of adjacent teeth after implant placement can cause esthetic problems [21-23]. The disharmonious levels of the gingival margins resulting from infra-positioned implant restorations are an evident disadvantage in patients with a high smile line. Thus, 'gummy smile', or patients who show the gingival margins, is in our opinion a contraindication for implant substitution of the upper incisors [5].

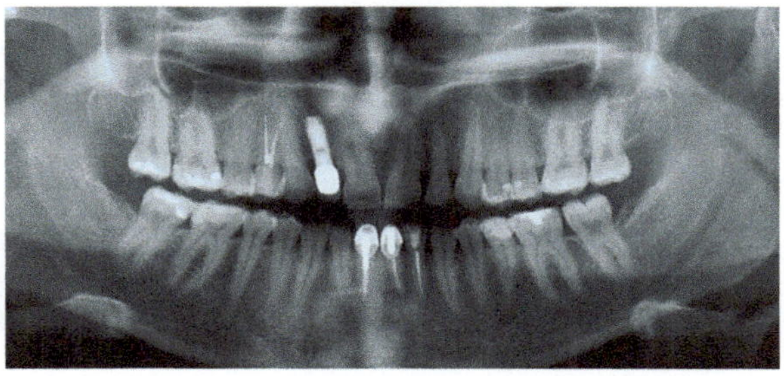

Figure 5 Panoramic radiograph of the same patient 5 years after implant insertion.

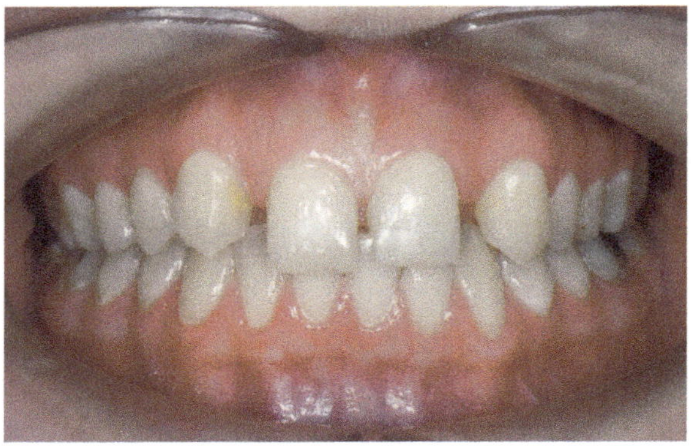

Figure 6 A patient with missing maxillary lateral incisors.

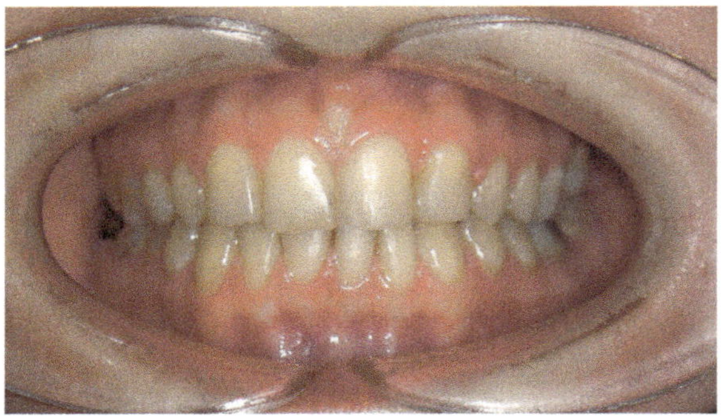

Figure 8 The same patient 5 years after orthodontic space closure.

Implant substitution could have other disadvantages. It has been shown that most implant crowns show some lack of interdental papillary fill, particularly on the distal papilla [24]. Furthermore, blue coloring of the labial gingiva has been reported in above more than 50% of single-implant crowns at 4-year follow-ups [25]. Peri-implantitis, gingivitis, increased probing depth, bleeding on probing, and progressive loss of marginal bone support at the buccal aspect of the implant have also been reported in implants [22,24,26,27].

Finally, the biggest disadvantage of the implant alternative is that adolescents must wait many years after orthodontic treatment before the implant insertion. During this interim time, patients must use temporary restorations that often create many different problems and replacements. Nevertheless, the comparatively shorter and easier treatment makes implants a favorable treatment option for substituting missing teeth.

In contrast to the abovementioned disadvantages related to implants, orthodontic space closure is a viable and safe procedure that could provide better long-term results [9]. Moreover, none of the abovementioned disadvantages have been noticed in orthodontic space closure [28,29]. Nevertheless, the applicability of orthodontic space closure for missing incisors is sometimes questioned. Concerns may be expressed related to the treatment complexity, the risk for space reopening, the questioned increased functional load on the first premolar roots, and the quality of the esthetic result especially in the case of a lateral incisor's root supporting the larger crown of a central incisor [30].

The main advantages of the space closure alternative compared to implants can be highlighted as follows:

- Treatment is finished immediately after orthodontics. This is for crucial interest when treating adolescent patients.
- Periodontal problems will not develop in space closure because the tooth has moved along with its bone and surrounding tissues.
- Space closure provides patients with better long-term esthetic results in the transition area, due to lack of bone loss and periodontal problems.
- Prosthetic replacement of the lost incisor also by partial denture or bonded bridges could need further treatments to replace the restorations or to fix possible periodontal breakdown.

Allocation of patients in this study and comparing their treatment effects could be considered as one of the weaknesses of the current study because the patients were allocated to the implant or the OSC group based on the space between their teeth. However, it should be considered that the results of the current study can assist in treatment

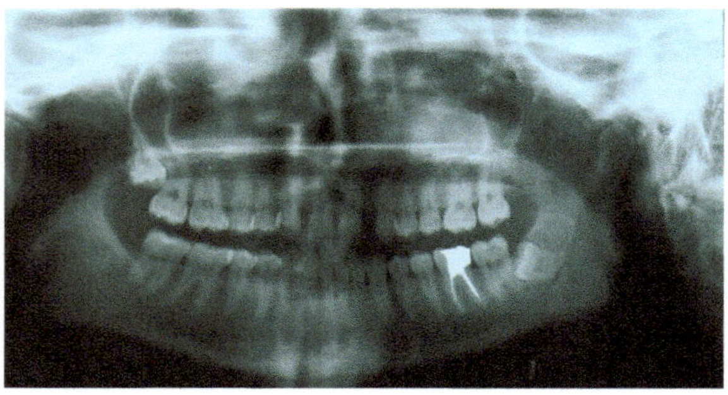

Figure 7 Panoramic radiograph of the same patient with missing maxillary lateral incisors.

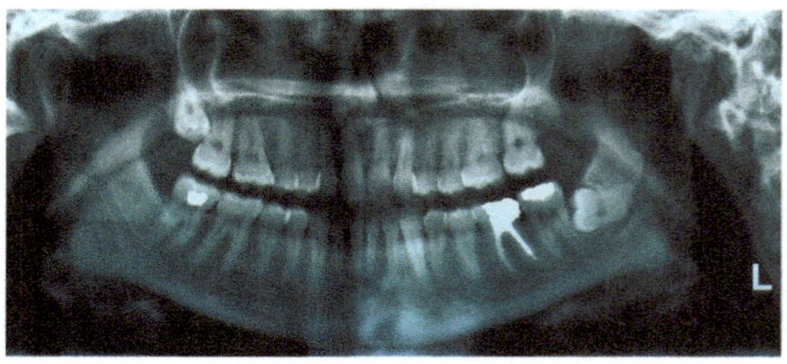

Figure 9 Panoramic radiograph of the same patient 5 years after orthodontic space closure.

planning for borderline cases who could be treated by either implant insertion or orthodontic space closure.

Conclusions

Five years after treatment, orthodontic space closure and implant substitution of missing maxillary incisors produced similar satisfactory esthetic results. Neither of the treatments impaired temporomandibular joint function. However, orthodontic space closure patients had better periodontal health in comparison with implant substitution patients. Furthermore, infraocclusion more than 1 mm was noticed in all the implant patients.

Competing interests

The authors declare that they have no competing interests.

Authors' contributions

AJ was responsible for the study design, administration, recruitment and treatment, drafting, writing and revising the report, critical revision, and final approval of the article. MR and LP were responsible for the study concept, analysis, data interpretation, critical revision, and final approval of the article. AJ is the guarantor. All authors read and approved the final manuscript.

Author details

[1]Department of Orthodontics, Dental Branch, Craniomaxillofacial Center Islamic Azad University, No 2713, Vali Asr St., Tehran 1966843133, Iran. [2]Post Graduate Orthodontic Program, Department of Orthodontics, Second University of Naples, Via bellini, 44 80135, Naples, Italy. [3]Post-graduate School in Orthodontics, Insubria University, P.za della Mostra, 19 38122, Trento, Italy.

References

1. Rupp RP, Dillehay JK, Squire CF. Orthodontics, prosthodontics, and periodontics: a multidisciplinary approach. Gen Dent. 1997;45(3):286–9.
2. Ghassemi M, Jamilian A, Fritz U, Riediger D, Ghassemi A. Orthodontic treatment after autotransplantation. Angle Orthod. 2011;81(4):721–5. doi:10.2319/102210-617.1.
3. Zachrisson BU, Stenvik A, Haanaes HR. Management of missing maxillary anterior teeth with emphasis on autotransplantation. Am J Orthod Dentofacial Orthop. 2004;126(3):284–8. doi:10.1016/S0889540604005244.
4. Rosa M, Olimpo A, Fastuca R, Caprioglio A. Perceptions of dental professionals and laypeople to altered dental esthetics in cases with congenitally missing maxillary lateral incisors. Prog Orthod. 2013;14:34. doi:10.1186/2196-1042-14-34.
5. Zachrisson BU, Rosa M, Toreskog S. Congenitally missing maxillary lateral incisors: canine substitution. Point. Am J Orthod Dentofacial Orthop. 2011;139(4):434, 436, 438 passim. doi:10.1016/j.ajodo.2011.02.003.
6. Showkatbakhsh R, Jamilian A. Opening or closing space for replacing upper incisors. Two case reports. Rev Esp Orthod. 2010;40:181–5.
7. Johal A, Katsaros C, Kuijpers-Jagtman AM, Angle Society of Europe membership. State of the science on controversial topics: missing maxillary lateral incisors–a report of the Angle Society of Europe 2012 meeting. Prog Orthod. 2013;14:20. doi:10.1186/2196-1042-14-20.
8. Zachrisson BU. Planning esthetic treatment after avulsion of maxillary incisors. J Am Dent Assoc. 2008;139(11):1484–90.
9. Nordquist GG, McNeill RW. Orthodontic vs. restorative treatment of the congenitally absent lateral incisor–long term periodontal and occlusal evaluation. J Periodontol. 1975;46(3):139–43. doi:10.1902/jop.1975.46.3.139.
10. Robertsson S, Mohlin B. The congenitally missing upper lateral incisor. A retrospective study of orthodontic space closure versus restorative treatment. Eur J Orthod. 2000;22(6):697–710.
11. Mombelli A, van Oosten MA, Schurch Jr E, Land NP. The microbiota associated with successful or failing osseointegrated titanium implants. Oral Microbiol Immunol. 1987;2(4):145–51.
12. Quigley GA, Hein JW. Comparative cleansing efficiency of manual and power brushing. J Am Dent Assoc. 1962;65:26–9.
13. Turesky S, Gilmore ND, Glickman I. Reduced plaque formation by the chloromethyl analogue of victamine C. J Periodontol. 1970;41(1):41–3. doi:10.1902/jop.1970.41.41.41.
14. Sharma AA, Park JH. Esthetic considerations in interdental papilla: remediation and regeneration. J Esthet Restor Dent. 2010;22(1):18–28. doi:10.1111/j.1708-8240.2009.00307.x.
15. Conti A, Freitas M, Conti P, Henriques J, Janson G. Relationship between signs and symptoms of temporomandibular disorders and orthodontic treatment: a cross-sectional study. Angle Orthod. 2003;73(4):411–7. doi:10.1043/0003-3219(2003)073<0411:RBSASO>2.0.CO;2.
16. O'Neill K, Harkness M, Knight R. Ratings of profile attractiveness after functional appliance treatment. Am J Orthod Dentofac Orthop. 2000;118(4):371–6. doi:10.1067/mod.2000.109492; discussion 7.
17. Schabel BJ, McNamara Jr JA, Franchi L, Baccetti T. Q-sort assessment vs visual analog scale in the evaluation of smile esthetics. Am J Orthod Dentofac Orthop. 2009;135(4 Suppl):S61–71. doi:10.1016/j.ajodo.2007.08.019.
18. Bernard JP, Schatz JP, Christou P, Belser U, Kiliaridis S. Long-term vertical changes of the anterior maxillary teeth adjacent to single implants in young and mature adults. A retrospective study. J Clin Periodontol. 2004;31(11):1024–8. doi:10.1111/j.1600-051X.2004.00574.x.
19. Kuijpers MA, de Lange J, van Gool AV. [Maxillofacial growth and dental implants in the maxillary anterior region]. Ned Tijdschr Tandheelkd. 2006;113(4):130–3.
20. Jemt T, Ahlberg G, Henriksson K, Bondevik O. Changes of anterior clinical crown height in patients provided with single-implant restorations after more than 15 years of follow-up. Int J Prosthodont. 2006;19(5):455–61.
21. Spear FM, Mathews DM, Kokich VG. Interdisciplinary management of single-tooth implants. Semin Orthod. 1997;3(1):45–72.
22. Thilander B, Odman J, Lekholm U. Orthodontic aspects of the use of oral implants in adolescents: a 10-year follow-up study. Eur J Orthod. 2001;23(6):715–31.
23. Oesterle LJ, Cronin Jr RJ. Adult growth, aging, and the single-tooth implant. Int J Oral Maxillofac Implants. 2000;15(2):252–60.
24. Chang M, Wennstrom JL, Odman P, Andersson B. Implant supported single-tooth replacements compared to contralateral natural teeth. Crown and soft tissue dimensions. Clin Oral Implants Res. 1999;10(3):185–94.
25. Dueled E, Gotfredsen K, Trab Damsgaard M, Hede B. Professional and patient-based evaluation of oral rehabilitation in patients with tooth agenesis. Clin Oral Implants Res. 2009;20(7):729–36. doi:10.1111/j.1600-0501.2008.01698.x.
26. Fransson C, Wennstrom J, Tomasi C, Berglundh T. Extent of peri-implantitis-associated bone loss. J Clin Periodontol. 2009;36(4):357–63. doi:10.1111/j.1600-051X.2009.01375.x.
27. Paolantonio M, D'Ercole S, Pilloni A, D'Archivio D, Lisanti L, Graziani F, et al. Clinical, microbiologic, and biochemical effects of subgingival administration of a Xanthan-based chlorhexidine gel in the treatment of periodontitis: a randomized multicenter trial. J Periodontol. 2009;80(9):1479–92. doi:10.1902/jop.2009.090050.
28. Rosa M, Zachrisson BU. Integrating space closure and esthetic dentistry in patients with missing maxillary lateral incisors. J Clin Orthod. 2007;41(9):563–73. quiz 424.
29. Thordarson A, Zachrisson BU, Mjor IA. Remodeling of canines to the shape of lateral incisors by grinding: a long-term clinical and radiographic evaluation. Am J Orthod Dentofac Orthop. 1991;100(2):123–32.
30. Czochrowska EM, Skaare AB, Stenvik A, Zachrisson BU. Outcome of orthodontic space closure with a missing maxillary central incisor. Am J Orthod Dentofac Orthop. 2003;123(6):597–603. doi:10.1016/S0889540603000544.

17

Sagittal and vertical effects of transverse sagittal maxillary expander (TSME) in three different malocclusion groups

Cinzia Maspero[1], Guido Galbiati[1], Lucia Giannini[1] and Giampietro Farronato[2,3*]

Abstract

Background: The aim of this retrospective study was to cephalometrically evaluate the skeletal and dental effects of the transverse sagittal maxillary expander (TSME), for the correction of sagittal and transverse maxillary deficiency in class I, II, and III malocclusions.

Methods: The sample for this retrospective study included 45 patients (mean age, 8.4 years; 26 females, 19 males; 15 skeletal class I subjects, 15 skeletal class II subjects, and 15 skeletal class III subjects) with maxillary bilateral cross-bite.

For each patient, a lateral cephalogram was obtained before treatment and at the end of the retention period. Changes in the groups during the observation period were calculated, compared, and statistically analyzed with a *t*-test.

Results: The cephalometric values before T0 and T1 showed significant changes.

Conclusions: The TSME can produce skeletal changes due to the transverse force and sagittal effects on the maxillary alveolar process. These modifications have benefic effects in classes I, II, and III. The data obtained in this study permit us to underline the fact that TSME can be used in all of the skeletal classes, with good vertical and sagittal results.

Keywords: Rapid maxillary expansion; Maxillary hypoplasia; Hyrax expander; Transverse sagittal maxillary expander

Background

Rapid maxillary expansion (RME) is widely used when transverse maxillary deficiency is diagnosed [1-3]. RME not only separates the midpalatal suture but also affects the circumzygomatic and circummaxillary sutural system [3,4]. It has been reported that opening of the midpalatal suture has vertical and sagittal effects on both of the jaws [3]. In 1970, Haas showed marked alteration in growth direction and facial morphology as a result of orthopedic therapy [5]. Many authors found that [5-8] the maxilla is frequently displaced downward and forward during maxillary expansion, while others found only an anterior movement after RME [9,10].

Da Silva et al. confirmed that the maxilla did not show any statistically significant modifications in the sagittal position over the period of activation of the appliance, while it displayed a tendency to rotate downward and backward, increasing the SN-PP angle value [1]. However, Wertz and Dreskin found no significant change in the angulations of the palate with RME therapy [8]. Cleall found unfavorable effects in patients with a well-positioned maxilla reporting that in the retention period it generally returns to its original position [11]. McNamara, in 1993, stated that widening the maxilla led to a spontaneous forward posturing of the mandible during the retention period, correcting the mild class II relationship. He held that it is important to consider the transverse plane prior to the diagnosis of a class II malocclusion [12,13]. The relationship between the transverse

* Correspondence: giampietro.farronato@unimi.it
[2]Maxillo-Facial and Odontostomatology Unit Fondazione Cà Granda IRCCS Ospedale Maggiore Policlinico, University of Milan, 20122 Milan, Italy
[3]UOC Chirurgia Maxillofacciale e Odontostomatologia, Fondazione IRCCS Cà Granda - Ospedale Maggiore Policlinico, University of Milan, Commenda 10, Milano 20122, Italy
Full list of author information is available at the end of the article

dimension and the correction of class II malocclusion was described in 1971 by Reichenbach and Taatz that prove the relationship between the improvement in transverse palatal diameter and the correction of sagittal intermaxillary relationships [14]. In 1889, Kingsley underlined this phenomenon, pointing out how the transverse expansion could favor mandible advancement [15]. This example allows to understand how palatal transverse expansion solves spontaneous mandible repositioning in a forward position, solving or improving sagittal malocclusion. Some authors underlined that in comparing skeletal class I patients with skeletal class II division II patients who have not been orthodontically treated, the second group presents a maxillary and mandible transverse diameter reduction [16].

Many authors observed that maxillary expansion has different effects in class I, II, and III malocclusions [3,17-22]. In the retrospective studies of Farronato et al. on 15 growing subjects with maxillary hypoplasia, the effects of RME in the three planes of space were investigated. The cephalometric tracings were analyzed before and after treatment and at the end of the retention period. The results of their study confirmed widening of the maxilla in the transverse plane and an increase in the floor of the nose. In the sagittal plane, different effects were observed in class I, II, and III subjects [23,24]. In class I patients, ANB angle was slightly affected, while in all class II subjects, it decreased due to forwarding positioning of the mandible, confirming that orthopedic force to the maxillary complex during the early phase of growth can contribute to the correction of class II malocclusions.

The aim of this retrospective study was to cephalometrically evaluate the skeletal and dental effects of the transverse sagittal maxillary expander (TSME), for the correction of sagittal and transverse maxillary deficiency in class I, II, and III malocclusions [25].

Methods

The sample for this retrospective study included 45 patients (mean age, 8.4 years; 26 females, 19 males; 15 skeletal class I subjects, 15 skeletal class II subjects, and 15 skeletal class III subjects) with maxillary bilateral cross-bite in mixed or permanent dentition.

The inclusion criteria were as follows:

- Caucasian ethnicity;
- No history of orthodontic treatment;
- Growing patients;
- Pretreatment and posttreatment lateral X-ray with excellent contrast;
- Transverse maxillary deficiency (at least 8 mm);
- Sagittal maxillary hypoplasia
- Presence of bilateral posterior cross-bite.

Exclusion criteria were as follows:

- Congenital anomalies;
- Previous orthodontic treatment;
- Dental anomalies

Lateral cephalograms were taken by the same technician [C.R.] with the same machine and manually traced by one operator [L.G.] and verified for landmark location and anatomic contours by a second operator [C.M.]. Any disagreements were solved by retracing the landmark or structure to the mutual satisfaction of both operators.

To exclude intra-operator error, each measurement was repeated by the same operator after a period of 7 days.

The method error was determined using Dahlberg's formula $ME = \sqrt{\Sigma d^2/2n}$, where n is the number of subjects and d is the difference between the two measures. The method error did not exceed 0.1 mm for the linear measurements and 0.2° for angular measurements.

Lateral cephalograms were traced by using acetate papers. A lateral cephalogram was taken before treatment (T0) and a second one was taken after retention (T1).

The assessment of the skeletal relationship was based on SNA-SNB, ANB SN^SNP.SNA, SN^GO.GN, S^GO, SNP.SNA^GO.GN, I^SN, and I^FH angles. N-Me and SNP-A were also analyzed.

Class I patients were considered if their ANB angles were between 0° and 4°, class II patients were considered if their ANB angles were greater than 4°, and class III patients were considered if their ANB angles were less than 0°.

All the patients were treated by a TSME (Figure 1), a modification of the Hyrax RME, to correct the transverse and sagittal dimensions [25].

The TSME is a fixed device designed to develop arch form in patients with constricted dental arches. It is specifically designed for transverse and anteroposterior arch development. The TSME consists of two bands cemented to the right and left I maxillary molars, a Hyrax-type transverse expansion screw, two .045′′ stainless steel wires extending to the palatal surfaces of the central incisors, and two 8-mm Hyrax-type screws attached to these wires between the molar bands and the incisors. The appliance may also be worn in association with extraoral devices.

The appliance was worn from 8 to 12 months. The protocol of activation consisted in the first phase of activation of the transverse screw one quarter turn twice a day until the desired amount of transverse diameter was obtained. In the second phase, the sagittal screws were activated one quarter turn every 15 days for 6 to 8 months. Then, the appliance was left in place for 4 months of passive retention.

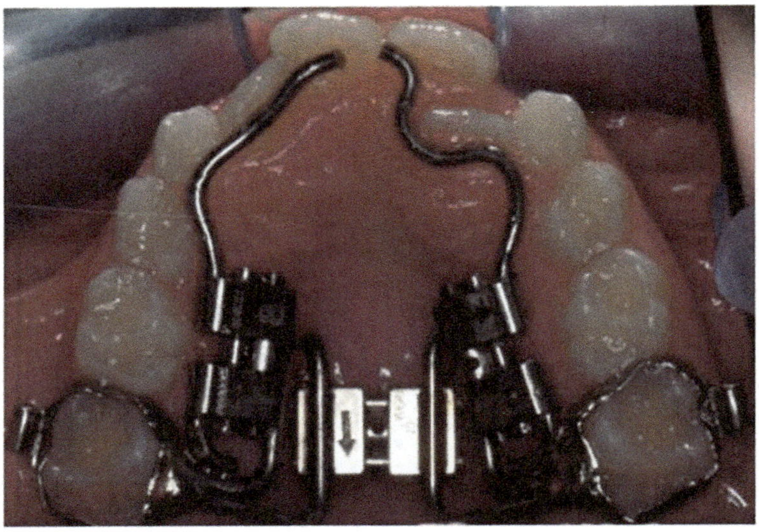

Figure 1 TSME appliance.

Changes in the cephalometric values during the observation period were calculated and compared.

Descriptive statistics included means and standard deviations (SD). The mean differences in cephalometric measurements before treatment (T0) and after retention period (T1) were examined.

No other treatment took place during the period from T0 to T1 which was the entire first phase treatment.

Statistical analysis has been done using *t*-test for paired samples after checking the normality of the distribution of the data and equality of variances. Statistical significance has been considered for $p < 0.05$.

Results

Measurements from T0 and T1 in lateral cephalograms for each group are shown in Tables 1, 2, and 3. The cephalometric values before T0 and T1 showed significant changes.

Changes in class I patients

The TSME procedures induced statistically significant modifications in the following cephalometric measurements:

- SNA (+0.10)
- SNB (+0.63)
- SN-SNP.SNA (+0.70)
- SNP.A (+2.26)
- I-SN (+2.55)
- I-FH (+2.97)

SNA increased as a result of an anterior movement of the dentoalveolar maxillary process.

The increase in SNB was due to a forward position of the mandible.

The increase of SN-SNP.SNA resulted in a downward and backward rotation of the palatal plane. SNP-A showed a statistically significant increase as well as the I^SN and I^FH angles. These results were obtained by the activation of the lateral screws during active growth which contribute to the forward movement of the dentoalveolar process and the labial movement of the incisors. SN-Go.Gn and N-Me did not show relevant modifications.

Changes in class II patients

In class II patients, the TSME procedures induced statistically significant modifications in the following measurements:

- SNB (+1.73)
- ANB (−1.36)
- SN-SNP.SNA (+1.02)
- S.GO (+0.53)
- SNP.A (+3.04)
- I-SN (+3.20)
- I-FH (+3.11)

The increase in SNB was due to a forward position of the mandible. The ANB angle decreased statistically as a result of the forward position of the mandible, improving the skeletal class, and the backward rotation of the palatal plane. In fact, as described for class I patients, the increase in SN-SNP.SNA resulted in a downward and backward rotation of the palatal plane. No increase in the anterior vertical dimension was noted, but a mild decrease in N-Me was noted (20.24) (Table 2). SNP-A, I^SN, and I^FH angles showed a statistically significant increase indicating that the dentoalveolar maxillary process moved anteriorly, because of the force delivered

Table 1 Changes in class I patients

	Pre										Post									
	SNA (°)	SNB (°)	ANB (°)	SN-SNPSNA (°)	SN-GOGN (°)	N.Me	S.GO	SNP.A	I.SN (°)	I.FH (°)	SNA	SNB	ANB	SN-SNPSNA	SN-GOGN	N.Me	S.GO	SNP.A	I.SN (°)	I.FH (°)
Average	80.16	78.06	2.1	9.73	33	111.01	64.63	46.34	99.87	112.04	80.26	78.7	1.73	10.43	33.36	111.35	65.02	48.6	102.41	115.01
st.dev.	1.41	1.54	0.89	1.7	4.42	4.28	4.69	4.14	4.32	2.28	1.79	1.75	1.22	1.88	4.23	2.87	4.25	2.05	115.01	2.03
st.anal.	S	S	NS	S	NS	NS	NS	S	S	S										

st.dev., standard deviation; st.anal., statistical analysis; S, significant; NS, not significant.

Table 2 Changes in class II patients

	Pre										Post									
	SNA (°)	SNB (°)	ANB (°)	SN-SNPSNA (°)	SN-GOGN (°)	N.Me	S.GO	SNP.A	I.SN (°)	I.FH (°)	SNA	SNB	ANB	SN-SNPSNA	SN-GOGN	N.Me	S.GO	SNP.A	I.SN (°)	I.FH (°)
Average	79.6	73.93	5.66	9.91	31.23	111.91	65.02	45.56	100.03	110.4	79.96	75.66	4.3	10.93	32.01	110.62	65.55	48.6	103.23	113.51
st.dev.	1.84	1.9	0.77	2.08	2.55	3.67	1.4	3.11	4.82	4.02	1.56	1.27	1.44	1.85	2.54	3.56	1.49	2.98	2.67	3.2
st.anal.	NS	S	S	S	NS	NS	S	S	S	S										

st.dev., standard deviation; st.anal., statistical analysis; S, significant; NS, not significant.

Table 3 Changes in class III patients

	Pre										Post									
	SNA (°)	SNB (°)	ANB (°)	SN-SNPSNA (°)	SN-GOGN (°)	N.Me	S.GO	SNP.A	I.SN (°)	I.FH (°)	SNA	SNB	ANB	SN-SNPSNA	SN-GOGN	N.Me	S.GO	SNP.A	I.SN (°)	I.FH (°)
Average	78.33	81.36	−3.03	9.4	34.26	111.48	64.31	43.26	100.07	109.4	79.2	79.86	−0.66	10.46	34.53	111.71	64.66	47.21	103.07	113.3
st.dev.	2.15	1.83	1.32	2.33	2.32	1.96	2.14	1.83	3.87	2.37	2.23	2.09	1.47	2.22	4.37	1.54	2.21	3.08	2.52	2
st.anal.	S	S	S	S	NS	NS	NS	S	S	S										

st.dev., standard deviation; st.anal., statistical analysis; S, significant; NS, not significant.

by the sagittal screws and the labial movement of the incisors during active growth.

Changes in class III patients

The TSME procedures induced statistically significant alterations in the following cephalometric measurements:

- SNA (+0.87)
- SNB (−1.50)
- ANB (+2.37)
- SN-SNP.SNA (+1.06)
- SNP.A (+3.95)
- I-SN (+3.00)
- I-FH (+3.90)

SNA increased as a result of an anterior movement of the dentoalveolar maxillary process.

SNB decreased as a result of the downward and backward rotation of the mandible. The increase in SNA angle and the decrease in SNB angle contributed to the improvement of ANB, which increased in a statistically significant manner. A downward and backward displacement of the palatal plane (SN-SNP.SNA) was observed. A mild increase in the anterior total facial height, N-Me, was also noted, but not statistically, and this caused the downward and backward rotation of the mandible (Table 3). SNP-A and I^SN and I^FH showed a statistically significant increase due to the forward movement of the dentoalveolar process and the labial movement of the incisors.

Comparison between the three groups

In all of the three groups, SNP-A, I^SN, and I^FH angles showed a statistically significant increase. These results were obtained by the activation of the lateral screws which contribute to the forward movement of the dentoalveolar process and the labial movement of the incisors. Also, SN-SNP.SNA angle increases in all the groups.

ANB showed a different statistically significant variation among the groups.

In class II patients, ANB decreased, while in class III patients, it increased. No statistically significant modifications were found in class I.

SNA increased in a statistically significant manner in class I and III patients.

SNB increased in a statistically significant manner in class II patients and decreased in class III patients. No statistically significant modifications were found for class I.

No statistically significant differences were found in the anterior (N-Me, SN-Go.Gn, and SNP.SNA-GoGn) vertical dimension in any of the three groups.

The posterior vertical dimension (S-Go) remained stable in classes I and III and increased in class II.

Discussion

Maxillary expansion is indicated in subjects with maxillary narrowness, and it is generally used to increase arch length. Sagittal arch development is indicated when the arch form is constricted since it helps resolve anterior crowding and proclination of the incisors. Labial movement of the anterior teeth may be combined with transverse development of the buccal segments where indicated [26,27].

The TSME is specifically designed for antero-posterior and transverse development. In this study, sagittal and vertical modifications in class I, II, and III growing patients were found after TSME procedures.

Significant modifications were found in the antero-posterior position of the maxillary alveolar process. This change occurred as a result of opening of the mid-palatal suture, bending and movement of the alveolar process anteriorly, and tipping of the incisors [28,29].

In this study, in class II patients, a statistically significant decrease in the ANB angle was obtained during treatment as a result of a statistically significant increase in the SNB angle. These data indicate that in skeletal class II subjects, the constricted maxillary bone impedes physiological sagittal mandibular growth. When the maxillary bone cannot develop normally in the transverse plane as a result of an anomalous function (tongue position, oral breathing), it enhances its development in the vertical plane, with a consequent backward and downward position of the mandible and insufficient and abnormal growth of the nasal septum, which is often deviated. Palatal expansion increases transverse maxillary diameter and releases the mandible, which gains a correct sagittal position. In addition, also the vestibular movement of the upper incisors permits a greater amount of mandibular advancement [30].

The data permit us to underline that class II malocclusions have a strong transverse component. In fact, the expansion of the maxilla disrupts the occlusion determining a slight forward position of the mandible, improving the sagittal occlusal relationship. McNamara suggested that the teeth themselves act as an endogenous functional appliance, encouraging a change in mandibular posture and subsequently a change in the maxillary-mandibular occlusal relationship [12]. According to the same author, this phenomenon usually happens during the first 6 to 12 months of the post-RME period as a result of the gradual repositioning of the lower jaw. Data obtained in this study confirm this theory. In a recent study, Volk et al. concluded that maxillary expansion does not predictably improve dental class II relationship. However, in the study in which 13 class II patients treated by RME were considered, 7 of them improved the dental class II occlusion as well (if not in a statistically significant manner) [27]. The discrepancy between the results obtained in our study and those of Volk et al. is due to the distinct methodologies used. The study of Volk et al. considered the occlusal relationship, in which cast models were mounted in the articulator in centric occlusion and in maximum intercuspation. In skeletal class III patients, a significant anterior movement of the maxilla was found. In fact, after a rapid palatal expansion, thanks to the activation of the circummaxillary suture, a maxillary movement downward and forward can be observed. This translation allows for correction of the skeletal class III occlusion with maxillary retrusion. A slight mandible clockwise rotation aids in the resolution of the sagittal discrepancy. It is important to underline that the correction of skeletal class III occlusion happens during the active phase of therapy, while the correction of skeletal class II occlusion happens during the retention phase [31,32]. This change agrees with the findings in the studies of Wertz [7], Cleall [11], Linder-Aronson and Lingren [21], Davis and Kronman [33], Hicks [34], and Gardner and Kronman [35].

Gardner and Kronman underlined that opening the spheno-occipital synchondrosis could be responsible for the forward displacement of the maxilla [35]. This change happens in the active phase of treatment. The ANB increased by 2.16°; this could be related to the anterior displacement of the maxilla (SNA increased by a statistically significant measure of +0.81°) and the posterior rotation of the mandible. This is in agreement with the findings of Haas [6] and Wertz [7,8]. However, Haas reported that after treatment the maxilla will partially or completely return to its original position. In this group of patients, a slight, but not statistically significant, increase in the mandibular plane angle (SN-Go.Gn) was found [6]. These data agree with the findings of Wertz, who noted that the increase in the mandibular plane angle could be accompanied by a decrease in the SNB angle. A downward and backward displacement of the apical base (SNB) results in a statistically significant rotation of the palatal plane (SN-SNP.SNA) and a slight but not statistically significant rotation of the mandibular plane (Sn- Go.Gn) [7,8]. The increase in the mandibular plane is responsible for the increase in anterior facial height, N-Me, in this group of patients. In class I patients, a slight but statistically significant decrease in the ANB angle and an increase in the palatal plane were found. The difference between the modification in classes I, II, and III of SNA and SNB angles may be due to the amount of transverse expansion needed that is higher in classes II and III in respect to class I. No other statistically significant modifications of the cephalometric measurements studied were found. In all of the patients in each group, SN-SNP.SNA increased as a result of a downward and backward displacement of the palatal plane. The mandibular plane did not show a statistically significant change after TSME procedures, as did the anterior (N-Me) and posterior vertical dimension (S-Go) in all of the groups [36].

The study which has begun from this work can be widened out comparing the data obtained with a control group and increasing the samples size.

Conclusions

The TSME can produce skeletal changes due to the transverse force and sagittal effects on the maxillary alveolar process. These modifications have benefic effects in classes I, II, and III. The data obtained in this study permit us to underline the fact that TSME can be used in all of the skeletal classes, with good vertical and sagittal results.

Competing interests

The authors declare that they have no competing interests.

Authors' contributions

GF and GG conceived of the study and participated in its design and coordination and helped to carry out the bibliographic research and to draft the manuscript. LG traced lateral cephalograms, and CM verified for landmark location and anatomic contours. LG and CM helped to draft the manuscript. All authors read and approved the final manuscript.

Author details

[1]U.O.C. Chirurgia Maxillo-facciale ed Odontostomatologia (dir: AB. Giannì) Fondazione Cà Granda IRCCS Ospedale Maggiore Policlinico, University of Milan, 20122 Milan, Italy. [2]Maxillo-Facial and Odontostomatology Unit Fondazione Cà Granda IRCCS Ospedale Maggiore Policlinico, University of Milan, 20122 Milan, Italy. [3]UOC Chirurgia Maxillofacciale e Odontostomatologia, Fondazione IRCCS Cà Granda - Ospedale Maggiore Policlinico, University of Milan, Commenda 10, Milano 20122, Italy.

References

1. Da Silva OG, Villas Boas MC, Capelozza L. Rapid maxillary expansion in the primary and mixed dentitions: a cephalometric evaluation. Am J Orthod. 1991;100:171–81.
2. Farronato G, Giannini L, Galbiati G, Maspero C. RME: influences on the nasal septum. Minerva Stomatol. 2012;61(4):125–34.
3. Farronato G, Giannini L, Galbiati G, Maspero C. Sagittal and vertical effects of rapid maxillary expansion in class I, II, and III occlusions. Angle Orthod. 2011;81(2):298–303.
4. Starnbach H, Bayne D, Cleall J, Subtelny JD. Facioskeletal and dental changes resulting from rapid maxillary expansion. Angle Orthod. 1966;36:152–64.
5. Haas AJ. Palatal expansion: just the beginning of dentofacial orthopaedics. Am J Orthod. 1970;57:219–55.
6. Haas AJ. Rapid expansion of the maxillary dental arch and nasal cavity by opening the midpalatal suture. Angle Orthod. 1961;31:73–90.
7. Wertz RA. Skeletal and dental changes accompanying rapid midpalatal suture opening. Am J Orthod. 1970;58:41–66.
8. Wertz R, Dreskin M. Midpalatal suture opening: a normative study. Am J Orthod. 1977;71:367–81.
9. Isaacson RJ, Murphy TD. Some effects of rapid maxillary expansion in cleft lip and palate patients. Angle Orthod. 1964;34:143–54.
10. Akkaya S, Lorenzon S, Ucem TT. A comparison of sagittal and vertical effects between bonded rapid and slow maxillary expansion procedures. Eur J Orthod. 1999;21:175–80.
11. Cleall CF. Dentofacial orthopaedics. Am J Orthod. 1974;66:237–50.
12. McNamara Jr JA. Orthodontic and orthopedic treatment in the mixed dentition. Ann Arbor, MI: NeedhamPress, Inc.; 1993.

13. Cozza P, Giancotti A, Petrosino A. Rapid palatal expansion in mixed dentition using a modified expander: a cephalometric investigation. J Orthod. 2001;28:129–34.
14. Reichenbach E, Taatz K. Kieferorthopaedische Klinik und Therapie. Leipzig, Germany: JA Barth Verl; 1971.
15. Kingsley N. A treatise on oral deformities as a branch of mechanical surgery. New York, NY: Appleton and Co.; 1880.
16. Bishara SE, Hoppens BJ, Jakobsen JR, Kohout FJ. Changes in the molar relationship between the deciduous and permanent dentitions: a longitudinal study. Am J Orthod Dentofacial Orthop. 1988;93:19–28.
17. Farronato G, Giannini L, Galbiati G, Grillo E, Maspero C. Occlus-o-Guide® versus Andresen activator appliance: neuromuscular evaluation. Prog Orthod. 2013;14:4.
18. Nienkemper M, Wilmes B, Pauls A, Drescher D. Maxillary protraction using a hybrid hyrax-facemask combination. Prog Orthod. 2013;14:5.
19. Durão AR, Pittayapat P, Rockenbach MI, Olszewski R, Ng S, Ferreira AP, et al. Validity of 2D lateral cephalometry in orthodontics: a systematic review. Prog Orthod. 2013;14:31.
20. Chung CH, Font B. Skeletal and dental changes in the sagittal, vertical, and transverse dimensions after rapid palatal expansion. Am J Orthod Dentofacial Orthop. 2004;126:569–75.
21. Linder-Aronson S, Lindgren J. The skeletal and dental effects of rapid maxillary expansion. Br J Orthod. 1979;6:25–9.
22. Gautam P, Valiathan A, Adhikari R. Stress and displacement patterns in the craniofacial skeleton with rapid maxillary expansion: a finite element method study. Am J Orthod Dentofacial Orthop. 2007;132:1–11.
23. Farronato G, Giannini L, Galbiati G, Maspero C. Upper midline deviation: modified Hyrax expander. Eur J Paediatric Dent. 2014;15(2):174–6.
24. Farronato GP, G Salvato A. Disgiunzione rapida del palato. II parte: risultati clinici. Mondo Ortod. 1983;6:49–56.
25. Farronato G, Maspero C, Esposito L, Briguglio E, Farronato D, Giannini L. Rapid maxillary expansion in growing patients. Hyrax versus transverse sagittal maxillary expander: a cephalometric investigation. Eur J Orthod. 2011;33(2):185–9.
26. Farronato G, Giannini L, Galbiati G, Maspero C. A 5-year longitudinal study of survival rate and periodontal parameter changes at sites of dilacerated maxillary central incisors. Prog Orthod. 2014;15:3.
27. Clark WJ. Transforce lingual appliances for arch development. J Clin Orthod. 2005;39:137–42.
28. Kiriakou J, Pandis N, Madianos P, Polychronopoulou A. Developing evidence-based dentistry skills: how to interpret randomized clinical trials and systematic reviews. Prog Orthod. 2014;15:58.
29. Volk T, Sadowsky C, Begole EA, Boice P. Rapid palatal expansion for spontaneous class II correction. Am J Orthod Dentofacial Orthop. 2010;137:310–5.
30. MacGinnis M, Chu H, Youssef G, Wu KW, Machado AW, Moon W. The effects of micro-implant assisted rapid palatal expansion (MARPE) on the nasomaxillary complex–a finite element method (FEM) analysis. Prog Orthod. 2014;15:52.
31. Perillo L, De Rosa A, Iaselli F, d'Apuzzo F, Grassia V, Cappabianca S. Comparison between rapid and mixed maxillary expansion through an assessment of dento-skeletal effects on posteroanterior cephalometry. Prog Orthod. 2014;15:46.
32. Farronato G, Giannini L, Galbiati G, Stabilini SA, Maspero C. Orthodontic-surgical treatment: neuromuscular evaluation in open and deep skeletal bite patients. Prog Orthod. 2013;14:41.
33. Davis MW, Kronman JH. Anatomical changes induced by splitting of the midpalatal suture. Angle Orthod. 1969;39:126–32.
34. Hicks EP. Slow maxillary expansion. A clinical study of the skeletal versus dental response to low-magnitude force. Am J Orthod. 1978;73:121–41.
35. Gardner GE, Kronman JH. Cranioskeletal displacements caused by rapid palatal expansion in the rhesus monkey. Am J Orthod. 1971;59:146–55.
36. Perillo L, Femiano A, Palumbo S, Contardo L, Perinetti G. Skeletal and dental effects produced by functional regulator-2 in pre-pubertal class II patients: a controlled study. Prog Orthod. 2013;14:18.

18

Psychological impact of visible differences in patients with congenital craniofacial anomalies

Varun Pratap Singh[1*] and Timothy P Moss[2]

Abstract

Background: Patients with craniofacial anomalies often have appearance concerns and related social anxiety which can affect their quality of life. This study assessed the psychological impact of facial and dental appearance in patients with craniofacial anomalies in comparison to a general population control group.

Methods: The study involved 102 adult patients (51% male) with congenital craniofacial anomalies and 102 controls (49% male). Both groups completed the Nepali version of Derriford Appearance Scale (DAS) and the Psychological Impact of Dental Aesthetic Questionnaire (PIDAQ) in a clinical setting to assess appearance-related distress, avoidance, and anxiety.

Results: There was a significant difference between patients and controls on both PIDAQ (mean score for patients 33.25 ± 9.45 while for controls 27.52 ± 5.67, $p < 0.001$) and DAS59 scores (mean score for patients 159.16 ± 31.54 while for controls 77.64 ± 6.57, $p < 0.001$), indicating that patients experienced greater negative psychological impact of living with their appearance (PIDAQ) and more appearance-related distress (DAS) than controls. DAS scores were not associated with gender. There was no association of the place of residence (rural vs. urban) with PIDAQ or DAS59 scores.

Conclusions: There is a significant psychological impact of altered facial and dental appearance in patients with craniofacial anomalies compared to controls. There was no effect of locality (rural/urban) on the psychological impact of facial and dental appearance in patients.

Keywords: Craniofacial anomalies; Dental aesthetics; Facial aesthetics; Orthodontic; Psychosocial; Derriford

Background

Craniofacial anomalies can be defined as the conditions that encompass all congenital deformities of the cranium and face. More specifically, however, the term has come to imply congenital deformities of the head and face that interfere with physical and mental well-being [1].

The spectrum of craniofacial anomalies is very diverse, and the most common conditions include (but not restricted to) cleft lip and/or palate, craniosynostosis (which may be associated with Crouzon's syndrome or Apert's syndrome), otomandibular anomalies (Treacher Collins syndrome), CHARGE associations, holoprosencephaly, Stickler syndrome, and fetal alcohol syndrome [2,3]. The clinical features include a spectrum of deformities of the craniofacial region including cranium and cranial sutures, and deformity of skull shape and facial bones including the maxilla, mandible, zygomatic arches, nose, eyes, ears, lips, and teeth [4-10].

Patients with abnormal facial appearance often have to face social discrimination. Individuals with abnormal facial appearance are typically considered to be less attractive and are often stereotypically considered as less capable, less intelligent, and less honest. Their facial appearance interferes with personal life, employability, and social interaction. Many investigations have shown that these disfiguring conditions can lead to various psychosocial problems such as high level of social anxiety and social avoidance, and poorer quality of life [11-13].

The potential problems in this patient group are further compounded by an increased prevalence of dental anomalies and malocclusion [14-18]. The best treatment

* Correspondence: varundc@gmail.com
[1]Department of Orthodontics and Dentofacial Orthopedics, Nobel Medical College and Teaching Hospital, Kanchanbari, Biratnagar 56700, Nepal
Full list of author information is available at the end of the article

approach is multidisciplinary, which includes teamwork and support from various specialties. During almost all phases of treatment, dental services are needed and orthodontists are almost always needed from early treatment until late adult life [19]. Good facial and dental aesthetics may have a beneficial role on behavior and self-esteem. Clinicians are expected to produce evidence of the quality of care they deliver. To this end, it is necessary to use standardized, valid, and reliable psychological as well as clinical measures to evaluate outcomes [20-22].

The research in this area is somewhat conflicting and suffers various lacunae for methodological reasons. These include inconsistency in psychometric scales and constructs used, the lack of validity and reliability in many of the measures, small sample sizes, and no subcategorization of anomalies among other methodological errors [23]. Investigators have highlighted the need to move towards a 'social science model' from a 'medical model' [24-27].

This study was undertaken to assess the impact of psychological adjustment due to altered facial and dental appearance in patients with craniofacial anomalies utilizing the Derriford Appearance Scale [28] and Psychological Impact of Dental Aesthetic Questionnaire (PIDAQ) [20] which are specially designed for evaluating the psychological adjustment in people with visible differences in appearance. There are few such studies utilizing the Derriford Appearance Scale [29] and no study studying the psychological impact of facial and dental aesthetics together.

There is a strong *prima facie* case for comparing rural and urban populations with regard to appearance satisfaction in Nepal. There are known differences in healthcare access, service utilization, and geographic distribution of providers and services in healthcare in Nepal, with rural communities typically experiencing greater difficulties than urban comparators [30]. Given the potential for increased social isolation on one hand, but possibility of reduced prevalence of contemporary appearance pressures in more isolated communities on the other, and the likely relation between this and appearance expectations and outcomes, we included an exploratory investigation of rural versus urban populations within this study.

The objectives of this study were therefore:

1. To assess the psychological impact of facial and dental appearance in patients with craniofacial anomalies in comparison to a general population sample.
2. To explore the relationship between urban and rural residence in relation to psychosocial impact of facial and dental anomalies.

The following hypotheses were put forward:

- H1 - There is a psychosocial impact of facial and dental appearance on patients with craniofacial anomalies.
- H2 - There is a difference in psychosocial impact of facial and dental appearance of rural and urban patients.

Methods

This study was conducted in two steps. The first step included translation and validation of the instruments - PIDAQ and DAS59 in the target population. This part is described in detail as published data elsewhere [31,32]. The second step included assessment of patients with craniofacial anomalies reporting for orthodontic treatment using these validated instruments.

The study was conducted in the Department of Orthodontics, BP Koirala Institute of Health Sciences, Dharan, Nepal, from 1 February 2011 to 30 October 2012. Ethical clearance was obtained from Institutional Ethical Committee, B.P. Koirala Institute of Health Sciences, Dharan, Nepal, reference no. Acd/216/068/069, and principles from the Declaration of Helsinki were followed. The study population consisted of adult patients with congenital craniofacial anomalies visiting the Department of Orthodontics during the above said period. The study also included similar patients who were referred/or reported to the orthodontic OPD during 2005 to 2010 and did not undergo orthodontic treatment and patients from the waiting list for whom treatment had not started. The inclusion criteria were adult patients with congenital craniofacial anomalies aged 18 to 30 years. Patients with acquired or traumatic facial disfigurement and history of orthodontic treatment, people who did not have the capacity to offer informed consent, and people who could not read the test booklet unaided were excluded.

Table 1 Classification of patients who participated in the study according to the diagnosis of craniofacial anomalies

Serial number	Craniofacial anomalies	Number (102)
1.	Isolated cleft lip/palate	45
2.	Isolated craniosynostosis	22
3.	Hemifacial microsomia	10
4.	Ectodermal dysplasia	4
5.	Cleidocranial dysplasia	3
6.	Treacher Collins syndrome	6
7.	Pierre Robin syndrome	4
8.	Crouzon's syndrome	4
9.	Apert's syndrome	4

There were 112 patients satisfying the inclusion and exclusion criteria. All were invited to participate, and 102 (91%) agreed to participate in the study. Written informed consent was obtained from all the participants. There were 52 males and 50 females with a mean age of 24.78 years (s.d. = 2.5). Forty-six were from rural areas and 56 from urban. Details regarding the classification of patients according to the craniofacial anomalies are presented in Table 1. A similar number of controls, 50 males and 52 females (mean age 24.99 years, s.d. = 2.73), were selected as a convenience sample from the university students and employees who have no acquired or congenital facial deformity. Thirty-nine were from rural areas and 63 from urban. Participants with severe malocclusion as assessed by an orthodontist were not included. The exclusion criteria were the same as those of the case groups.

The questionnaire pack consisted of

1. An introductory section with basic demographic information including age, sex, and place of residence in terms of rural and urban.
2. Nepali version of DAS consisting of 59 items. Each item response is marked based on a Likert scale from 1 to 4, with 1 indicating 'almost never' and 4 indicating 'almost always'.
3. Nepali version of PIDAQ consisting of 23 items arranged in four domains. Each item response is marked based on a Likert scale from 0 to 4, with 0 indicating 'not at all' and 4 indicating 'very strongly.'

These questionnaires were administered to the participants by one author who is well trained in this procedure. The patients were seated in a private room, in the

Table 2 Differences between the DAS 59 and PIDAQ scores for patients and controls

Items	Group	Mean	Standard deviation	*p* value
General self-consciousness	Cases	49.29***	10.8	<0.001
	Controls	21.84***	3.2	
Social self-consciousness	Cases	58.23***	14.17	<0.001
	Controls	22.8***	2.40	
Sexual and bodily self-consciousness	Cases	24.26***	5.98	<0.001
	Controls	8.77***	2.09	
Negative self-concept	Cases	9.65***	3.16	<0.001
	Controls	16.91***	1.17	
Facial self-consciousness	Cases	12.02***	2.50	<0.001
	Controls	4.66***	1.06	
Physical	Cases	5.71***	1.60	<0.001
	Controls	2.65***	0.99	
Total DAS score	Cases	159.16***	31.54	<0.001
	Controls	77.64***	6.57	
Dental self-confidence	Cases	12.84***	3.10	<0.001
	Controls	11.11***	2.91	
Social impact	Cases	7.2**	3.36	0.004
	Controls	6.1**	1.72	
Psychological impact	Cases	6.33***	2.86	<0.001
	Controls	5.03***	1.92	
Aesthetic concern	Cases	6.88***	2.76	<0.001
	Controls	5.28***	1.62	
Dental self-consciousness	Cases	8.56***	4.20	<0.001
	Controls	6.65***	1.99	
Total PIDAQ score	Cases	33.25***	9.45	<0.001
	Controls	27.52***	5.67	

* correlation is significant at the 0.05 level.
** correlation is significant at the 0.01 level.
***correlation is significant at the 0.001 level.

Department of Orthodontics, and were asked to fill the questionnaire pack without the aid of the investigators, minimizing the likelihood of demand characteristics biasing responses. Participants were paid legitimate expenses incurred in attending the session but otherwise offered no incentive to participate. Payment was entirely independent of participants' responses and, as such, unlikely to induce any bias in responding. Furthermore, the level of remuneration was such that participants did not profit from participation and such were not induced to a particular response set.

Statistical procedures

Descriptive statistics was calculated for the demographic data. Independent *t* tests were used to evaluate the differences between cases and controls for scores of DAS59 and PIDAQ scales. Independent *t* tests were used to assess the effect of gender (male vs. female) and locality (rural vs. urban) on PIDAQ and DAS59 scores in both cases and controls. Bonferroni corrections were applied to the results to correct for type 1 errors resulting from multiple comparisons.

Results

There was a significant difference between patients and controls on PIDAQ (mean score for patients = 33.25, s.d. = 9.45; mean for controls = 27.52, s.d. = 5.67; $p < 0.001$) and DAS59 scores (mean score for patients = 159.16, s.d. = 31.54; mean for controls = 77.64, s.d. = 6.57; $p < 0.001$) (Table 2). The patients' scores were significantly higher than those of controls on both the PIDAQ and DAS59 scales.

Gender

There was no effect of gender except for sub-domains of PIDAQ 'psychological impact' and 'aesthetic

Table 3 Effect of gender on PIDAQ and DAS59 scores in patients

Domain	Sex	Mean	Standard deviation	Standard error mean	*p* value
General self-consciousness	Male	49.29	10.815	1.5	0.996
	Female	49.3	10.998	1.555	
Social self-consciousness	Male	58.73	14.096	1.955	0.715
	Female	57.7	14.379	2.033	
Sexual and bodily self-consciousness	Male	24.44	5.992	0.831	0.762
	Female	24.08	6.037	0.854	
Negative self-concept	Male	9.52	3.032	0.421	0.68
	Female	9.78	3.328	0.471	
Facial self-consciousness	Male	12.23	2.51	0.348	0.388
	Female	11.8	2.507	0.355	
Physical	Male	5.85	1.638	0.227	0.372
	Female	5.56	1.58	0.223	
Total DAS	Male	160.06	31.585	4.38	0.77
	Female	158.22	31.799	4.497	
Dental self-confidence	Male	12.69	2.86	0.397	0.62
	Female	13	3.369	0.476	
Social impact	Male	6.98	3.006	0.417	0.512
	Female	7.42	3.709	0.525	
Psychological impact	Male	5.44***	2.2	0.305	0.001
	Female	7.26***	3.18	0.45	
Aesthetic concern	Male	6.13**	2.385	0.331	0.005
	Female	7.66**	2.939	0.416	
Dental self-consciousness	Male	8.17	4.218	0.585	0.348
	Female	8.96	4.204	0.595	
Total PIDAQ score	Male	31.25*	7.963	1.104	0.028
	Female	35.34*	10.458	1.479	

* correlation is significant at the 0.05 level.
** correlation is significant at the 0.01 level.
***correlation is significant at the 0.001 level.

Table 4 Effect of gender on PIDAQ and DAS59 scores in controls

Domain	Sex	Mean	Standard deviation	Standard error mean	*p* value
General self-consciousness	Male	21.84	3.046	0.431	0.992
	Female	21.85	3.438	0.477	
Social self-consciousness	Male	22.7	2.667	0.377	0.67
	Female	22.9	2.135	0.296	
Sexual and bodily self-consciousness	Male	8.92	2.311	0.327	0.494
	Female	8.63	1.869	0.259	
Negative self-concept	Male	16.98	1.22	0.173	0.566
	Female	16.85	1.127	0.156	
Facial self-consciousness	Male	4.56	0.812	0.115	0.371
	Female	4.75	1.266	0.176	
Physical	Male	2.58	0.883	0.125	0.506
	Female	2.71	1.091	0.151	
Total DAS	Male	77.58	6.843	0.968	0.932
	Female	77.69	6.379	0.885	
Dental self-confidence	Male	11.18	2.833	0.401	0.808
	Female	11.04	3.016	0.418	
Social impact	Male	6	1.702	0.241	0.575
	Female	6.19	1.749	0.243	
Psychological impact	Male	5.22	1.93	0.273	0.328
	Female	4.85	1.914	0.265	
Aesthetic concern	Male	5.5	1.681	0.238	0.19
	Female	5.08	1.557	0.216	
Dental self-consciousness	Male	6.84	1.707	0.241	0.34
	Female	6.46	2.236	0.31	
Total PIDAQ score	Male	27.9	5.319	0.752	0.509
	Female	27.15	6.024	0.835	

concern,' where females had higher scores than males (mean, M = 5.44 (s.d. = 2.2), F = 7.26 (s.d. = 3.18), $p = 0.001$; M = 4.27 (s.d. = 1.99), F = 5.32 (s.d. = 2.55), $p = 0.005$). However, the total PIDAQ score was significantly higher in females as compared to males (mean, M = 31.25 (s.d. = 7.96), F = 35.34 (s.d. = 10.45), $p = 0.02$). DAS scores were not differentiated by gender (Table 3). In controls, there was no difference in PIDAQ and DAS59 scores by gender (Table 4).

Rural versus urban

There was no difference in the place of residence (rural vs. urban) with either PIDAQ or DAS59 scores in patients (Tables 5 and 6), nor for subscales of each of these measures following Bonferroni control for multiple comparisons.

Discussion

In comparison to general population controls, craniofacial patients with orthodontic and orthognathic concerns showed greater appearance-related distress, according to valid and reliable psychometric scales. For general distress, there was also no difference between urban and rural participants. Females did not demonstrate more distress than males when assessed using the DAS59. However, on two of the dental-specific scales of the PIDAQ, 'psychological impact' and 'aesthetic concern,' female patients reported more distress than male patients.

Some studies and reviews suggest that there are few significant differences in overall psychological functioning of patients with craniofacial anomalies as compared to general population norms. However, these studies report some difficulty in a particular area of functioning [33-39]. There is substantial evidence of appearance concern due to dissatisfaction with facial appearance in patients with craniofacial anomalies [40-44]. This dissatisfaction with facial appearance may lead to behavioral difficulties [45-48].

Many studies point out that the adult population is at risk of psychosocial problems due to concerns regarding their facial appearance [49-52]. The results of this study

Table 5 Effect of locality (rural/urban) on PIDAQ and DAS59 scores in patients

Domain	Rural/urban	Mean	Standard deviation	Standard error mean	Significance
General self-consciousness	Rural	49.91	10.167	1.499	0.604
	Urban	48.79	11.447	1.53	
Social self-consciousness	Rural	59.07	13.401	1.976	0.59
	Urban	57.54	14.864	1.986	
Sexual and bodily self-consciousness	Rural	24.63	5.867	0.865	0.579
	Urban	23.96	6.12	0.818	
Negative self-concept	Rural	9.59	2.941	0.434	0.863
	Urban	9.7	3.368	0.45	
Facial self-consciousness	Rural	11.76	2.349	0.346	0.347
	Urban	12.23	2.628	0.351	
Physical	Rural	5.89	1.464	0.216	0.293
	Urban	5.55	1.715	0.229	
Total DAS	Rural	160.85	29.731	4.384	0.626
	Urban	157.77	33.165	4.432	
Dental self-confidence	Rural	12.7	3.595	0.53	0.666
	Urban	12.96	2.669	0.357	
Social impact	Rural	7.37	3.555	0.524	0.639
	Urban	7.05	3.216	0.43	
Psychological impact	Rural	6.13	2.841	0.419	0.519
	Urban	6.5	2.892	0.386	
Aesthetic concern	Rural	6.85	3.048	0.449	0.91
	Urban	6.91	2.539	0.339	
Dental self-consciousness	Rural	9.09	4.56	0.672	0.253
	Urban	8.13	3.885	0.519	
Total PIDAQ score	Rural	33.04	10.321	1.522	0.839
	Urban	33.43	8.761	1.171	

have supported the hypothesis that adults who have craniofacial anomalies have negative psychosocial impact due to facial and dental appearance. In the current study, both DAS and PIDAQ scores were significantly higher in patients than in controls, indicating that patients experienced negative psychological impact and more distress (Table 2).

In this study, it was shown that there were no significant differences in DAS59 scores for male versus female patients. This is in accordance with Kiyak and Bell [53], who stated that there were no gender differences on psychological variables in the pre-surgical assessment of patients needing orthognathic surgery, though counter to other evidence regarding self-consciousness of appearance, which typically shows more distress among female participants [28]. In the analysis of the PIDAQ, it was interesting that there was statistically significant difference for overall psychological impact of dental aesthetics on two PIDAQ subscales, though when a Bonferroni correction for multiple comparisons is applied to the data, the difference becomes non-significant. However, the specific psychological impact upon males and females assessed using PIDAQ subscales does significantly differ, with females having higher scores for both (Table 3). It may be hypothesized that females are socialized to be more concerned and dissatisfied by their dental appearance as compared to males and to socially evaluate their appearance to a greater degree than males [54]. While it remains to be further investigated in subsequent research, it is possible that patients with craniofacial conditions are more sensitized to appearance distress than controls, and in combination with social pressure associated with gender, more distress ensues.

Contrary to our expectations, there was no effect of area of residence (rural vs. urban) on the overall psychological impact of facial and dental appearance in patients or control participants following Bonferroni correction for type 1 errors. This may indicate that aesthetic norms and pressures are not decreased by living in a less populous urban environment and that these norms are

Table 6 Effect of locality (rural/urban) on PIDAQ and DAS59 scores in controls

Domain	Rural/urban	Mean	Standard deviation	Standard error mean	Significance
General self-consciousness	Rural	21.46	2.584	0.414	0.351
	Urban	22.08	3.58	0.451	
Social self-consciousness	Rural	22.92	2.559	0.41	0.695
	Urban	22.73	2.315	0.292	
Sexual and bodily self-consciousness	Rural	8.33	2.144	0.343	0.094
	Urban	9.05	2.027	0.255	
Negative self-concept	Rural	16.62*	1.206	0.193	0.044
	Urban	17.1*	1.118	0.141	
Facial self-consciousness	Rural	4.49	0.823	0.132	0.208
	Urban	4.76	1.187	0.15	
Physical	Rural	2.69	0.977	0.157	0.719
	Urban	2.62	1.007	0.127	
Total DAS	Rural	76.51	6.476	1.037	0.176
	Urban	78.33	6.594	0.831	
Dental self-confidence	Rural	11.31	3.262	0.522	0.588
	Urban	10.98	2.697	0.34	
Social impact	Rural	5.82	1.819	0.291	0.201
	Urban	6.27	1.648	0.208	
Psychological impact	Rural	5.44	1.917	0.307	0.093
	Urban	4.78	1.896	0.239	
Aesthetic concern	Rural	5.72*	1.701	0.272	0.033
	Urban	5.02*	1.529	0.193	
Dental self-consciousness	Rural	6.69	1.838	0.294	0.858
	Urban	6.62	2.098	0.264	
Total PIDAQ score	Rural	28.28	6.017	0.964	0.288
	Urban	27.05	5.446	0.686	

* correlation is significant at the 0.05 level.
** correlation is significant at the 0.01 level.
***correlation is significant at the 0.001 level.

pervasive. It also suggests that the availability of complex cosmetic dentistry in urban Nepal has not fundamentally shifted the discrepancy between perceived dental appearance ideals and actuality.

There are some methodological limitations inherent in this study which should be considered when generalizing findings. Firstly, the age of participants in both the experimental and control groups was low compared to a random sample of the general population. It is feasible that as people age beyond the age boundaries within this study, they will become differentially sensitive to differences of appearance due to craniofacial anomalies. A second limitation lies in the nature of the comparison group. As university students and employees, it is feasible that they are not directly equivalent to the patient group in cognitive and social domains. However, there is no *a priori* reason to assume that these differences would be related to subjective feelings or coping around appearance, and as such, the use of this comparison sample is justified. The comparison between rural and urban samples was not significant. This may, as described, reflect a genuine lack of difference. However, it is also worth reflecting on the categorization of these groups. For pragmatic reasons, current residence was used as the variable to code participants as 'urban' or 'rural.' What remains to be investigated in further work is the degree of stability of these categories. It may well be that those in the 'urban' category have been previously socialized in rural areas during formative periods of their development, and vice versa for those in the 'rural' category. If this were the case, differences between our groups would be less apparent than might be otherwise expected. In terms of the study instruments, both PIDAQ and DAS are robust measures. However, it is possible that there could be aspects of appearance sensitivity which are not identified in these measures.

Conclusions

1. There is a significant psychological impact of altered facial and dental appearance in patients with craniofacial anomalies.
2. There was no significant effect of gender on the psychological impact of facial appearance in patients; however, significant negative psychological impact of dental appearance was seen in female patients.
3. There was no effect of locality (rural/urban) on the psychological impact of facial and dental appearance.

Competing interests

The authors declare that they have no competing interests.

Authors' contributions

VPS conceived the study and VPS and TPM participated in study design, VPS carried out the study, VPS and TPM carried out statistical analysis, VPS and TPM prepared the manuscript. Both authors read and approved the final manuscript.

Author details

[1]Department of Orthodontics and Dentofacial Orthopedics, Nobel Medical College and Teaching Hospital, Kanchanbari, Biratnagar 56700, Nepal. [2]Department of Health Psychology, University of the West of England, Frenchary Campus, cold Harbour Lane, Bristol BS161QY, UK.

References

1. Marsh JL, Vannier MW. Comprehensive care for craniofacial deformities. 1st ed. CV Mosby: St. Louis; 1985.
2. World Health Organization. Addressing the global challenges of craniofacial anomalies. 2004. http://www.who.int/genomics/publications/CFA%20Completed%20text.pdf. Accessed on Friday, December 20, 2013.
3. World Health Organization. Global strategies to reduce the health-care burden of craniofacial anomalies. 2002. http://whqlibdoc.who.int/publications/9241590386.pdf. Accessed on Friday, December 20,2013.
4. Husu E, Hove H, Farholt S, Bille M, Tranebjaerg L, Vogel I, et al. Phenotype in 18 Danish subjects with genetically verified CHARGE syndrome. Clin Genet. 2013;83(2):125–34.
5. Stavropoulos D, Tarnow P, Mohlin B, Kahnberg KE, Hagberg C. Comparing patients with Apert and Crouzon syndromes – clinical features and cranio-maxillofacial surgical reconstruction. Swed Dent J. 2012;36(1):25–34.
6. Tuna EB, Orino D, Ogawa K, Yildirim M, Seymen F, Gencay K. Craniofacial and dental characteristics of Goldenhar syndrome: a report of two cases. J Oral Sci. 2011;53:121–4.
7. Kini U, Hurst JA, Byren JC, Wall SA, Johnson D, Wilkie AO. Etiological heterogeneity and clinical characteristics of metopic synostosis: evidence from a tertiary craniofacial unit. Am J Med Genet A. 2010;152(6):1383–9.
8. Chong DK, Murray DJ, Britto JA, Tompson B, Forrest CR, Phillips JH. A cephalometric analysis of maxillary and mandibular parameters in Treacher Collins syndrome. Plast Reconstr Surg. 2008;121(3):77–84.
9. Itthagarun A, Nair RG, Epstein JB, King NM. Fetal alcohol syndrome: case report and review of the literature. Oral Surg Oral Med Oral Pathol Oral Radiol Endod. 2007;103(3):20–5.
10. Lu DW, Shi B, Wang HJ, Zheng Q. The comparative study of craniofacial structural characteristic of individuals with different types of cleft palate. Ann Plast Surg. 2007;59(4):382–7.
11. Van den Elzen MEP, Versnel SL, Hovius SER, Passchier J, Duivenvoorden HJ, Mathijssen IMJ. Adults with congenital or acquired facial disfigurement: impact of appearance on social functioning. J Craniomaxillofac Surg. 2012;40(8):777–82.
12. Moss TP. The relationships between objective and subjective ratings of disfigurement severity, and psychological adjustment. Body Image. 2005;2(2):151–9.
13. Versnel SL, Duivenvoorden HJ, Passchier J, et al. Satisfaction with facial appearance and its determinants in adults with severe congenital facial disfigurement: a case-referent study. J Plast Reconstr Aesthet Surg. 2010;63:1642–9.
14. Da Silva DG, Costa B, Gomide MR. Prevalence of dental anomalies, ectopic eruption and associated oral malformations in subjects with Treacher Collins syndrome. Oral Surg Oral Med Oral Pathol Oral Radiol Endod. 2006;101(5):588–92.
15. Menezes R, Vieira AR. Dental anomalies as part of cleft spectrum. Cleft Palate Craniofacial journal. 2008;45(4):414–9.
16. Da Silva AP, Costa B, De Carvalho-Carrara CF. Dental anomalies of number in the permanent dentition of patients with bilateral cleft lip: radiographic study. Cleft Palate Craniofacial Journal. 2007;45(5):473–6.
17. Vettore MV, Sousa- Campose MV. Malocclusion characteristics of patients with cleft lip and/or palate. Eur J Orthod. 2011;33(3):311–7.
18. Tannure PN, Oliveira CA, Maia LC, Vieira AR, Granjeiro JM, de Castro CM. Prevalence of dental anomalies in nonsyndromic individuals with cleft lip and palate: a systematic review and meta-analysis. Cleft Palate Craniofacial Journal. 2012;49(2):194–200.
19. Lorenzzaoni D, Carcereri DL, Locks A. The importance of multi-professional, interdisciplinary care in rehabilitation and health promotion directed at patients with cleft lip/palate. Rev odonto cienc. 2010;25(2):198–203.
20. Klages U, Claus N, Wehrbein H, Zentner A. Development of a questionnaire for assessment of the psychosocial impact of dental aesthetics in young adults. Eur J Orthod. 2006;28(1):103–11.
21. Kenealy PM, Kingdon A, Richmond S, Shaw WC. The Cardiff dental study: a 20 year critical evaluation of the psychological health gain from orthodontic treatment. Br J Health Psychol. 2007;12:17–49.
22. Rappaport TG, Shalish MH, Gazil E. Psychosocial reward of orthodontic treatment in adult patients. Eur J Orthod. 2010;32(1):441–6.
23. Singh VP, Singh RK, Roy D, Baral DD, Vikram M. Guidelines and recommendations for studies on psychosocial aspects of patients with craniofacial anomalies. Mymensingh Med J. 2012;21(4):736–40.
24. Strauss R, Broder H. Directions and issues in psychosocial research and methods as applied to cleft lip and palate and craniofacial anomalies. Cleft Palate Craniofacial Journal. 1991;28(2):150–6.
25. Broder HL. Psychological research of children with craniofacial anomalies: review, critique and implications for the future. Cleft Palate Craniofacial Journal. 1979;34(5):402–4.
26. Speltz ML. Editorial: Progress and limitations in the psychological study of craniofacial anomalies. J Pediatr Psychol. 1997;22(4):433–8.
27. Endriga MC, Kapp- Simon KA. Psychological issues in craniofacial care: state of the art. Cleft Palate Craniofacial Journal. 1999;36(1):3–11.
28. Carr T, Harris D, James C. The Derriford Appearance Scale (DAS-59): a new scale to measure individual responses to living with problems of appearance. Br J Health Psychol. 2000;5:201–15.
29. Bessell A, Brough V, Clarke A, Harcourt D, Moss TP, Rumsey N. Evaluation of the effectiveness of Face IT, a computer-based psychosocial intervention for disfigurement-related distress. Psychol Health Med. 2012;17(5):565–77.
30. Rai SK, Rai G, Hirai K, Abe A, Ohno Y. The health system in Nepal - an introduction. Environ Health Prev Med. 2001;6(1):1–8.
31. Singh VP, Singh RK. Translation and validation of Nepalese version of PIDAQ. J Orthod. 2014;41:6–12.
32. Singh VP, Singh RK, Moss TP, Roy DK, Baral DD. Translation and validation of the Nepalese version of Derriford appearance scale (DAS-59). Modern Plastic Surgery. 2013;3:51–6.
33. McWilliams BJ. Social and psychological problems associated with cleft palate. Clin Plast Surg. 1982;9:317–26.
34. Richman LC, Eliason M. Psychological characteristics of children with cleft lip and palate: Intellectual, achievement, behavioral and personality variables. Cleft Palate Journal. 1982;19:249–57.
35. Madison LS. Psychologic aspects of cleft lip and palate. Ear Nose and Throat Journal. 1986;65:337–41.
36. Eliason MJ. Cleft lip and palate: developmental effects. J Pediatr Nurs. 1991;6(2):107–13.
37. Tobiasen JM, Hiebert JM. Clefting and psychosocial adjustment: influence of facial aesthetics. Clin Plast Surg. 1993;20:623–31.
38. Turner SR, Rumsey N, Sandy JR. Psychological aspects of cleft lip and palate. European Orthodontic Journal. 1998;20:407–15.
39. Thompson A, Kent G. Adjusting to disfigurement: processes involved in dealing with being visibly different. Clin Psychol Rev. 2001;21:663–82.

40. Lockhart E. The mental health needs of children and adolescents with cleft lip and/or palate. Clin Child Psychol Psychiatry. 2003;8:7–16.
41. Tyl J, Dytrych Z, Helclová H, Scüller V, Matějcěk Z, Beránková A. Psychic and social stress of children with cleft lip and palate. Cesk Pediatr. 1990;45:532–6.
42. Richman LC. Behavior and achievement of cleft palate children. Cleft Palate Journal. 1976;13:4–10.
43. Thomas PT, Turner SR, Rumsey N, Dowell T, Sandy JR. Satisfaction with facial appearance among subjects affected by cleft. Cleft Palate Craniofacial Journal. 1997;34(3):226–31.
44. Marcusson A. Adult patients with treated complete cleft lip and palate: methodological and clinical studies. Swed Dent J. 2001;145:1–57.
45. Marcusson A, Paulin G, Ostrup L. Facial appearance in adults who had cleft. lip and palate treated in childhood. Scand J Plast Reconstr Surg Hand Surg. 2002;36:16–23.
46. Clifford E. Parental ratings of cleft palate infants. Cleft Palate Journal. 1969;6:235–44.
47. Richman LC. Self-reported social, speech, and facial concerns and personality adjustment of adolescents with cleft lip and palate. Cleft Palate Journal. 1983;20:108–12.
48. Richman LC, Holmes CS, Eliason MJ. Adolescents with cleft lip and palate: self-perceptions of appearance and behavior related to personality adjustment. Cleft Palate Journal. 1985;22:93–6.
49. Ramstad T, Otten E, Shaw WC. Psychosocial adjustment in Norwegian adults who had undergone standardized treatment of complete cleft lip and palate. Part II. Self-reported problems and concerns with appearance. Scand J Plast Reconstr Surg Hand Surg. 1995;29:329–36.
50. Bernstein NR, Kapp K. Adolescents with cleft palate: body-image and psychosocial problems. Psychosomatics. 1981;22(8):697–703.
51. Cochrane VM, Slade P. Appraisal and coping in adults with cleft lip: associations with well-being and social anxiety. Br J Med Psychol. 1999;72(4):485–503.
52. Berk NW, Cooper ME, Liu YE, Marazita ML. Social anxiety in Chinese adults with oral-facial clefts. Cleft Palate Craniofac J. 2001;38(2):126–33.
53. Kiyak HA, Bell R. Psychosocial considerations in surgery and orthodontics. In: Proffit WR, White Jr RP, editors. Surgical-orthodontic treatment. St. Louis: Mosby Year Book; 1991. p. 71–91.
54. Tin-Oo MM, Saddki N, Hassan N. Factors influencing patient satisfaction with dental appearance and treatments they desire to improve aesthetics. BMC Oral Health. 2011;11:6. doi:10.1186/1472-6831-11-6.

19

Computational fluid dynamics analysis of the upper airway after rapid maxillary expansion: a case report

Ahmed Ghoneima[1,2*], Sahar AlBarakati[3], Feifei Jiang[4], Katherine Kula[1] and Tamer Wasfy[4]

Abstract

Background: Assessment of the upper airway volume, morphology, and mechanics is of great importance for the orthodontic patient. We hypothesize that upper airway dimensions have significant effects on the dynamics of the airway flow and that both the dimensions and mechanics of the upper airway are greatly affected by orthodontic and orthopedic procedures such as rapid maxillary expansion (RME). The aim of the current study was to assess the effect of RME on the airway flow rate and pattern by comparing the fluid dynamics results of pre- and post-treatment finite element models.

Methods: Customized pre- and post-treatment computational fluid dynamics models of the patient's upper airway were built for comparison based on three-dimensional computed tomogram. The inhalation process was simulated using a constant volume flow rate for both models, and the wall was set to be rigid and stationary. Laminar and turbulent analyses were applied.

Results: Comparisons between before and after RME airway volume measurements showed that increases were only detected in nasal cavity volume, nasopharynx volume, and the most constricted area of the airway. Pressure, velocity, and turbulent kinetic energy decreased after dental expansion for laminar and turbulent flow. Turbulent flow shows relatively larger velocity and pressure than laminar flow.

Conclusions: RME showed positive effects that may help understand the key reasons behind relieving the symptom of breathing disorders in this patient. Turbulence occurs at both nasal and oropharynx areas, and it showed relatively larger pressure and velocity compared to laminar flow.

Keywords: Finite element analysis; Palatal expansion technique; Airway resistance

Background

Rapid maxillary expansion (RME) is a dentofacial orthopedic procedure that is routinely used by dental clinicians and orthodontists to treat maxillary transverse discrepancies such as "posterior crossbites"; the same technique has been reported by some researchers to help expand the upper airway and improve breathing function in patients with nasal breathing disorders [1-3]. The main objective would be that correcting the existing posterior crossbite and widening of the maxillary dental arch is expected to reduce maxillary constriction and mouth breathing, thereby reliving the symptoms through decreasing the nasal resistance [1-5].

The human respiratory system can be divided into the upper and lower respiratory systems. The upper respiratory system consists of the nasal cavity, nasopharynx, oropharynx, and trachea. The shape and diameter of these passages determine the volume of air passing through them [6]. A patent airway and normal nasal breathing is considered crucial in the growth and development of craniofacial structures [7]. Reports have previously indicated that maxillary morphologic differences exist between individuals with normal airway systems and those with airway problems [6, 8, 9].

* Correspondence: aghoneim@iu.edu
[1]Department of Orthodontics and Oral Facial Genetics, Indiana University School Dentistry, 1121 West Michigan Street, Indianapolis, IN 46202, USA
[2]Department of Orthodontics, Faculty of Dental Medicine, Al-Azhar University, Cairo, Egypt
Full list of author information is available at the end of the article

Table 1 Definition of airway boundaries

	Anterior boundary	Posterior boundary	Superior boundary	Inferior boundary
Nasal cavity	Line connecting the ANS to the tip of the nasal bone	Line extending from S to the PNS	Line connecting N to S	Line extending from ANS to PNS
Nasopharynx	Line extending from S to the PNS	Line extending from S to the tip of the odontoid process	Line extending from S to the tip of the odontoid process	Line extending from PNS to the tip of the odontoid process
Oropharynx	Line extending from PNS to the tip of the epiglottis	Line extending from the tip of the odontoid process to the posterior superior border of CV4	Line extending from PNS to the tip of the odontoid process	Line extending from the base of the epiglottis to the posterior superior border of CV4
Hypopharynx	Line extending from the base of the epiglottis to the inferior border of the symphysis	Line extending from the posterior–superior corner of CV4 to the posterior–inferior corner of CV4	Line extending from the base of the epiglottis to the posterior superior border of CV4	Line extending from the posterior–inferior corner of CV4 to the inferior border of the symphysis

ANS anterior nasal spine, *PNS* posterior nasal spine, *S* sella, *N* nasion, *CV* cervical vertebrae

Computational fluid dynamics (CFD) is considered the most appropriate technique to simulate the internal flow dynamics of the upper airway. It also allows evaluation of the airflow in the nasal, nasopharynx, and oropharynx areas separately providing an accurate assessment tool [10, 11]. In addition, CFD also provides accurate simulation to the magnitudes of air pressure and velocity and thus more precise evaluation of the airway function [10]. Iwasaki et al. [11], in a CFD study, reported that in obstructive sleep apnea children, the pharyngeal airway pressure during inspiration decreases with the reduction of nasal resistance by RME [11].

Because of its impact on airway, maxillary expansion can potentially be used as a treatment option for airway constrictions. Multiple studies confirmed that RME increases airway widths and volumes [1-5]. However, there is lack of data on airway internal flow dynamics and patterns of airflow. The purpose of this study was to assess the effects of RME on the upper airway using CFD results of comparing pre- and post-treatment finite element models.

Methods

Ethical approval was obtained from the university's institutional review board committee (Indiana University), and informed consent was signed by the parents of the study subject. Pre- and post-treatment finite element models were constructed for a 9-year-old male with collapsed maxillary arch who suffer from improper nasal breathing. The patient was treated by RME as part of his comprehensive orthodontic treatment plan. He had no history of previous orthodontic or orthopedic treatment; no systemic diseases, craniofacial anomalies, or temporomandibular joint disorders; no tonsillectomy or adenoidectomy; no carious or periodontal lesions; and no metallic restorations.

The RME appliance used was a Hyrax appliance (Dentaurum, Ispringen, Germany), which included bands on the permanent first molars and first pre-molars. The patient was instructed to turn the expansion screw two times, twice daily (producing 0.8 mm of expansion daily) until the palatal cusps of the maxillary first molars contacted the buccal cusps of the mandibular first molars after about 2 weeks. Spiral computed tomography (CT) images were taken immediately before the RME and 3 months after the last activation of the appliance using the Xvision EX spiral machine (Toshiba Medical Systems, Otawara-Shi, Japan). Scans were made at 120 kV, 20 mA, and 0.4-mm voxel size, with a scanning time of 2 s per section and a 25-cm field of view. The window width was 2400 Hounsfield units. The machine's perpendicular light beam was used to adjust the head position in all three planes and thus allow comparison of the pre- and post-treatment scans.

On the three-dimensional (3D) CT scans, the airway volume was measured at the nasal cavity, nasopharynx, oropharynx, hypopharynx, and the most constricted area of the airway using Dolphin imaging software version 11.0 (Dolphin Imaging, Chatsworth, CA, USA). The anatomic boundaries and airway outlines used are identified in Table 1. The same software was used for orienting the pre- and post-treatment 3D images. The midsagittal plane was adjusted on the skeletal midline of the face, the axial plane was lined up with the Frankfort horizontal plane, and the coronal plane was adjusted to pass through the level of the furcation point of the right maxillary first molar.

In order to perform the fluid dynamics analysis of the upper airway, customized pre- and post-CFD finite element models of the upper airway of the patient were constructed. The inhalation process was simulated using

Table 2 Comparison between pre- and post-RME airway volume measurements

Parameters	Pre-RME	Post-RME	Change
Nasal cavity	32,746.8	36,585.1	3838.3
Nasopharynx	5499.6	6935.1	1435.5
Oropharynx	7680.5	7680.5	0
Hypopharynx	4557.8	4557.8	0
Most constricted area of the airway	112	127	15

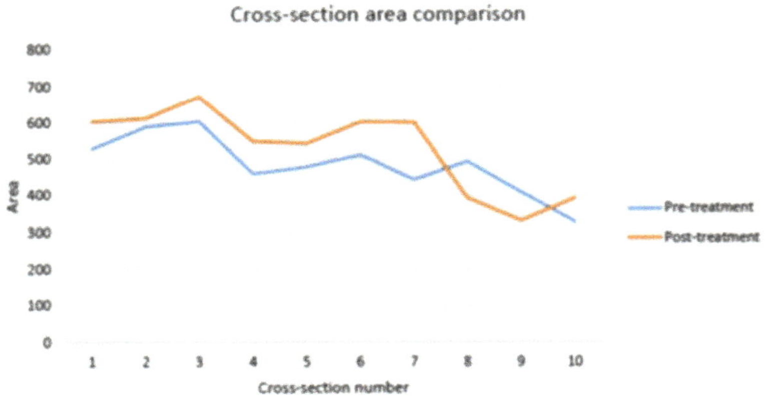

Fig. 1 Cross-sectional area (mm²) comparison of the most constricted area of the upper airway

a constant volume flow rate at the end of the airway for both models, and the wall was set to be rigid and stationary. Laminar and turbulent analyses were applied. Before and after RME models were evaluated using Mimics 13 (Materialise, Belgium) and ANSYS Workbench 12 (Canonsburg, PA, USA) softwares. The pressure, flow rate, and pattern of the upper airway were recorded and assessed. The software Mimics 13 (Materialise, Belgium) was used to process the scan images for upper airway segmentation. A threshold that best isolated the airway was set to segment the pre-treatment scan, and the same threshold was applied for the post-treatment scan. Manual modification was also applied after thresholding for detailed segmentation in the nasal area. The geometry of the airway was rebuilt after segmentation and then meshed in Mimics with a four-node tetrahedral element. The mesh

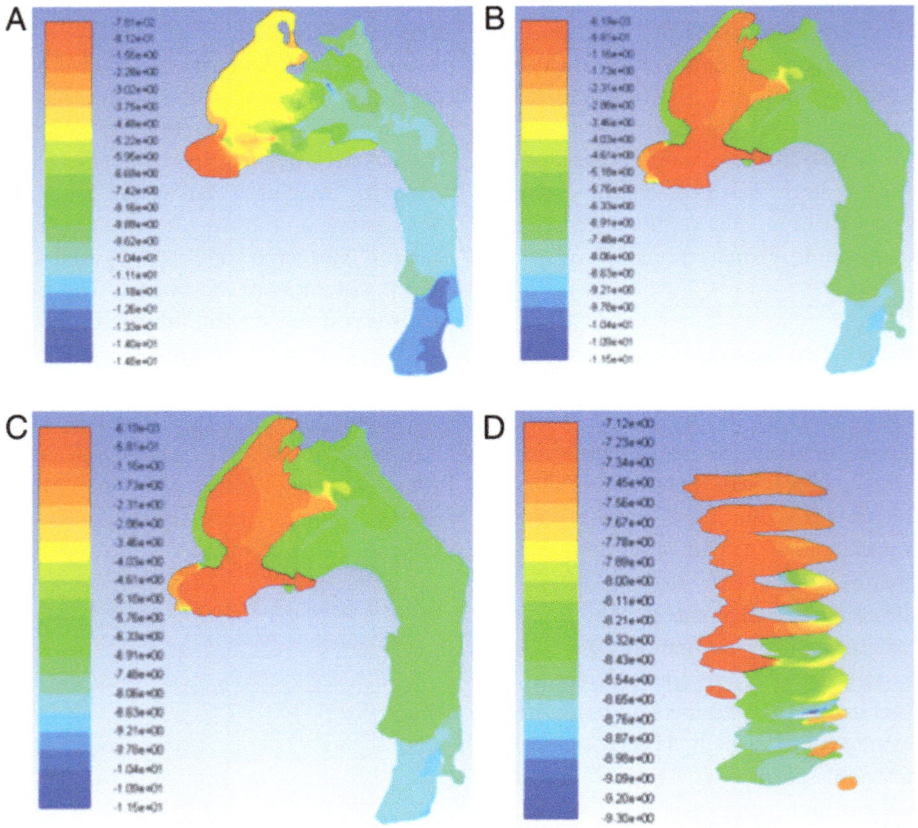

Fig. 2 Pressure on the wall of laminar flow **a** pre-RME and **b** post-RME; pressure at cross-sections of laminar flow **c** pre-RME and **d** post-RME (Pa)

was then exported to ANSYS Workbench 12 (Canonsburg, PA, USA). The geometrical changes were also measured after segmentation. Cervical vertebras (CV2 and CV5) were used as references to align pre- and post-treatment models. The most constricted area of the airway was selected and divided into ten cross-sections for comparison of finite element models.

The pressure at the nostrils was set to be zero at inlet, and the velocity at outlet was adjusted to match with the constant volume flow rate −300 mL/s [12]. Laminar and turbulent steady-state analyses (k-ε model) were applied for longitudinal comparison. Low level of under-relaxation factors from previous study was applied to stabilize the solution [13]. Pressure, velocity, geometrical change, and resistance of airway were compared to assess the effect of dental expansion. The resistance of airway is defined as:

$$\text{Resistance of airway} = \frac{\text{Presssure difference}}{\text{Flow rate}}$$

Results

Comparisons between before and after RME airway volume measurements showed that increases were only detected in nasal cavity volume, nasopharynx volume, and the most constricted area of the airway (Table 2).

For the element independence test, the element size was adjusted to be 3, 2, and 1 mm, and corresponding maximum velocity and pressure were recorded to show the independence. The result showed that 1-mm element size allowed accurate longitudinal comparison. The mesh comprised more than 158K nodes and 580K elements.

The geometry and cross-sectional area comparison of the most constricted area of the upper airway is presented in Fig. 1. The CFD results comparison of laminar flow analysis are shown in Figs. 2 and 3. Resistance of airway between the first and last cross-section was 6.3 Pa·s/L for pre-treatment and 2.3 Pa·s/L for post-treatment. The CFD results comparison of turbulent flow analysis are shown in Figs. 4, 5, and 6.

The pressure and velocity were compared at the cross-sections located in the same position. Pressure, velocity, and turbulent kinetic energy decreased after RME for laminar and turbulent flow, but they were similar for the integral and partial models. The pressure difference changed from 4.3 to 4.5 Pa, and the maximum velocity changed from 2.2 to 2.1 m/s. The variations were less

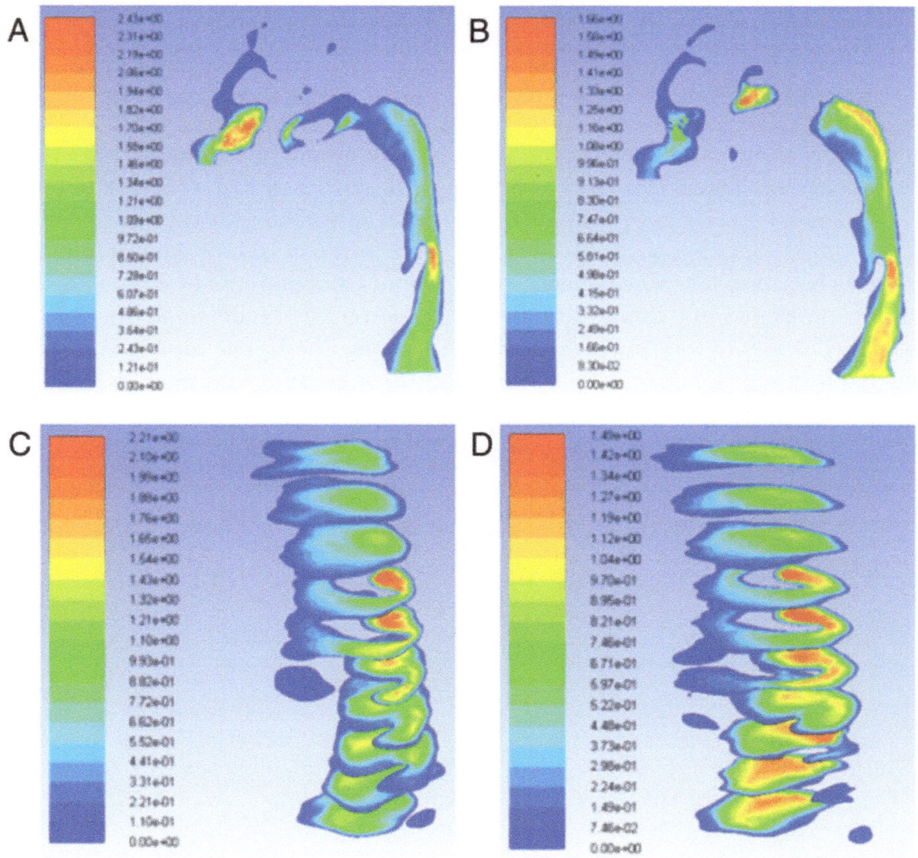

Fig. 3 Velocity of laminar flow **a** pre-RME and **b** post-RME; velocity at cross-sections of laminar flow **c** pre-RME and **d** post-RME (m/s)

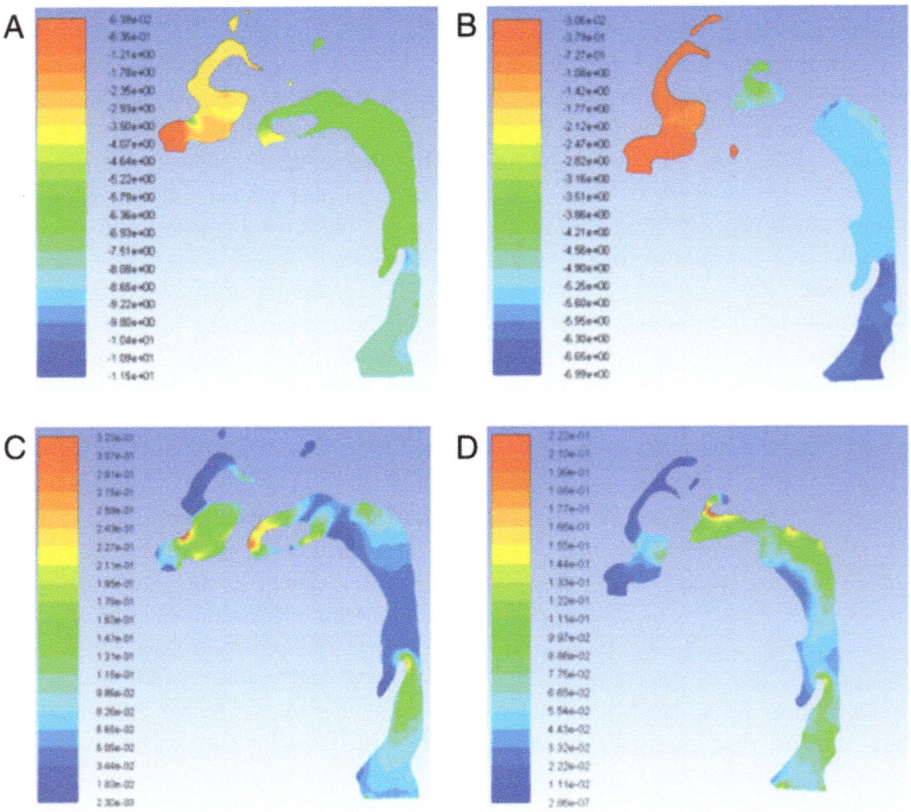

Fig. 4 Pressure of turbulent flow **a** pre-RME and **b** post-RME (Pa); turbulence kinetic energy **c** pre-RME and **d** post-RME (m^2/s^2)

than 5 %. Turbulent flow showed relatively larger velocity and pressure than laminar flow (Fig. 7).

Discussion

Evaluation of the airway is critical for those patients who suffer from breathing problems and airway disorders. RME is widely used by clinicians to treat maxillary transverse discrepancies and is sometimes associated with improvement in the breathing patterns in patients with airway disorders. Literatures have reported the impact of RME on dental and skeletal structures, tongue posture, nasal morphology, and airway volume [14-17]. However, there is lack of data on airway internal flow dynamics and patterns of airflow in relation to RME. It is important to understand the effect of RME and increasing the upper airway volume in relation to the airflow dynamics in order to explore the exact mechanisms involved in relieving the symptoms associated

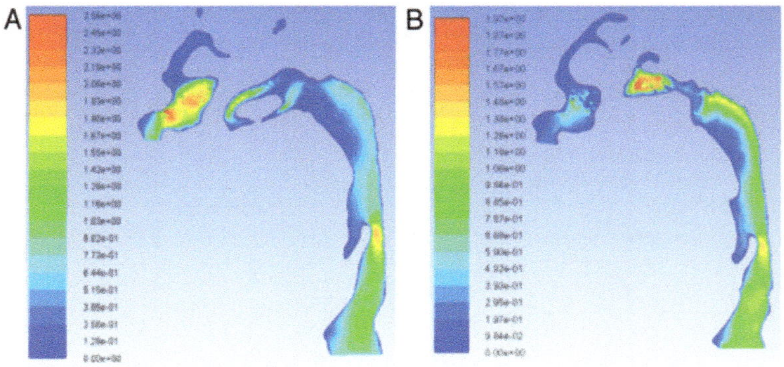

Fig. 5 Velocity of turbulent flow **a** pre-RME and **b** post-RME (m/s)

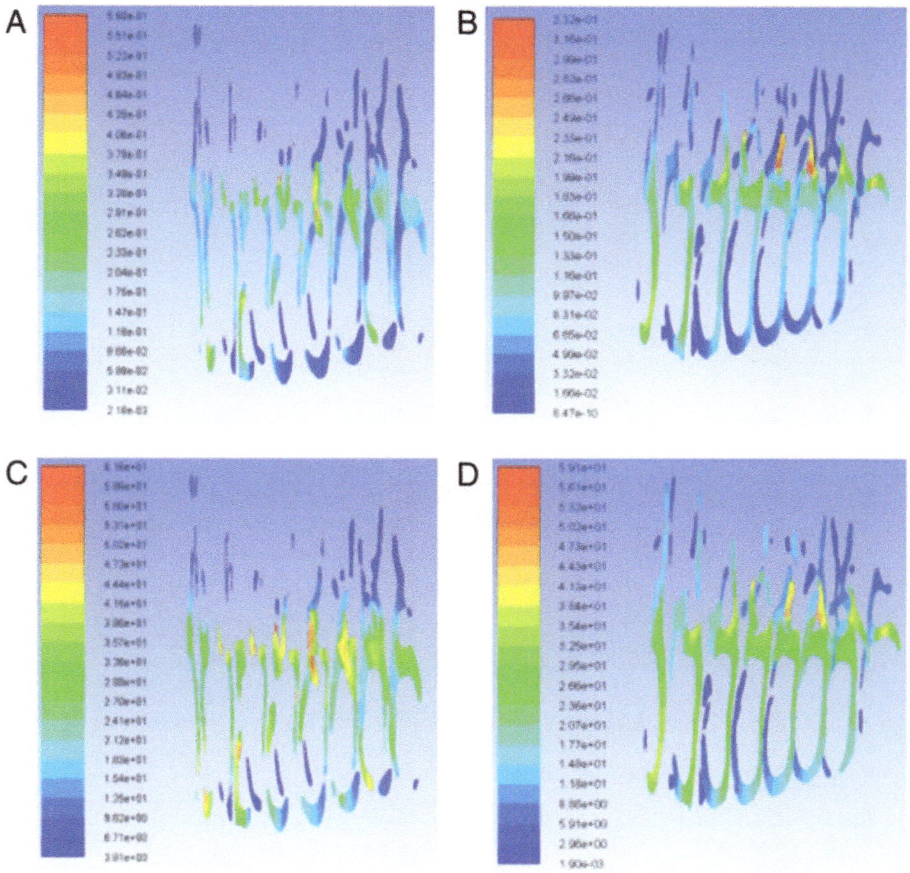

Fig. 6 Turbulence kinetic energy at nasal cross-sections **a** pre-RME and **b** post-RME (m^2/s^2); turbulent intensity at nasal cross-sections **c** pre-RME and **d** post-RME (%)

with breathing disorders. The purpose of this study was to assess the effects of RME on the upper airway using CFD results of comparing pre- and post-treatment finite element models.

CFD is a convenient, reliable, and non-invasive evaluating tool for simulating the internal flow dynamics of the upper airway [18-21]. In the present study, CFD was used to provide information about the internal flow dynamics and measure the pressure, velocity, and turbulent kinetic energy of the upper airway of a male patient with collapsed maxilla. Results were compared between before and after RME treatment of the same patient. Three-dimensional evaluation of the airway volume was performed after dividing the airway passage into the nasal cavity, nasopharynx, oropharynx, hypopharynx, and the most constricted area of the airway. The results showed that increases were only detected in nasal cavity volume, nasopharynx volume, and the most constricted area of the airway after RME.

CFD results indicated that the geometry of airway showed some changes that were especially located at the nasal area. For laminar flow, the pressure dropped from −14.6 to −9.3 Pa after RME. The velocity dropped from 2.2 to 1.5 m/s. The resistance of airway was reduced from 6.3 to 2.3 Pa·s/L between the first and last cross-sections. Most importantly, CFD assessment of airway showed increase in geometry of the most constricted area of the airway. Comparison of laminar and turbulent flow analysis before and after RME indicated that when air flowed at low velocity and through a wider structure, pressure decreased and thus air appeared to flow in a more straight line "laminar flow." Turbulence occurs at both nasal and oropharynx areas. Turbulent flow shows relatively larger pressure and velocity compared to laminar flow.

The pressure and velocity at the most constricted area of the airway decreased after RME for the laminar flow more than the turbulent flow although they both showed similar distribution patterns for the integral and partial models. The variations of both models were less than 5 %.

The results of the current study confirm the findings of Yu et al. [22] who investigated the effect of

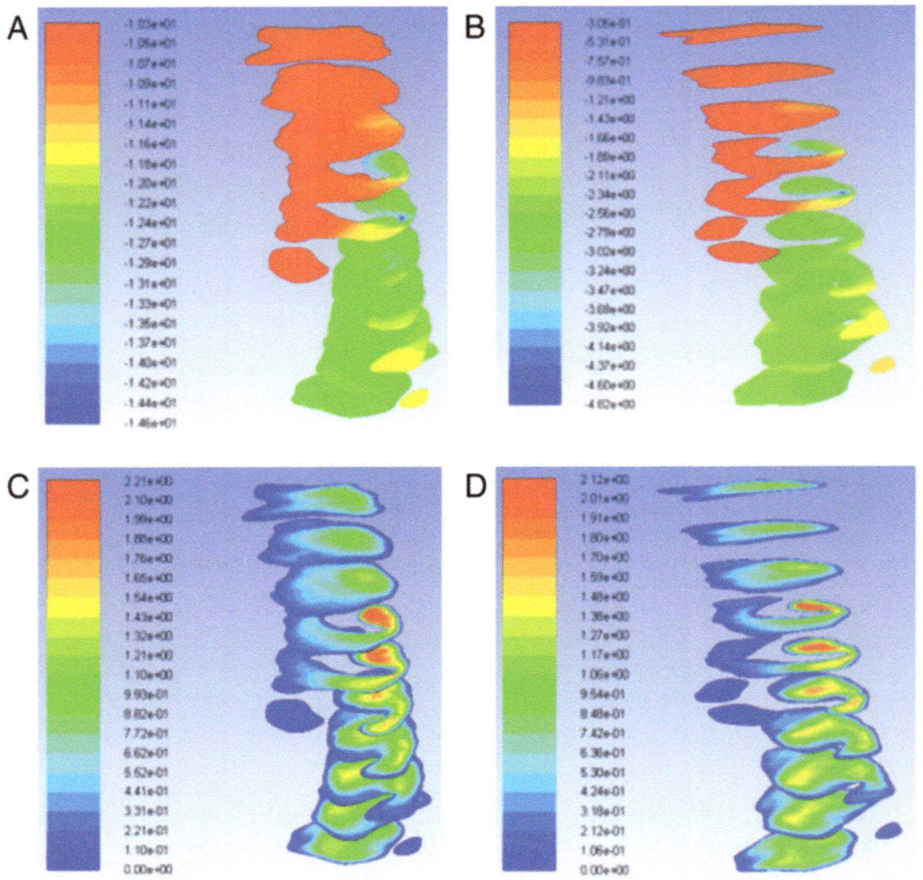

Fig. 7 Pressure at cross-sections of laminar flow **a** integral model and **b** partial model (Pa); velocity at cross-sections of laminar flow **c** integral model and **d** partial model (m/s)

maxillomandibular advancement on two obstructive sleep apnea (OSA) patients' upper airway flow dynamics using CFD. They indicated that the cross-sectional area of the narrowest part of the upper airway increased in all dimensions associated with decreased pressure gradient across the whole conduit during the passage of air. They stated that this was consistent with the clinical improvement and less breathing efforts reported for both cases. Similarly, Fan et al. [12], in their study, investigated the effect of surgical intervention on the size of the airway in an OSA patient using CFD. The results demonstrated significant pressure drop along the upper airway after the surgical procedure and suggested that this indicates decreasing collapsibility of the airway which will consequently improve the breathing function as well as the sleep quality.

Future studies are being planned with increased sample size and comparisons with gender- and age-matched control sample in order to overcome the current study sample size limitation.

Conclusions

- Comparisons between before and after RME airway volume measurements showed that increases were only detected in nasal cavity volume, nasopharynx volume, and the most constricted area of the airway.
- Turbulence occurs at both nasal and oropharynx areas, and it showed relatively larger pressure and velocity compared to laminar flow.
- RME showed positive effects in terms of reduction of pressure, velocity, and resistance of airway in this patient. This may help understand the key mechanisms behind relieving the symptom of breathing disorders as a result of treatment with RME.

Competing interest
The authors declare that they have no competing interests.

Authors' contributions
FJ and TW were responsible on construction of the finite element models and interpretation of the data. SA and KK participated in data analysis and drafted the manuscript. AG carried out the study conception and design,

participated in analysis of the 3D data, and revised the article for submission. All authors read and approved the final manuscript.

Acknowledgements

This research project was supported by a grant from the Center for Female Scientific and Medical Colleges, Deanship of Scientific Research, King Saud University, and Indiana University School of Dentistry (IUSD) 3D Imaging of the Craniofacial Complex Center.

Author details

[1]Department of Orthodontics and Oral Facial Genetics, Indiana University School Dentistry, 1121 West Michigan Street, Indianapolis, IN 46202, USA. [2]Department of Orthodontics, Faculty of Dental Medicine, Al-Azhar University, Cairo, Egypt. [3]Department of Pediatric Dentistry and Orthodontics, College of Dentistry, King Saud University, Riyadh, Saudi Arabia. [4]Department of Mechanical Engineering, Indiana University School of Engineering, Indianapolis, IN, USA.

References

1. Haas AJ. Long-term posttreatment evaluation of rapid palatal expansion. Angle Orthod. 1980;50:189–217.
2. Bishara SE, Staley RN. Maxillary expansion: clinical implications. Am J Orthod Dentofacial Orthop. 1987;91:3–14.
3. Doruk C, Sökücü O, Sezer H, Canbay EI. Evaluation of nasal airway resistance during rapid maxillary expansion using acoustic rhinometry. Europ J Orthod. 2004;26:397–401.
4. Timms DJ. The reduction of nasal airway resistance by rapid maxillary expansion and its effect on respiratory disease. J Laryngol Otol. 1984;98:357–62.
5. Matsumoto MA, Itikawa CE, Valera FC, Faria G, Anselmo-Lima WT. Long-term effects of rapid maxillary expansion on nasal area and nasal airway resistance. Am J Rhinol Allergy. 2010;24:161–5.
6. Wong ML, Sandham A, Ang PK, Wong DC, Tan WC, Huggare J. Craniofacial morphology, head posture, and nasal respiratory resistance in obstructive sleep apnoea: an inter-ethnic comparison. Eur J Orthod. 2005;27:91–7.
7. Moss-Salentijn L, Melvin L. Moss and the functional matrix. J Dent Res. 1997;76:1814–7.
8. Kilic N, Oktay H. Effects of rapid maxillary expansion on nasal breathing and some naso-respiratory and breathing problems in growing children: a literature review. Int J Pediatr Otorhinolaryngol. 2008;72:1595–601.
9. Gungor AY, Turkkahraman H. Effects of airway problems on maxillary growth: a review. Eur J Dent. 2009;3:250–4.
10. Iwasaki T, Saitoh I, Takemoto Y, Inada E, Kanomi R, Hayasaki H, et al. Improvement of nasal airway ventilation after rapid maxillary expansion evaluated with computational fluid dynamics. Am J Orthod Dentofacial Orthop. 2012;141:269–78.
11. Iwasaki T, Takemoto Y, Inada E, Sato H, Suga H, Saitoh I, et al. The effect of rapid maxillary expansion on pharyngeal airway pressure during inspiration evaluated using computational fluid dynamics. Int J Pediatr Otorhinolaryngol. 2014;78:1258–64.
12. Fan Y, Cheung LK, Chong MM, Chua HD, Chow KW, Liu CH. Computational fluid dynamics analysis on the upper airways of obstructive sleep apnea using patient-specific models. IAENG INT J Comp Sci. 2011;38:401–8.
13. Jeong SJ, Kim WS, Sung SJ. Numerical investigation on the flow characteristics and aerodynamic force of the upper airway of patient with obstructive sleep apnea using computational fluid dynamics. Med Eng Phys. 2007;29:637–51.
14. Kim YJ, Hong JS, Hwang YI, Park YH. Three-dimensional analysis of pharyngeal airway in preadolescent children with different anteroposterior skeletal patterns. Am J Orthod Dentofacial Orthop. 2010;137:306. e1–11.
15. Chaconas SJ, Caputo AA. Observation of orthopedic force distribution produced by maxillary orthodontic appliances. Am J Orthod. 1982;82:492–501.
16. Starnbach H, Bayne D, Cleall J, Subtelny JD. Facioskeletal and dental changes resulting from rapid maxillary expansion. Angle Orthod. 1966;36:152–64.
17. Iwasaki T, Saitoh I, Takemoto Y, Inada E, Kakuno E, Kanomi R, et al. Tongue posture improvement and pharyngeal airway enlargement as secondary effects of rapid maxillary expansion: a cone-beam computed tomography study. Am J Orthod Dentofacial Orthop. 2013;143:235–45.
18. De Backer JW, Vos WG, Gorle CD, Germonpre P, Partoens B, Wuyts FL, et al. Flow analyses in the lower airways: patient-specific model and boundary conditions. Med Eng Phys. 2008;30:872–9.
19. Xu C, Sin S, McDonough JM, Udupa JK, Guez A, Arens R, et al. Computational fluid dynamics modeling of the upper airway of children with obstructive sleep apnea syndrome in steady flow. J Biomech. 2006;39:2043–54.
20. Mihaescu M, Murugappan S, Gutmark E, Donnelly LF, Khosla S, Kalra M. Computational fluid dynamics analysis of upper airway reconstructed from magnetic resonance imaging data. Ann Otol Rhinol Laryngol. 2008;117:303–9.
21. Sung SJ, Jeong SJ, Yu YS, Hwang CJ, Pae EK. Customized three-dimensional computational fluid dynamics simulation of the upper airway of obstructive sleep apnea. Angle Orthod. 2006;76:791–9.
22. Yu CC, Hsiao HD, Lee LC, Yao CM, Chen NH, Wang CJ, et al. Computational fluid dynamic study on obstructive sleep apnea syndrome treated with maxillomandibular advancement. J Craniofac Surg. 2009;20:426–30.

20

Sagittal lip positions in different skeletal malocclusions: a cephalometric analysis

Merina Joshi[1*†], Li Peng Wu[1†], Surendra Maharjan[2] and Mukunda Raj Regmi[2]

Abstract

Background: The objectives of this paper are to (1) study use of soft tissue analyses advocated by Steiner, Ricketts, Burstone, Sushner and Holdway to develop soft tissue cephalometric norms as baseline data for sagittal lip position in Northeast Chinese adult population, (2) compare the sagittal lip positions in different skeletal malocclusions and (3) compare the sagittal lip positions in Northeast Chinese adults with other reported populations.

Methods: Lateral cephalometric radiographs of subjects were taken in natural head position. Radiographs were manually traced and five reference lines - Sushner, Steiner, Burstone, Holdway and Ricketts, were used. The linear distance between the tip of the lips and the five reference lines were measured. Statistical analysis was done using the Statistical Package for Social Sciences (SPSS) 21. Descriptive analysis was done for each variable for each subject. Coefficient of variation between lip positions as assessed by reference lines was determined. *Post hoc* Tukey's test was used for comparison of the mean cephalometric values of three skeletal malocclusions. The level of significance for the analysis was set at $p < 0.05$.

Results: The findings showed significant difference in the sagittal lip positions in different skeletal malocclusions. There was variation in consistent reference line in each skeletal malocclusion. The S2 line was the most consistent reference line in skeletal class I and class II group. The B line was the most consistent line in skeletal class III. In skeletal class II group, upper lips were the most protrusive and lower lips were retrusive than in skeletal class I and class III groups. In case of skeletal class III group, upper lips were retrusive and lower lips were more protrusive than in skeletal class I and class II groups.

Conclusions: The sagittal lip positions were found to be associated with the skeletal malocclusion pattern. Northeast Chinese population has protrusive upper and lower lip in comparison to Caucasians. Each skeletal malocclusion group showed different preferable reference lines for analysis of sagittal lip position.

Keywords: Northeast Chinese population; Skeletal class; Reference lines; Sagittal; Lip

Background

The soft tissue analysis has always been an integral part of diagnosis and treatment planning. The nose, lip and chin are the major components of soft tissue profile. Various soft tissue analyses have been developed to help clinicians to quantitatively evaluate the facial morphology. Among this, position of lips profoundly alters the choice of treatment. Moreover, orthodontic treatment plan can also alter the lip positions. Lip position has become one of the most important soft tissue analyses as it influences the occlusion, tooth stability and facial aesthetic [1]. The anteroposterior lip position can be evaluated by various reference lines such as Sushner's S2 line, Steiner's S1 line, Burrstone's B line, Ricketts E line and Holdway's H line (Figure 1).

These normative cephalometric values for soft tissue analyses are based on the studies carried out on Caucasians samples of European-American ancestry (Table 1). Many investigators have proved that there are vast differences among different ethnic and racial groups. They have developed cephalometric standards for different groups and should be treated according to their own characteristics [7]. The adaptation of facial tissues over underlying skeletal discrepancy varies among different races and population.

* Correspondence: merinajoshi1@hotmail.com
†Equal contributors
[1]Department of Stomatology, College of Stomatology, Jiamusi University, Street no. 522, Hongqi street, Jiamusi 154004, Republic of China
Full list of author information is available at the end of the article

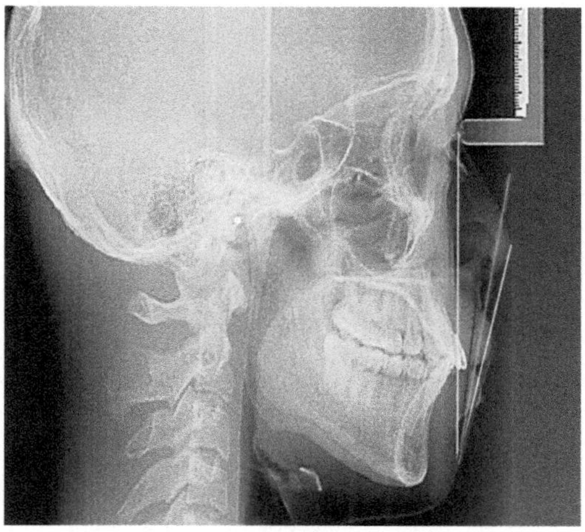

Color	Reference lines
Yellow	Burstone B line
Red	Sushner S2 line
Green	Steiner S1 line
White	Ricketts E line
Blue	Holdway H line

Figure 1 Lateral cephalometric radiograph representing the five reference lines.

This greatly influences the treatment planning and also the success of treatment. The cephalometric norms reported by these authors may not be suitable to serve as reference values for treatment planning in the Chinese population. Therefore, the objectives of this study are to (1) investigate use of soft tissue analyses advocated by Steiner, Ricketts, Burstone, Sushner and Holdway to develop soft tissue cephalometric norms as baseline data for sagittal lip position in Northeast Chinese adult population for orthodontic diagnosis and treatment planning, (2) compare sagittal lip position in different skeletal malocclusions and (3) compare the sagittal lip position in Northeast Chinese adults with other reported populations.

Methods

This retrospective study comprised of 150 randomly selected patients referred to the Jiamusi University Dental Department. The subjects were selected according to the following criteria:

1. Northeast Chinese population with Northeast Chinese grandparents,
2. Age between 18 and 25 years at the time of cephalometric radiograph,
3. Presence of all permanent teeth except third molars, no anterior or posterior cross bite,
4. No previous history of orthodontic and prosthodontic treatment,
5. No congenital abnormalities or trauma to face and
6. Good lateral cephalometric radiographs.

Consents were obtained from each patient. Lateral cephalometric radiographs were taken in natural head position with the eyes straight ahead, the teeth in centric occlusion and lips in relaxed contact. The same operator took all the lateral cephalometric radiographs. An acetate sheet of 0.003 mm was placed on top X-ray film and traced by 0.5-mm lead pencil. Soft tissue and hard tissue landmarks were traced on acetate sheets (Table 2 and Figure 2). Skeletal malocclusion was classified based upon the ANB (A point, nasion, B point) angle [3,8] and Wits value [9,10] which indicates the positional relationship of the maxilla and mandible Table 3.

The patients were categorized into three skeletal malocclusions classes and each skeletal malocclusion class having 50 patients. The linear distances between the tips of the lips and the five reference lines were measured using digital vernier caliper. When lips were positioned in front of reference line, they were denoted by positive

Table 1 Normal values for the five reference lines [1-6]

Reference lines	Sushner's S2 line	Burstone's B line	Steiner's S1 line	Holdway H line	Ricketts E line
Normal values in mm	Female	3.5 ± 1.4 UL	Lips should touch the reference line	LL should touch the reference or line −1 to +2	3 to 4 UL
	8.8 UL	2.2 ± 1.6 LL			−2 LL
	6.7 LL				
	Male				
	10.3 UL				
	7.8 LL				

UL, upper lips; LL, lower lips.

Table 2 Cephalometric soft tissue landmarks [11]

Soft tissue landmarks	Description
Soft tissue nasion (Ns)	The point of deepest concavity of the soft tissue contour of the root of the nose
Pronasale (Pn)	The most prominent point of the nose
Subnasale (Sn)	The point where the lower border of the nose meets the outer contour of the upper lip
Labial superius (Ls)	The median point in the upper margin of the upper membranous lip
Labial inferius (Li)	The median point in the lower margin of the lower membranous lip
Soft tissue pogonion (Pos)	The most prominent point on the soft tissue contour of the chin

sign; when behind the reference line, they were denoted by negative sign; and zero when lips were on the reference line.

Statistical analysis

Statistical analysis was done using the Statistical Package for Social Sciences (SPSS) version 21. Descriptive analysis was carried out for each variable for each subject. Coefficient of variation between lip positions as assessed by reference lines was determined. *Post hoc* Tukey's test was used for comparison of the mean cephalometric values of the three skeletal malocclusions. The level of significance for the analysis was set at $p < 0.05$.

All the radiographic tracing and measurements were performed by one investigator. To avoid observer bias, each radiograph was coded with a number so that the observer was blinded to the skeletal pattern of the subject. To evaluate the presence of any error with digitization and measurement, 30 randomly selected radiographs were again traced and measured by the same investigator 1 week after the initial measurements.

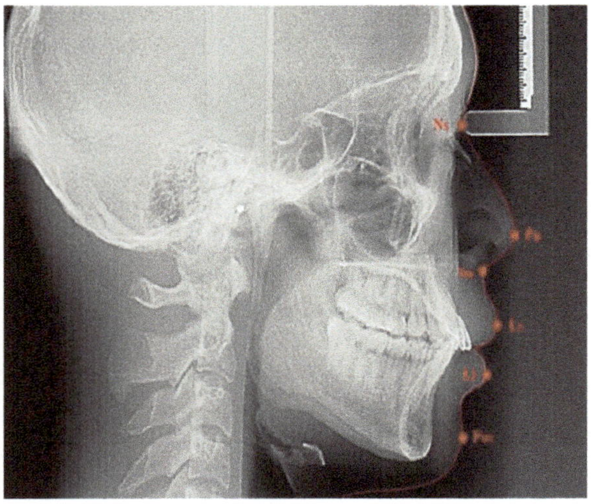

Figure 2 Cephalometric radiograph showing soft tissue landmarks.

Table 3 Normal values of ANB angle and Wits appraisal for different skeletal malocclusions

Skeletal malocclusions	Class I	Class II	Class III
ANB angle	0° to 4°	>4°	<0°
Wits value	0 and −3 mm	≥−1 mm	≤−4 mm

Results

Table 4 shows the statistical analysis along with the mean and standard deviation of skeletal class I, class II and class III groups. The coefficient of variation in skeletal class I was the least in relation to S2 line in both the upper lip (UL) (coefficient of variation (CV) = 25.41%) and the lower lip (LL) (CV = 27.897%). The E line showed the greatest variation in both UL and LL (UL = 196.04% and LL = 194.05% of CV). In skeletal class II, S2 line related to both UL (CV = 19.89%) and LL (CV = 34.38%) and had the least CV. The H line showed the greatest variation in LL (477.46%). In both UL and LL, E line showed low variation (UL = 117.44% and LL = 356.86% of CV). The CV in skeletal class III was the least in case of B line related to both UL (CV = 17.76%) and LL (CV = 19.75%). The E line showed greatest variation in both UL and LL (UL = 170.87% and LL = 41.22% of CV).

An analysis of variance (ANOVA) test was performed, and it showed all lines are different in all the skeletal malocclusions. *Post hoc* Tukey's test was used for comparison of the mean cephalometric values of the three skeletal malocclusions. The level of significance for the analysis was set at $p < 0.05$. Table 4 shows mean and standard deviation and result for *post hoc* test (Tukey's HSD) showing the difference between skeletal classes. Additional data of Post Hoc Tukey Test showing the difference between each skeletal class are shown in Additional file 1: Table S1.

Sushner's S2 line

Comparison was done among the skeletal classes to access the sagittal lip position using five reference lines. In

Table 4 Mean standard deviation and result for *post hoc* test (Tukey's HSD) showing the difference between skeletal classes

	Class I	Class II	Class III
UL to S2 line	11.81^{a}(±3.00)	13.75^{a}(±2.73)	10.42^{a}(±1.95)
LL to S2 line	9.04^{a}(±2.52)	8.70^{b}(±2.99)	11.42^{ab}(±2.30)
UL to B line	6.66^{a}(±2.00)	7.48^{b}(±2.07)	6.87^{c}(±1.22)
LL to B line	5.74^{a}(±2.31)	4.85^{b}(±2.25)	7.77^{ab}(±1.53)
UL to S1 line	4.32^{a}(±2.03)	5.35^{a}(±1.68)	4.55^{b}(±1.20)
LL to S1 line	4.22^{a}(±2.32)	3.47^{b}(±2.29)	5.83^{ab}(±1.29)
LL to H line	1.48^{a}(±1.36)	0.49^{a}(±2.37)	3.58^{a}(±1.01)
UL to E line	1.11^{a}(±2.19)	2.14^{b}(±2.51)	0.82^{b}(±1.40)
LL to E line	1.07^{a}(±2.09)	0.75^{b}(±2.70)	3.44^{ab}(±1.41)

Mean values with same letter ("a" or "b") in superscript are statistically different ($p < 0.05$). Mean (±SD), n = 50.

skeletal class I group, S2 line showed slightly more protrusive UL (11.81 ± 3.00 mm) and LL (9.042 ± 2.52 mm) than norms given by Sushner (UL 8.8/10.3 mm and LL 6.7 to 7.8 mm). In skeletal class II group, ULs (13.75 ± 2.73 mm) were more protruded and LLs (8.70 ± 2.99 mm) were retrusive than skeletal class I and class III groups. In the case of skeletal class III group, the ULs (10.42 ± 1.95 mm) were retrusive and LLs (11.42 ± 2.30 mm) were protrusive in comparison to class I and class II. There were statistically significant differences between the skeletal classes in S2 to UL. In the case of S2 to LL, there were statistically significant difference between class I and class III and class II and class III.

Burstone's B line

When using B line, the UL (6.66 ± 2.00 mm) and the LL (5.74 ± 2.31 mm) in skeletal class I group were protrusive than the normal values given by Burstone. In the case of skeletal class II group, UL (7.48 ± 2.07 mm) were more protrusive and LL (4.85 ± 2.25 mm) were retrusive than skeletal class I and class III groups. Skeletal class III group showed most protruded LL (7.77 ± 1.53 mm) than class I and class II. There were no statistically significant differences between the skeletal classes in case of B line to UL ($p > 0.05$). However, there were statistically significant differences between class I and class III and class II and class III in the case of B line to LL.

Steiner's S1 line

In skeletal class I group, S1 line showed protrusive UL (4.32 ± 2.03 mm) and LL (4.22 ± 2.32 mm) than norms given by Steiner. In skeletal class II group, UL (7.03 ± 3.66 mm) were more protrusive and LL (5.77 ± 1.18 mm) were retrusive than in skeletal class I and class III groups. In skeletal class III, the UL (4.55 ± 1.20 mm) were retrusive in comparison to skeletal class II and LL were slightly protrusive (5.83 ± 1.29 mm) in comparison to skeletal class I and class II. There were statistically significant differences between class I and class II in the case of S1 line with UL and between class I and class II in the case of S1 line with LL.

Ricketts E line

In skeletal class I group, both UL (1.11 ± 2.19 mm) and LL (1.07 ± 2.09 mm) were protrusive than norms provided by Ricketts. In skeletal class II group, LL (2.14 ± 2.51 mm) was more protruded than in skeletal class I and class III groups. In the case of skeletal class III, ULs (0.82 ± 1.40 mm) were retrusive and LLs (3.44 ± 1.41 mm) were protrusive in comparison to class I and class II. There were statistically significant differences between class II and class III in the case of E line with UL and between class II and class III and class I and class II in the case of E line with LL.

Holdway's H line

Comparing the lower lip with reference to the H line, it was found that the LL (1.48 ± 1.36 mm) in skeletal class I was protrusive than the norms. LLs in skeletal class III were protrusive than in skeletal class I and class II. There were statistically significant differences between class I and class III and class II and class III.

Discussion

This study is designed to determine the sagittal lip positions in relation to the five reference lines in three different skeletal malocclusions. The sample included adult subjects of age 18 to 25 years as the majority of facial growth is usually completed by 16 to 17 years of age [12]. The subjects were selected from those individuals who had a lateral cephalometric radiograph taken for diagnosis purposes. The selection criteria for many studies are mostly excellent class I molar in relation with good intercuspation, pleasing facial profiles [13,14]. Assessment based on pleasing profiles and satisfactory occlusion is subjective and introduces biases. Also, they do not represent the randomized representation of the particular population. Hence, it is important to analyse these reference lines in different skeletal malocclusions to determine which reference line is more reliable in each skeletal malocclusion.

Erbay et al. found that soft tissue analysis differs according to population. Every race has its one nose and chin characteristics [15]. Sushner developed his norms for black population. Ricketts norms are applied to Caucasians and not to all ethical and racial groups. Thus, using soft tissue norms of one population would be unreliable in diagnosis and treatment planning for another population. It would be helpful to assess the reliability of these reference lines in Northeast Chinese adult population. This would serve as the baseline data for orthodontic diagnosis and treatment planning.

In this study, five reference lines were used because these reference lines are most frequently used during diagnosis and treatment.

Consistency of reference lines in different skeletal classes

There was variation in consistency of reference line in each skeletal malocclusion. S2 line had the smallest coefficient of variation and provided the narrowest dispersion in skeletal class I and class II groups. In the case of skeletal class III group, B line had the smallest CV. Hence, S2 line and B line can be considered to be the best reference lines in terms of judging the sagittal lip position in skeletal classes. The possible cause for the S2 line and the B line to be the most consistent lines may be the fact that these lines do not transverse any anatomical landmarks of the nose and also the lines are close to skeletal structure.

E line had the largest CV in both skeletal class I and class III groups and had low CV in skeletal class II. On the other hand, H line was the least reliable in the case of skeletal class II. Therefore, E line and H line can be considered as less reliable to judge sagittal lip position in skeletal malocclusions. From a clinical point of view, if the reference line is located closer anteroposteriorly to the lips, it is convenient to judge the lip position. From this point of view, the E and the H lines are more reliable. The less consistency of the E line and the H line may be because these lines pass through nose and UL, respectively. In the Taiwanese, B line was also the best line in terms of consistency. However, E line is of great value because its anterior location makes it convenient for the clinician to use it, but the B line appears the best from the perspective of the value of reference [16]. Ninety-six Anatolian Turkish adult's horizontal lip position was analysed cephalometrically using the soft tissue analyses of Steiner, Ricketts, Burstone, Sushner, Holdway and Merrifield. The study indicates that in Anatolian Turkish adults, the UL and the LL were retrusive according to the norms of Steiner and Ricketts. The UL was protrusive and the LL was retrusive according to Sushner line and was within normal range according to Burstone's B line. The LL was similar to the standard proposed by Holdway [15]. Ricketts norms for lips closely resembled to the value found for the attractive profile [17].

Comparison of skeletal class I with Caucasian norms and other populations

Our study revealed that both the UL and the LL in skeletal class I were more protrusive than normative values of Ricketts, Burstone, Sushner and Steiner. This is due to the fact that the craniofacial morphology between individuals with typical Chinese and Caucasian ancestry shows significant difference. Chinese samples exhibited significantly protrusive UL and LL than Caucasians and also less obtuse nasolabial angle than Caucasian. The protrusion of LL on the profile of Chinese population was associated with significant labial inclination of lower incisors. Another possible explanation for this difference is may be the Chinese adults have less prominent nasal tips and steeper nasal bridge [18].

In our study, the LL in skeletal class I was 0.92 mm less protrusive than the UL with respect to B line. This can be considered as a consistent result. With respect to S1 line in skeletal class I group, UL and LL were more protrusive. This is in contrast to the result given by Steiner. The UL (4.32 mm) was slightly more protrusive than the LL (4.22 mm).

Additionally, the H line reported for the Northeast Chinese population was protrusive than the normal range. Lew compared H angle between Chinese and Caucasians and found that the Chinese samples had more protrusive lips, a more anteriorly placed maxilla than Caucasian and lips that were not harmonious with the H line [13].

There are few previous cephalometric studies of this kind done on Chinese population. P. Yeong and J. Huggare's research on craniofacial morphology of Singaporean Chinese found significantly greater protrusion of the UL and LL [19]. Lew also studied the Singaporean Chinese adults with aesthetically pleasing profiles and found Chinese facial profile to be less convex compared to Caucasians, with the maxilla more posteriorly located in Chinese. The UL was more protrusive and at a less obtuse nasolabial angle [13]. He also found that Chinese subjects had UL and LL protrusion of 3.4 mm and 3.5 mm, respectively, with ANB angle to be 2.4° [20]. In one of the studies conducted on the Cantonese Chinese male with pleasing or acceptable profile showed both the UL and the LL protruded beyond the Ricketts' aesthetic planes and also the lips were more protrusive than those described by Burstone's B line [14].

Adult Nigerian population showed more protrusive UL and LL than the normative values reported for Caucasians [21]. The Korean population is also reported to have greater degree of UL and LL protrusion when compared to a European American sample [22].

Craniofacial cephalometric analysis of Bangladeshi females had significantly more protruded lip positions when compared with the Caucasian group. When compared with the Japanese females, Bangladeshi females had significantly less protrusion. In the case of males, there was no significant difference in lip protrusion [23] (Table 5). Mean and standard deviation of sagittal lip positions in different populations are shown in Additional file 1: Table S2.

These variation in lip position of different populations reinforce the fact that soft tissue features are specific for each given race and ethnicity. And also this comparison with Caucasian and other population group must be interpreted with caution because of variations in sample sizes and also differences in the population.

Comparison among different skeletal classes

Overall, we can observe that in the case of skeletal class II group, all the reference lines showed the upper lips to be the most protrusive and the lower lips to be retrusive compared to skeletal class I and class III groups. In the case of skeletal class III group, upper lips were retrusive than in skeletal class I and class II and the lower lips more protrusive than in skeletal class I and class II groups.

Statistically significant correlation was found in case of upper lip with S2 line among all three skeletal classes. In the case of lower lip, H line showed significant statistical differences between all skeletal classes. Upper lip sagittal position can be better assessed by S2 line in different

Table 5 Summary of different reported populations

Study	Sample population	Age in years	Sample size	Sample selection	Soft tissue analysis	Conclusion
2012	Nigerian population	18 to 25	100	Class I molar and canine relationship, a symmetrical face	Steiner, Rickets, Burstone, Merrifield and Holdway	More protrusive upper and lower lip as compared to normative values reported for Caucasians
2002	Kwangju sample (Korean population)	18 to 20	60	Normal occlusion, class I molar and canine relationship	Steiner, Rickets, Merrifield and Holdway	Greater degree of lip protrusion in comparison to European-American samples
2004	Singapore Chinese children	Mean 12.5 girls, 12.7 boys	81	Class incisor relationship (British standards institute, 1983)	Rickets E line	Boys had more protrusive lips than Malaysian Chinese and less protrusive lips than Hong Kong Chinese
1992	Chinese adult	18 to 24	72	Harmonious facial profiles with presence of intact dentition, no difference was made between orthodontic treated and non-treated subjects	Legan and Burstone analysis, Holdway analysis	Upper and lower lip not in balance with H line, upper and lower lip were positioned more anteriorly
1972	Males of Kwangtung province origin (Cantonese Chinese)	18 to 33	30	Clinically excellent occlusion, class I molar, pleasing profile	E line and B line	Lips protruded beyond E line
2013	Bangladeshi population	23.2 to 14.6	98	Class I occlusion	B line	Females had more protrude lips compared to Caucasians and less protruded lips than Japanese, males no significant difference between Caucasian and Japanese

The relevant soft tissue analysis and conclusions are only mentioned in brief.

skeletal malocclusions. In the case of lower lip sagittal position, H line is the line of choice. This finding may be due to the fact that S2 line is close to skeletal structure and not influenced by the nose. As the lower lip is closely influenced by the upper lip position, H line can be considered as the best line in assessing lower lip position. In the present study, statistically significant difference for all the reference lines in assessing sagittal lip position among all skeletal classes were not observed. The reason behind could be variation in dentoalveolar structures especially the upper and lower incisors.

Surprisingly, there were no significant differences found between class II and class III groups in the case of E line, and also there was no statistically significant difference between skeletal classes in case of B line when assessing the upper lip. E line is influenced by the nose, but in our study, we did not include assessment of the nose. However, if samples had been based on cephalometric values like large ANB differences, incisor relations or profile assessment, we could have seen significant differences between all the skeletal classes. If soft tissue thickness at various points like nasion, subnasion and pogonian and lip thickness and lip strain were considered during analysis, we could have achieved more precise results.

Factors affecting lip position

Cephalometric measurements of face in terms of aesthetics can be difficult and misleading due to various factors. Several studies had shown that soft and hard tissue changes are highly correlated. Altemus LA, in his study, found that facial balance and harmony are often in compromised or compensated in relationship with skeletal, dental and soft tissue component of the face [24]. Dental factors, such as the inclination of upper and lower anterior relative to the palatal and mandibular plane, respectively, affects the lip positions. The movement of the cervical point of the upper incisor or the incisor retraction with translator movement greatly influenced changes in the UL position in the horizontal plane [25]. As many of the reference lines used for facial analysis pass through the nose and chin, growth and morphology of the nose and chin would greatly affect the lip position. Ricketts E line should be read in relation to the nose and chin. Ricketts E line is influenced by the growth of the nose. Whereas Steiner's S1 line eliminates half of the changes in integument profile due to the growth of the nose. Nasal growth is eliminated in H line, B line and Sushner line. The relation of the lip with the B line depends on the thickness of the lip and correct position of lips. When lips are equally thick, B line is more reliable. Both chin and nasal position influence the horizontal lip position [16,26,27]. In Turkish adult, significant differences in soft tissue thickness among skeletal malocclusions were observed for the labrale superius, stomion and labrale inferius sites. Moreover, soft tissue thickness at all sites was greater in men than in women [28].

The two main treatment approaches extraction and non-extraction have been highly controversial issues, and it mainly depends upon the patient profile. This controversy becomes even greater when dealing with borderline cases. When planning treatment for class I cases, the extraction decision mainly depends on lower anterior crowding, lower lip to E line, upper crowding and overjet. These four key orthodontic measurements will possibly vary if we take different populations [29].

There are a number of limitations to our study. First, this study utilized a small sample. Second, the gender differentiation was not done. It is difficult to find detailed information regarding each subjects when doing retrospective study. Third, China having the largest population in the world and also having many sub ethnic groups makes it difficult to collect the sample representing the Chinese population.

The growth and development of soft tissue profile is a result of complex changes within hard and soft tissue. Thus, aging factors had to be considered when evaluating soft tissue profile in adults [30]. Most importantly, it is difficult to make a valuable comparison between findings of our study and others since a limited number of studies have been published on this subject. In the future, we can extend our study to broader geographical area and give quantitative data to represent the norms for each skeletal class.

Conventional cephalometric approach encounters several limitations. Cone-beam computed tomography (CBCT) offers the possibility of accurate localization and quantification of even minor asymmetries without distortion and hence much more precise cephalometric analyses [31,32]. In the future, we can extend our study to a broader geographical area and use the latest CBCT technology to give more precise quantitative data to represent the norms for each skeletal class.

Conclusions

On the basis of lateral cephalometric records from a sample of 150 Northeast Chinese people examined, the following conclusions can be drawn:

1. UL and LL in skeletal class I group are protrusive than norms on all reference lines.
2. Skeletal class II group have the most protrusive UL and retrusive LL in comparison to skeletal class I and class III on all the reference lines.
3. Skeletal class III group has the most protrusive LL in comparison to skeletal class II and class I on all reference lines.
4. In the case of skeletal class I and class II, S2 line is the line of choice to judge the sagittal position of lips in profile analysis.
5. In the case of skeletal class III, B line is the line of choice to judge the sagittal position of lips in profile analysis.

Abbreviation

B line: Burstone's line; CV: coefficient of variation; CBCT: cone-beam computed tomography; E line: Ricketts line; H line: Holdway line; LL: lower lip; S1 line: Steiner's line; S2 line: Sushner's line; UL: upper lip.

Competing interests

All the authors declare that they have no competing interests.

Authors' contributions

MJ and LW designed the study and carried out the cephalometric studies. SM performed the statistical analysis and helped in collection of data. MRR participated in design and coordination and helped to draft the manuscript. All authors read and approved the final manuscript.

Author details

[1]Department of Stomatology, College of Stomatology, Jiamusi University, Street no. 522, Hongqi street, Jiamusi 154004, Republic of China.
[2]Department of Health Services, Teku, Kathmandu 44600, Nepal.

References

1. Burstone CJ. Lip posture and its significance in treatment planning. Am J Orthod. 1967;53(4):262–84.
2. Sushner NI. A photographic study of the soft-tissue profile of the Negro population. Am J Orthod. 1977;72(4):373–85.
3. Steiner CC. The use of cephalometrics as an aid to planning and assessing orthodontic treatment: report of a case. Am J Orthod. 1960;46(10):721–36.
4. Holdaway RA. A soft-tissue cephalometric analysis and its use in orthodontic treatment planning. Part II Am J Orthod. 1984;85(4):279–93.
5. Ricketts RM. Planning treatment on the basis of facial pattern and an estimate of its growth. Angle Orthod. 1957;27(1):14–37.
6. Holdaway RA. A soft-tissue cephalometric analysis and its use in orthodontic treatment planning. Part I Am J Orthod. 1983;84(1):1–28.
7. Faruk Ayhan Basciftci TU, Buyukerkmen A. Determination of Holdaway soft tissue norms in Anatolian Turkish adults. Am J Orthod Dentofacial Orthop. 2003;123(4):395–400.
8. Taylor CM. Changes in the relationship of nasion, point A, and point B and the effect upon ANB. Am J Orthod. 1969;56(2):143–63.
9. Jacobson A. The 'Wits' appraisal of jaw disharmony. Am J Orthod. 1975;67(2):125–38.
10. Jacobson A. Application of the 'Wits' appraisal. Am J Orthod. 1976;70(2):179–89.
11. Athanasiou AE. Orthodontic cephalometry. Maryland Heights, MI, USA: Mosby-Wolfe; 1995.
12. Oliver MLJRG. W&H orthodontic notes. J Orthod. 2000;28:1. K.M.Varghese Co.
13. Kenneth KK, Lew KKH, Keng SB, Ho KH. Soft tissue cephalometric norms in Chinese adults with esthetic facial profiles. J Maxillofac Oral Surg. 1992;50(11):1184–9.
14. Chan GK-H. A cephalometric appraisal of the Chinese (Cantonese). Am J Orthod. 1972;61(3):279–85.
15. Elif F, Erbay CMC, Şevket K, Erbay. Soft tissue profile in Anatolian Turkish adults: part I. Evaluation of horizontal lip position using different soft tissue analyses. Am J Orthod Dentofacial Orthop. 2002;121(1):57–64.
16. Hsu BS. Comparision of five analytic reference lines of the horizontal lip position;their consistency and sensitivity. Am J Orthod Dentofacial Orthop. 1993;104(4):355–60.
17. Erbay EF, CMC. Soft tissue profile in Anatolian Turkish adults: part II. Evaluation of horizontal lip position using different soft tissue analyses. Am J Orthod Dentofacial Orthop. 2002;121(1):65–72.

18. Yan Gu JAM, Lauren M, Sigler Tiziano B. Comparison of craniofacial characteristics of typical Chinese and Caucasian young adults. Eur J Orthod. 2011;33(2):205–11.
19 Yeong JH P. Morphology of Singapore Chinese. Eur J Orthod. 2004;26(6):605–12.
20. Lew KKK. Cephalometric ideals in Chinese, Malay and Indian ethnic groups. Asian J Aesthetic Dent. 1994;2(1):35–8.
21. Gerald Ikenna Isiekwe OO, Michael Chukwudi I. A cephalometric invesigation of horizontal lip position in adult Nigerians. J Orthod. 2012;39(3):160–9.
22. Hyeon-Shik Hwang W-SK, James A, McNamara. Ethnic differences in the soft tissue profile of korean and European American adults with normal occlusion and well balanced faces. Angle Orthod. 2002;72(1):72–80.
23. Ali Ahsan MY, Zakir H, Isao S. Craniofacial cephalometric analysis of Bangladeshi and Japanese adults with normal occlusion and balanced faces: a comparative study. J Orthodont Sci. 2013;21(11):7–15.
24. Altemus LA. Cephalofacial relationships. Angle Orthod. 1968;38(3):175–84.
25. Adilson Luiz Ramos MTS, Ary Dos Santos P, Jay Bowman S. Upper lip changes correlated to maxillary incisor retraction - a metallic implant study. Angle Orthod. 2005;75(4):499–505.
26. Hee Soo Oh EL, Xiaoyun Z, Yan L, Tianmian X, Robert B, Sheldon B. Correlations between cephalometric and photographic measurements of facial attractiveness in Chinese and US patients after orthodontic treatment. Am J Orthod Dentofacial Orthop. 2009;136(6):762.e761–14.
27. Luka Cala SS, Martina S, Marina Varga L, Mladen S. Facial profile preferences :differences in the perception of children with and without orthodontic history. Am J Orthod Dentofacial Orthop. 2010;138(4):442–50.
28. Hasan Kamak MC. Facial soft tissue thickness among skeletal malocclusions: is there a difference? Korean J Orthod. 2012;42(1):25–31.
29. Dimitrios Konstantonis CA. Margarita Makou. Extraction decision and identification of treatment predictors in Class I malocclusions Prog Orthod. 2013;14:47.
30. Lino Torlakovic EF. Age -related changes of soft tissue profile from second to fourth decades of life. Angle Orthod. 2011;81(1):50–7.
31. Sanders TKC, Uribe FA, Rigali PH, Nanda R. Quantification of skeletal asymmetries in normal adolescents: cone-beam computed tomography analysis. Prog Orthod. 2014;15:26.
32. Farronato GSS, Nolet F, Zoia A, Farronato D. Assessment of inter- and intra-operator cephalometric tracings on cone beam CT radiographs: comparison of the precision of the cone beam CT versus the latero-lateral radiograph tracing. Prog Orthod. 2014;15:1.

21

Functional evaluation in orthodontic surgical treatment: long-term stability and predictability

Giampietro Farronato*, Lucia Giannini, Guido Galbiati, Santo Andrea Stabilini, Michele Sarcina and Cinzia Maspero

Abstract

Background: The introduction of electromyographic and kinesiographic technology in orthodontics allows to obtain objective data regarding the functional aspects of the mandibular movements and the masticatory muscular activity. It is then important to be able to correlate the data obtained by instrumental activity with the clinical ones. The aim of this study consists to analyse the post ortodontic surgical stability through instrumental evaluation of the masticatory muscles and mandibular movements.

Method: 30 patients undergo electromyographic and kinesiographic evaluations through all the surgical orthodontic iter and were than followed during other 4 years. JMP software was used to analyze and correlate the electromyographic and knesioographic data during treatment and during the follow up.

Results: A linear correlations between some functional objective values collected from the examinations at the beginning and during therapy and the follow up one has been demonstrated.

Conclusion: It is important to submit patients in surgical ortodontic treatment to instrumental analysis which can evidence how masticatory function and mandibular movements are performed. It is also important to highlight some functional values also from the beginning of the treatment because an alteration of such values can be related to a better or worse postsurgical rehabilitation.

Background

During the last decades, the electromyographic and kinesiographic technology has allowed dentists to study the homeostatic response of the body to the physiological and pathological alterations of the stomatognathic system [1–3].

This has permitted to obtain quantitative data which consequently has improved the overall diagnostic process. In fact, such measurements can be statistically evaluated and are considered important not only during the diagnostic and therapeutic phases of the treatment but also during the follow-up [4, 5].

Post-orthodontic stability is guaranteed if the occlusion obtained is in harmony with the oral cavity functions and in particular with the activity of the masticatory muscles [6, 7].

Hence, it is essential to make a correct diagnosis and define a treatment plan which is based on the clinical and instrumental data obtained taking into account the functional aspect of the oral cavity [8–12].

In literature, many authors believe that an inappropriate functioning of the neuromuscular system can cause important malocclusions [4, 7, 10].

Nowadays, an electromyographic evaluation has become essential for the diagnostic process in patients undergoing combined surgical-orthodontic treatment as both electromyographic and kinesiographic assessments allow to diagnose neuromuscular problems. They permit to assess the benefits of the therapy and maintenance during the follow-up phase as they are important markers for a possible relapse. Furthermore, these diagnostic tools allow to evaluate the time interval required for the functional and kinesiological parameters to return to the preoperative values [13–23].

At the end of treatment, it is essential that the muscles which are mainly involved in the masticatory movements are relaxed and painless with no spasm. If the muscles are

* Correspondence: giampietro.farronato@unimi.it
Maxillo-Facial and Odontostomatology Unit (Head: prof. AB. Giannì), Fondazione Cà Granda IRCCS Ospedale Maggiore Policlinico, Milan, Italy

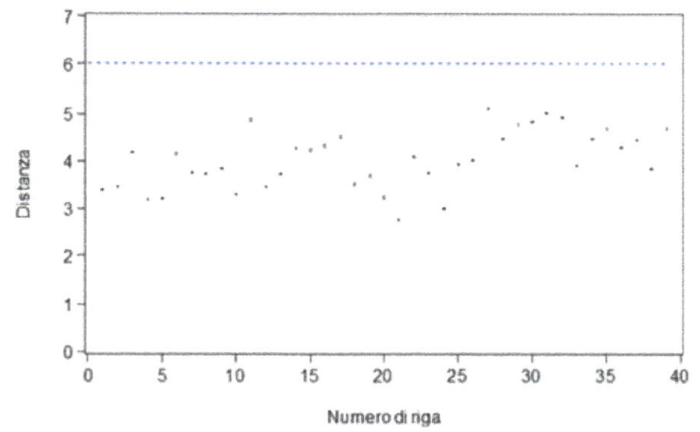

Fig. 1 Mahalanobis distances

fatigued or are in a condition of spasm, they must recruit more motor units to maintain the same function. Hence, these will register a higher electromyographic activity.

The aim of this study was to investigate, from an electromyographic and kinesiographic point of view, muscular functionality and the mandibular kinesiology of patients undergoing orthodontic-surgical treatment. Such assessment was carried out from the diagnostic phase to the end of treatment and follow-up with the aim of identifying whether there was a predictive model of correlation between such measurements.

In particular, this retrospective study focused on determining whether there was a correlation model between electromyographic values recorded after 4 years from the end of the orthodontic-surgical therapy and the measurements made at the beginning, during, and at the end of the treatment.

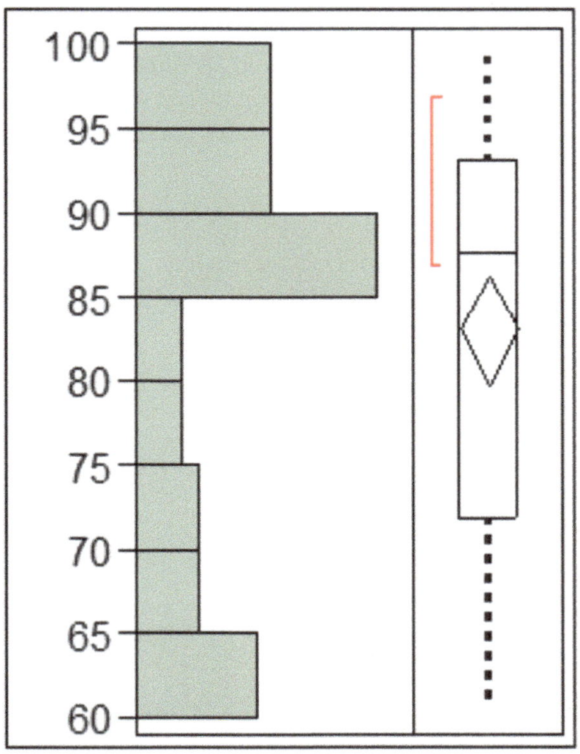
Fig. 2 Fundamental measure expressed in percentage

Methods

Selection of the sample and research procedure

This study involved 98 adult patients attending the Orthodontic department of the University of Milan.

All patients included in the study were diagnosed with a specific malocclusion and were hence eligible to receive orthodontic-surgical treatment.

Therefore, the patients have been followed from the electromyographic and kinesiographic point of view during all the therapeutic orthodontic-surgical phases starting from the diagnosis to follow-up (follow-up average = 4.3 ± 0.1 years after the end of the therapy).

Out of 98 adult patients, 30 have been selected, 12 males and 18 females, aging between 19 and 54 years old (average age 31.18 ± 7.63).

For the selection of the 30 patients, the inclusion criteria were as follows:

- Adult age (≥18 years).
- Presence of a dentoskeletal discrepancy and the need for combined surgical orthodontic treatment. The choice of surgical treatment was related to every single case. Some of them were bimaxillary surgical operations, and others involved only one maxillary bone.
- Electromyographic and kinesiographic exams during the following stages:
  - Diagnosis (to obtain additional information to the clinical and radiographic methods evaluations)
  - Before bonding
  - Every 2 months during the pre-surgical orthodontic phase and monthly immediately before and after surgery
  - The day before surgery
  - Before the intermaxillary fixation phase
  - After the intermaxillary fixation phase
  - During the post-surgical orthodontic phase
  - At the removal of the surgical bite
  - At the de-bonding phase
  - In follow-up controls
- Presence of a post-treatment follow-up of at least 4 years.

Patients who did not satisfy all inclusion criteria were excluded.

Data collection involved a questionnaire which included information on age, weight, job, sex, previous orthodontic treatment, and temporo-mandibular disorders.

The assessments were performed by a single operator in order to eliminate operator variability.

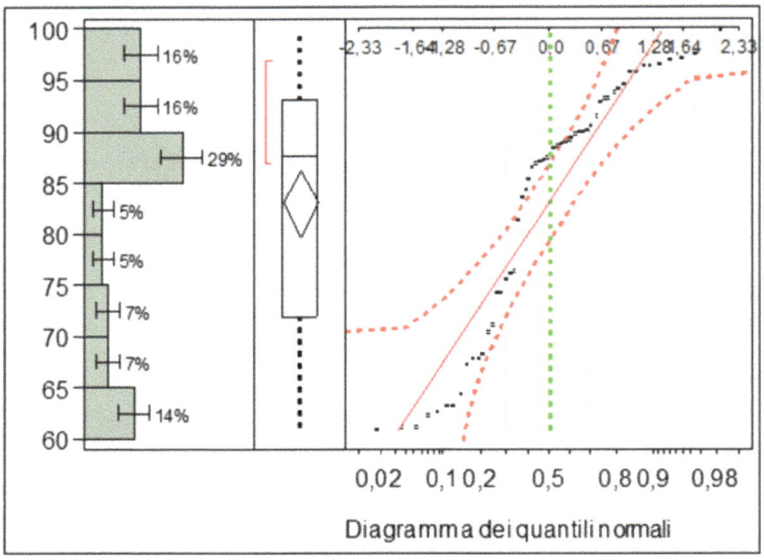

Fig. 3 Normal quantile diagram of the fundamental measure

No ethical approval or ethical review board judgment was necessary because the electromyographic tests were not invasive and represent an important part of the diagnostic phase.

Equipment

The de Gotzen electromyograph Freely and Myotronics electromyography and kinesiography K6-I was used on all patients.

Each patient underwent an electromyographic and a kinesiographic exam performed with the K6-I equipment during all phases of the orthodontic-surgical treatment and in particular during the diagnostic phase, at the bonding, during the pre-surgical treatment, the day before surgery, during the intermaxillary fixation period, at the de-bonding, and in the follow-up phases.

Analysis and data interpretation

The statistical analysis of this study has been performed using JMP statistical discovery software (2010).

This program allows to calculate correlation predictive models through multiple linear regression methods in which a series of data known as dependent variables (which we have referred to as fundamental measure) is related to a series of independent variables.

The aim was to highlight a significant correlation between the electromyographic values obtained at 4 years

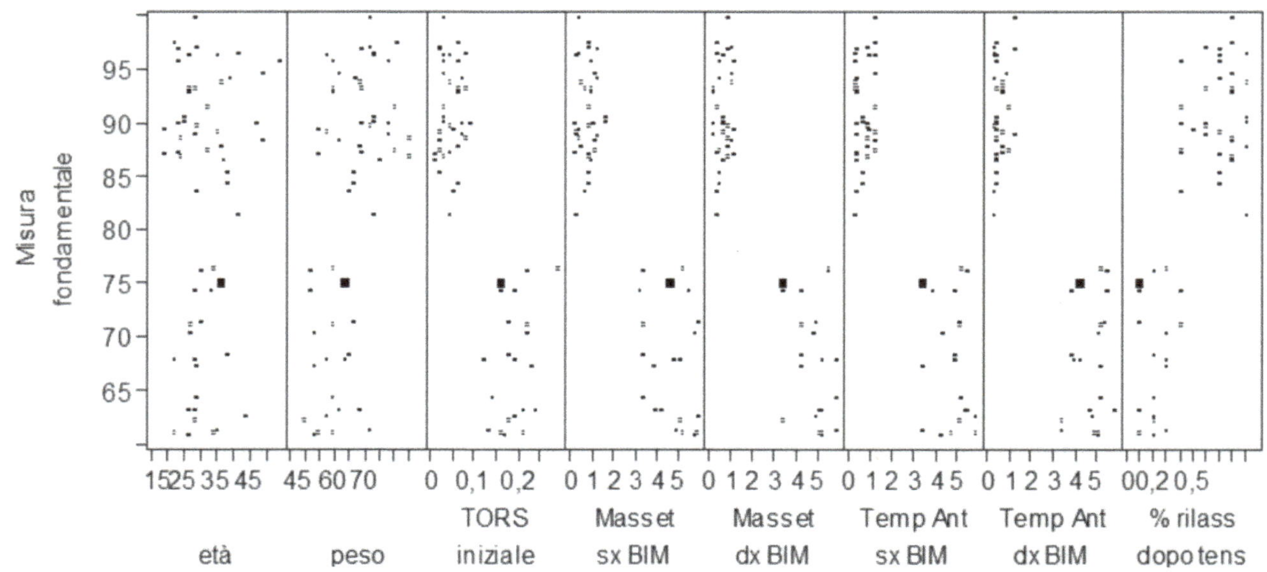

Fig. 4 Release matrix graphic ABOVE

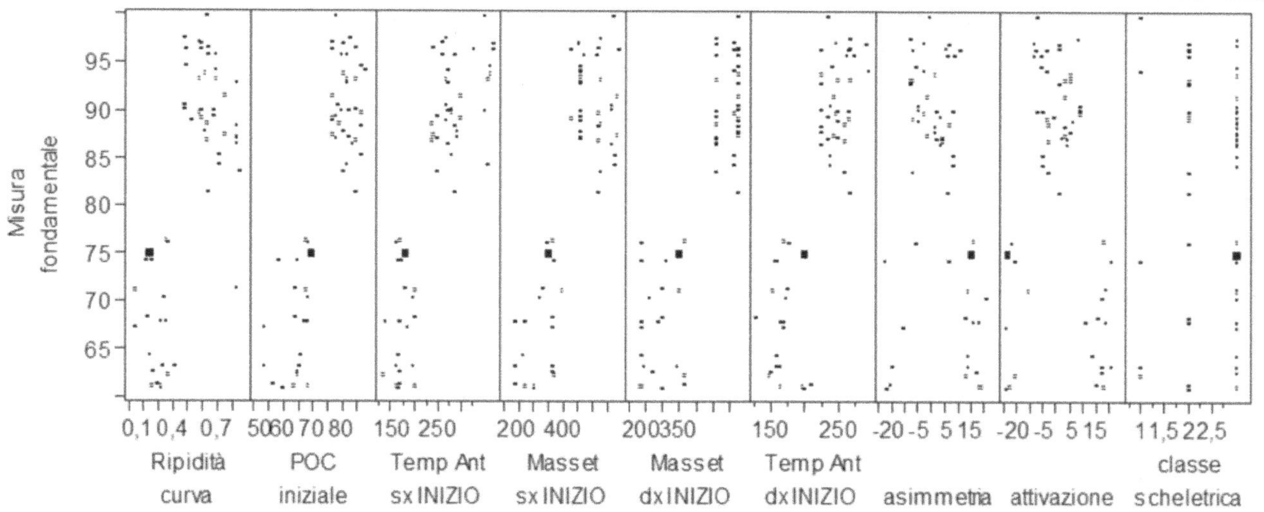

Fig. 5 Release matrix graphic BELOW

after the orthodontic-surgical treatment and the values obtained at the beginning and during the therapy.

The JMP software is able to establish a correlation between the electromyographic evaluation undertaken after 4 years of the end of treatment and the previous evaluations made at the beginning, during, and at the end of treatment.

Concerning the electromyographic index obtained from the exams made before and during treatment, the following parameters have been assessed:

- The TORS at the beginning of treatment
- The value expressed in micronvolts of the right masseter muscle activity in maximum voluntary clench (MVC) at the beginning of treatment
- The value expressed in micronvolts of the left masseter muscle activity in MVC at the beginning of treatment
- The value expressed in micronvolts of the anterior left temporal muscle activity in MVC at the beginning of treatment
- The value expressed in micronvolts of the anterior right temporal muscle activity in MVC at the beginning of treatment
- The percentage overlapping coefficient (POC) value at the beginning of treatment
- The asymmetry value at the beginning of treatment
- The activation value at the beginning of treatment
- The relaxing percentage of the muscle pairs after transcutaneous electrical neuromuscular stimulation (TENS) at the beginning of treatment
- The value expressed in micronvolts of the right masseter muscle activity at rest during the intermaxillary block
- The value expressed in micronvolts of the left masseter muscle activity at rest during the intermaxillary block
- The value expressed in micronvolts of the anterior left temporal muscle activity at rest during the intermaxillary block
- The value expressed in micronvolts of the anterior right temporal muscle activity at rest during the intermaxillary block
- The steepness of the recovery curve after surgery
- The age
- The sex
- The weight

In addition, the following information was included:

- Previous orthodontic treatment
- Temporo-mandibular disorders
- The skeletal class
- The type of surgery (maxillary, mandibular, and maxillary and mandibular ones)

Through the distance method of Mahalanobis, we have identified and excluded the outlier values which must be excluded in the evaluation of the linear regression model.

Once the outlier values were eliminated, it was necessary to identify which of the independent variables taken as reference in the sample was to be included in the model. To do this, the linear correlation coefficient between the selected couple of dependent and independent variables was assessed.

In case of two variables, the linear correlation coefficient is given by the ratio between the co-variance and the product of the corresponding deviations. This coefficient ranges between −1 and +1.

Where the coefficient is equal to +1, there is a directly proportional positive linear correlation.

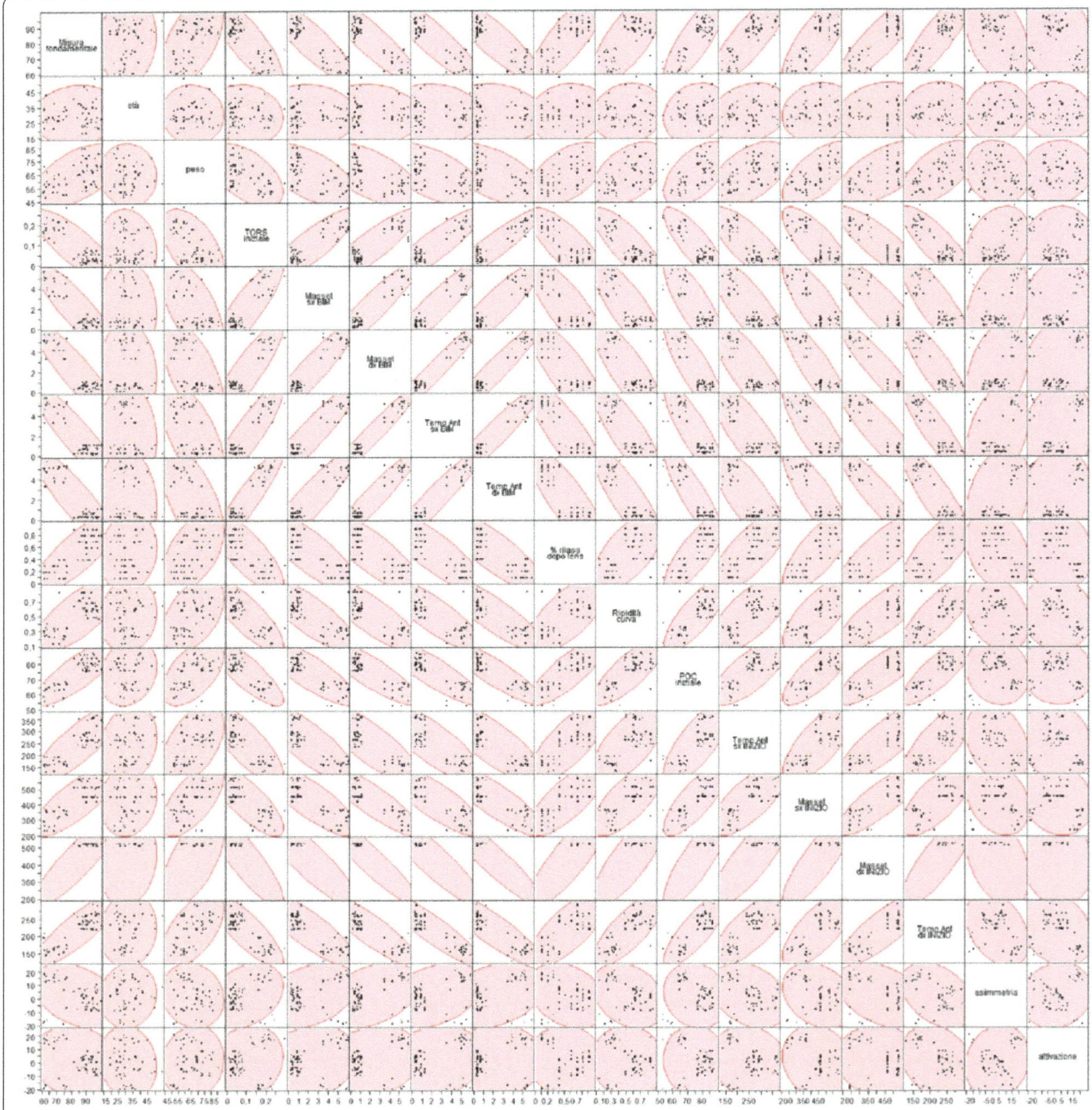

Fig. 6 Matrix of correlations

Where the coefficient is equal to −1, there is a directly proportional negative linear correlation.

If the coefficient is equal to 0, there is no correlation.

The JMP software allows to evaluate the linear correlation coefficient between the couple of variables identified.

In cases where the coefficient was equal to 0 between an independent variable and a dependent one, the assumption was that for the dependent value there was no correlation and hence it was to be excluded from the model.

If the linear correlation coefficient between two dependent variables was equal to +1, we assumed that there was binding co-linearity between the two dependent variables. In such cases, only one of the two was included in the model.

Regression analysis is a technique of multivariate statistical analysis which aims at identifying the relationship between a variable (dependent var iable) and the ensemble of explanatory variables (independent variables) through a correlation model obtained by a linear regression procedure. A *t*-test for each

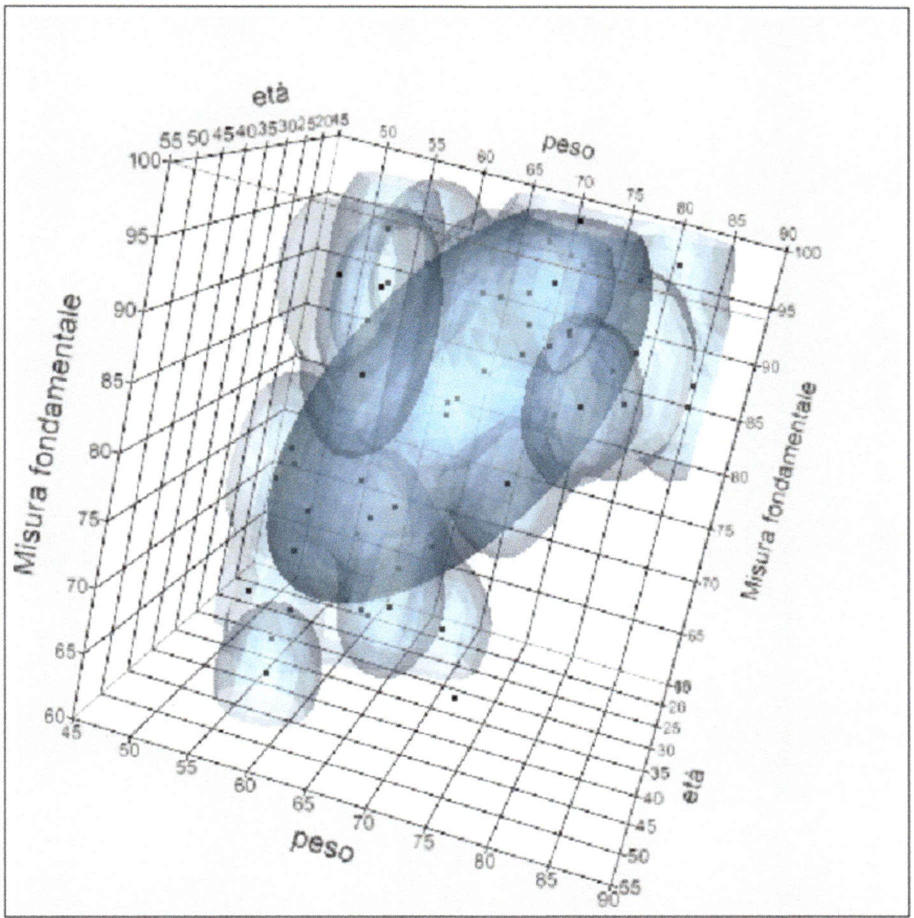

Fig. 7 Correlation between fundamental measure, age, and weight

independent variable is performed to verify if the parameter b is different from 0 (i.e. if there is a statistically significant correlation).

Thereby, if the test was significant, there was a linear dependence between the dependent variable and the independent ones selected. Therefore, all independent variables, for which the test was not significant, were removed. The Fisher test was then applied which allows to check if the number of independent variables is sufficient to describe the dependent variable.

The variables in which the test was less significant were removed.

If one or more variables were not significant, the less significant variable was eliminated. The model was then simplified, and the procedure was repeated until all variables were maintained.

Results

From the analysis of the clinical cases considered, 16 independent variables were selected to correlate with the fundamental measure. For each of the variables, the distribution has been displayed both graphically and statistically through the evaluation of the quantiles, average, and standard deviation.

The distribution analysis allows to exclude the presence of an anomalous value. According to the Mahalanobis distances method, the results of which are shown in Fig. 1, it was highlighted that all the data was below the critical value.

None of the data included in the study reach the critical value established by the Mahalanobis technique; hence, all patient data were acceptable.

Analyzing graphically the distribution of the fundamental measure and the independent variables, the following were observed:

- The fundamental measure ranges from a minimum of 60.95 to a maximum of 99.75 with an average value of 83.13. Such value is considered optimal.
- The data concerning the fundamental measure was distributed randomly with a high number of patients with a fundamental measure between 85 and 90.
- In relation to the age, the variable was between 19 and 54 years with an average age of 30.98.

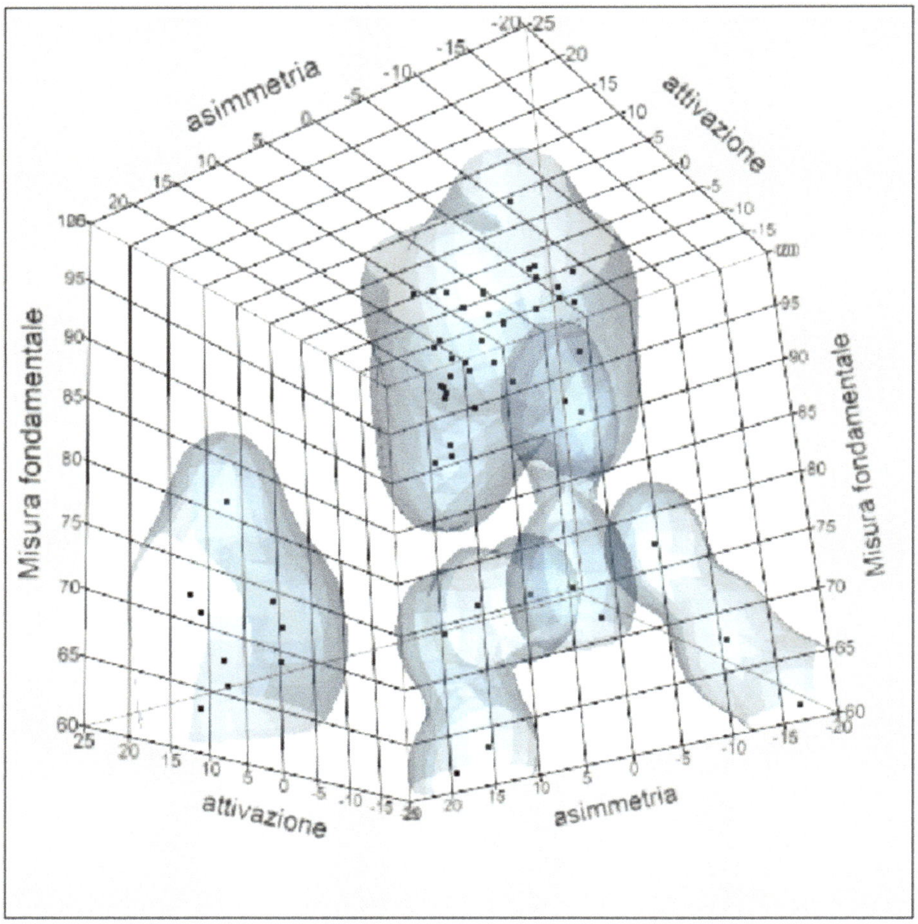

Fig. 8 Correlation between fundamental measure, asymmetry, and activation

- Only one case over the age of 50 was registered
- The mean age was between 25 and 30 years old (Figs. 2 and 3).

After isolating the patients that had a fundamental measure between 85 and 90 %, we noted the following:

- They were not represented by a precise age.
- They were not represented by a specific body weight.
- They showed an initial torsion index (TORS) value lower than 10 %, therefore, considered standard.
- They had an initial percentage overlapping coefficient (POC) value higher than 75 %.
- They had the masseter muscle values in micronvolts at the beginning of treatment higher than 400 μV.
- They had the temporal muscle values in micronvolts at the beginning of treatment higher than 200 μV.
- They had an asymmetrical value between −10 and 10 %, considered physiological.
- They had an activation value between −10 and 10 %, considered physiological.
- Relaxing after TENS was lower than 40 %, reaching the 99 % value.
- The steepness curve is higher than 50 %.

By isolating the patients who had a fundamental measure higher than 95 %, the following were noted:

- There was no specific age.
- There was no specific body weight.
- The initial TORS value was lower than 10 %, hence, considered standard.
- The initial POC value was between 75 and 85 %.
- The masseter muscle value in micronvolts obtained at the beginning of treatment was higher than 400 μV.
- The temporal muscle value in micronvolts obtained at the beginning of treatment was higher than 200 μV.
- The asymmetrical value obtained was between −10 and 15 %, which is considered physiological.
- The activation value obtained was between −10 % and 10 %, which is considered physiological.
- The relaxation value after TENS was lower than 40 %.
- The steepness curve was higher than 50 %.

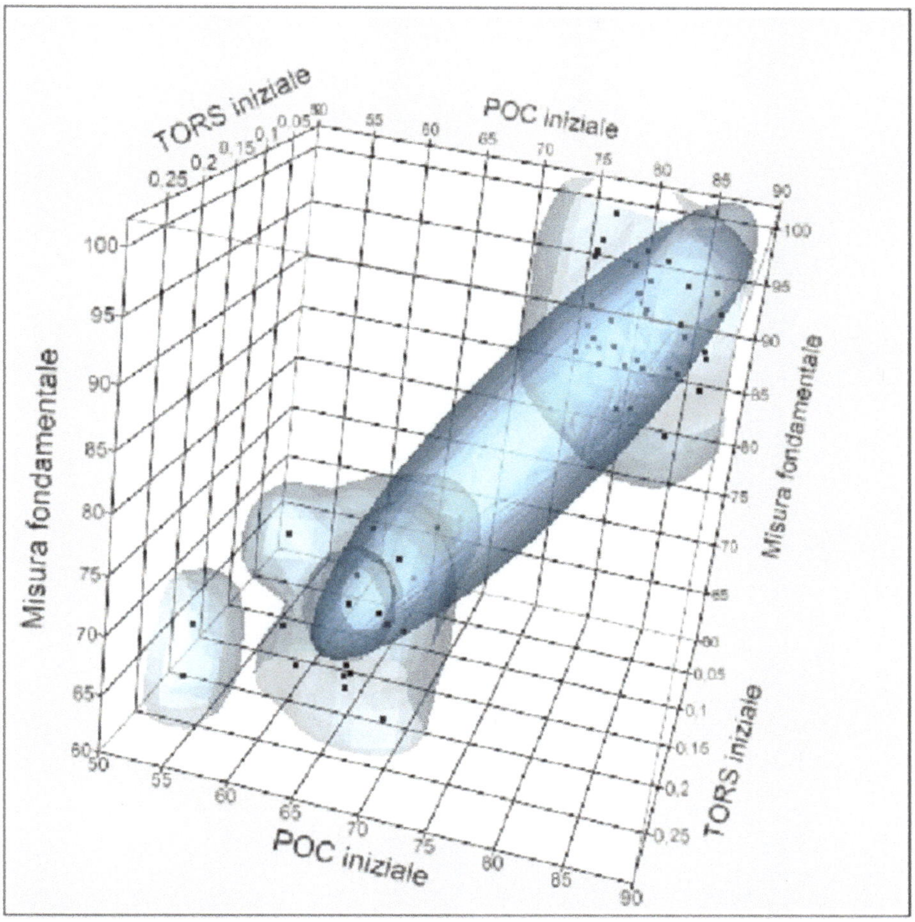

Fig. 9 Correlation between fundamental measure and initial POC and TORS

Such findings were also highlighted by the scatter graph and from the matrix of the scatter graph. Particularly, high values of the fundamental measure corresponded to the following:

- A low value of the initial TORS compared to the total.
- A high value of the temporal and masseter muscle contraction at the beginning of treatment compared to the total.
- A high value of the masseter muscle contraction at the beginning of treatment compared to the total.
- A lower and higher value compared to the standard values for what concerned the asymmetrical and activation index.
- A high value of the initial POC.
- A low value of the masseter and temporal muscles during the intermaxillary block.
- A high value of the steepness curve and of the relaxing value after TENS.
- There were no correlations with weight, age, and skeletal class.

Instead, the following corresponded to the low values of the fundamental measure:

- A high value of the initial TORS compared to the total.
- A low value of the temporal and masseter muscles contraction at the beginning of treatment compared to the total.
- A low value of the masseter muscle contraction at the beginning of treatment compared to the total.
- Within the standard values for what concerns the asymmetrical and activation index.
- A low value of the initial POC.
- A high value of the masseter and temporal muscles during the intermaxillary block.
- A low value of the steepness curve and muscle relaxation after TENS.
- There were no correlations with weight, age, and skeletal class (Figs. 4 and 5).

From the analysis of the correlation chart in which are listed the linear correlation coefficients, it was noted that the relationship between fundamental measure and

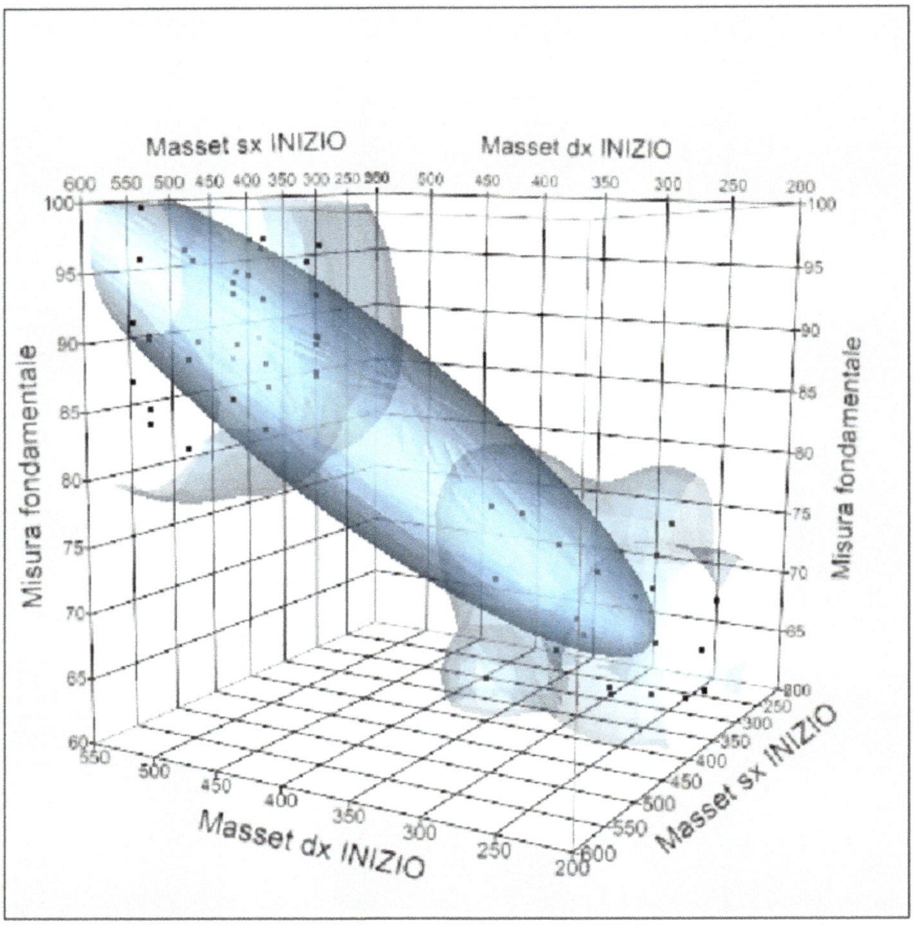

Fig. 10 Correlation between fundamental measure and the masseter values expressed in micronvolts at the beginning of treatment

age, weight, asymmetry, and activation was weak. A strong and positive relationship was observed between the relaxation percentages after TENS, the steepness of the post-surgery rehabilitation curve, and the initial POC for the values in micronvolts of the right and left temporal at the beginning of treatment and the right and left masseter at the beginning of treatment.

The relationship between the fundamental measure and initial TORS, the right and left masseter at rest during the intermaxillary block, and the right and left temporal during the intermaxillary block was strong and negative.

The same type of relationship is shown in the chart in which we have reported the data through a dispersion contained in the correlation ellipses. If the ellipses are flattened and facing downwards, the correlation is strong and negative, whilst if they are flattened and facing upwards, the correlation is strong and positive. In cases where the ellipses are close to the circle shape, there is no correlation (Fig. 6).

The correlations assessed were between the fundamental measure and the following:

- Weight and age
- Asymmetry and activation
- POC and TORS at the beginning of treatment
- Right and left masseter in MVC at the beginning of treatment
- Right and left temporal in MVC at the beginning of treatment
- Right and left temporal at rest during the intermaxillary block
- Right and left masseter at rest during the intermaxillary block
- Relaxing post-TENS and curve steepness
- Skeletal class and surgery
- Previous orthodontic treatment and temporomandibular disorders

There was no correlation between the fundamental measure and age-weight and asymmetry activation (Figs. 7 and 8).

From the chart, a correlation between the initial POC and TORS and the fundamental measure is observed. In addition, from the chart, it is highlighted that as the

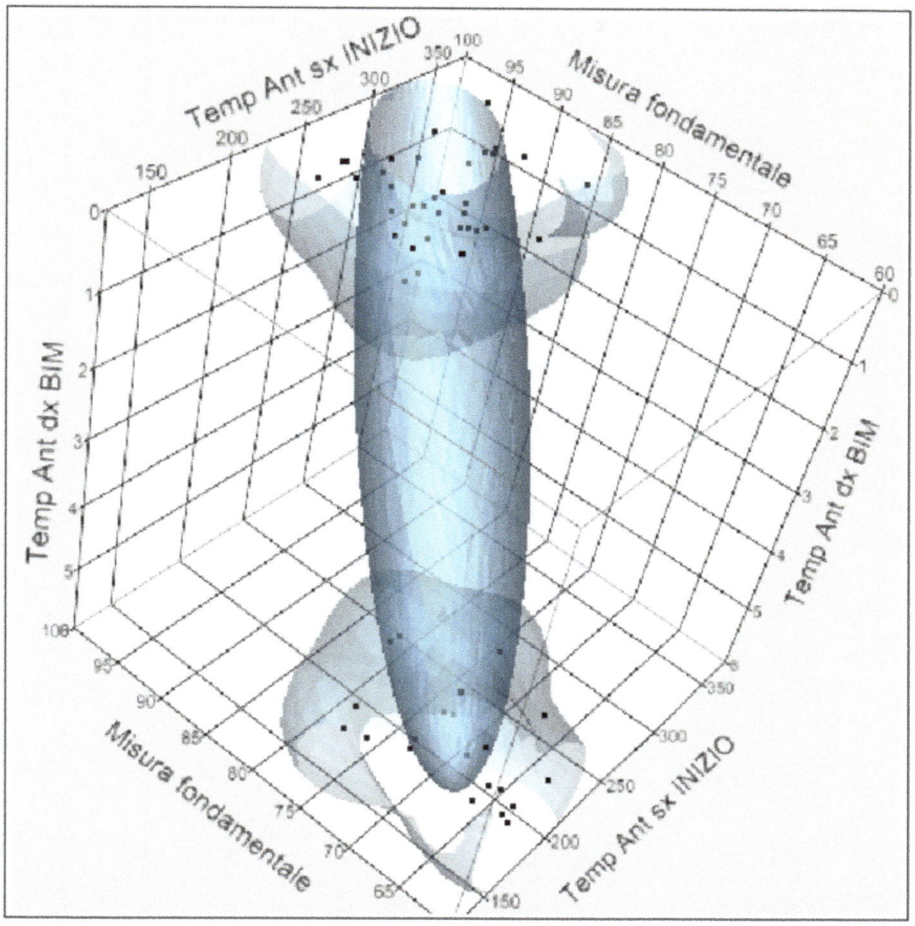

Fig. 11 Correlation between fundamental measure and the temporal values expressed in micronvolts at the beginning of treatment

initial TORS index increases, the value of the fundamental measure decreases, and as the initial POC index increases, the fundamental value increases.

Therefore, for the POC index, there is a positive type of correlation, whilst for the TORS index, the correlation is negative (Fig. 9).

Regarding the correlation between the value expressed in micronvolts of the right and left masseter in MVC at the beginning of treatment, it is noticeable that there is a positive correlation. In fact, with the increase of the masseter muscle activity, the value of the fundamental measure increases.

Therefore, patients who have a high masseter muscle activity at the beginning of treatment will probably have a high fundamental measure after a long period of time (Fig. 10).

Concerning the correlation between the value expressed in micronvolts of the right and left temporal in MVC at the beginning of treatment and the fundamental measure, a positive correlation is noticeable. In fact, as the activity of the temporal muscle increases, the fundamental value increases. Hence, patients who have a high activity of the temporal muscles at the beginning of treatment will have a high fundamental measure after a long period of time (Fig. 11).

Analyzing the correlation model between the value expressed in micronvolts of the right and left masseter muscle at rest during the intermaxillary block and the fundamental measure, a negative correlation is noticeable (when this value increases, the fundamental measure decreases). In fact, patients who have a high masseter muscle activity at rest during the intermaxillary block have a low fundamental measure at the long term follow-up.

Analyzing the correlation model between the value expressed in micronvolts of the right and left temporal muscle at rest during the intermaxillary block and the fundamental measure, a negative correlation is noticeable; hence, when this value increases, the fundamental measure decreases (Fig. 12).

The relationship between the fundamental measure and the percentage of muscle relaxation post-TENS proved a positive correlation, i.e., the higher is the muscular relaxation post-TENS, the higher is the level of the fundamental measure at the long-term follow-up.

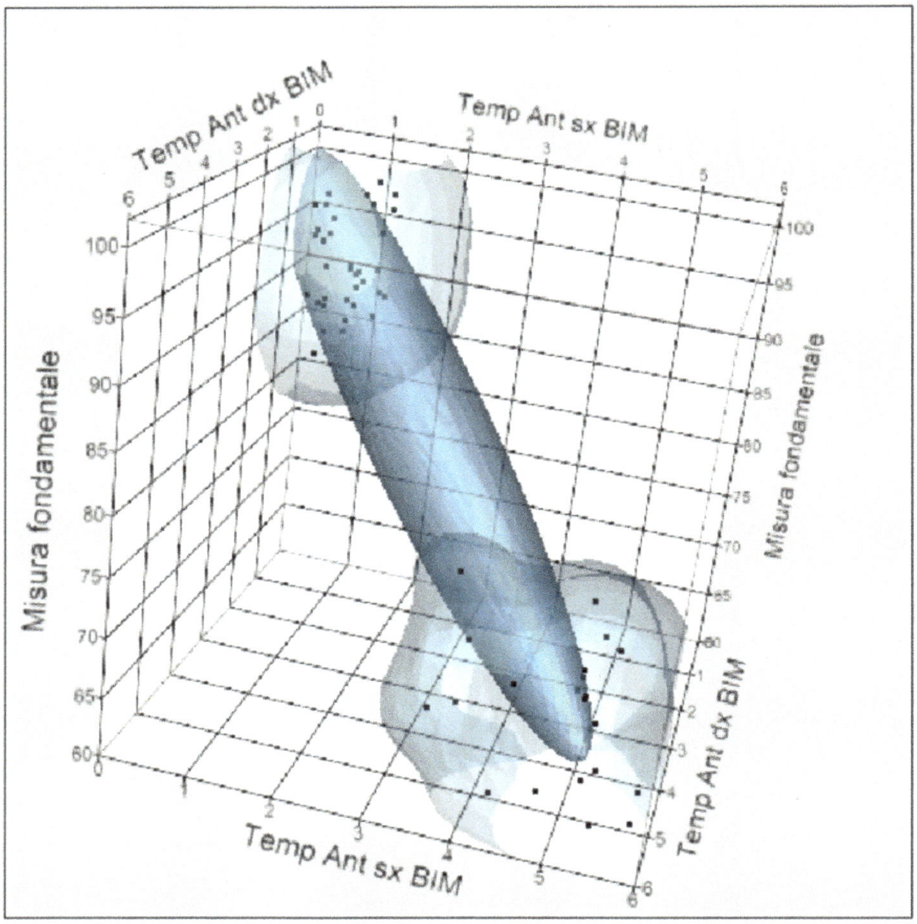

Fig. 12 Correlation between fundamental measure and the temporal values expressed in micronvolts during the intermaxillary block

There also is a positive correlation between the steepness curve and the fundamental measure; hence, the steeper is the post-surgery rehabilitation curve, the higher is the fundamental measure. This implies that patients who have a fast neuro-muscular post-surgery recovery will have the best electromyographic values at the long-term follow-up (Fig. 13).

Once the correlations were identified, we proceeded to the evaluation of the multivariate linear correlation model using the 16 independent variables. The variables for which the evaluation of the estimation parameter was not equal to the student test were eliminated.

It was assumed that in the fundamental hypothesis of the test (H), the correlation parameter was 0, i.e., there was no correlation. If the t value was higher than the limit value evaluated with a significance threshold of 5 %, we rejected the H hypothesis and hence we considered it as a significant correlation. Once the variables were removed, the model remained with nine variables which all passed the student test.

Once the p value concerning Fisher's F test was lower than 0.0001, Fisher's test was passed. Consequently, the variables were sufficient to describe the relationship between the fundamental measure and the independent variables selected. The graph shows the comparison between the values of the fundamental measure expected and the ones observed. It is highlighted that all values are found on a 45° straight line.

This data proves that the values expected by the model are close to the actual observed values.

In particular, the value of the R chart is high and equal to 0.871 which is considered excellent as it is close to 1.

Complete model

From the variance analysis, there is a Fisher distribution p value lower than 0.0001 (Fig. 14 and Table 1).

Variance analysis

The p value of the Student t-test distribution was lower than 5 % (Tables 2, 3, and 4).

From the residual analysis, it is noticeable that they are uniformly distributed around 0 which shows how the linear correlation hypothesis is acceptable (Fig. 15).

In the graphs are reported the leverage coefficient values for each of the dependent variables.

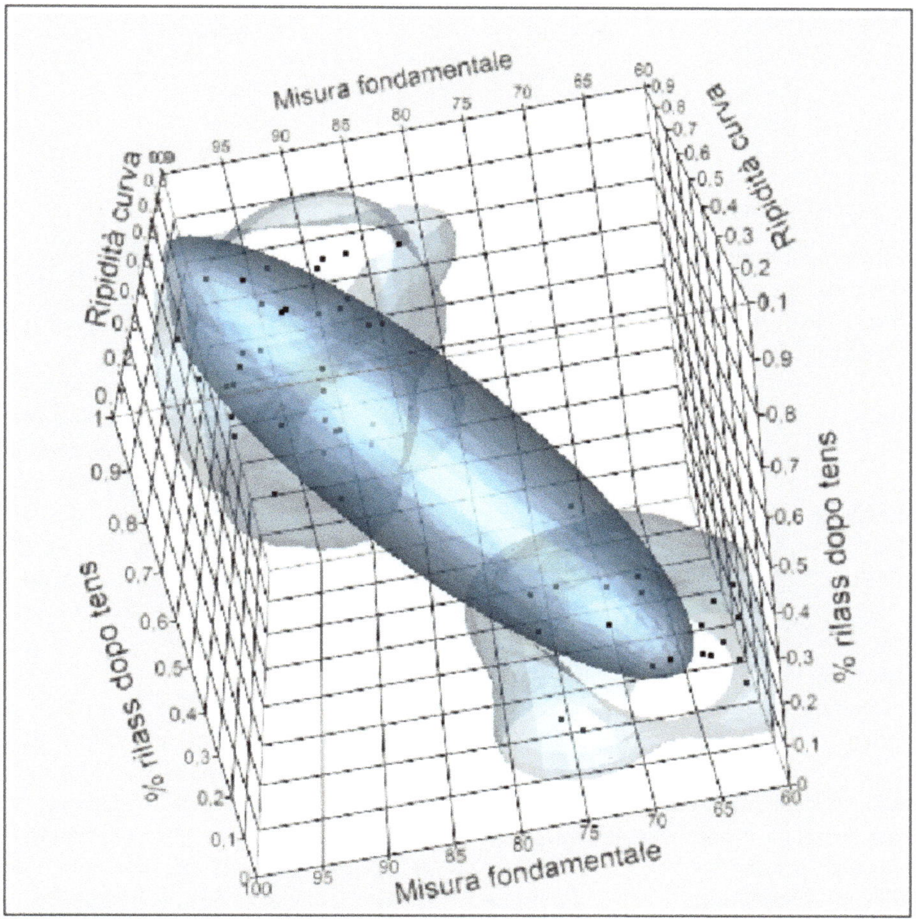

Fig. 13 Correlation between fundamental measure and relaxing percentage post-TENS and the curve steepness

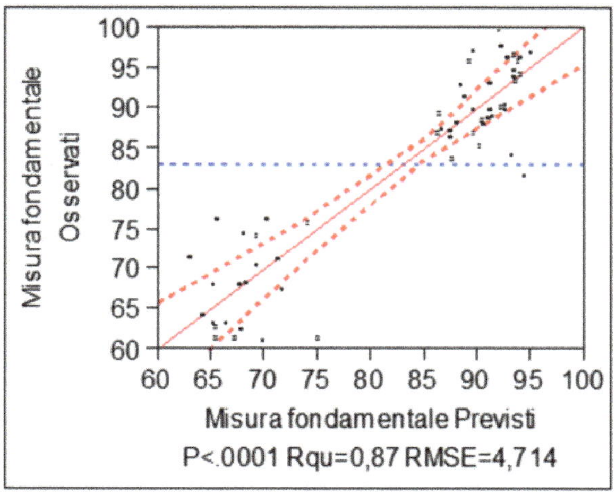

Fig. 14 Ex graph of the observed answers compared to the expected ones

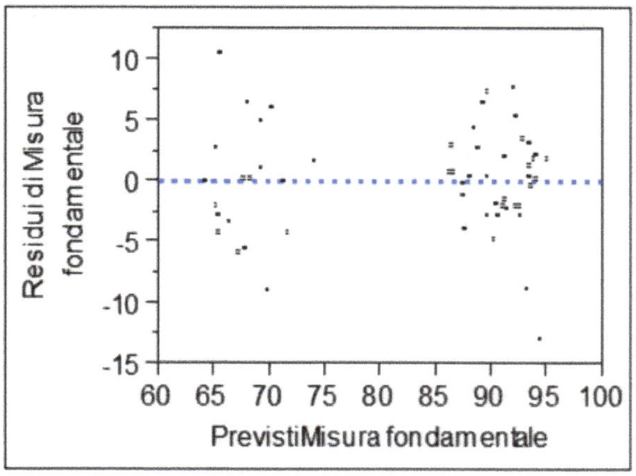

Fig. 15 Residual

Table 1 Estimate summary

R-squared	0,871829
Correct R-squared	0,846752
Mean Square Deviatio	4,713992
Average of Results	83,13625
Weighted Addition	30

The leverage coefficient (stimulus, influence) that varies between 0 and 1 is a measure of how much a given value of the independent variable deviates from its average.

Finally, we deduced the prevision model.

Prevision expression

Initial TORS
Left temp intermaxillary fixation (BIM)
Right temp BIM
Relaxing % after TENS
Steepness curve
Left temp beginning
Left masseter beginning
Right masseter beginning
Right temp beginning

From this formula, it is highlighted that some values for which a previous correlation had been shown proved to be not statistically significant.

Statistically significant correlations have been proved between the fundamental measure and the following:

- The TORS at the beginning of treatment
- The values expressed in micronvolts of the temporal and masseter muscles in MVC at the beginning of treatment
- The relaxing percentage after TENS
- The temporal muscle values at rest during the intermaxillary block
- The steepness value of the rehabilitation curve in the post-surgical phase

Therefore, the values of the masseter muscles expressed in micronvolts during the intermaxillary block and the POC initial value are not correlated to the fundamental measure in a statistically significant way.

To give more authenticity to the correlations obtained, we assumed to have no data of the fundamental measure and tried to deduce them from the previous electromyographies. Hence, we tried to predict the electromyography values at the follow-up on the basis of the previous data obtained.

From the graph of the observed values (actually registered) and the expected ones, it is highlighted how the model is able to foresee the data at both high values and low value of the fundamental measure.

This allows to deduce that the model is predictive (Figs. 16 and 17).

Table 2 Variance analysis

Origin	DF	Addition of squares	Quadratic means	F ratio
Model	9	6953,0949	772,566	34,7663
Error	46	1022,1992	22,222	Prob > F
C. total	55	7975,2941		<,0001*

Table 3 Missed estimate

Origin	DF	Addition of squares	Quadratic means	F ratio
Miss Evaluation	45	1022,1984	22,7155	28394,40
Neat Error	1	0,0008	0,0008	Prob > F
Total Error	46	1022,1992		0,0047*
				Max. r-square
				1,0000

Discussion

The data collected and analyzed in this study allowed to reach a few conclusions on the functional post-surgery rehabilitation in patients receiving combined surgical-orthodontic treatment and concerning the presence of correlations between the patients' neuromuscular situation at the beginning of treatment and in the follow-up [24–37].

It was possible, in fact, to deduce that patients receiving surgical-orthodontic treatment had indices that allowed to formulate a prognosis, i.e., to estimate the neuromuscular function and measure at the follow-up.

From a first data analysis, we considered all electromyographic and kinesiographic values collected from the diagnostic phase to the follow-up [38, 39].

The values that were not statistically significantly correlated between themselves have been rejected. In particular, the kinesiographic values have been rejected

Table 4 Estimates and parameters

Term	Evaluation	Std error	T - error	Prob>|t|
Intercept	54,118739	14,92805	3,63	0,0007*
Initial TORS	14,607324	22,73505	0,64	0,0005*
Temp Ant sx BIM	−1,493326	1,248338	−1,20	0,0009*
Temp Ant dx BIM	−1,149171	1,382826	−0,83	0,0003*
% relax after tens	3,8688461	4,69093	0,82	0,0002*
Rake curve	−8,1938	6,524735	−1,26	0,0007*
INITIAL Temp Ant sx	0,0328983	0,018219	1,81	0,0004*
INITIAL Masset sx	0,0080032	0,013443	0,60	0,0007*
INITIAL Masset dx	0,0212825	0,017359	1,23	0,0007*
INITIAL Temp Ant dx	0,0658332	0,035948	1,83	0,0004*

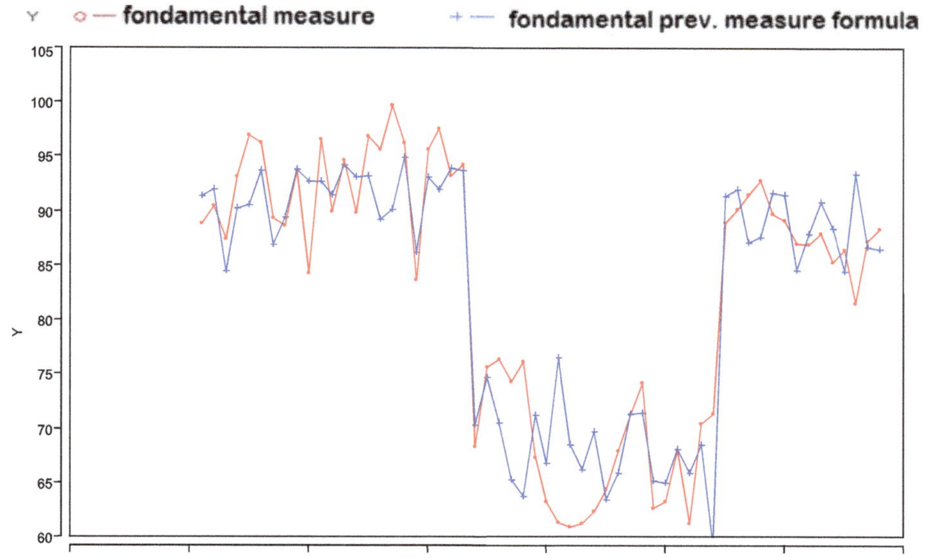

Fig. 16 Overlaid graph between expected and observed data

both because they were not significantly correlated and because it is known from the studies of Tate et al. and Throckmorton et al. that the long-term kinesiographic rehabilitation is not so quick and satisfying as the electromyographic one [24, 25, 34].

By selecting the data, we have obtained 16 indexes, or independent variables, obtained from the electromyographies made before and during treatment. Among these, some data was specific to the patient (weight and age), some referred to the electromyographies at the beginning of treatment (initial POC and TORS, values expressed in micronvolts for the four muscles at the beginning of treatment, asymmetry, and activation values), other data referred to the pre-surgical phase (relaxing % after TENS), and others referred to the intermaxillary block phase (values at rest for the four muscles) and the post-surgical phase (steepness of the rehabilitation curve in the post-surgical period).

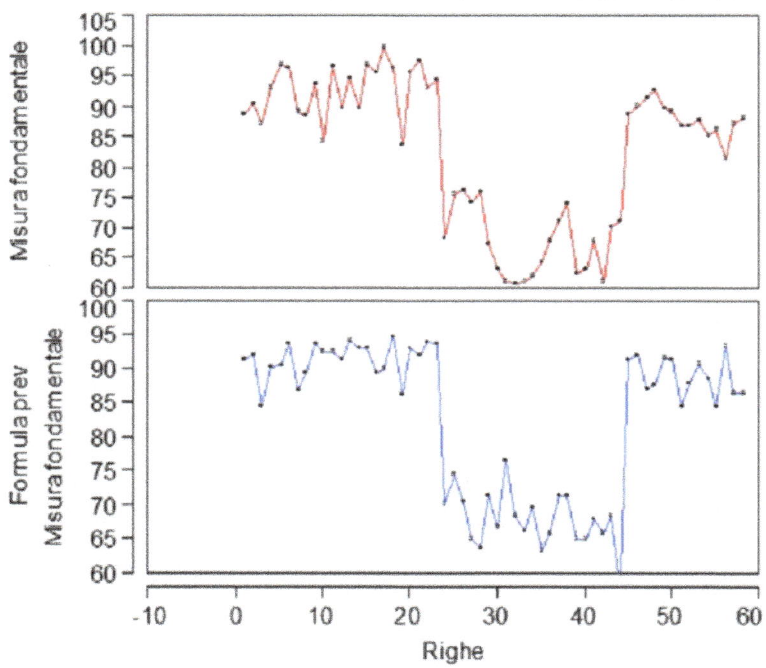

Fig. 17 Overlaid graph between expected and observed data divided in two diagrams

From the distribution's analysis, we noted that patients with high, medium, or low fundamental measure values had specific characteristics both at the beginning and during treatment. The statistical model utilized allowed the elimination of values which did not correlate (backward elimination). Therefore, the values less correlated were the first ones to be excluded until only highly correlated values were obtained.

These last values obtained are then subjected to further statistical analysis which allows to find the values which correlate to the fundamental measure.

This correlation model allows, at the end of treatment, to obtain indices statistically correlated to the fundamental measure. In this study, these indices were the initial TORS, the values expressed in micronvolts for the four muscles at the beginning of treatment, the temporal muscle values during the intermaxillary block, the relaxing percentage after TENS, and the steepness of the curve during post-surgery.

This model can be useful to estimate, during the treatment phase, the post-surgical rehabilitation level of the patient.

In literature, there are no studies that show the same correlation. One study in 2011 [39] had shown that high values of the temporals' activity at rest during the intermaxillary block were a negative prognostic index.

Conclusions

It is important that the combined surgical-orthodontic treatment is planned taking into consideration the functional needs. The surgical repositioning of the bone bases determines alterations of both the anatomy and function and of the relationship of the various anatomical structures. Hence, a functional evaluation is essential [40–46].

This study highlights the importance of monitoring patients in the long term, especially several years after the end of treatment [47–50].

In literature, many authors have published works similar to this; however, there are still many doubts and uncertainties.

In particular, there is no evidence on studies that have correlated the values obtained at the end of treatment with those collected during treatment.

In conclusion, each patient responds to treatment differently, and therefore, there is a big individual variability in terms of neuromuscular and functional response to the orthodontic-surgical therapy. However, it is possible to make correlations between electromyographic evaluations made at the follow-up and those made before and during treatment. In fact, we have reached a linear correlation between the electromyographic values obtained before and during therapy and those registered at the follow-up which could allow to make predictive evaluations of the neuromuscular stability in the long term.

Competing interests
The authors declare that they have no competing interests.

Authors' contributions
CM, GG, and LG carried out the electromyographic and kinesiographic procedure of selected patients at the beginning, during, and at the end of the orthodontic-surgical therapy. GF chose the correct sample of patients. SAS participated in the design of the study and performed the statistical analysis. MS conceived of the study and participated in its design and coordination and helped to draft the manuscript. All authors actively participated to all phases of the manuscript. All authors read and approved the final manuscript.

References

1. Throckmorton GS. Oral food processing and digestive efficiency in the herbivorous lizards Iguana iguana and Uromastix aegyptius. PhD Thesis. Chicago: University of Chicago; 1974.
2. Throckmorton GS. Oral food processing in two herbivorous lizards Iguana iguana (Iguanidae) and Uromastix aegyptius (Agamidae). J Morph. 1979;160:195–208.
3. Throckmorton GS. The chewing cycle in the herbivorous lizard Uromastix aegyptius (Agamidae). Achs Oral Biol. 1980;25:225–33.
4. Farronato G, Giannini L, Galbiati G, Sesso G, Maspero C. Orthodontic-surgical treatment: neuromuscular evaluation in skeletal Class II and Class III patients. Prog Orthod. 2012;13(3):226–36.
5. Farronato G, Giannini L, Galbiati G, Mortellaro C, Maspero C. Presurgical orthodontic planning: predictability. J Craniofac Surg. 2013;24(2):e184–6.
6. Dickers C, Giannini L, Esposito L, Maspero C, Bellincioni F, Farronato G. Neuromuscolar effects caused by orthopedic-functional therapy. Mondo Ortodontico. 2009;34(5):245–53.
7. Ghiglione V, Maspero C, Maiorana C. Importanza dello studio elettromiografico nella diagnosi e nella terapia ortognatodontica. Descrizione di un caso clinico. Monte Carlo: IV Congresso Internazionale odontostomatologico; 1994.
8. Farronato G, Giannini L, Galbiati G, Maspero C. Sagittal and vertical effects of rapid maxillary expansion in Class I, II, and III occlusions. Angle Orthod. 2011;81(2):298–303.
9. Farronato G, Giannini L, Galbiati G, Consonni D, Maspero C. Spontaneous eruption of impacted second molars. Prog Orthod. 2011;12(2):119–25.
10. Farronato G, Giannini L, Riva R, Galbiati G, Maspero C. Correlations between malocclusions and dyslalias. Eur J Paediatr Dent. 2012;13(1):13–8.
11. Maspero C, Giannini L, Riva R, Tavecchia MG, Farronato G. Valutazione del ciclo nasale di dieci giovani soggetti: indagine rinomanometrica. Mondo Ortodontico. 2009;5:263–8.
12. Farronato G, Giannini L, Galbiati G, Maspero C. Modified Hyrax expander for the correction of upper midline deviation: a case report. Minerva Stomatol. 2011;60(4):195–204.
13. Jankelson B. Neuromuscular aspects of occlusion: effects of occlusal position on the physiology and dysfunction of the mandibular muscolature. Dent Clin N Am. 1979;23(2):157–68.
14. Tate GS, Ellis E, Throckmorton GS. Bite forces in patients treated for mandibular angle fractures implications for fixation recommendations. J Oral Maxillofac Surg. 1994;52:734–8.
15. Throckmorton GS, Buschang BH, Hayasaki H, Phelan T. The effects of chewing rates on mandibular kinematics. J Oral Rehabil. 2001;28:328–34.
16. Throckmorton GS, Buschang PH, Hayasaki H, Pinto AS. Changes in the masticatory cycle following treatment of posterior unilateral crossbite in children. Am J Orthod Dentofacial Orthop. 2001;120:521–9.
17. Throckmorton GS, Dean JS. The relationship between jaw-muscle mechanical advantage and activity levels during isometric bites in humans. Arch Oral Biol. 1994;39:429.
18. Throckmorton GS, Teenier TJ, Ellis E. Reproducibility of mandibular motion and muscle activity levels using a commercial computer recording system. J Prosthet Dent. 1992;68:348.
19. Throckmorton GS, Throckmorton LS. Quantitative calculations of temporomandibular joint reaction forces. The importance of the magnitude of the jaw muscle forces. J Biomech. 1985;18:445.
20. Miralles R, Hevia R, Contreras L, Carvajal R, Bull R, Manns A. Patterns of electromyographic activity in subjects with different skeletal facial types. Angle Orthod. 1991;61(4):277–84.

21. Miralles R, Santander H, Ide W, Bull R. Influence of mucosal mechanoreceptors on elevator muscle activity in healthy subjects. J Prosthet Dent. 1991;65(3):431–5.
22. Miralles R, Valenzuela S, Ramirez P, Santader H, Palazzi C, Ormeno G, et al. Visual input effect on EMG activity of sternocleidomastoid and masseter muscles in healthy subjects and in patients with myogenic cranio-cervical-mandibular dysfunction. Cranio. 1998;16(3):168–84.
23. Miralles R, Zuniga C, Santander H, Manns A. Influence of mucosal mechanoreceptors on anterior temporalis EMG activity in patients with craniomandibular dysfunction a preliminary study. Cranio. 1992;10(1):21–7.
24. Tate GS, Throckmorton GS, Ellis III E, Sinn DP, Blackwood DJ. Estimated masticatory force in patients before orthognathic surgery. J Maxillofac Surg. 1994;52:130–6.
25. Tate GS, Throckmorton GS, Ellis III E, Sinn DP. Masticatory performance muscle activity and occlusal force in preorthognathic surgery patients. J Oral Maxillofac Surg. 1994;52:476–81.
26. Throckmorton GS, Ellis III E, Hayasaki H. Jaw kinematics during mastication after unilateral fractures of the mandibular condylar process. Am J Orthod Dentofacial Orthop. 2003;124(6):695–707.
27. Zarrinkelk HM, Throckmorton GS, Ellis 3rd E, Sinn DP. Functional and morphologic changes after combined maxillary intrusion and mandibular advancement surgery. J Oral Maxillofac Surg. 1996;54(7):828–37.
28. Throckmorton GS, Buschang PH, Ellis 3rd E. Improvement of maximum occlusal forces after orthognathic surgery. J Oral Maxillofac Surg. 1996;54:1080–6.
29. Throckmorton GS, Buschang PH, Ellis 3rd E. Morphological and biomechanical determinants in the selection of orthognathic surgery procedures. J Oral Maxillofac Surg. 1999;57:1044–57.
30. Farronato G, Giannini L, Galbiati G, Stabilini SA, Maspero C. Orthodontic-surgical treatment: neuromuscular evaluation in open and deep skeletal bite patients. Prog Orthod. 2013 Oct 29;14:41.
31. Throckmorton GS, Ellis 3rd E, Buschang PH. Morphologic and biomechanical correlates with maximum bite forces in orthognathic surgery patients. J Oral Maxillofac Surg. 2000;58:515–24.
32. Throckmorton GS, Ellis III E, Sinn DP. Functional characteristics of retrognathic patients before and after mandibular advancement surgery. J Oral Maxillofac Surg. 1995;53:898–908.
33. Throckmorton GS, Ellis III E. The relationship between surgical changes in dentofacial morphology and changes in maximum bite force. J Oral Maxillofac Surg. 2001;59:620–7.
34. Throckmorton GS, Johnston CP, Gonyea WJ. A preliminary study of biomechanical changes produced by orthognathic surgery. J Prosthet Dent. 1984;51(2):252–61.
35. Pepato AO, Palinkas M, Regalo SC, de Medeiros EH, de Vasconcelos PB, Sverzut CE, et al. Effect of surgical treatment of mandibular fracture: electromyographic analysis, bite force, and mandibular mobility. J Craniofac Surg. 2014 Sep;25(5):1714-20.
36. Farronato G, Maspero C, Giannini L, Farronato D. Occlusal splint guides for presurgical orthodontic treatment. J Clin Orthod. 2008;42(9):508–12.
37. Farronato G, Giannini L, Galbiati G, Mortellaro C, Maspero C. Presurgical virtual three-dimensional treatment planning. J Craniofac Surg 2015;26(3):820-3.
38. Miralles R, Berger B, Bull R, Manns A, Carvajal R. Influence of the activator on electromyographic activity of mandibular elevator muscles. Am J Orthod Dentofac Orthop. 1988;94:97–103.
39. Giannini L, Maspero C, Batia C, Galbiati G. Valutazione elettromiografica ed elettrognatografica del trattamento ortodontico chirurgico. Mondo ortodontico. 2011;36(1):12–28.
40. Li JL, Kau C, Wang M. Changes of occlusal plane inclination after orthodontic treatment in different dentoskeletal frames. Prog Orthod. 2014;15(1):41.
41. Konstantonis D, Anthopoulou C, Makou M. Extraction decision and identification of treatment predictors in Class I malocclusions. Prog Orthod. 2013;14:47.
42. Farronato G, Salvadori S, Giannini L, Maspero C. Congenital macroglossia: surgical and orthodontic management. Prog Orthod. 2012;13(1):92–8.
43. Throckmorton GS, Ellis III E, Hayasaki H. Masticatory motion after surgical or nonsurgical treatment for unilateral fractures of the mandibular condylar process. J Oral Maxillofac Surg. 2004;62:127–38.
44. Throckmorton GS, Ellis E. Recovery of mandibular motion after closed and open treatment of unilateral mandibular condylar process fractures. Int J Oral Maxillofac Surg. 2000;29:421–7.
45. Throckmorton GS, Finn RA, Bell WH. Biomechanics of differences in lower facial height. Am J Orhod. 1980;77:410.
46. Throckmorton GS, Talwar RM, Ellis III E. Changes in masticatory patterns after bilateral fracture of the mandibular condylar process. J Oral Maxillofac Surg. 1999;57:500–8.
47. Farronato G, Giannini L, Galbiati G, Maspero C. Long term results of open reduction management of condylar fracture: a 20 years follow-up. Case report. Minerva Stomatol. 2012;61(10):457–65.
48. Farronato G, Carletti V, Giannini L, Farronato D, Maspero C. Juvenile idiopathic arthritis with temporomandibular joint involvement: functional treatment. Eur J Paediatr Dent. 2011;12(2):131–4.
49. Grippaudo C, Oliva B, Greco AL, Sferra S, Deli R. Relationship between vertical facial patterns and dental arch form in class II malocclusion. Prog Orthod. 2013;14:43.
50. Borzabadi-Farahani A. A review of the evidence supporting the aesthetic orthodontic treatment need indices. Prog Orthod. 2012;13(3):304–13.

22

Anchorage onto deciduous teeth: effectiveness of early rapid maxillary expansion in increasing dental arch dimension and improving anterior crowding

Sabrina Mutinelli[1*], Mario Manfredi[2], Antonio Guiducci[3], Gloria Denotti[4] and Mauro Cozzani[5]

Abstract

Background: Anchorage onto permanent dentition is a common procedure in rapid maxillary expansion. However, replacing first permanent molars with the second deciduous molars seems to be an option to reduce some negative side effects during orthodontic treatment. The purpose of this study was to evaluate the dental effect of rapid maxillary expansion with anchorage exclusively onto deciduous teeth performed in the first period of transition.

Methods: Twenty patients with a lateral cross-bite treated exclusively by a Haas expander in early mixed dentition were retrospectively analyzed before treatment, at appliance removal, and at 21 months out of retention. The sagittal and transverse dimensions, together with the inter-canine arch and irregularity index, were digitally measured on scanned images of dental casts. The patients were compared with three balanced control groups (in total, 60 individuals) matched for gender. Two control groups had the same canine dental class as the treated group at T1, were in the inter-transitional period, and either had or lacked a lateral cross-bite. The last control group was comprised of adolescents in permanent dentition with a dental class I. The statistical analysis was performed by means of repeated-measures ANOVA for paired data and one-way ANOVA, the Kruskal-Wallis test, and the Mann-Whitney test for independent measures (α-level $p < 0.05$).

Results: At the end of follow-up (inter-transitional period of dentition), the dental arch dimensions of treated patients were similar to those of adolescents with a dental class I and significantly wider than those of patients with a lateral cross-bite. Also, the anterior irregularity index was lower among patients who had undergone expansion treatments than in all untreated study participants.

Conclusions: The Haas expander anchored to the deciduous teeth is effective in increasing the dental arch width in patients with a lateral cross-bite. The dimensions of the dental arch were modified earlier toward the values of the permanent dentition.

Keywords: Rapid maxillary expansion; Early mixed dentition; Dental arch changes; Irregularity index

* Correspondence: sabrinamutinelli@orthodontics.it

[1]Private practice, via Brennero 260/B, 38121 Trento, Italy

Full list of author information is available at the end of the article

Background

Rapid maxillary expansion (RME) is a widely used method to treat transverse deficiency [1], by opening the mid-palatal suture [2–4] during the period of skeletal growth [5, 6].

The Haas appliance [7] is a tooth-/tissue-borne device, anchored to the first molars and premolars by bands and to the palatal vault by an acrylic body. Some authors [8–11] have demonstrated the effectiveness of a modified Haas device, anchored onto the deciduous teeth (canines and second deciduous molars), in producing expansion of the transverse diameters of the upper arch. Moreover, there appears to be less relapse in the anterior area if the expansion is carried out in the first period of transition, that is, before the permanent lateral incisor will have fully erupted, and in the presence of a lateral cross-bite [12].

The anchorage onto deciduous teeth could be a viable option for preventing root resorption [2, 13–15], bone loss [16, 17], gingival recession [18], and white-spot lesions [19] on permanent dentition.

The purpose of the present study was to investigate the clinical relevance of changes in dental arch dimensions and irregularity produced by a Haas appliance anchored onto the deciduous dentition and to compare young treated patients with homogeneous untreated individuals.

Methods

The study group was comprised of 20 Caucasian children (13 females and 7 males) in the first period of transition (mean age, 7 years and 1 month; SD, 11 months) with a mono- or bilateral cross-bite. Fifteen of the 20 patients had a canine class II.

The study group was selected retrospectively and sequentially in the clinical archives of two orthodontists who followed the same treatment protocol.

The Haas appliance was anchored to the second deciduous molars and deciduous canines (Fig. 1) and was activated once or twice per day; each activation was 0.2 mm, with a maximum allowable total expansion of 10 mm.

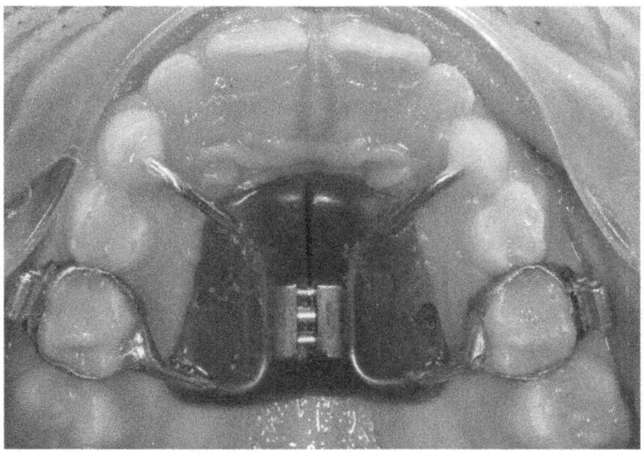

Fig. 1 The Haas RME anchored onto the deciduous dentition

The patients were monitored weekly, and the expansion was terminated when the cross-bite was corrected (mean, 20 days) [9]. The appliance was kept *in situ* as retention for 12 months (SD, 4 months), after the screw was fixed.

For each patient, the dental casts before expansion (T1; mean age, 7 years and 1 month; SD, 11 months), after the appliance was removed (T2; mean age, 8 years and 1 month; SD, 10 months), and at 21 months (SD, 9 months) out of retention, during the inter-transitional period of the dentition (T3; mean age, 9 years and 10 months; SD, 1 year and 4 months), were collected.

Three control groups were selected from among the patients sequentially checked during either the orthodontic consult or the periodic check-up for caries. For two groups, the inclusion criteria were the same canine dental class and the male-to-female ratio as the study group. The dental age coincided with the inter-transitional period [12]. Patients in one of the two groups had a lateral cross-bite (mean age, 9 years; SD, 11 months), and those in the other were without a lateral cross-bite (mean age, 9 years and 2 months; SD, 1 year and 1 month). The last control group, adolescents in permanent dentition (mean age, 14 years and 4 months; SD, 2 years and 5 months), was in normal occlusion, presented the same male-to-female ratio as the study group, and had a full natural dental arch up to the first or second molars. Impressions were taken for each patient. The case-control study design diagram is shown in Fig. 2.

The scanned images of the dental casts of all treated and non-treated individuals were measured by a computerized method described previously [20].

The mesial and distal points and the tips of the cusps of each tooth and the inter-incisive point were digitally identified. If the central incisors had not erupted, the landmark of the inter-incisive point was marked with respect to the insertion of the frenulum. The measurements for each dental cast were as follows (Fig. 3):

- inter-canine width (between cusp tips of the left and right canines),
- inter-canine arch (elliptical arch between cusp tips of the left and right canines),
- inter-molar width (between mesio-buccal cusps of the left and right first molars),
- inter-molar arch depth (distance between the inter-incisive point and inter-molar width), and
- the Little irregularity index [21] applied to the upper arch.

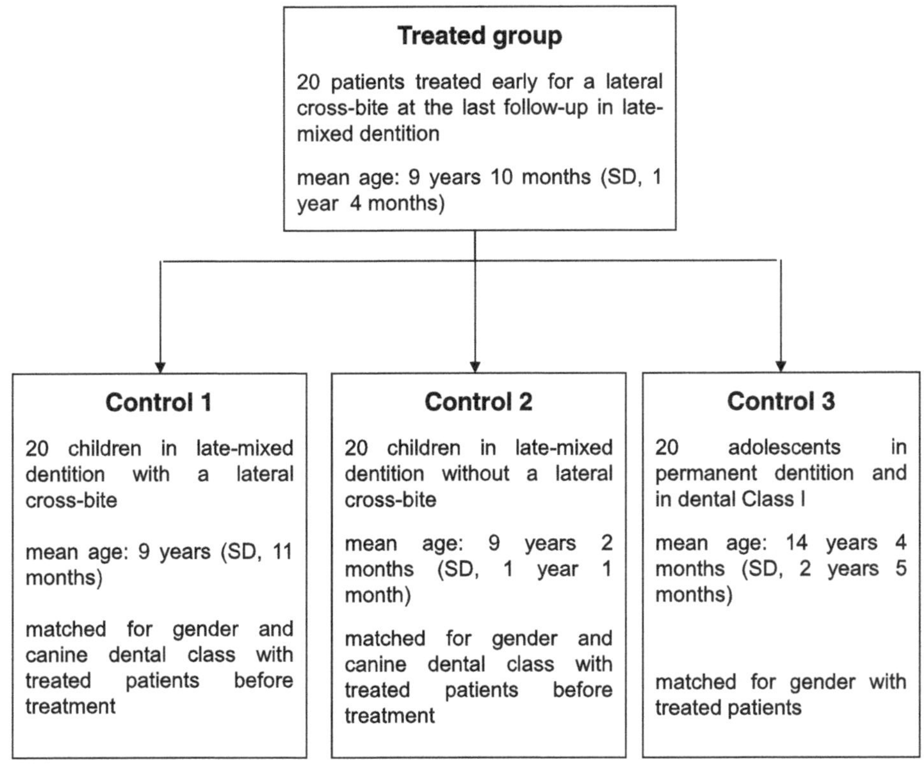

Fig. 2 Case-control study design diagram

Statistical analysis

The normal distribution of variables was tested with a graphical visualization and the Shapiro-Wilk test. The data from the treated patients were analyzed by comparison of the values measured at T1, T2, and T3 with the repeated-measures ANOVA and the Tukey test (α level, 0.05). The null hypothesis stated that there was no difference in the dimensions of the dental arch before and after treatment.

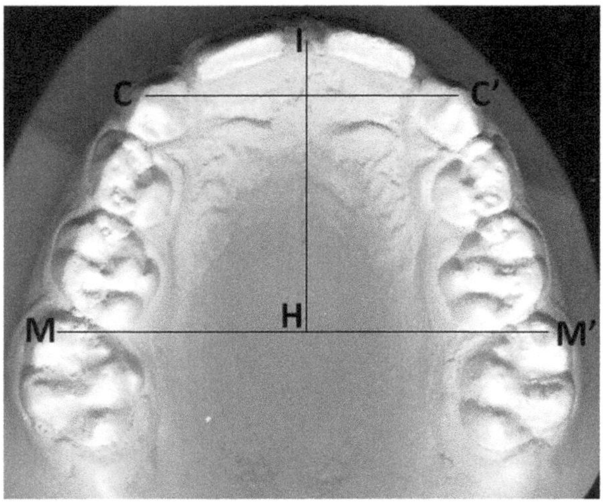

Fig. 3 Distances drawn on an image of scanned dental cast. *C–C'* is inter-canine width, *M–M'* is inter-molar width, and *I–H* is inter-molar depth

The patients undergoing expansion were matched with the members of each control group with respect to gender for adolescents in normal occlusion and on the basis of gender and canine dental class for those in malocclusion (Fig. 2). The comparison of the measures correlated to the deciduous canines was performed only among the groups in the inter-transitional period.

The applied statistics were the one-way ANOVA and the Bonferroni test for normally distributed data and the Kruskal-Wallis equality-of-populations rank test and the Mann-Whitney test for not normally distributed variables. The null hypothesis was the equality in the dimensions of the dental arches of the treated and untreated individuals, with a significance level of $p < 0.05$.

The reliability of the operator in identifying the points on the scanned images of dental casts was calculated by the intraclass correlation coefficient (ICC). The same operator repeated the identification of landmarks of 20 patients 1 week after the first examination. The outcome was non-significant (ICC, 99.95 %), and therefore, the reliability was confirmed.

All data were statistically analyzed with STATA12 (StataCorp LP, College Station, TX, USA).

Results

Study group

The statistical analysis of the variations in the study group showed, at T3, a significant increase ($p < 0.001$) in the inter-canine width (mean, 4.2 mm; SD, 2.0) and arch (mean, 6.2 mm; SD, 3.8), in the inter-molar width (mean, 4.7 mm; SD, 2.0), and in the inter-molar depth (mean, 0.8 mm; SD, 1.1). The relapse from T2 to T3 was significant ($p < 0.001$) in the inter-canine width (mean, −2.2 mm; SD, 2.0) and arch (mean, −4.1 mm; SD, 3.6) (Tables 1 and 2).

Study group vs control groups

Inter-canine width

The inter-canine width of the patients who had undergone expansion, at T3 (mean, 32.2 mm; SD, 2.0), was significantly higher than the value for children in the inter-transitional period with a lateral cross-bite (mean, 30.3 mm; SD, 3.1; $p = 0.042$) (Table 3).

Inter-molar width

The inter-molar width of the treated group (mean, 49.6 mm; SD, 2.3) was significantly higher than that of children with a lateral cross-bite (mean, 44.5 mm; SD, 2.4; $p < 0.001$) but was not higher than that of children without a lateral cross-bite (mean, 47.9 mm; SD, 2.9; $p = 0.264$). There was no difference between adolescents with a normal occlusion (mean, 50.6 mm; SD, 2.8) and treated patients ($p = 0.938$). Inter-molar width in adolescents was wider than that in children with ($p < 0.001$) and without a lateral cross-bite ($p = 0.005$) (Table 3).

Inter-molar depth

The value of the inter-molar depth was significantly lower in the treated group (mean, 29.8 mm; SD, 1.7) than in the children with (mean, 31.8 mm; SD, 2.2; $p = 0.006$) and without a lateral cross-bite (mean, 32.1 mm; SD, 2.0; $p = 0.001$). In the same manner, the difference was significant between adolescents with a normal occlusion (mean, 29.0 mm; SD, 1.6) and children with ($p < 0.001$) and without a lateral cross-bite ($p < 0.001$). There was no difference between the adolescents with a normal occlusion and the treated patients (Table 3).

Anterior irregularity index

The irregularity index was significantly higher in untreated children in malocclusion, whether with (median, 3.2 mm; interquartile range, 2.9; $p = 0.0094$) or without (median, 4.0 mm; interquartile range, 4.0; $p = 0.0080$) a lateral cross-bite, compared with that of the treated group (median, 2.4 mm; interquartile range, 1.4) (Table 3).

Discussion

This research confirms the efficacy of the Haas expander anchored to the deciduous teeth in modifying the dental arch width in a group of patients with a lateral cross-bite, treated in the first period of transition. The dimension of the inter-molar width maintained a stable measure not different from that of older individuals during adolescence and in normocclusion.

In previous studies, many authors evaluated the timing of rapid maxillary expansion during growth. Sari et al. [22] found that the increase in the inter-molar and inter-canine

Table 1 Descriptive statistics and statistical analysis of the treated sample recorded at T1, T2, and T3

	Time			Comparisons		
	T1	T2	T3	T1 vs T2	T1 vs T3	T2 vs T3
	$n = 20$	$n = 20$	$n = 20$			
Inter-canine width						
mean (SD), mm	28.0(1.9)	34.4(2.4)	32.2(2.0)	S*	S*	S*
95 % CI	27.1 to 28.9	33.3 to 35.6	31.3 to 33.1			
Inter-canine arch						
mean (SD), mm	30.7(3.2)	41.1(4.7)	37.0(3.6)	S†	S†	S†
95 % CI	29.2 to 32.3	38.7 to 43.3	35.3 to 38.7			
Inter-molar width						
mean (SD), mm	44.8(2.5)	49.7(1.9)	49.6(2.3)	S‡	S‡	NS‡
95 % CI	43.7 to 46.0	48.7 to 50.5	48.5 to 50.6			
Inter-molar depth						
mean (SD), mm	29.8(1.7)	30.9(2.1)	30.6(1.9)	S§	S§	NS§
95 % CI	29.0 to 30.6	30.0 to 31.9	29.7 to 31.4			

S is the significant result of the Tukey test performed after the repeated-measures ANOVA *($F_{(2,21)} = 17.21$; $p < 0.001$; power of the test = 100 %); †($F_{(2,21)} = 11.67$; $p < 0.001$; power of the test = 100 %); ‡($F_{(2,21)} = 18.79$; $p < 0.001$; power of the test = 100 %). §*S* is the significant result and *NS* is the non-significant result of the Tukey test performed after the repeated-measures ANOVA ($F_{(2,19)} = 17.13$; $p < 0.001$; power of the test = 99 %)

Table 2 Mean difference and 95 % CI in the measurements of the treated patients at time points T1, T2, and T3

	Differences between measurements at time-points T1, T2, and T3		
	T2–T1	T3–T1	T3–T2
	$n = 20$	$n = 20$	$n = 20$
Inter-canine width			
mean, mm	6.4*	4.2*	−2.2*
95 % CI	5.7 to 7.2	3.3 to 5.1	−3.1 to −1.3
Inter-canine arch			
mean, mm	10.3*	6.2*	−4.1*
95 % CI	8.6 to 12.1	4.4 to 8.0	−5.8 to −2.4
Inter-molar width			
mean, mm	4.8*	4.7*	−0.1
95 % CI	4.2 to 5.4	3.8 to 5.7	−0.9 to 0.7
Inter-molar depth			
mean, mm	1.1*	0.8*	−0.4
95 % CI	0.6 to 1.7	0.2 to 1.3	−0.8 to −0.04

*Significant difference

widths was equally significant in the mixed and the permanent dentition. In contrast, Bacetti et al. [23] found that the modification in the maxillary inter-molar width was more pronounced in the patients who underwent expansion before the pubertal peak.

In the present study, the treated group was retrospectively selected following the timing for expansion reported in the paper by Mutinelli et al. [10] and corresponding to the first period of transition. The comparison at the final follow-up with three control groups allowed for evaluation of the change in treated patients with respect to that in untreated individuals. One limit of this analysis is the evaluation of the inter-canine width. The last available record for the treated patients was the dental cast in mixed dentition with the deciduous canines. Therefore, it was not possible to perform any comparison of inter-canine width between treated children in late-mixed dentition and adolescents in permanent dentition and in dental class I. Moreover, there was no follow-up of the control groups during the growth period; three groups were analyzed at two different dental ages. However, the matching of patients controlled the effects of the two well-known confounding variables, gender [24] and dental class II [25]. In addition, canine class II [26, 27] and lateral cross-bite [6] do not self-correct during dental arch growth, which is completed with the eruption of permanent canines [12, 24, 28, 29]. Therefore, it could be hypothesized that the control groups well represented the dental arch dimension of children, homologous to the treated group, at the late-mixed dentition with or without a lateral cross-bite but not treated with a rapid maxillary expansion. Further, deciding not to treat a patient with a lateral cross-bite and to follow that individual as a control is not feasible for ethical reasons. Therefore, a randomized controlled trial is difficult to implement.

The expander anchored to the deciduous teeth had, as a transverse effect, a significant increase at T3 in inter-

Table 3 Descriptive statistics and statistical analysis of the treated patients at T3 and the control groups

	Groups				Comparison among groups
	Treated group	Children *with* a lateral cross-bite	Children *without* a lateral cross-bite	Adolescents with a normal occlusion	*p* value
	$n = 20$	$n = 20$	$n = 20$	$n = 20$	
Mean age (SD), years	9.8(1.3)	9.0(0.9)	9.2(1.1)	14.3(2.4)	
Inter-canine width					
mean (SD), mm	32.2(2.0)	30.3(3.1)	31.8(2.0)	-	0.0353*
95 % CI	31.3 to 33.1	28.8 to 31.7	30.9 to 32.7		
Inter-molar width					
mean (SD), mm	49.6(2.3)	44.5(2.4)	47.9(2.9)	50.6(2.8)	<0.001†
95 % CI	48.5 to 50.6	43.3 to 45.6	46.5 to 49.2	49.4 to 52.1	
Inter-molar depth					
mean (SD), mm	29.8(1.7)	31.8(2.2)	32.1(2.0)	29.0(1.6)	
95 % CI	29.0 to 30.6	30.8 to 32.9	31.2 to 33.0	28.3 to 29.8	<0.001‡
Irregularity index					
median (Iqr)§, mm	2.4(1.4)	3.2(2.9)	4.0(4.0)	-	0.0094‡

*One-way ANOVA ($F_{(2,57)} = 3.55$; power of the test = 98 %; rho = 0). Significant pair differences (Bonferroni test): treated group vs children with a lateral cross-bite ($p = 0.042$). †One-way ANOVA ($F_{(3,76)} = 21.60$; power of the test = 100 %; rho = 0). Significant pair differences (Bonferroni test): treated group vs children with a lateral cross-bite ($p < 0.001$) and adolescents with a normal occlusion vs both children with a lateral cross-bite ($p < 0.001$) and children without a lateral cross-bite ($p = 0.005$). ‡One-way ANOVA ($F_{(3,76)} = 12.86$; power of the test = 99 %; rho = 0). Significant pair differences (Bonferroni test): treated group vs both children with a lateral cross-bite ($p = 0.006$) and children without a lateral cross-bite ($p = 0.001$); adolescents with a normal occlusion vs both children with a lateral cross-bite ($p < 0.001$) and children without a lateral cross-bite ($p < 0.001$). §Iqr is interquartile range. ‡Kruskal-Wallis equality-of-populations rank test. Significant pair differences (two-sample Wilcoxon rank-sum test): treated patients vs children with a lateral cross-bite ($p = 0.0094$) and children without a lateral cross-bite ($p = 0.0080$)

canine width in 4.2 mm and inter-canine arch in 6.2 mm. The inter-molar diameter maintained 4.6 mm of the initial expansion (96 %) at 21 months post-retention (T3). Furthermore, the final value was no different from the values of the adolescent control group in normal occlusion. No statistically significant variation in inter-molar arch depths was recorded.

Spillane and McNamara [30] demonstrated, on average, 5 mm of residual expansion in the inter-molar width 2.4 years after expansion. Lima et al. [31] reported 4.5 mm (81.1 % of the initial expansion) 4 years after the end of activation. In an equal period of observation, this amounted to 84 % (3.7 mm) in the findings of Wong et al. [32], but these authors followed the SME and not the RME protocol of activation. The final dimension was no different from that of the control group with normal growth. At least 1 year out of retention, the residual expansion was 3.8 mm (79 %) for Mutinelli et al. [10] and 3.7 mm (90.2 %) for Cozzani et al. [9].

Schiffman and Tuncay [33] found a mean loss of 40 % of expansion in the inter-molar width within 5 years after the end of treatment. The net increase was between 3 and 4 mm in the long term, similar to the amount of normal growth in the period of time between the stages of the late-mixed and the permanent dentition. The authors did not consider that amount of increase a success, as Turpin [34] discussed in his editorial, if the aim of the treatment was to achieve a larger increase. Also, in this study, in which the global effect of the RME on the dental arch was analyzed, it can be concluded that the patients in the inter-transitional period showed sagittal and transverse dimensions no wider than those of adolescents in canine dental class I. The inter-molar arch depths were not influenced directly by the expansion, but at T3, the values were significantly lower than those in individuals at the same dental age. Normally, the upper arch modifies until the full eruption of the permanent dentition [12, 24] and has a tendency to become wider and shorter [12, 24, 35]. Further, expansion improved the transverse deficiency connected to the presence of a canine class II [27, 35]. Another important outcome was the value of the anterior irregularity index. In treated patients, it was significantly lower than in untreated individuals in malocclusion at the same dental age. Therefore, the choice to treat in the first transitional period and not later can have the goal of creating conditions conducive for development of the upper dental arch toward the dimensions of a patient in normal occlusion and not toward wider dimensions. Moreover, increasing the inter-canine arch length before the end of eruption of the permanent incisors, as reported by other authors [10, 32], can be a treatment option in middle and non-severe crowding, because the mean available space at T3 was 6.2 mm. A better alignment of the anterior teeth, a correct arrangement of the transseptal fibers, and a consequent reduction of risk in severe rotation [36] can be hypothesized. Similarly, this might confirm the results reported by Canuto et al. [37] that the RME applied later in the permanent dentition did not influence long-term maxillary anterior alignment stability.

Moreover, the option to anchor the appliance to the deciduous teeth can avoid the side effects of periodontal problems [16–18], root resorption [2, 13, 14], and white-spot lesions [19].

Further long-term studies based on a bigger sample size, more representative of the orthodontic population, are necessary to confirm these results.

Conclusions

Rapid maxillary expansion performed in the first period of transition is effective in the treatment of patients with a lateral cross-bite. The dental arch increases in dimensions earlier toward the values of the permanent dentition stage, in comparison with dimensions in homogeneous untreated individuals. As a result, the increase in arch length can improve the alignment of the upper anterior teeth in patients with low or moderate crowding.

Therefore, early treatment with a Haas expander anchored to the primary dentition could be a satisfactory procedure for lateral cross-bite resolution and for anterior crowding improvement, due to simplicity of appliance design, ease of treatment management, and low risk of side effects.

Competing interests

The authors declare that they have no competing interests.

Authors' contributions

SM participated in the design of the study, carried out the case selection and data acquisition, performed the statistical analysis, and helped to draft the manuscript. MM participated in dental cast digital analysis, in data acquisition and in the manuscript correction. AG treated the patients and participated in the design of the study. GD participated in the design of the study and in the manuscript correction. MC treated the patients, participated in the design of the study and in the manuscript correction. All authors read and approved the final manuscript.

Author details

[1]Private practice, via Brennero 260/B, 38121 Trento, Italy. [2]Private practice, via Monte Cauriol 10, 38068 Rovereto, Italy. [3]Private practice, viale Stazione 94, 54100 Massa, Italy. [4]University of Cagliari Department of Pedodontics and Interceptive Orthodontics, via Ospedale 54, 09123 Cagliari, Italy. [5]University of Cagliari School of Dental Medicine, IRCCS "G. Gaslini" and Hospital "Galliera" (Genova), Via Fontevivo 21 N, 19125 La Spezia, Italy.

References

1. Bishara SE, Staley RN. Maxillary expansion: clinical implication. Am J Orthod Dentofacial Orthop. 1987;91:3–14.
2. da Silva Filho OG, Montes LA, Torelly LF. Rapid maxillary expansion in the deciduous and mixed dentition evaluated through posteroanterior cephalometric analysis. Am J Orthod Dentofacial Orthop. 1995;107:268–75.

3. Lione R, Franchi L, Cozza P. Does rapid maxillary expansion induce adverse effects in growing subjects? Angle Orthod. 2013;83:172–82.
4. Perillo L, De Rosa A, Iaselli F, d'Apuzzo F, Grassia V, Cappabianca S. Comparison between rapid and mixed maxillary expansion through an assessment of dento-skeletal effects on posteroanterior cephalometry. Prog Orthod. 2014;15:46.
5. Melsen B. Palatal growth studied on human autopsy material. A histologic microradiographic study. Am J Orthod. 1975;68:42–54.
6. Thilander B, Wahlund S, Lennartsson B. The effect of early interceptive treatment in children with posterior cross-bite. Eur J Orthod. 1984;6:25–34.
7. Haas AJ. Palatal expansion: just the beginning of dentofacial orthopaedics. Am J Orthod. 1970;57:219–55.
8. Cozzani M, Rosa M, Cozzani P, Siciliani G. Deciduous dentition-anchored rapid maxillary expansion in crossbite and non-crossbite mixed dentition patients: reaction of the first permanent molar. Prog Orthod. 2003;4:15–22.
9. Cozzani M, Guiducci A, Mirenghi S, Mutinelli S, Siciliani G. Arch width changes with a rapid maxillary expansion appliance anchored to the primary teeth. Angle Orthod. 2007;77:296–302.
10. Mutinelli S, Cozzani M, Manfredi M, Bee M, Siciliani G. Dental arch changes following rapid maxillary expansion. Eur J Orthod. 2008;30:469–76.
11. Mutinelli S, Cozzani M. Rapid maxillary expansion in early-mixed dentition: effectiveness in increasing arch dimension with anchorage to deciduous teeth. Eur J Ped Dent. 2015;16:115–22.
12. van der Linden FP, Duterloo HS. Development of the human dentition: an atlas. Hagerstown, MD, USA: Harper & Row; 1976.
13. Vardimon AD, Graber TM, Pitaru S. Repair process of external root resorption subsequent to palatal expansion treatment. Am J Orthod Dentofacial Orthop. 1993;103:120–30.
14. Baysal A, Karadede I, Hekimoglu S, Ucar F, Ozer T, Veli I, et al. Evaluation of root resorption following rapid maxillary expansion using cone-beam computed tomography. Angle Orthod. 2012;82:488–94.
15. Chugh T, Ganeshkar SV, Revankar AV, Jain AK. Quantitative assessment of interradicular bone density in the maxilla and mandible: implications in clinical orthodontics. Prog Orthod. 2013;14:38.
16. Pangrazio-Kulbersh V, Jezdimir B, de Deus HM, Kulbersh R, Wine P, Kaczynski R. CBCT assessment of alveolar buccal bone level after RME. Angle Orthod. 2013;83:110–6.
17. Brunetto M, Andriani Jda S, Ribeiro GL, Locks A, Correa M, Correa LR. Three-dimensional assessment of buccal alveolar bone after rapid and slow maxillary expansion: a clinical trial study. Am J Orthod Dentofacial Orthop. 2013;143:633–44.
18. Vanarsdall RL, Secchi AG. Periodontal-orthodontic interrelationships current principle and techniques. In: Graber TM, Vanarsdall RL, Vig KWL, editors. Orthodontics. Philadelphia: Elsevier Mosby; 2012. p. 810–3.
19. Shungin D, Olsson AI, Persson M. Orthodontic treatment-related white spot lesions: a 14-year prospective quantitative follow-up, including bonding material assessment. Am J Orthod Dentofacial Orthop. 2010;138:136.e1–e8.
20. Mutinelli S, Cozzani M, Manfredi M, Siciliani G. Dental arch analysis system. Progr Orthod. 2004;5:200–8.
21. Little RM. The irregularity index: a quantitative score of mandibular anterior alignment. Am J Orthod. 1975;68:554–63.
22. Sari Z, Uysal T, Usumez S, Basciftci FA. Rapid maxillary expansion. Is it better in the mixed or in the permanent dentition? Angle Orthod. 2003;73:654–61.
23. Bacetti T, Franchi L, Cameron CG, McNamara JA. Treatment timing for rapid maxillary expansion. Angle Orthod. 2001;71:343–50.
24. Thilander B. Dentoalveolar development in subjects with normal occlusion. A longitudinal study between the ages of 5 and 39 years. Eur J Orthod. 2009;31:109–20.
25. Bishara SE, Bayati P, Jakobsen JR. Longitudinal comparisons of dental arch changes in normal and untreated class II, division 1 subjects and their clinical implications. Am J Orthod Dentofacial Orthop. 1996;110:483–9.
26. Moyers RE, van der Linden FP, Riolo ML, McNamara JA. Standards of human occlusal development. Monograph No. 5, Craniofacial Growth Series. Ann Arbor, MI, USA: University of Michigan, Center for Human Growth and Development; 1976.
27. Guest SS, McNamara Jr JA, Baccetti T, Franchi L. Improving Class II malocclusion as a side-effect of rapid maxillary expansion: a prospective clinical study. Am J Orthod Dentofacial Orthop. 2010;138:582–91.
28. Sillman JH. Dimensional changes of the dental arches: longitudinal study from birth to 25 years. Am J Orthod. 1964;50:824–42.
29. Bishara SE, Jakobsen JR, Treder J, Nowak A. Arch width changes from 6 weeks to 45 years of age. Am J Orthod Dentofacial Orthop. 1997;111:401–9.
30. Spillane LM, McNamara JA. Maxillary adaptation to expansion in the mixed dentition. Semin Orthod. 1995;1:176–87.
31. Lima AL, Lima Filho RMA, Bolognese AM. Long-term clinical outcome of rapid maxillary expansion as the only treatment performed in Class I malocclusion. Angle Orthod. 2005;75:416–20.
32. Wong CA, Sinclair PM, Keim RG, Kennedy DB. Arch dimension changes from successful slow maxillary expansion of unilateral posterior cross-bite. Angle Orthod. 2011;81:616–23.
33. Schiffman PH, Tuncay OC. Maxillary expansion: a meta analysis. Clin Orthod Res. 2001;4:86–96.
34. Turpin DL. Dealing with posterior crossbite in young patients. Am J Orthod Dentofacial Orthop. 2004;126:531–2.
35. Moorrees CFA, Grøn A-M, Lebret LML, Yen PKJ, Fröhlich FJ. Growth studies of the dentition: a review. Am J Orthod. 1969;55:600–16.
36. Kusters ST, Kuijpers-Jagtman AM, Maltha JC. An experimental study in dogs of transseptal fiber arrangement between teeth which have emerged in rotated or non-rotated positions. J Dent Res. 1991;70:192–7.
37. Canuto LF, de Freitas MR, Janson G, de Freitas KMS, Martins PP. Influence of rapid palatal expansion on maxillary incisor alignment stability. Am J Dentofacial Orthop. 2010;137:164.e1–e6.

23

Development of a standardized testing system for orthodontic sliding mechanics

Maryam Fathimani[1], Garrett W Melenka[2], Dan L Romanyk[3], Roger W Toogood[2], Giseon Heo[3], Jason P Carey[2] and Paul W Major[4*]

Abstract

Background: The primary objective of this study was to develop a computer-controlled three-dimensional friction measuring system, the orthodontic friction simulator (OFS). A clinically-based in vitro experiment considering wet and dry friction for conventionally and self-ligated brackets is presented to elucidate debate surrounding sliding mechanics and illustrate capabilities of the OFS.

Methods: The OFS was designed and manufactured using sound engineering principles and with the primary concern of being able to measure all forces and moments generated during sliding mechanics. This required the implementation of a six-axis load cell. A variety of translation and rotation stages were also incorporated to allow for precise positioning of the bracket relative to the archwire. Once designed and built, the OFS was then used to compare conventional and self-ligation methods in both the wet and dry state. Damon Q brackets and 0.018″ × 0.025″ stainless steel wires were used for all tests with a sample size of $n = 65$ for each ligation method. Archwires were pulled at a speed of 0.1 mm/s in 11 increments of 0.1 mm. At each increment, the bracket would be rotated 0.5° resulting in a total archwire travel of 1.1 mm and a second-order bracket angle range of 0°–5°. A repeated measures ANOVA was conducted to determine if ligation method and/or addition of moisture effected resulting orthodontic loads.

Results: The developed equipment for studying orthodontic sliding mechanics was able to measure forces and moments in all three directions; a capability not previously realized in the literature. Additionally, it was found that passive ligation significantly reduced resistance to sliding, $P \leq 0.05$, while the dry/wet state did not.

Conclusions: The OFS certainly proved to be an adequate instrument for the scientific evaluation of orthodontic sliding mechanics. It is capable of measuring loads generated in all directions and is a fully automated apparatus allowing for simple and repeatable friction tests to be conducted. Furthermore, the addition of saliva was not found to significantly influence the loads generated during sliding mechanics regardless of ligation method.

Keywords: Resistance to sliding; Friction; Orthodontics; Archwire/bracket interaction

Background

Resistance to sliding (RS), or friction, in bracket-archwire interaction is of clinical interest in sliding mechanics. In the past, many studies were conducted on this subject [1–5]. Although this has been partly in response to marketing claims of new orthodontic appliances, interest in friction was present [1] long before these appliances were available. Despite this interest, there have been no proposed or adopted standards to measure or evaluate RS, in the oral or laboratory environment. This has contributed to a spirited discussion [6, 7] about the fundamental nature of friction and, separately, its role in the clinical environment.

The complicated frictional interaction, hence the friction coefficient, between two sliding surfaces cannot be deduced theoretically from first principles of physics. A numerical model [2] showed good agreement with experimental phenomena including time dependence of static friction, stick–slip, velocity weakening, and others that are relevant in orthodontic

* Correspondence: major@ualberta.ca
[4]Faculty of Medicine and Dentistry, 5-478, Edmonton Clinic Health Academy (ECHA), University of Alberta, 11405-87 Avenue NW, Edmonton, AB T6G 1C9, Canada
Full list of author information is available at the end of the article

biomechanics. This model, however, must be adapted in an ad hoc manner to produce satisfactory results as experimental parameters are not known beforehand. For the present, knowledge of the friction interaction in any specific situation must be obtained by physical experiment.

An ongoing and common misconception [3] is that the force of friction is a constant fraction of the normal force. This is usually expressed as $F = \mu N$, where F is the friction force, N is the normal force, and μ is an experimentally determined friction coefficient. This is true only under conditions of either impending or relative motion. For impending motion when the surfaces are on the verge of sliding, $\mu = \mu_s$ is the coefficient of static friction, and $F = F_{max}$ is the static friction limit. During relative motion when surfaces slide relative to each other, $\mu = \mu_k$ is the coefficient of kinetic friction, and typically $\mu_k < \mu_s$. Throughout the majority of treatment, however, there is minimal relative motion of the archwire and bracket. The friction, including its direction, is determined by conditions of equilibrium of all the forces acting on the tooth-bracket-archwire complex and will be less than the limiting value (e.g. $0 \le F \le \mu_s N$).

Clinically, the complete set of forces acting on the tooth is not known, therefore friction is also unknown. However, it is experimentally possible to determine the limiting value of friction since it is a property of the two surfaces involved. This is presumably the value that must be exceeded to allow relative motion between the archwire and bracket. The static limit is difficult to determine and recourse is made to measure μ_k, with the understanding that it represents a lower bound on the static limit.

Nanda [4] listed over 20 variables and factors that affect this interaction in the mouth. Because of this complexity, measures of friction in the oral environment are very difficult and therefore extremely rare. Recourse has been made to in vitro experiments to examine key interactions. Previous bench-top studies have explored the effects of wire and bracket geometry [5, 8], material properties [9, 10], ligation method [11–15], tooth angulation [16–19], position of adjacent teeth [20, 21], effect of saliva [22–25], perturbation [26–28], and others. RS is the combination of several different effects, which become dominant at different angles of second-order rotation.

For the coordinate system (CSYS) attached to the bracket in Fig. 1, tip, or second-order angulation, is the angle θ. Kusy and Whitley [5, 9] suggested that RS is a combination of simple (classical) friction (FR), binding (BI), and/or notching (NO), expressed as, Eq. (1):

$$\text{RS} = \text{FR} + \text{BI} + \text{NO} \quad (1)$$

FR occurs at low tip angles due to the force pressing the wire onto one of the sides or back of the slot wall or due to the gripping of the wire by the ligation. For low angulation, *FR* is only mildly affected by the tip angle.

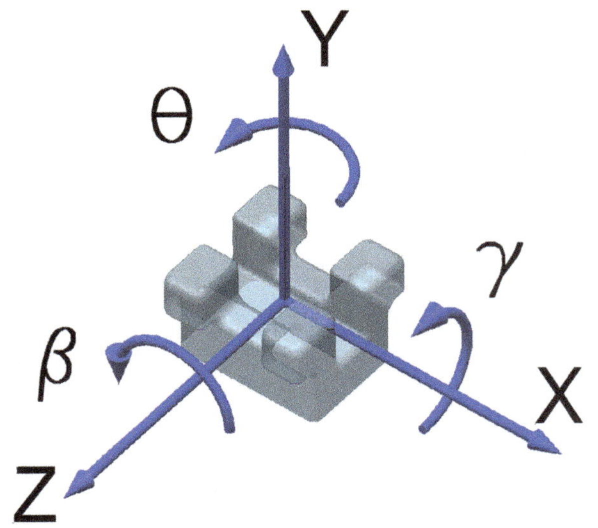

Fig. 1 The bracket coordinate system CSYS and positive direction of forces, moments, and displacements

When the tip angle exceeds some critical value θ_c [5], BI is the dominant interaction. The wire contacts opposite (medial-distal) edges at each end of the slot such that there are opposing contact forces in the ±Z direction. The two opposing normal forces produce a couple M_y. If the opposing forces are equal, there is no net force in the Z direction. Non-equal opposing forces will yield a net force and friction, thus *FR* is still present. The large opposing forces on the corners of the bracket will cause a frictional resistance parallel to the slot even if the net force is zero. The friction at these contact points is therefore related to the magnitude of the couple; if the wire is linearly elastic (for example, stainless steel (SS)), the friction increase is proportional to the tip angle of the bracket beyond θ_c. For a given couple M_y, the friction force will increase for narrower brackets [29]. That is, if M_y remains constant but the bracket width decreases, then the normal force must increase. As friction is proportional to the normal force, it follows that friction will also increase in this scenario.

At sufficiently high angles of tip, physical interlocking of the wire and slot edges caused by plastic (i.e., permanent) deformation of the wire or bracket and/or other surface damage will cause very high, non-friction-based resistance; this is called notching (*NO*). Above the critical notching angle θ_z, *RS* increases unpredictably and very quickly to the extent that sliding likely ceases. For this reason, the *NO* phenomenon is not of great clinical interest.

The vast majority of laboratory experiments investigating orthodontic friction only record one-dimensional (1D) frictional data (i.e., the force required to pull the wire; nominally F_x). As such, the component breakdown of forces at the bracket is not understood, nor are any couples generated during sliding. The apparatus of Kusy and Whitley [5] measured the applied normal force perpendicular to the back wall of the slot at the same time as F_x. The extreme variability of experimental methods used in the literature makes it difficult to compare results between friction studies. With no standardized test equipment or methods, often the results can be used only to draw qualitative conclusions within the limitations of the tests conducted (e.g., wire/bracket combination A versus combination B).

It was proposed by Kamelchuk and Rossouw [30] that an apparatus was required to obtain a more complete picture of orthodontic friction and "would allow a high standard of basic hypothesis testing, product development, quality control, and product performance evaluation with relative ease. (Kamelchuk and Rossouw [30])". A series of design specifications included simultaneous control of velocity and acceleration of both linear wire position and angular bracket position and high-speed digital data acquisition. However, their prototype device [30] was capable only of measuring F_x, as a uniaxial testing machine was used. The device did allow tensioning of the wire which affects its stiffness and therefore, ultimately, *RS*. By testing only a single bracket without lateral constraints on the wire caused by adjacent brackets, the important effect of interbracket distance was not included.

No apparatus measuring three-dimensional (3D) forces and moments on the bracket during friction tests has been published. Devices do exist that measure the 3D loads during other orthodontic treatment protocols; however, this is the first exclusively focusing on sliding mechanics. An understanding of loads in 3D space is essential [31] to effectively analyze tooth movements. There is certainly a relation between the normal forces and moments (caused either by ligation or wire stiffness) and RS; however, these other force and moment components have not been reported.

This paper describes the first published apparatus for measuring the complete 3D six components of force and moment (i.e., F_x, F_y, F_z, M_x, M_y, and M_z) system applied to the bracket during simulated retraction of a canine tooth in an extraction case. The apparatus supports the study of the following variables: bracket and wire geometry, materials, ligation method, dry/wet tests, direct force between wire and slot surface, and second-order angulation, or tip, of the tooth. With minor modifications, the apparatus can also support study of third-order rotation, or torque, buccal/lingual and coronal/apical misalignment, and interbracket distance. Since it is small and portable, the apparatus can be placed within an environment chamber to assess effects of temperature. The apparatus will be demonstrated here by exploring the effects of second-order angulation on forces and moments on conventional and self-ligating brackets in the dry and wet states.

Methods

The orthodontic friction simulator (OFS) is shown in Figs. 2 and 3. Since forces involved are low, design goals were high precision, stiffness of the system, and portability.

The bracket is mounted on a stainless steel dowel inserted into an adaptor mounted on a six-axis load cell (Nano17® force transducer, ATI Industrial Automation, Apex, NC, USA). The dowel can be beveled to accommodate the torque prescription of the bracket, resulting in alignment of the bracket CSYS with the load cell. The sliding movement of an archwire through the bracket is achieved using a programmable motorized micrometer (microactuator) (M230.10 DC-Mike Actuator, Physik

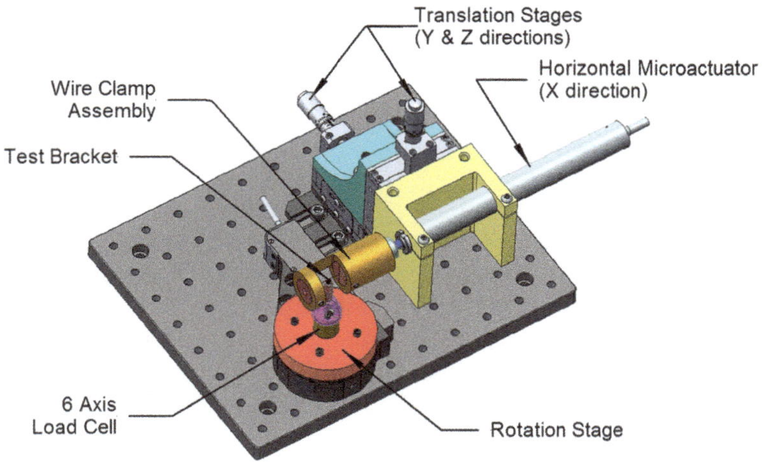

Fig. 2 Orthodontic friction simulator (OFS) general view

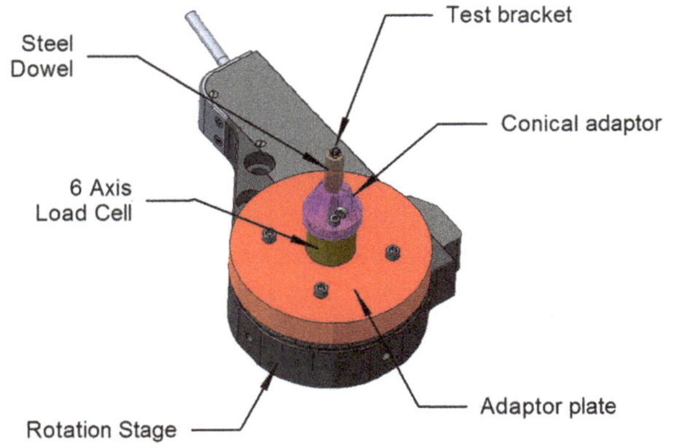

Fig. 3 Detailed schematic of the bracket holder assembly and rotational stage

Instrumente (PI) GmbH & Co., Karlsruhe, Germany) and motor controller (C-863.10 Mercury TM DC motor controller, Physik Instrumente (PI) GmbH & Co., Karlsruhe, Germany) connected to a computer via a universal serial bus (USB) cable. The tip orientation of the bracket relative to the wire is obtained using a programmable rotating stage (PRM1Z8E, Rotation Mount with motor driver, Thorlabs, Newton, NJ, USA). Two manual translating stages (PT1, Translation Stage, Thorlabs, Newton, NJ, USA) are utilized to control the Y and Z position of the wire in the slot and hence either the wire offset or direct normal force applied by the wire on the bracket. The wire movement and bracket angulation are controlled digitally (acceleration, maximum velocity, and incremental move).

There are three significant differences between the device presented here and the one previously developed by Kamelchuk and Rossouw [30]. In the current apparatus, all six components of force and moment acting on the bracket are measured instead of only the pull force, F_x. Previously, the wire was free on either side of the test bracket so that interbracket distance was not included [30]; this is incorporated in the present work. Finally, in previous work [30], the wire could be held under tension during the test and the amount of wire that could be pulled through the bracket was not limited. This is not implemented in the present apparatus, nor was it deemed necessary, as the wire tension in the oral environment is unknown.

A customized configuration file for each bracket contained settings determined by the testing protocol. These include motion settings for the actuators (linear and rotary) and for the data acquisition (NI-DAQ 6215, National Instruments, TX, USA) system (sampling speed and averaging settings, etc.). A custom computer program (LabWindows/ CVI, National Instruments, TX, USA) was written with a graphical user interface allowing for experiment automation and for real-time display of the experiment. Data is transformed from the load cell coordinate system to the bracket coordinate system and saved for later processing (Fig. 4).

Sample preparation

Brackets were mounted on stainless steel cylindrical (1/4″ diameter, 1–1/4″ length) dowel pins (McMaster-Carr) using a porcelain conditioner (Reliance), primer (Ortho-Solo, Universal Bond Enhancer), and composite resin application (Transbond XT, 3M Unitek). The top of the dowel was beveled at the manufacturer specified angle to compensate for any third-order torque prescription in the bracket; however, there was no compensation for other angular prescriptions, namely the first-order bracket angle of 5° for the Damon Q brackets. The rotation prescription for these brackets is 0°, and thus compensation is not required for this angle. Each dowel was machined with a locating flat surface in order to repeatedly maintain the orientation of the bracket and dowel relative to the load cell measurement coordinate system.

A CCD camera (Bausch & Lomb) captured three orthogonal views (Fig. 5) of each bracket/dowel pair. The image scales were approximately 0.005 mm/pixel. Custom software was used to determine the offset of the bracket CSYS relative to the coordinate system of the load cell at the base of the dowel. The (x, y, z) offset values and (θ, γ, β) bracket orientation angles for each bracket/dowel pair are stored in each bracket's configuration file. This data was used to calculate the correct transformation of force/moment data from the load cell to the bracket coordinate system.

To prevent contamination of surfaces, ethanol was used to clean each bracket and archwire, and nitrile gloves were used throughout testing procedure. A new archwire was used for each bracket to avoid the introduction of wire surface damage or distortions caused by testing. For tests using elastic ligatures, a Straight Shooter Ligature Gun (TP Orthodontics) was used to standardize the force and stretching as much as possible. Because a new elastic was used for each bracket, effects of elastic stretch and aging were minimized.

Once the dowel was mounted in the load cell adaptor, a dissection microscope was used to precisely align the archwire in the center of the bracket slot using the manual translation stages. In addition to visualization of the archwire relative to the slot, the load cell data can be viewed in real time to ensure loads are negligible in the passive state. This adjustment also allows presetting the interaction force between the archwire and bracket if desired. The bracket was then ligated. For wet tests, 50 μL of human saliva was deposited on the bracket before and after wire ligation using a micro pipette for a total of 100 μL.

Wire speeds up to 1.2 mm/s are possible with the OFS, however, testing was conducted at 0.1 mm/s. All

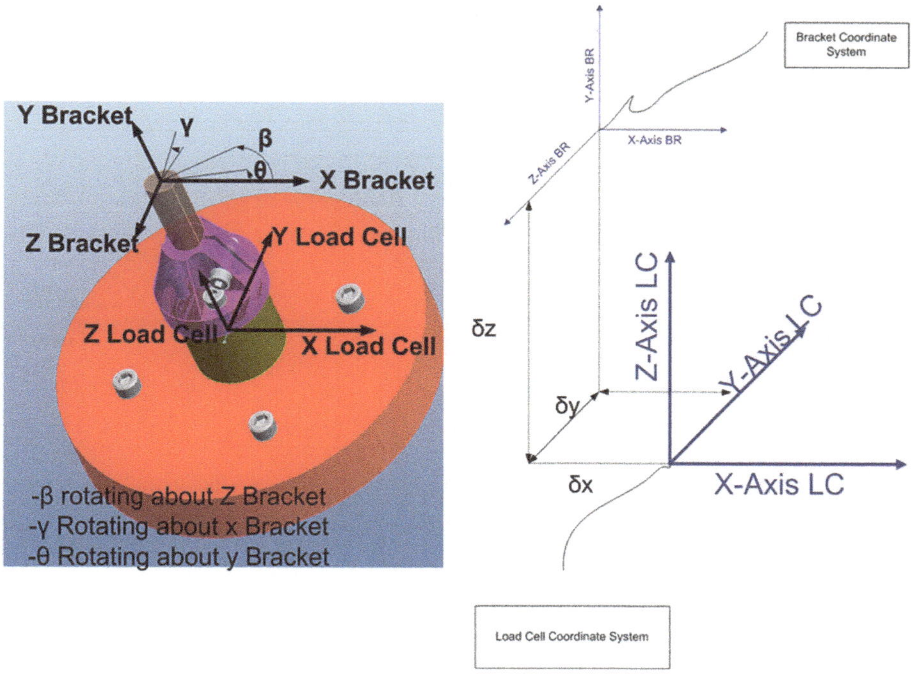

Fig. 4 Representation of the coordinate system transformation from load cell to the bracket

tests occurred over a distance of 1.1 mm. Bracket tip angle θ was incremented by 0.5° from 0° up to 5°. At each angle, the wire was moved 0.1 mm, travel time 1 s, during which force and moment data was collected at a sampling rate of 2000 Hz (50 samples/channel and with three channels each for forces and moments). This data was then averaged over every 50 samples and recorded in a log file for later processing.

The Damon Q (Ormco) left maxillary canine bracket with 0.018″ × 0.025″ stainless steel wires (Ormco) were used for this study. Damon Q brackets were used for both passive and elastomer ligation so that slot geometry remained consistent between trials. A sample size of 65 for elastic and self-ligating brackets in both the wet and dry state, yielding a total sample of 130, was used in this study. A new bracket, ligature (if required), and wire segment were used for each trial to remove any possible effects of wear and/or permanent deformation. Size 0.120 Power O Module (Ormco) elastic ligatures were used in this study. Brackets were randomly assigned to either be passively or elastically ligated prior to any testing, and the order of experiments was also randomized to remove bias.

Error analysis

The potential system errors of the testing apparatus were quantified. With a 16-bit DAQ system, the resolution for the load cell was 0.003 N for force and 0.008 Nmm for moment. Errors could also arise in the transformation from the measured values at the load cell to the computed bracket values. With worst case offset errors, the overall transformation error was less than 0.8 % for F_x, F_z, and M_y and between 1.9–2.8 % for F_y, M_x, and M_z. These marginal errors were acceptable.

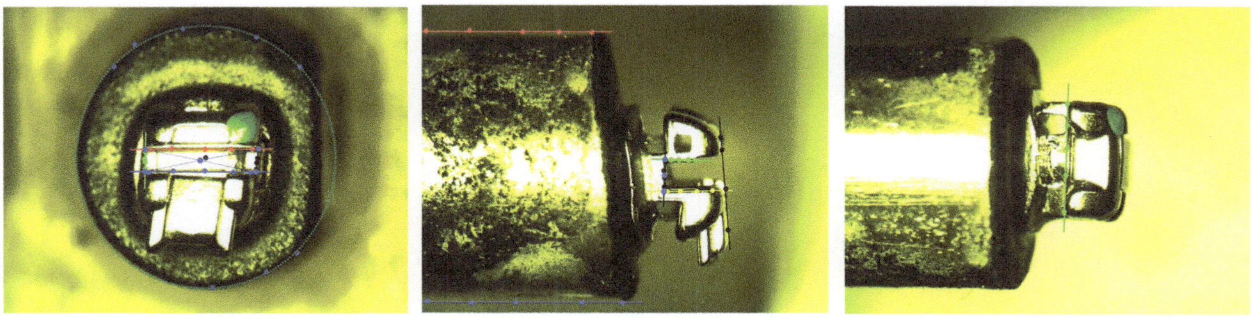

Fig. 5 Top (left), side (middle), and front (right) views of a test bracket showing offset measurements

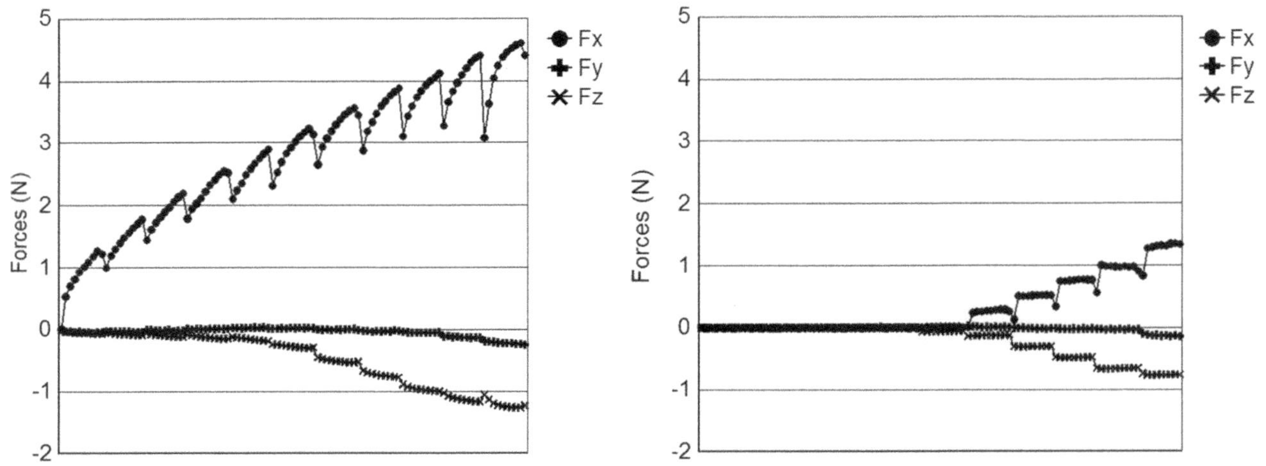

Fig. 6 Typical force (N) versus wire travel (mm) plots from the OFS for elastic (left) and self-ligation (right) methods

Although manufacturing variations of brackets and wires exist, they are generally unknown to the clinician. Using Damon Q self-ligating bracket (slot = 0.022″, width = 0.110″) and 0.018″ × 0.025″ stainless steel archwire, the approximate theoretical θ_c is 2.08°. Manufacturing tolerance errors of 0.0005″ for archwire width, 0.0005″ for slot width, and 0.002″ for bracket width would produce θ_c in the range from 1.54° to 2.65°, contributing significantly to the variability in results. The variations in measured data are therefore more likely to arise from variations in bracket and wire geometry and elastic ligation force than from system errors in the friction apparatus itself.

Results

Typical raw data sets for force, Fig. 6, and moment, Fig. 7, are presented considering only the dry state. The form of this data is typical of all tests. The horizontal axis represents the linear movement of the wire, and the stepped nature of the graphs corresponds to the incrementally changing tip angle. Of particular note in Fig. 6, however, is that for elastic ligation, the current test utilizing short incremental translations of the wire does not allow the forces (especially F_x) to be fully expressed. Observing the test through a microscope, the stretching of the elastic during the test and a mild relapse at the end of each motion increment were noted. This means that the elastic ligation force is not constant through the test and has not reached its maximum. The measured force and moment components are therefore an underestimate of what might be considered a steady state value. This may be an advantage here since long continuous motion of the archwire does not occur clinically, and the ability of the elastic to "rebound" between incremental moves is probably closer to clinical reality.

Figure 8 shows the averaged data for all tests ($N = 65$ for both elastic and self-ligation). The general shape of

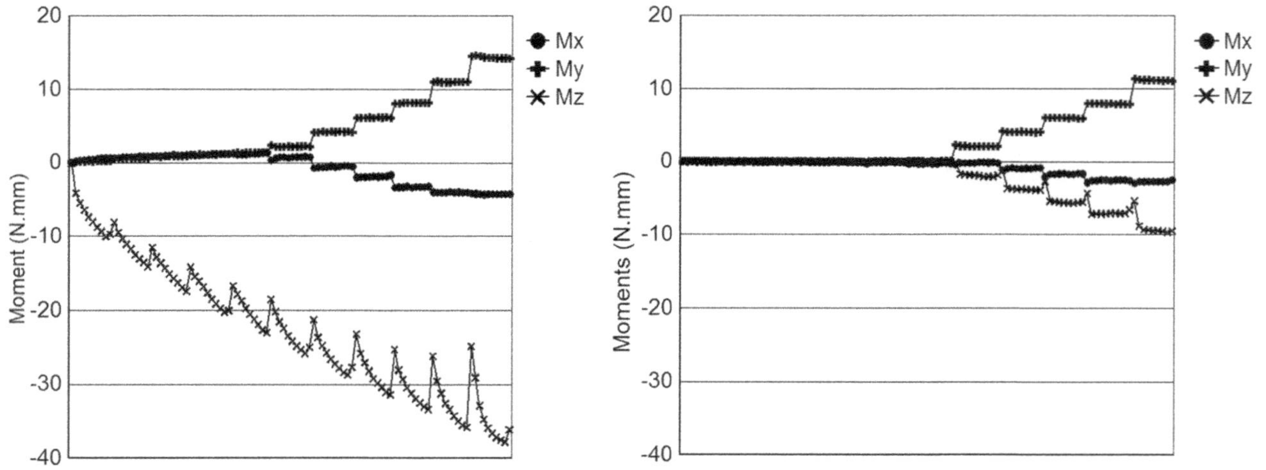

Fig. 7 Typical moment (Nmm) versus wire travel (mm) plots from the OFS for elastic (left) and self-ligation (right) methods

these curves is the same as for the individual test data shown in Figs. 6 and 7, without the "stretching elastic" effect. It can be noticed that the magnitude of M_z increased throughout the experiment. This result is suspected to be due to the lack of bracket prescription compensation on the dowel in the first-order rotation direction. The minor change in M_x is also likely due to this factor as well.

The wire pull direction is initially aligned with the bracket slot. As the bracket rotates, the wire pull direction is no longer purely in the X direction and a force component in the Z direction of the bracket will be generated (Fig. 9). Therefore, since RS is the total force in the nominal direction of the wire, it is calculated as Eq. (2):

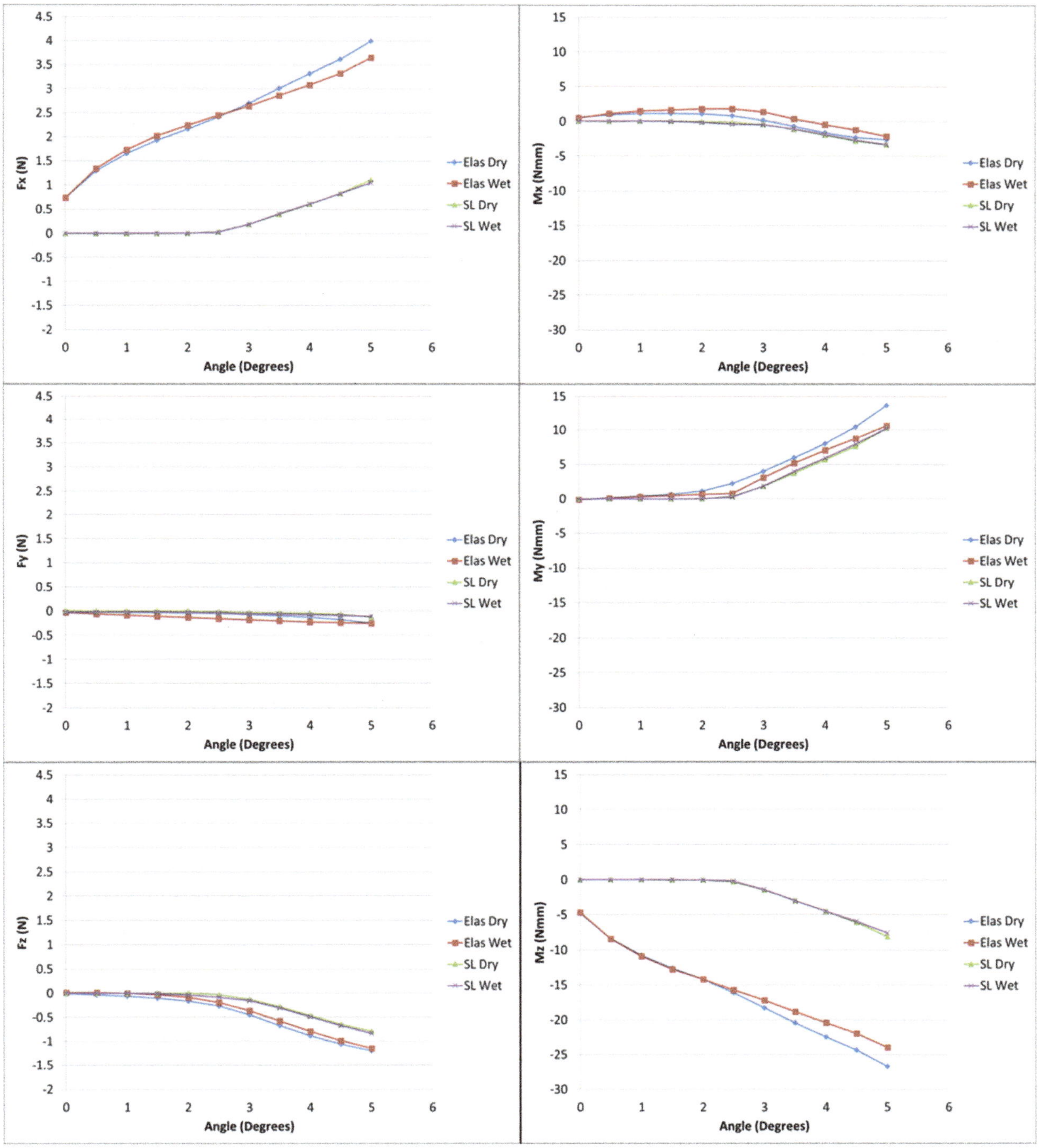

Fig. 8 Average force components (left, top = X, middle = Y, bottom = Z) and moment components (right, top = X, middle = Y, bottom = Z) for all tests

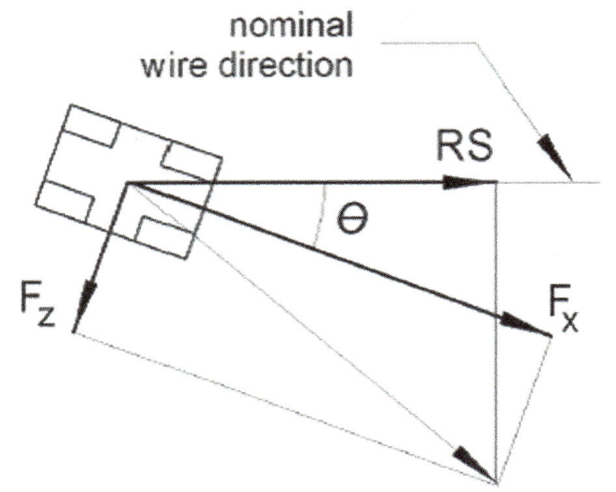

Fig. 9 Definition of RS with positive values of Fx and Fz assumed

$$RS = Fx * \cos\theta - Fz * \sin\theta \quad (2)$$

Note that the F_z components in Figs. 6, 7, and 8 are negative and so will actually increase *RS*. Although F_y is present, it is more-or-less perpendicular to the XZ plane and of very small magnitude; therefore, its contribution to *RS* is ignored. The combined average and standard deviation values of *RS* for all tests are shown in Fig. 10. The standard deviation of data tended to increase with angle. Note that the variation of the elastic ligation data is substantially greater than for self-ligation, undoubtedly due to variations in the ligation force of the elastics.

Using data only for angulation above the critical contact angle for binding (2°), Fig. 11 illustrates M_y to be a linear function of F_x for both ligation methods. Since $M_y = N^*w$, and using $F_x = 2^*\mu_k{}^*N$ (because there are two contact points), the relationship between M_y and F_x can be expressed as Eq. (3):

$$My = (w/2 * \mu k) * Fx \quad (3)$$

From linear regression of Fig. 11, μ_k values were determined and reported in Table 1.

A repeated measures ANOVA was conducted (Table 2) to study the effect of state and ligation method on F_x and M_y values for angulations of 0° and 5°. When conducting experiments, five bracket de-bonded from the dowels and two additional brackets were omitted due to severe data corruption; thus, a total of 123 samples remained for statistical analysis. From the analysis, ligation method had a significant effect ($P < 0.05$) on F_x and M_y for both angles. Interestingly, the wet/dry state was found to have little effect on either value at 0° but made a significant contribution at 5°.

Discussion

OFS performance

From the results presented in this manuscript, it is immediately apparent that the OFS improves upon existing experimental methods. Namely, this device is able to measure all the forces and moments acting at the bracket. At best, previous work was able to measure two components of force during friction tests. Through this capability, a relationship was derived relating F_x and M_y through the coefficient of kinetic friction, μ_k. Previously, this would not have been possible as M_y at the bracket was not measureable.

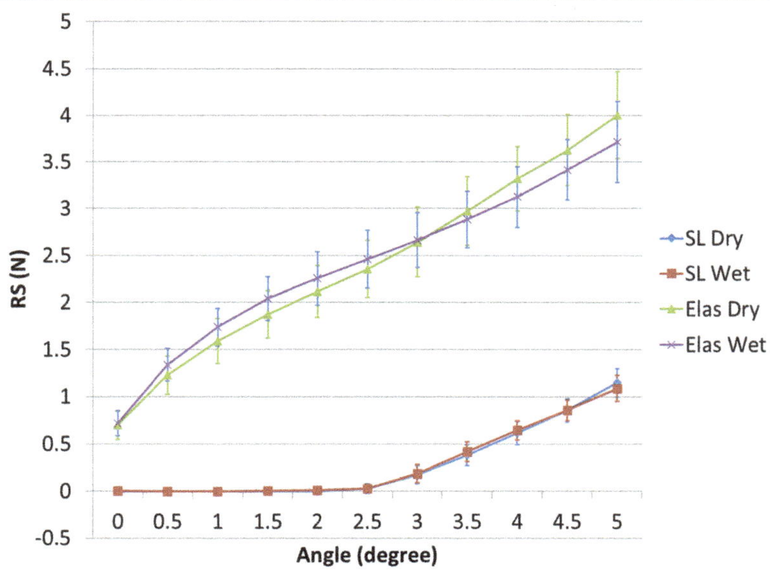

Fig. 10 Average resistance to sliding (RS) and standard deviation for all test conditions

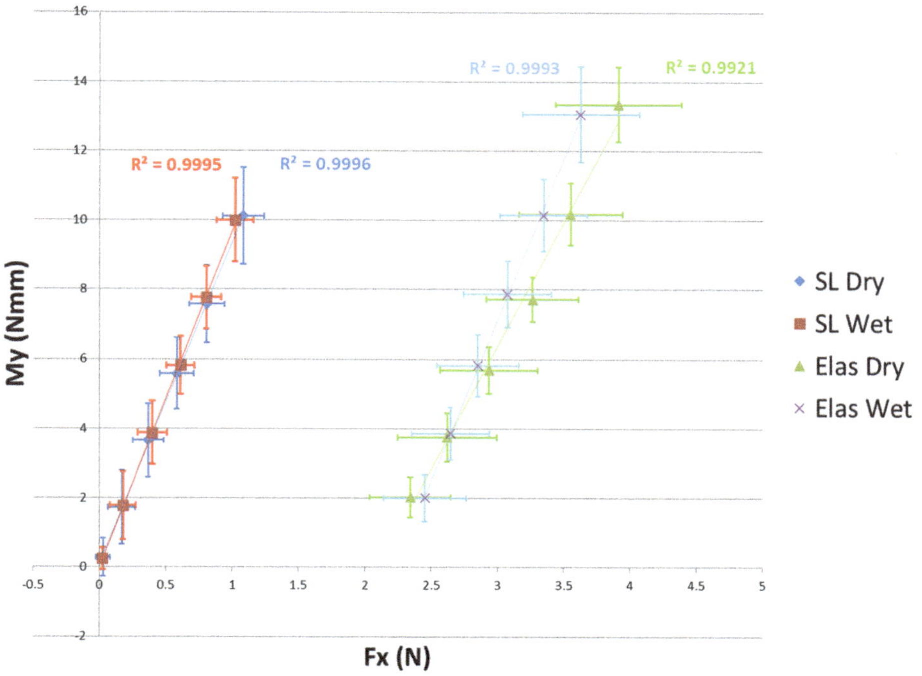

Fig. 11 Relationship between My and Fx for binding, their correlation coefficients (R2), and respective standard deviations

Through the developed and programmable user interface, operators are able to easily and accurately control many test variables such as velocity, acceleration, and bracket rotation (in this case second-order rotation). This allows for a variety of experimental procedures to be set up quickly and performed repeatedly with minimal training. Given the amount of variables that may be manipulated with this apparatus, it was imperative that the controls remained as simple and straight forward as possible.

Finally, the OFS can be readily adapted to accommodate a variety of future hypotheses and experiments. For instance, by slightly offsetting the dowel and mounting the bracket on the side instead of on top, the effect of first-order rotation may be explored. In addition, by machining the tops of the dowels at various angles using the existing bracket position, the influence of third-order torque can be considered. Indeed, a number of future studies can be considered with only minimal adjustments to the OFS presented here.

Effect of ligation method and dry/wet state

Based on the retrieved data, it is apparent that for self-ligation, since the wire is initially aligned with the slot, force and moment components are essentially zero until the onset of binding at approximately 2°. Once binding has occurred in self-ligating brackets, the force and moment values increased in a linear fashion with angle. This is in contrast to F_y and M_x, however, which showed little variation with angulation, ligation method, or dry/wet state.

Table 1 Coefficient of friction determined from binding data

	Coefficient of kinetic friction	
	Self-ligation	Elastic ligation
Dry	0.15	0.21
Wet	0.14	0.16

When considering elastic ligation, *FR* was not constant as expected due to the incremental stretching and rebound of the elastics. That is, the elastic tests never really reached a steady state. It is not clear, in fact, if that state would actually occur in vivo. Additionally, variations in measured forces and moments were considerably higher with elastic ligation than with self-ligation, undoubtedly due to inconsistency and variability in the elastomers or application technique.

While only *RS* has been analyzed by previous researchers, the role of binding illustrated by M_y can now be explored. It is evident that binding affects M_y for both self-ligated and elastically ligated brackets in a similar way: onset occurs at the binding angle and the rate of increase is similar for both types. Thus, the "uprighting moment" that is opposing the continued tip of the tooth is the same for both ligation methods. This has not been previously shown.

The differences due to dry versus wet testing were not significant in general based on the data. Using Fig. 11, there is negligible difference in μ_k values between dry and wet conditions for self-ligating brackets. Based on the results in Table 2, the state of the experiment had no

Table 2 Repeated measures ANOVA for each outcome and mean differences from pairwise comparisons ($n = 123$)

Outcome	Effects	F	*P*	η_p^2	Mean difference[a]
Fx 0°	State	0.001	0.982	4.0×10^{-6}	NS
	State + elastomer	0.033	0.856	2.7×10^{-4}	NS
	Elastomer	2904.2	<0.001*	0.96	0.74 N
Fx 5°	State	23.6	<0.001*	0.16	0.21 N
	State + elastomer	11.3	0.001*	0.09	0.30 N
	Elastomer	4281.9	<0.001*	0.97	2.74 N
My 0°	State	2.3	0.134	0.02	NS
	State + elastomer	0.2	0.685	0.001	NS
	Elastomer	4.0	0.047*	0.03	−0.05 Nmm
My 5°	State	3.9	0.050*	0.03	0.33 Nmm
	State + elastomer	3.7	0.056	0.03	NS
	Elastomer	282.3	<0.001*	0.70	3.12 Nmm

Degrees of freedom (1, 121) for each effect
F F statistic, η_p^2 partial eta squared, *NS* not significant
*$P \leq 0.05$ was significant
[a]If *P* is significant, mean differences recorded from pairwise comparisons for state (dry–wet), elastomer (yes–no), and interaction of state + elastomer

effect on F_x or M_y at 0° angulation but did have a significant effect at 5°. While this would imply that the introduction of saliva could impact sliding mechanics at some point, in general, it was found to have negligible effect. The coefficient of kinetic friction for self-ligating bracket in this study was 0.15 (dry) and 0.14 (wet), which is comparable to 0.14 (dry) reported by Thorstenson and Kusy [10].

It is well known that interbracket distance has an effect on *RS* due to a change in effective stiffness of the wire [32]. The present system used an interbracket distance of approximately 6 mm, defined as the distance from the edge of the bracket to the edge of the clamp. This value varied slightly during the test due to the clamping system for the wire. In the current setup, the varying interbracket distance and wire misalignment could have contributed to the higher than expected observed F_z values. The ability to set a fixed desired interbracket distance as a test parameter is recommended for the next-generation 3D OFS. A more secure wire clamp design would ensure no rotational or lateral wire movements contributing to moment effects. A modified load cell adaptor would produce a smaller offset from the load cell to the bracket, which would allow a broader range of test conditions to be explored without overloading the load cell.

Clinical significance

The presented study serves to explore fundamental relationships that exist both in the lab and in vivo. It is questionable whether informative lab experiments could be devised that involves all 20+ factors listed by Nanda [4]. This data is not available through any form of in vivo testing, nor would such testing be advisable since exploring the full range of variables would undoubtedly interfere with clinical treatment. It is desirable to maintain as many conditions fixed while varying only a few parameters in order to expose the correlation between those parameters. This sort of control is not available in vivo.

Laboratory findings, therefore, are meant to provide the underlying fundamentals that may then be considered in the expected clinical context. Only four of the many variables contributing to *RS* are explored with this system. These data, however, show the direct link between two of the force/moment components and the second-order tip. The critical contact angle is confirmed, as is a method for determining the effective coefficient of friction between the wire and the bracket.

Of particular note is the result that the couple M_y resulting from binding is the same for both elastic and self-ligation. This is the important uprighting moment that occurs during retraction in sliding mechanics.

This system measures kinetic friction on an isolated bracket in a steady state environment. Though clinical conditions are complicated to simulate, future studies evaluating both static and kinetic friction on a bracket experiencing oral functions, such as vibrations or vertical displacements, would be insightful. Similarly, since the compliance of the tooth mounted in the PDL will interact with the stiffness of the wire and hence the forces applied to the bracket, a future enhancement of the apparatus should include a method to simulate the PDL. An adjustable and constant interbracket distance would also be a desirable enhancement.

Conclusions

The results reported here support Kusy and Whitley's model for *RS* as composed of *FR* and *BI* components.

The experimental θ_c value agreed with the theoretical equation based on bracket and wire geometry. Similar to Kusy and Whitley's work for F_x, above θ_c, *RS* increased linearly with angulation for both self-ligation and elastic ligation. There was minimal effect of saliva in changing the frictional behavior of self-ligating bracket, while a small reduction in friction was observed under wet conditions with elastic ligation. Examination of all force and moment components acting on the bracket leads to additional insights into this complex interaction which was not previously possible. Current testing did not extend into the notching (*NO*) region due to issues with overloading the load cell.

The novelty of this 3D friction device includes measuring forces and moments in the X, Y, and Z directions applied on the bracket. These unique results, in addition to the marginal data errors, strengthen the utilization of this 3D device. Indeed, 3D simulations should be the standard protocol for understanding the friction phenomenon, as current 1D methods are limited in scope of information and application. The methodological variability between research teams makes comparisons between studies difficult or nearly impossible. As the interest in friction for orthodontic tooth movement continues, a goal of the research community should entail more standardized testing methods. This may include collaboration between research groups to use the same device and/or protocols.

Abbreviations

RS: resistance to sliding; F: friction force; N: normal force; μ: general coefficient of friction; μs: static coefficient of friction; μk: kinetic coefficient of friction; CSYS: coordinate system located at the bracket; FR: simple, or classical, friction; BI: binding; NO: notching; Θ: second-order angle of the bracket; θ_C: critical angle where the wire contacts bracket edges; OFS: orthodontic friction simulator.

Competing interests

The authors declare that they have no competing interests.

Authors' contributions

MF participated in design of the experimental procedure, performed all experiments, conducted data analysis, and contributed to drafting and editing of the manuscript. GM contributed significantly to development of the orthodontic friction simulator (OFS), designing the experimental protocol, assisting in use of the OFS, and editing the manuscript. DR participated in data analysis as well as drafting and editing the manuscript. RT was primarily involved in developing the OFS, guiding experimental procedures, and drafting and editing the manuscript. GH provided significant guidance in the statistical analysis of experimental results and participated in editing of the manuscript. Finally, JC and PM provided engineering and clinical guidance, respectively, in regards to developing the experimental protocol and ensuring its clinical relevancy, as well as editing the manuscript. All of the authors have read and approved the manuscript.

Author details

[1]Orthodontic Department, School of Dentistry, University of Alberta, Edmonton, AB, Canada. [2]Department of Mechanical Engineering, University of Alberta, Edmonton, AB, Canada. [3]School of Dentistry, University of Alberta, Edmonton, AB, Canada. [4]Faculty of Medicine and Dentistry, 5-478, Edmonton Clinic Health Academy (ECHA), University of Alberta, 11405-87 Avenue NW, Edmonton, AB T6G 1C9, Canada.

References

1. Stoner M. Force control in clinical practice. Am J Orthod. 1960;46(3):163–8.
2. Al-Bende F, Lampaert V, Swevers J. A novel generic model at asperity level for dry friction force dynamics. Tribol Lett. 2004;16(1):81–93.
3. Braun S, Bluestein M, Moore K, Benson G. Friction in perspective. Am J Orthod Dentofacial Orthop. 1999;115(6):619–27.
4. Nanda R. Biomechanical considerations in sliding mechanics in biomechanics in clinical orthodontics. WB Saunders; 1997.
5. Kusy RP, Whitley JQ. Influence of archwire and bracket dimensions on sliding mechanics: derivations and determinations of the critical contact angles for binding. Euro J Orthod. 1999;21(2):199–208.
6. Rossouw PE, Kamelchuk LS, Kusy RP. A fundamental review of variables associated with low velocity frictional dynamics. Semin Orthod. 2003;9(4):223–35.
7. Burrow III SJ. Critical appraisal of in vitro steady-state frictional resistance studies. Semin Orthod. 2010;16(4):244–8.
8. Tecco S, Tetè S, Festa F. Friction between archwires of different sizes, cross-section and alloy and brackets ligated with low-friction or conventional ligatures. Angle Orthod. 2009;79(1)):111.
9. Kusy RP, Whitley JQ. Friction between different wire-bracket configurations and materials. Semin Orthod. 1997;3(3):166–77.
10. Thorstenson GA, Kusy RP. Effect of archwire size and material on the resistance to sliding of self-ligating brackets with second-order angulation in the dry state. Am J Orthod Dentofacial Orthop. 2002;122(3):295–305.
11. Ehsani S, Mandich M, El-Bialy TH, Flores-Mir C. Frictional resistance in self-ligating orthodontic brackets and conventionally ligated brackets. A systematic review Angle Orthod. 2009;79(3):592–601.
12. Khambay B, Millett D, McHugh S. Evaluation of methods of archwire ligation on frictional resistance. Euro J Orthod. 2004;26(3):327–32.
13. Chimenti C, Franchi L, Di Giuseppe MG, Lucci M. Friction of orthodontic elastomeric ligatures with different dimensions. Angle Orthod. 2005;75(3):421–5.
14. Franchi L, Baccetti T, Camporesi M, Barbato E. Forces released during sliding mechanics with passive self-ligating brackets or non-conventional elastomeric ligatures. Am J Orthod Dentofacial Orthop. 2008;133(1):87–90.
15. Thorstenson GA, Kusy RP. Effects of ligation type and method on the resistance to sliding of novel orthodontic brackets with second-order angulation in the dry and wet states. Angle Orthod. 2003;73(4):418–30.
16. Hamdan A, Rock P. The effect of different combinations of tip and torque on archwire/bracket friction. Euro J Orthod. 2008;30(5):508–14.
17. Thorstenson GA, Kusy RP. Resistance to sliding of orthodontic brackets with bumps in the slot floors and walls: effects of second-order angulation. Dent Mater. 2004;20(9):881–92.
18. Articolo L, Kusy RP. Influence of angulation on the resistance to sliding in fixed appliances. Am J Orthod Dentofacial Orthop. 1999;115(1):39–51.
19. Kusy RP, Whitley JQ. Influence of archwire and bracket dimensions on sliding mechanics: derivations and determinations of the critical contact angles for binding. Euro J Orthod. 1999;21(2):199–208.
20. Matarese G, Nucera R, Militi A, Mazza M, Portelli M, Festa F, et al. Evaluation of frictional forces during dental alignment: an experimental model with 3 nonleveled brackets. Am J Orthod Dentofacial Orthop. 2008;133(5):708–15.
21. Baccetti T, Franchi L, Camporesi M, Defraia E. Orthodontic forces released by low-friction versus conventional systems during alignment of apically or buccally malposed teeth. Euro J Orthod. 2011;33(1):50–4.
22. Downing A, Mccabe JF, Gordon PH. The effect of artificial saliva on the frictional forces between orthodontic brackets and archwires. Brit J Orthod. 1995;22(1):41–6.
23. Al-Mansouri N, Palmer G, Moles DR, Jones SP. The effects of lubrication on the static frictional resistance of orthodontic brackets. Aus Orthod J. 2011;27(2):132–8.
24. Kusy RP, Whitley JQ, Prewitt MJ. Comparison of the frictional coefficients for selected archwire-bracket slot combinations in the dry and wet states. Angle Orthod. 1991;61(4):293–302.
25. Thorstenson GA, Kusy RP. Resistance to sliding of self-ligating brackets versus conventional stainless steel twin brackets with second-order angulation in the dry and wet (saliva) states. Am J Orthod Dentofacial Orthop. 2001;120(4):361–70.

26. Liew CF, Brockhurst P, Freer TJ. Frictional resistance to sliding archwires with repeated displacement. Aus Orthod J. 2002;18(2):71–5.
27. Olson JE, Liu Y, Nickel JC, Walker MP, Iwasaki LR. Archwire vibration and stick-slip behavior at the bracket-archwire interface. Am J Orthod Dentofacial Orthop. 2012;142(3):314–22.
28. Sirisaowaluk N, Kravchuk O, Ho CT. The influence of ligation on frictional resistance to sliding during repeated displacement. Aus Orthod J. 2006;22(2):141–6.
29. Tidy DC. Frictional forces in fixed appliances. Am J Orthod Dentofacial Orthop. 1989;96(3):249–54.
30. Kamelchuk L, Rossouw P. Development of a laboratory model to test kinetic orthodontic friction. Semin Orthod. 2003;9(4):251–61.
31. Kusy R. Influence of force systems on archwire-bracket combinations. Am J Orthod Dentofacial Orthop. 2005;127(3):333–42.
32. Creekmore T. The importance of interbracket width in orthodontic tooth movement. J Clin Orthod. 1976;10(7):530–4.

24

Three-dimensional assessment of teeth first-, second- and third-order position in Caucasian and African subjects with ideal occlusion

Luca Lombardo*, Alessandro Perri, Angela Arreghini, Michele Latini and Giuseppe Siciliani

Abstract

Background: The aim of this study was to provide an updated version of Andrews' seminal study by exploiting 3D software to analyse the tip, torque and in-out values of two groups of different racial and ethnic background.

Methods: The analysis was conducted on one Caucasian group (30 individuals) and one of African origin (29). All subjects were adult, in normal occlusion and had no previous history of orthodontic treatment. Rhinoceros™ 3D modelling software was used to identify anatomical reference points, planes and axes and to make the appropriate measurements.

Results: Compared to Andrews' measurements, we found more positive coronal tip values in both African and Caucasian subjects, while the torque values we measured tended to be less negative in the posterior sectors than those reported by Andrews. We measured greater tip values in the lower jaw of Caucasian with respect to African subjects, particularly in the middle sectors.

Conclusions: Race and ethnicity have a strong influence on values of tip, torque and in-out. This is translated as a more positive tip in Caucasian subjects and a more positive torque in those of African descent (greater proclination of the incisors). Finally, with respect to the values reported by Andrews, we found a tendency to more positive mean tip (except for at the upper second molars and lower incisors) and less negative torque in the posterior sectors.

Keywords: Tip; Torque; In-out; Straight-wire prescription; Andrews

Background

Andrews was the first to put forward the hypothesis that the ideal occlusion of untreated patients could serve as the target of orthodontic treatment [1]. However, despite Andrews' undeniable influence on orthodontics as we know it today, several authors [1–6] have identified sources of bias in this seminal study, in both the method Andrews adopted for making his measurements—ascribable to the instruments he used—and the sample he selected—North American subjects of Caucasian origin. Nevertheless, only Sebata [2], Watanabe [3], Currim [4] and Doodamani [5] have since replicated Andrews' study using different samples (Japanese in the first two, Indians in the latter two) and a modified method. As could be expected from the different approaches used and samples considered in these investigations, all four produced results that were significantly different from those of Andrews.

In spite of the many advances in orthodontics since Andrews' proposed his pre-programmed appliance, the majority of devices on the market still feature prescriptions based on his measurements. This means that, generally speaking, not enough attention is paid to the position of the roots. In reality, there is a strong correlation between the tip and torque and the tooth root position, as there are variations in coronal morphology, incongruencies between the inclination of the roots and the crown, and a disproportion between the height of the crown and the length of the root of the same tooth [7].

That being said, measurement of the angulation and inclination of the roots relies on 3D imaging, which has only been available in recent years following the development of such diagnostic tool technology. In this regard, the

* Correspondence: lulombardo@tiscali.it
Department of Orthodontics, University of Ferrara, Via montebello, 31, Ferrara 44100, Italy

Table 1 Inclusion criteria

Adult age (not less than 18 years)	No previous orthodontic treatment
Regular arch form with little or no crowding	Complete dentition to second molars
No bridges or implants	Centred midlines
No gingival recession	No joint or muscle pathologies
No ectopic teeth	No supernumerary teeth or tooth agenesis
At least four of Andrews' six keys with bilateral molar and canine class I occlusion always present	Presence of minimal diastems and/or small premolar rotation or little irregularity (Little's index less than 3) at incisors in some individuals
Overbite and overjet within normal limits 2 mm ± 1 mm	No anterior or posterior cross-bite
No markedly visible intra-oral or extra-oral symmetry	

study by Tong [8] was a real innovation; its aim was to analyse the tip and torque of the teeth in patients in normal, or nearly normal, occlusion by means of CBCT. The only flaw in that study was the fact that it was carried out on a small sample of single ethnicity (13 Caucasians).

Huanca Ghislanzoni et al. [9] have validated a method for the analysis of 3D virtual casts, which allow to identify the values of the first, second and third order of teeth with great intra- and inter-operator reproducibility. This confirms the potential of new technologies in obtaining reliable data for clinical diagnosis and the tooth position.

As mentioned, to date, no researcher has attempted to replicate Andrews' work exploiting the potential of today's technology, which provides a far greater degree of accuracy and reproducibility than can be obtained by the manual methods available in his time. Hence, we set out to compare the values manually measured by Andrews with those, based on the same anatomical reference points and planes, obtained using digital technology to determine whether Andrews' values are still relevant or whether significant differences indicate that digital measurements provide us with better reference values. We also extended the study to two ethnic groups.

Methods

Sample selection

The study was conducted on a sample made up of two groups of adults in ideal occlusion with no previous history of orthodontic treatment, one of Caucasian and one of African origin. Thirty Caucasian subjects (14 males and 16 females) were recruited from among patients presenting for general dentistry procedures or routine check-up at various private practices in Italy, and 29 African subjects (14 males and 15 females) were recruited from among the students of the Eduardo Mondlane University in Inhambane, Mozambique. Subject selection was performed according to the inclusion criteria noted in Table 1.

Precision impressions of the dental arcades of each patient were taken using the dual-phase putty and light body (Elite HD+ Fast Set, Zhermack, Rovigo, Italy) technique. Bite registrations of each patient's dentition were taken in maximum intercuspidation. Silicone was chosen as the impression material due to its precision and dimensional stability [10]. Each subject's impressions were placed in an orthodontic 3D scanner (3Shape D700/710, Copenhagen, Denmark) to obtain virtual 3D renderings in stereolithography (STL) format (Fig. 1). The anatomical reference points, axes and planes on these renderings were marked using Rhinoceros™ 4.0 3D modelling software (Robert McNeel & Associates, Seattle, USA), which was also used to make the measurements detailed below.

Measurements taken

Tip and torque: two operators performed measurements. Both operators used Rhinoceros™ software to make the measurements, which were based on the anatomical reference points described by Andrews. The occlusal plane was identified on each 3D rendering and used as a plane of reference. This plane, described by Rhinoceros as the "C-plane", was made to pass through three anatomical points: the inter-incisal point and the halfway points on

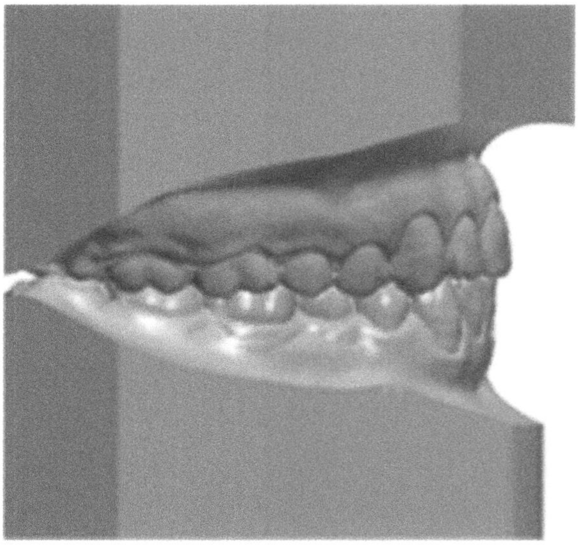

Fig. 1 Three-dimensional model

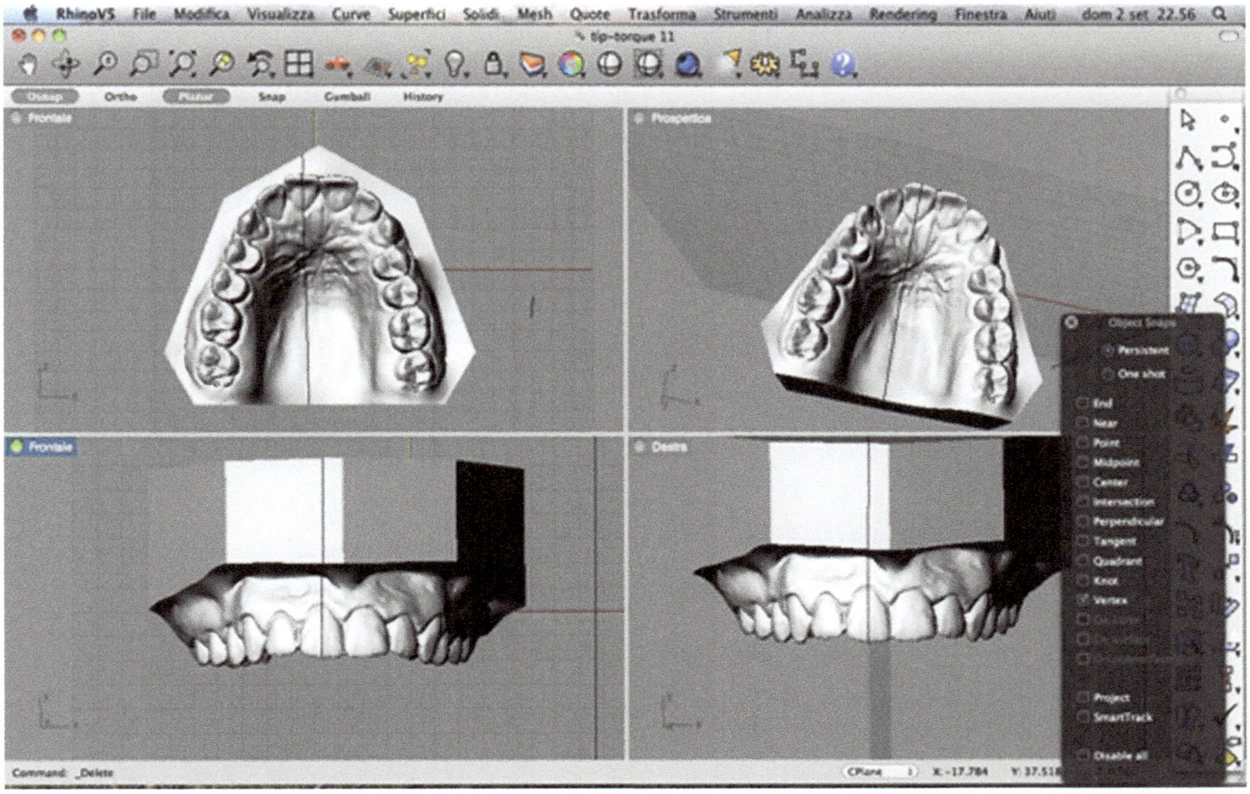

Fig. 2 Measuring the FACC

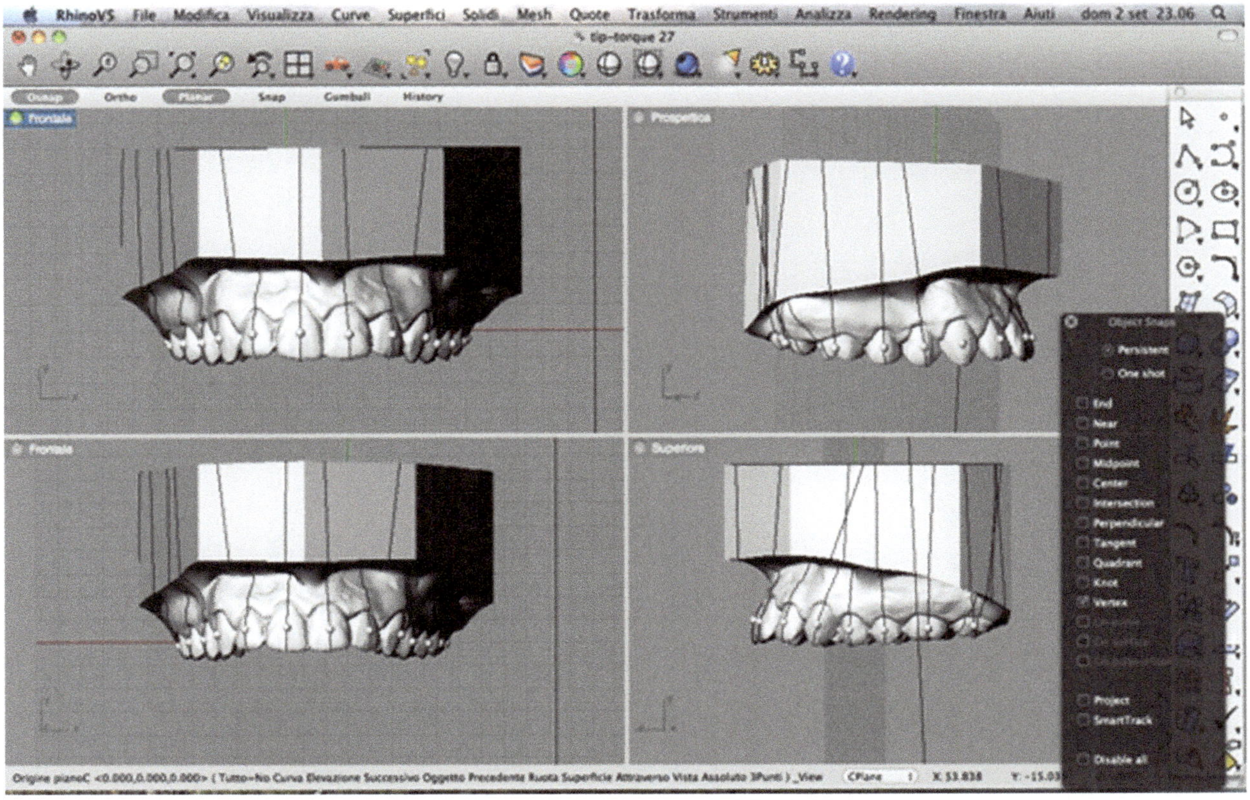

Fig. 3 Creation of virtual spheres around FA points

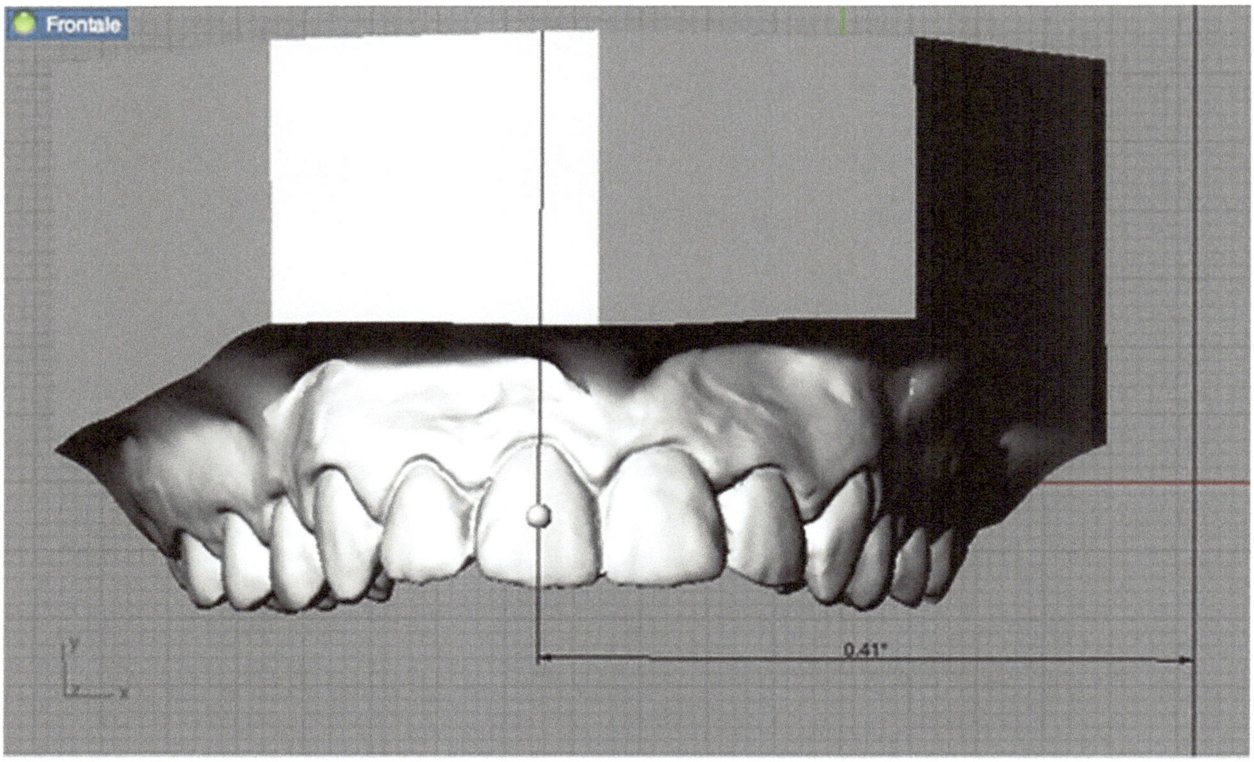

Fig. 4 Calculating the upper central incisor tip

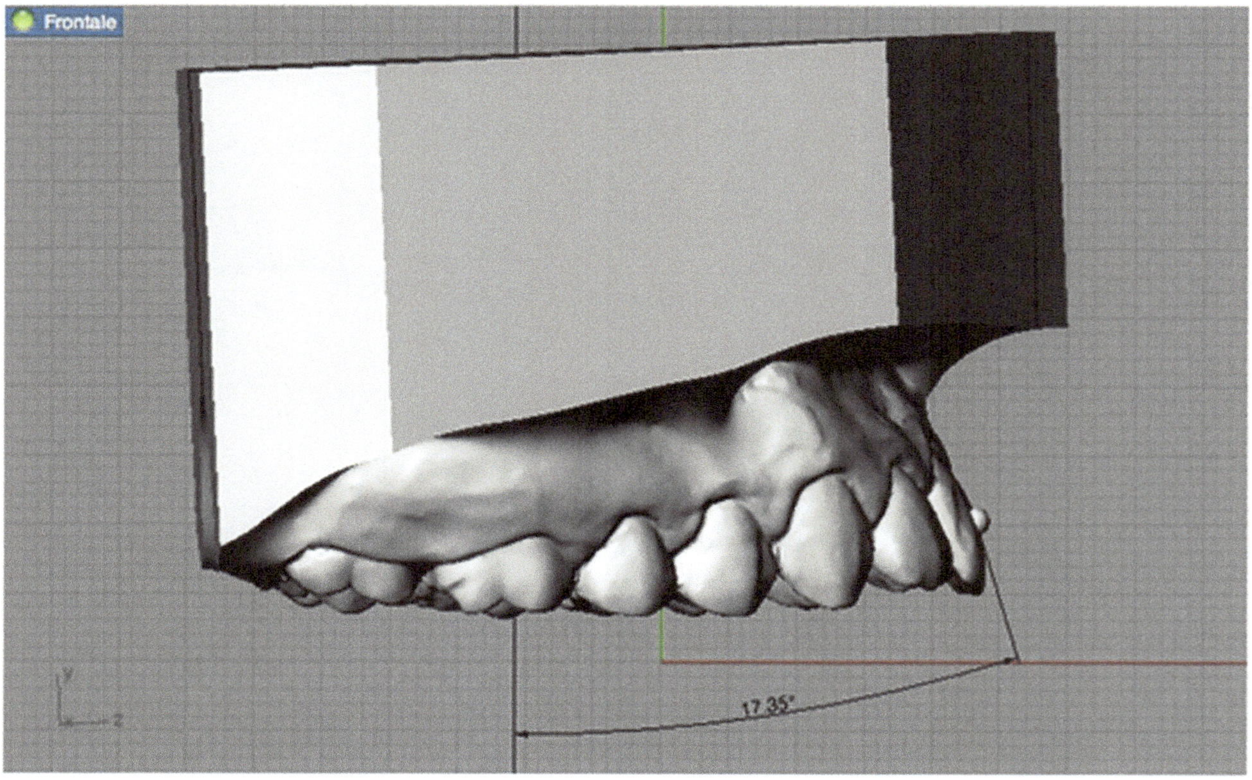

Fig. 5 Calculating the upper central incisor torque

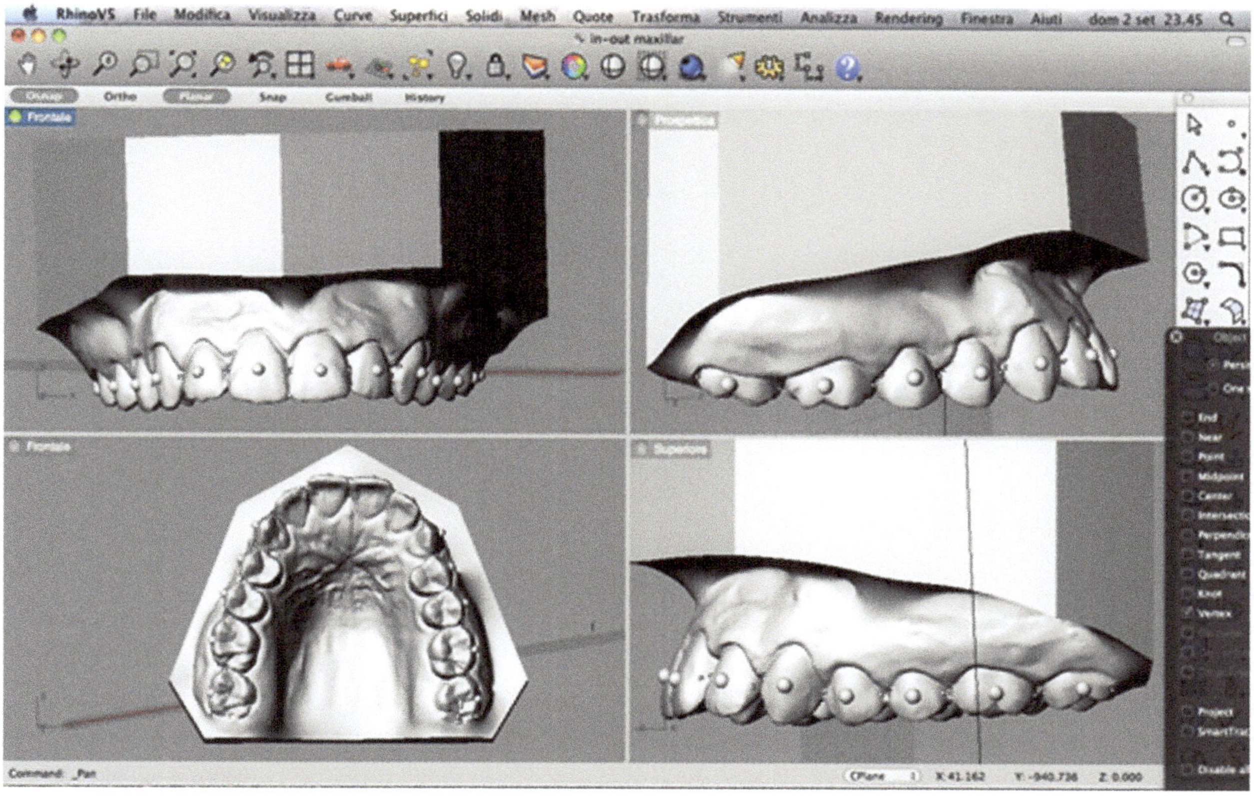

Fig. 6 Determining contact points

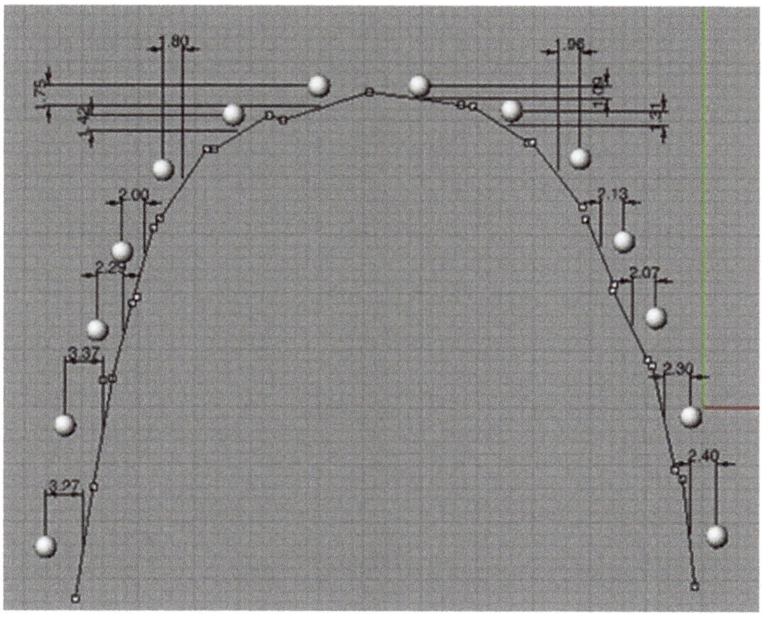

Fig. 7 Calculating the in-out

Table 2 Comparison of tip values measured for the two groups

Africans—tip				Caucasians—tip			Comparison	
	n	Mean	Standard deviation	*n*	Mean	Standard deviation	*t* test	*p* level
TIP U7	58	−3.06	6.78	60	−3.88	10.60	0.51	ns
TIP U6	58	9.48	3.53	60	10.26	5.54	−0.98	ns
TIP U5	58	5.96	5.84	60	9.64	4.16	−3.93	<0.001
TIP U4	58	3.29	4.45	60	7.67	4.28	−5.45	<0.001
TIP U3	58	8.23	5.20	60	9.96	4.81	−1.87	ns
TIP U2	58	9.23	3.87	60	9.99	3.69	−1.10	ns
TIP U1	58	3.68	3.55	60	4.53	2.84	−1.44	ns
TIP L7	58	12.65	5.83	60	14.20	6.47	−1.37	ns
TIP L6	58	6.30	5.36	60	10.99	2.78	−5.95	<0.001
TIP L5	58	3.60	4.02	60	6.90	3.09	−4.99	<0.001
TIP L4	58	2.95	3.89	60	6.06	3.36	−4.63	<0.001
TIP L3	58	3.478	4.850	60	5.91	3.98	−2.98	0.004
TIP L2	58	−0.26	3.01	60	0.14	4.46	−0.57	ns
TIP L1	58	−1.13	3.30	60	0.00	4.46	−1.57	ns

ns not significant.

the distal marginal crest of each second molar. After the occlusal plane was aligned visually, the line perpendicular to it was traced. The facial axis of each tooth crown (FACC) was marked using the "section" tool, in all cases making sure that the C-plane was aligned correctly. To make the facial axis (FA) point visible, this was placed in the centre of a virtual 1-mm sphere whose centre lay on the previously traced axis (Figs. 2 and 3). Once these anatomical reference points had been marked on the renderings, the tip and torque of each tooth were measured. The tip was taken as the angle between the FACC and the line perpendicular to the occlusal plane, using the "Evaluate/angle" function (Fig. 4). To calculate the torque, a tangent line was drawn perpendicular to the surface of each tooth, passing through the FA point (i.e. the centre of the virtual sphere) on a mesiodistal view of each tooth (therefore positioned at 90° with respect to the FACC), the angle between this line and the occlusal reference plane was calculated (Fig. 5).

Table 3 Comparison of torque values measured for the two groups

Africans—torque				Caucasians—torque			Comparison	
	n	Mean	Standard deviation	*n*	Mean	Standard deviation	*t* test	*p* level
TORQUE U7	58	−12.79	10.11	60	−5.50	12.23	−3.54	<0.001
TORQUE U6	58	−10.98	9.75	60	−6.26	10.24	−2.56	0.013
TORQUE U5	58	−4.00	8.43	60	−3.54	6.42	−0.33	ns
TORQUE U4	58	−4.49	8.38	60	−5.35	5.64	0.65	ns
TORQUE U3	58	−2.03	7.95	60	−3.35	7.15	0.95	ns
TORQUE U2	58	7.41	8.14	60	6.23	6.31	0.88	ns
TORQUE U1	58	11.41	6.28	60	7.41	6.19	3.49	<0.001
TORQUE L7	58	−32.51	10.93	60	−33.26	11.69	0.36	ns
TORQUE L6	58	−23.50	9.57	60	−29.24	9.29	3.31	0.003
TORQUE L5	58	−11.39	8.52	60	−17.43	7.98	3.97	<0.001
TORQUE L4	58	−9.23	7.02	60	−14.96	7.69	4.23	<0.001
TORQUE L3	58	−1.95	7.49	60	−9.01	5.74	5.73	<0.001
TORQUE L2	58	5.50	8.26	60	−1.36	6.89	4.90	<0.001
TORQUE L1	58	9.68	9.18	60	2.19	7.11	4.94	<0.001

ns not significant.

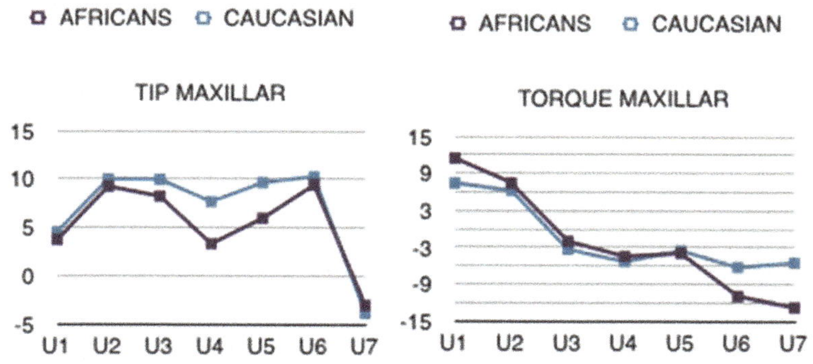

Fig. 8 Comparing African and Caucasian tip and torque values for the upper jaw

In-out: a plane parallel to the occlusal plane, passing through the FA point of each tooth, was identified, and the mesial, the distal and the most vestibular point of every tooth was selected (Fig. 6). These points were joined together by a line whose perpendicular distance from the FA point (i.e. the centre of the virtual sphere) was taken as the in-out value of that crown. These values were calculated using the "'Evaluate/Distance" ! ?/"Evaluate/Length" ! ?' software tool (Fig. 7).

Statistical analysis

The mean, standard deviation and standard error of each value obtained above were calculated. The Shapiro-Wilk test was performed to assess the normal distribution of the studied samples. Student's t test for independent samples (significance level $p < 0.05$) was used to compare the group mean values for every tooth. To verify the repeatability of the measurements performed, 10 renderings of the upper arcade and 10 of the lower were selected at random from each ethnic sample. The measurements were then repeated by the other operator, and the second set of measurements was compared with the first by means of measurement systems analysis (MSA) conducted using the t test for paired data.

Results

African sample

The measurements taken of the upper jaw highlight positive tip values for all the teeth except for the second molars (Table 2). The tip values in the lower jaw tended to be more positive in an anteroposterior direction (Table 2), whereas the torque on both the upper and lower teeth tended to get more negative in an anteroposterior direction (Table 3); only the central and lateral incisors displayed positive torque.

Caucasian sample

With the exception of the second molar, tip values in the upper jaw were all positive, displaying a tendency to decrease from the anterior to the posterior sectors (Table 2). The lower tip values were all positive, but tended to increase in an anteroposterior direction (Table 2). As for torque, in the upper jaw, this showed a tendency to increase in negativity in an anteroposterior direction, being positive at the incisors and negative in the canines, premolars and molars (Table 3). In the lower jaw, increasingly negative torque values were measured in an anteroposterior direction. Only the central incisors had a positive torque while the most negative torque was seen at the second molars (Table 3).

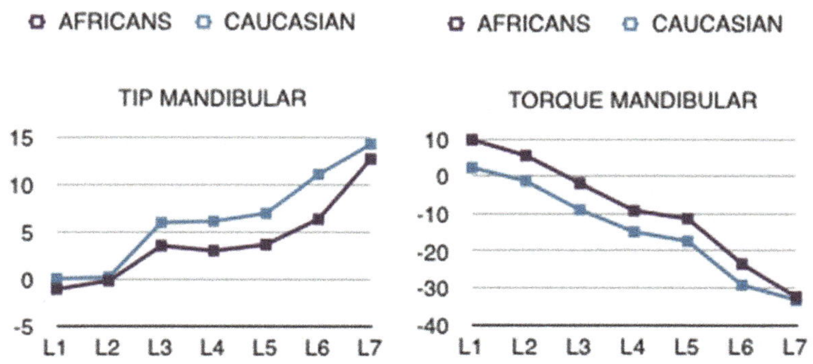

Fig. 9 Comparing African and Caucasian tip and torque values for the lower jaw

Table 4 Comparison of our African tip values with those measured by Andrews

Africans—tip				Andrews' values			Comparison	
	n	Mean	Standard deviation	*n*	Mean	Standard deviation	*t* test	*p* level
TIP U7	58	−3.06	6.78	240	.39	5.69	−3.58	<0.001
TIP U6	58	9.43	3.53	240	5.73	1.90	7.71	<0.001
TIP U5	58	5.96	5.84	240	2.82	1.52	4.07	<0.001
TIP U4	58	3.29	4.45	240	2.65	1.69	1.07	ns
TIP U3	58	8.23	5.20	240	8.40	2.97	−.24	ns
TIP U2	58	9.23	3.87	240	8.04	2.80	2.20	0.031
TIP U1	58	3.68	3.55	240	3.59	1.65	.18	ns
TIP L7	58	12.65	5.83	240	2.94	2.05	12.50	<0.001
TIP L6	58	6.30	5.36	240	2.03	1.14	6.03	<0.001
TIP L5	58	3.60	4.02	240	1.54	1.35	3.84	<0.001
TIP L4	58	2.95	3.89	240	1.28	1.90	3.19	0.002
TIP L3	58	3.478	4.850	240	2.48	3.28	1.49	ns
TIP L2	58	−.26	3.01	240	.38	1.47	−1.57	ns
TIP L1	58	−1.13	3.30	240	.53	1.29	−3.77	<0.001

ns not significant.

Measurement system analysis

From the analysis of the measurement method, in results that there are no statistically significant differences (significance (two-tailed) <0.05) between the values of tip and torque measured by the two operators, both in the Caucasian and the African groups.

Comparison of tip and torque of African and Caucasian groups

A comparison of the mean tip and torque values obtained for each ethnic sample was performed using Student's t test for independent samples. This showed that, in terms of tip values in the upper teeth, there were only significant differences between the two groups at the premolars, whose mean tip in the Caucasian samples was roughly 4° more positive than that in the African group. In the lower jaw, comparable values were only found at the incisors, whereas the tip at the canines, premolars and molars was significantly more positive in the Caucasian sample, at 2.5°, 3° and 4° greater, respectively (Table 2).

Statistically significant differences were also found in the torque values measured for the upper arch, this time at the central incisors and both sets of molars. In each case, absolute torque values were greater in the African subjects, with a torque 4° more positive at the central incisors and roughly 5° and 7°, respectively, at the first and second molars (Table 3). Among the lower teeth, only the second molar torque of the two groups was comparable; all the other teeth displayed more positive torque in the African group, reaching statistical significance in the canines, premolars and first molars. In particular, the

Table 5 Comparison of our Caucasian tip values with those measured by Andrews

Caucasians—tip				Andrews' values			Comparison	
	n	Mean	Standard deviation	*n*	Mean	Standard deviation	*t* test	*p* level
TIP U7	60	−3.88	10.60	240	.39	5.69	−3.02	0.004
TIP U6	60	10.26	5.54	240	5.73	1.90	6.24	<0.001
TIP U5	60	9.64	4.16	240	2.82	1.52	12.49	<0.001
TIP U4	60	7.67	4.28	240	2.65	1.69	8.91	<0.001
TIP U3	60	9.96	4.81	240	8.40	2.97	2.40	0.019
TIP U2	60	9.99	3.69	240	8.04	2.80	3.83	<0.001
TIP U1	60	4.53	2.84	240	3.59	1.65	2.46	0.017
TIP L7	60	14.20	6.47	240	2.94	2.05	13.32	<0.001
TIP L6	60	10.99	2.78	240	2.03	1.14	24.47	<0.001
TIP L5	60	6.90	3.09	240	1.54	1.35	13.12	<0.001
TIP L4	60	6.06	3.36	240	1.28	1.90	10.60	<0.001
TIP L3	60	5.913	3.980	240	2.48	3.28	6.18	<0.001
TIP L2	60	.14	4.46	240	.38	1.47	−.41	ns
TIP L1	60	.00	4.46	240	.53	1.29	−.90	ns

ns not significant.

Table 6 Comparison of our African torque values with those measured by Andrews

Africans—torque				Andrews' values			Comparison	
	n	Mean	Standard deviation	*n*	Mean	Standard deviation	*t* test	*p* level
TORQUE U7	58	−12.79	10.11	240	−8.10	5.63	−3.41	0.001
TORQUE U6	58	−10.98	9.75	240	−11.53	3.91	.42	ns
TORQUE U5	58	−4.00	8.43	240	−8.78	4.13	4.20	<0.001
TORQUE U4	58	−4.49	8.38	240	−8.47	4.02	3.52	<0.001
TORQUE U3	58	−2.03	7.95	240	−7.25	4.21	4.84	<0.001
TORQUE U2	58	7.41	8.14	240	4.42	4.38	2.70	0.009
TORQUE U1	58	11.41	6.28	240	6.11	3.97	6.14	<0.001
TORQUE L7	58	−32.51	10.93	240	−36.03	6.57	2.35	0.030
TORQUE L6	58	−23.50	9.57	240	−30.67	5.90	5.46	<0.001
TORQUE L5	58	−11.39	8.52	240	−23.63	5.58	10.41	<0.001
TORQUE L4	58	−9.23	7.02	240	−18.95	4.96	9.96	<0.001
TORQUE L3	58	−1.95	7.49	240	−12.73	4.65	10.48	<0.001
TORQUE L2	58	5.50	8.26	240	−3.24	5.37	7.68	<0.001
TORQUE L1	58	9.68	9.18	240	−1.71	5.79	9.02	<0.001

ns not significant

torque on the central and lateral incisors was, respectively, roughly 7° and 6° more positive in the African sample. Analogously, the canines displayed roughly 7° less negative torque in the African sample, and approximately 6° less negative torque was measured at the premolars and first molars (Table 3) (Figs. 8 and 9).

Comparison of tip and torque of African and Caucasian groups with values reported by Andrews

Statistically significant differences with respect to values reported by Andrews were found in terms of the tip values measured in the upper jaw of both African and Caucasian subjects [10] (Tables 4 and 5). In the African sample, only the tip measured at the upper central incisors, canines and first premolars was comparable with values reported by Andrews (differences of <1°) (Table 4). In the Caucasian subjects, all upper crowns had angulation values significantly different to those measured in Andrews' original sample of North American subjects. The greatest differences were seen at the molars and premolars, and in our Caucasian sample, only the second molars had a negative tip (Table 5). A similar discrepancy was found in the lower jaw (Table 4); in the African group, substantial differences were noted at the lower incisors, which presented negative tip, at the first and second premolars and in particular at the first and second molars, which both had considerably greater angulation values in our sample, the difference being as much as 10° at the second molars. Likewise, in our Caucasian group, lower tip values were markedly different to those reported by Andrews, especially in the posterior

Table 7 Comparison of our Caucasian torque values with those measured by Andrews

Caucasians—torque				Andrews' values			Comparison	
	n.	Mean	Standard deviation	*n*	Mean	Standard deviation	*t* test	*p* level
TORQUE U7	60	−5.50	12.23	240	−8.10	5.63	1.60	ns
TORQUE U6	60	−6.26	10.24	240	−11.53	3.91	3.92	<0.001
TORQUE U5	60	−3.54	6.42	240	−8.78	4.13	6.02	<0.001
TORQUE U4	60	−5.35	5.64	240	−8.47	4.02	4.04	<0.001
TORQUE U3	60	−3.35	7.15	240	−7.25	4.21	4.05	<0.001
TORQUE U2	60	6.23	6.31	240	4.42	4.38	2.10	0.040
TORQUE U1	60	7.41	6.19	240	6.11	3.97	1.54	ns
TORQUE L7	60	−33.26	11.69	240	−36.03	6.57	1.77	ns
TORQUE L6	60	−29.24	9.29	240	−30.67	5.90	1.14	ns
TORQUE L5	60	−17.43	7.98	240	−23.63	5.58	5.68	<0.001
TORQUE L4	60	−14.96	7.69	240	−18.95	4.96	3.83	<0.001
TORQUE L3	60	−9.01	5.74	240	−12.73	4.65	4.66	<0.001
TORQUE L2	60	−1.36	6.89	240	−3.24	5.37	1.97	ns
TORQUE L1	60	2.19	7.11	240	−1.71	5.79	3.93	<0.001

ns not significant.

sectors, in which the crowns displayed a more positive tip (Table 5).

As regards the torque in the upper arcade, we found a greater positive tendency in the African subjects with respect to Andrews' measurements. This was true of all teeth except for the second molars, which had a more negative inclination in our sample (Table 6). The only upper teeth in which there were no statistically significant differences in the Caucasian group were the central incisors and second molars; the torque on the upper lateral incisors and first premolars was roughly 2–3° lower, and this discrepancy reached 4–5° at the canines, second premolars and first molars (Table 7). In the lower jaw, the torque values we measured in African subjects were in all cases more positive than those reported by Andrews. Differences were statistically significant in all cases, from a minimum of roughly 5° at the second molar, up to approximately 12° at the second premolar (Table 6). In the Caucasians we studied, the torque on the lower molars and lateral incisors was comparable to Andrews' measurements, while the torque we measured at the two premolars was less negative. In contrast to the other teeth, the central incisors displayed a positive torque (Table 7).

Analysis of in-out values

In both jaws of our African sample (Table 8), there is an observable tendency for the in-out values to increase progressively from the lateral incisor to the second molar. The same was true for the Caucasian subjects we measured (Table 8). However, a comparison of our ethnic groups revealed that the in-out values were greater in all teeth of the African upper jaw except for the second molars (Table 8). In the lower jaw, we found statistically significant differences at both sets of incisors and the second premolars, whose torque values were greater in the African group. In contrast, the second molar had a greater prominence, roughly 0.6 mm

Table 8 Comparison of African and Caucasian in-out values

	Africans—in-out			Caucasians—in-out			Comparison	
	n	Mean	Standard deviation	*n*	Mean	Standard deviation	*t* test	*p* level
U1	58	1.62	.30	58	1.48	.30	2.60	0.012
U2	58	1.25	.24	58	1.15	.24	2.11	0.039
U3	58	1.65	.31	58	1.66	.34	−.30	ns
U4	58	1.89	.33	58	1.61	.24	5.20	<0.001
U5	58	1.85	.29	58	1.66	.29	3.60	<0.001
U6	58	2.29	.40	58	2.01	.47	3.35	0.001
U7	58	2.47	.56	58	2.75	.62	−2.51	0.015
L1	58	1.18	.21	58	1.01	.32	3.42	0.001
L2	57	1.16	.19	58	.93	.32	4.65	<0.001
L3	58	1.36	.28	58	1.38	.27	−.41	ns
L4	58	2.01	.38	58	1.93	.28	1.30	ns
L5	56	2.06	.45	58	1.91	.32	2.06	0.044
L6	58	2.53	.37	58	2.66	.38	−1.96	ns
L7	56	2.22	.65	58	2.83	.72	−4.76	<0.001

ns not significant.

Table 9 Comparison of our African in-out values with those measured by Andrews

	Africans—in-out			Andrews—in out			Comparison	
	n	Mean	Standard deviation	*n*	Mean	Standard deviation	*t* test	*p* level
U1	58	1.62	.30	240	2.01	.32	−8.73	<0.001
U2	58	1.25	.24	240	1.84	.30	−15.82	<0.001
U3	58	1.65	.31	240	2.67	.39	−21.40	<0.001
U4	58	1.89	.33	240	2.54	.35	−13.36	<0.001
U5	58	1.85	.29	240	2.48	.36	−14.22	<0.001
U6	58	2.29	.40	240	2.88	.40	−10.17	<0.001
U7	58	2.47	.56	238	3.00	.51	−6.58	<0.001
L1	58	1.18	.21	240	1.59	.27	−12.61	<0.001
L2	58	1.16	.19	240	1.64	.32	−14.63	<0.001
L3	58	1.36	.28	240	2.37	.40	−22.57	<0.001
L4	58	2.01	.38	240	2.72	.43	−12.52	<0.001
L5	56	2.06	.45	240	2.60	.34	−8.49	<0.001
L6	58	2.53	.37	240	3.02	.40	−9.00	<0.001
L7	58	2.22	.65	236	2.79	.47	−6.22	<0.001

Table 10 Comparison of our Caucasian in-out values with those measured by Andrews

	Caucasians—in-out			Andrews—in-out			Comparison	
	n	Mean	Standard deviation	*n*	Mean	Standard deviation	*t* test	*p* level
U1	60	1.48	0.30	240	2.01	0.32	−11.88	<0.001
U2	60	1.15	0.24	240	1.84	0.30	−18.36	<0.001
U3	60	1.66	0.34	240	2.67	0.39	−19.75	<0.001
U4	60	1.61	0.24	240	2.54	0.35	−24.19	<0.001
U5	60	1.66	0.29	240	2.48	0.36	−18.53	<0.001
U6	60	2.01	0.47	240	2.88	0.40	−12.86	<0.001
U7	60	2.75	0.62	238	3.00	0.51	−2.85	0.006
L1	60	1.01	0.32	240	1.59	0.27	−12.97	<0.001
L2	60	0.93	0.32	240	1.64	0.32	−14.98	<0.001
L3	60	1.38	0.27	240	2.37	0.40	−22.91	<0.001
L4	60	1.93	0.28	240	2.72	0.43	−17.36	<0.001
L5	60	1.91	0.32	240	2.60	0.34	−14.55	<0.001
L6	60	2.66	0.38	240	3.02	0.40	−6.37	<0.001
L7	60	2.83	0.72	236	2.79	0.47	0.37	ns

ns not significant.

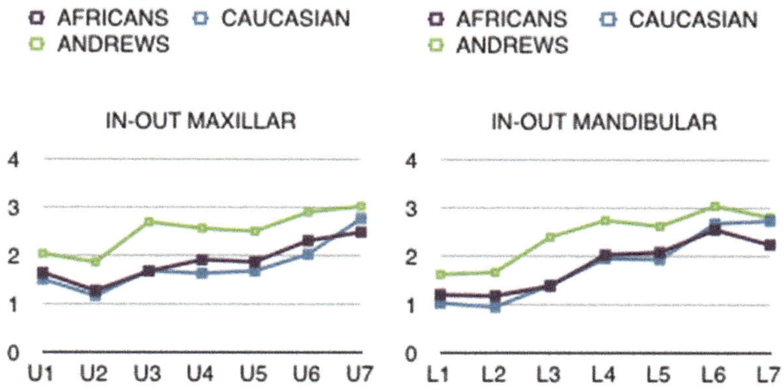

Fig. 10 A comparison of in-out values we measured with those of Andrews

(statistically significant), in our Italian Caucasian sample (Table 8).

Both of our samples were significantly different from that of Andrews in terms of in-out. In both of our samples, the mean prominence was greater than in Andrews' North American group at all teeth (Tables 9 and 10).

Discussion

On the whole, our findings from this part of the study are in line with those previously reported in the literature [2–5, 8], namely that ethnic background appears to play a significant role in determining the angulation and inclination of the teeth in both arcades. In certain circumstances, these ethnic differences can be great enough (i.e. greater than 3°) to take on clinical relevance.

Indeed, although our sample size was relatively small, if our measurements were taken as reference values, orthodontic bracket prescription would need to be altered or bends made in the wire to obtain optimal finishing in the Mozambican population.

When comparing the values we measured in our Italian sample with those reported by Andrews, it became clear that on the whole, their teeth had a more positive tip (i.e. a greater mesiodistal angulation). Similarly, torque values were larger on the whole in our sample. Hence, the results of this part of the study also agree with the literature, showing that individuals of the same race have different tip and torque values, depending on their ethnic background. Indeed, a similar picture was seen in two different Japanese [2] and Indian [4] samples, as well as Andrews' North American Caucasians.

As regards the in-out measurements, those taken on our sample showed that the lateral incisors had the smallest values, whereas the molars were the most prominent. We also revealed a similar trend in both samples for the in-out values to progressively increase in an anteroposterior direction from the central incisor to the second molar. The African sample generally (incisors, premolars and first molars) presented greater in-out values than the Caucasian group in the upper jaw. In the lower jaw, the vestibular prominence of the tooth crowns was essentially similar in African and Caucasian subjects. With respect to Andrews' values, however, we did notice a difference, as we revealed a tendency for the in-out values to increase towards the posterior sectors, where, according to the American author, there is none. Moreover, many of the values in our sample were smaller than those measured by Andrews, which may suggest that the coronal prominence in an anteroposterior direction is lower in Africans and Italian Caucasians than in North American Caucasians (Fig. 10).

Furthermore, the standard deviation values that emerged in our statistical analysis of the two samples were significant in some cases, thereby demonstrating that there is a considerable dispersion around the mean measurements for each tooth, especially in terms of torque. This finding, in agreement with previous studies [1–4, 6, 11–13], must be interpreted as a consequence of the biological variation in the inclination and angulation of the teeth, the variation in profile of the clinical crown, and variations in the inclination of the occlusal plane.

Conclusion

- The measurement system used on our sample is repeatable.
- There is great dispersion around the mean values measured for each tooth (especially torque).
- Race and ethnicity greatly influence tip, torque and in-out values.
- Caucasians have more positive tip values and Africans, more positive torque values, with greater proclination of the incisors.
- In-out values were slightly greater in the African sample than in the Caucasian group, especially in the upper arch.
- Both Caucasian and African groups differ from Andrews' sample in tip, torque and in-out values.

Competing interests

The authors declare that they have no competing interests.

Authors' contributions

LL designed the research protocol, AP carried out the measurements, AA drafted the manuscript, ML carried out the data processing and statistical analysis, GS supervised the research. All authors read and approved the final manuscript.

References

1. Sebata E. An orthodontic study of teeth and dental arch form on the Japanese normal occlusions. The Shikwa Gakuho. 1980;80:945–69.
2. Watanabe K, Koga M, Yatabe K, Motegi E, Isshiki Y. A morphometric study on setup models of Japanese malocclusions. The Shikwa Gakuho. 1996;96:209–22.
3. Currim S, Wadkar PV. Objective assessment of occlusal and coronal characteristics of untreated normals: a measurement study. Am J Orthod Dentofacial Orthop. 2004;125(5):582–8.
4. Doodamani GM, Khala AS, Manohar M, Umashankar. Assessment of crown angulations, crown inclinations, and tooth size discrepancies in a South Indian population. Contemp Clin Dent. 2011;2(3):176–81.
5. Ferrario VF, Sforza C, Colombo A, Ciusa V, Serrao G. Three-dimensional inclination of the dental axes in healthy permanent dentitions—a cross sectional study in a normal population. Angle Orthod. 2001;71(4):257–64.
6. Lombardo L, Fattori L, Mirabella D, Molinari C, Siciliani G. Dental and alveolar arch forms in a Caucasian population compared with commercially available archwires. Int Orthod. 2013;115:1–33.
7. Balut N, Klapper L, Sandrik J, Bowman D. Variations in bracket placement in the preadjusted orthodontic appliance. Am J Orthod Dentofacial Orthop. 1992;102:62–7.
8. Tong H, Kwon D, Shi J, Sakai N, Enciso R, Sameshima GT. Mesiodistal angulation and faciolingual inclination of each whole tooth in 3-dimensional space in patients with near-normal occlusion. Am J Orthod Dentofacial Orthop. 2012;141(5):604–17.
9. Huanca Ghislanzoni LT, Lineberger M, Cevidanes LH, Mapelli A, Sforza C, McNamara Jr JA. Evaluation of tip and torque on virtual study models: a validation study. Prog Orthod. 2013;14:19.
10. Caputi S, Varvara G. Dimensional accuracy of resultant casts made by a monophase, one-step and two-step, and a novel two-step putty/light-body impression technique: an in vitro study. J Prosthet Dent. 2008;99(4):274–81.
11. Andrews LF 1993: Straight wire. Masson Spa Milano
12. Vardimon AD, Lambertz W. Statistical evaluation of torque angles in reference to straight-wire appliance (SWA) theories. Am J Orthod. 1986;89:56–66.
13. Uğur T, Yukay F. Normal faciolingual inclinations of tooth crowns compared with treatment groups of standard and pretorqued brackets. Am J Orthod Dentofacial Orthop. 1997;112(1):50–7.

25

Smile analysis in different facial patterns and its correlation with underlying hard tissues

Neha Grover[1*], DN Kapoor[2], Santosh Verma[3] and Preeti Bharadwaj[4]

Abstract

Background: The subject's inherent growth pattern can be an effective factor in characteristics of smile. More vertical growth in the posterior maxilla than in the anterior maxilla could result in a changed relationship between the occlusal plane and the curvature of the lower lip upon smile. In order to broaden the understanding of how smile gets affected by growth pattern and the underlying hard tissues, the present study was undertaken to compare smile in various growth patterns, to determine sexual dimorphism, if any; as well as to correlate smile with underlying hard tissues.

Methods: One hundred and fifty subjects were selected amongst the students in the Dental Institute and from the outpatient department of Department Orthodontics and Dentofacial Orthopedics. Sample selected for the study ranged in the age group of 17 to 25 years. Selected individuals were subjected to lateral head cephalometric radiography in the Department of Oral Medicine and Radiology and videography. Cephalograms were traced and the subjects were divided into horizontal, average, and vertical growth pattern on the basis of GoGn-SN, lower anterior facial height, and Jaraback's ratio. The video clip was downloaded to obtain frame of posed smile. Cephalometric and photographic measurements were recorded and subjected to statistical analysis.

Results: The mean values of smile parameters were significantly higher in males as compared to females irrespective of the growth pattern. The mean incisal display, interlabial gap, lower lip to incisal edge distance, upper vertical lip length, and occlusal plane angle was highest in both males and females of vertical facial growth pattern group; whereas, the smile index, posterior corridor (left and right) were less in vertical facial growth pattern group in both males and females. Thus, the parameters in vertical dimension were increased in vertical growers whereas, the parameters in transverse dimension decreased.

Conclusions: The facial growth pattern has significant influence on the parameters of smile along with definite sexual dimorphism. The angular and linear parameters, except saddle angle and lower incisor to NB (linear and angular), influenced smile.

Background

The smile is one of the most important facial expressions and is essential in expressing friendliness, agreement, and appreciation. A smile when pleasing and attractive to observers enriches not only the one who smiles but also those who view it. An attractive or pleasing smile clearly enhances the acceptance of an individual in the society by improving the initial impression in interpersonal relationships [1]. The esthetic considerations are paramount in treatment planning; however, rigid rules cannot be applied to this process because almost an infinite variety of faces could be esthetic [2].

There are two forms of smiles—the enjoyment or Duchenne smile and the posed or social smile. The posed smile is voluntary and not elicited by an emotion. In other words, it is reliably reproducible and can be sustained [3]. Posed smiles, therefore have importance in orthodontic diagnosis and treatment planning. The unposed or social smile, however, is involuntary and is induced by joy or mirth. It is a natural response as it expresses authentic human emotion. Unlike the posed smiles, these smiles are not sustained.

The vertical aspects of smile anatomy are the degree of maxillary anterior tooth display (Morley ratio), upper lip

* Correspondence: Ortho.neha@gmail.com
[1]Nora Medical Polyclinics, Tower 4. Marks and Spencer Building, No. 106, Abu Dhabi, United Arab Emirates
Full list of author information is available at the end of the article

drape, and gingival display. In a youthful smile, 75–100 % of the maxillary central incisors should be positioned below an imaginary line drawn between the commissures [4]. Both skeletal and dental relationships contribute to these smile components. The present study was undertaken to compare smile in various growth patterns, to determine sexual dimorphism, if any; as well as to correlate smile with underlying hard tissues.

Methods

In this cross-sectional study, a total of 150 subjects were selected amongst the students studying in Dental College and the outpatient department of the College. Selected individuals ranged in age of 17–25 years had class I molar relation, well aligned anterior teeth, presence of all permanent teeth except third molars, no gross facial asymmetry, with no previous orthodontic treatment, and no history of facial trauma, plastic surgery, or orthognathic surgery.

Selected subjects were first taken for videography using Sony digital camera (DSC-H20, Sony Corp. Japan). Signed consent of the subjects was taken on using video for research purpose. The method used for videography here was as described by Sarver and Ackerman [2, 5, 6]. The subjects were instructed to hold their head in natural head position by looking straight into an imaginary mirror [7]. The camera lens was adjusted parallel to the apparent occlusal plane and focussed only on the dentofacial complex (corresponding to the area from the nose to the chin) (Fig. 1). Included in the captured area were two rulers with millimeter markings. These two rulers were made to fit perpendicular to each other in order to help minimize any error. If the subject was unable to hold the ruler perpendicular in one dimension to the angle in which the dynamic record was taken, the second ruler would still be perpendicular to the camera.

Recording was started about 1 s before the subject began to smile and continued till the end of the smile. The video clip was downloaded to laptop (Dell, Inspiron) and uploaded to video-editing software program (DVD VideoSoft Studio) (Figs. 3 and 4) to obtain frames of smile. Each frame was analyzed and the frame showing the subjects' widest commissure to commissure was chosen as posed smile. These frames were converted into a JPEG file using the same video-editing software program (DVD VideoSoft Studio) (Fig. 2). The approval was taken from Institute Ethics Committee whose students were involved in the study.

The lateral head cephalogram of the selected subjects were taken with radiograph machine Villa (Italy, Strato 2000) using a standardized technique.

The cephalometric tracings were carried out, and the following cephalometric landmarks and planes were used in the study (Figs. 3 and 4). The parameters used to classify subjects in different groups are shown in Table 1.

Based on these three parameters, the subjects were divided into six groups:

A. Group 1: Males with average growth pattern
B. Group 2: Females with average growth pattern
C. Group 3: Males with horizontal growth pattern
D. Group 4: Females with horizontal growth pattern
E. Group 5: Males with vertical growth pattern
F. Group 6: Females with vertical growth pattern

Standardization of image

Each JPEG file of the selected subjects were opened in Adobe Photoshop CS2 (Adobe Systems, San Jose, California) and was adjusted by using the ruler option in the frame. The method used to standardize the image was as described by Desai et al [8]. First, the resolution was changed to 300 pixels per inch by going to "image > image size." Then, the ruler function was chosen and set to millimeter which can measure a minimum of 0.1 mm length. On the parallel end of the ruler, a 10-mm area, close to the smile, was measured. That number was divided into 10 (10/measurement on JPEG file) and multiplied by the width value found in image size screen (image > image

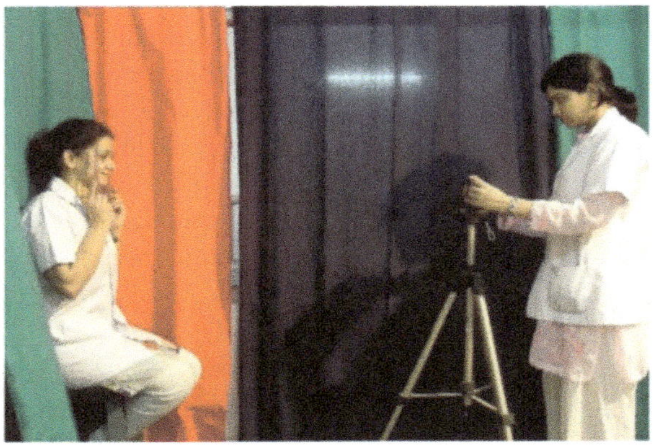

Fig. 1 Video camera set on a tripod at 4 ft distance from the subject in sitting position

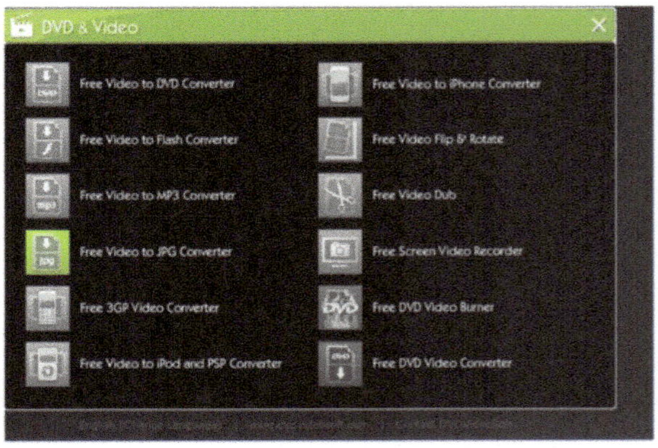

Fig. 2 Video to JPEG converter

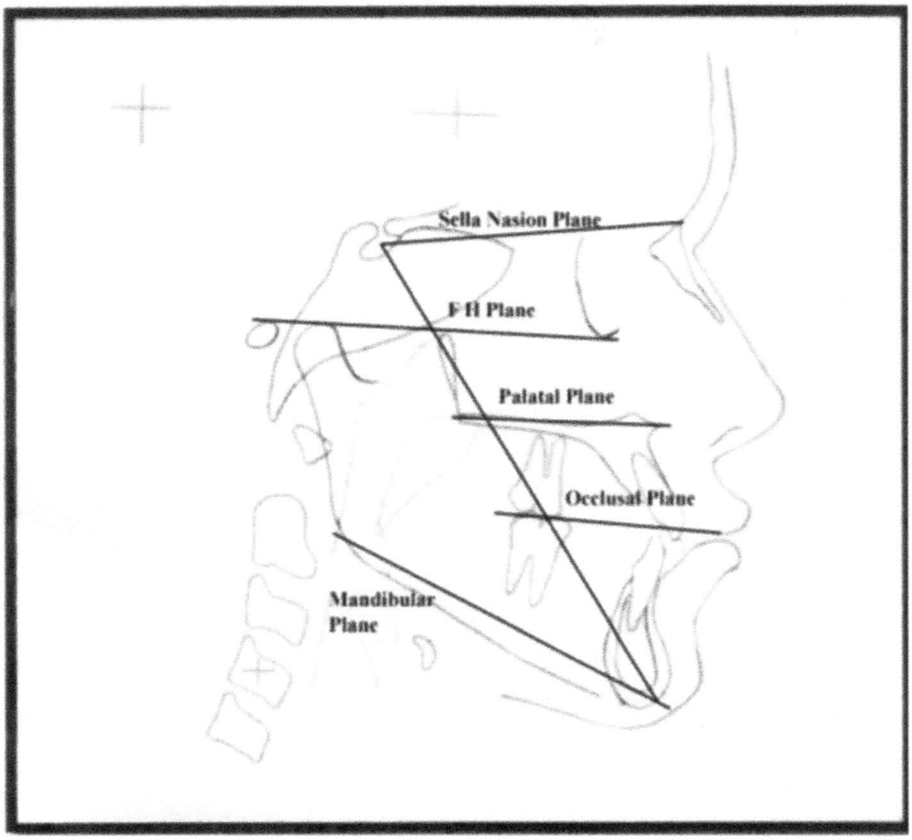

Fig. 3 Cephalometric planes

size). The resulting number was copied and pasted in place of the width reading, and the changes were applied to the JPEG file (Fig. 5).

In Adobe Photoshop, the following parameters of the selected subjects were measured and entered into Microsoft Excel to evaluate smile:

1. Maximum incisor exposure [9]: the amount of vertical display of the maxillary right central incisor (Fig. 6).
2. Lower lip to maxillary incisor [9]: vertical distance from the deepest midline point on the superior margin of the lower lip to the maxillary right central incisor edge (Fig. 7).
3. Interlabial gap [9]: the distance between the most inferior portion of the tubercle of the upper lip and the deepest midline point on the superior margin of the lower lip (Fig. 8).
4. Maxillary intercanine width [9]: the distance from the distal aspect of the right canine to the distal aspect of the left canine (Fig. 9).
5. Width of all visible maxillary teeth [9]: the distance from the distal aspect of the most posterior visible tooth on the right to the most posterior visible tooth on the left side of the maxilla (Fig. 10).
6. Smile width [9]: the distance from outer commissure to outer commissure on smile (Fig. 11).
7. Smile index [9]: smile width/interlabial gap (Fig. 12).
8. Right and left buccal corridors [9]: the horizontal distance from the distal aspect of the canine to the respective outer commissure (Fig. 13).
9. Right and left posterior corridors [9]: the horizontal distance from the distal aspect of the most posterior tooth visible on smile to the respective outer commissure (Fig. 14).
10. Buccal corridor ratio [9]: intercanine width/smile width (Fig. 15).
11. Posterior corridor ratio [9]: visible maxillary teeth width/smile width (Fig. 16).
12. Upper vertical lip thickness [9]: the vertical distance from the most superior peak of the lip to the most inferior portion of the tubercle of the upper lip (Fig. 17).
13. Lower vertical lip thickness [9]: the vertical distance from the deepest midline point on the superior margin of the lower lip to the most inferior portion of the lower lip (Fig. 18).

Double determination for assessment of inherent error in measurements was done on 20 random photographs

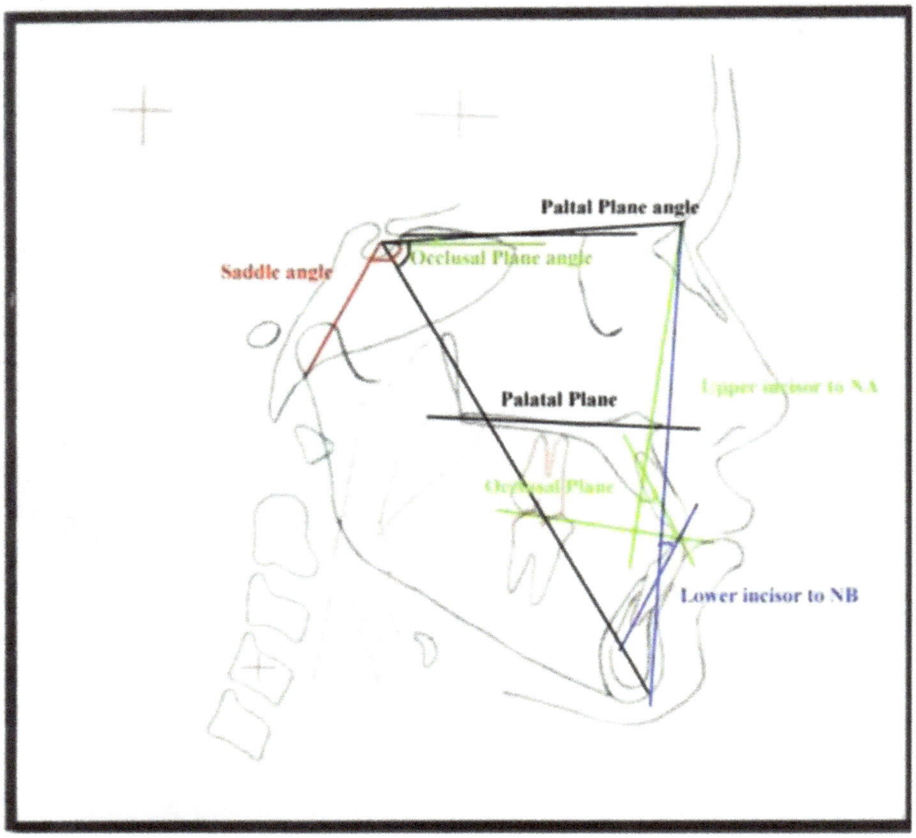

Fig. 4 Cephalometric parameters (angular and linear)

and cephalometric measurements. The variability was found to be statistically insignificant.

Results

The smile parameters of male and female were compared in all three growth patterns as shown in Tables 2, 3, and 4.

As seen in Table 2, lower lip to maxillary incisor distance, interlabial gap, total width of visible teeth, posterior corridor ratio, and lower vertical lip thickness were significantly higher in males as compared to females in average growth pattern group.

According to Table 3, total width of visible teeth, smile width, buccal corridors left and right and lower vertical lip thickness were significantly higher in males as compared to females in horizontal growth pattern group.

Table 4 shows upper incisor exposure, interlabial gap, inter canine width, total width of visible teeth, posterior corridors left and right, and lower vertical lip thickness were significantly higher in males as compared to females in vertical growth pattern group.

Comparison of males in average group with horizontal growth pattern group and vertical growth pattern group was done separately as shown in Tables 5 and 6, respectively. Also comparison of females in average growth pattern group with horizontal growth pattern group and vertical growth pattern group was done separately as shown in Tables 7 and 8, respectively.

According to Table 5, upper incisor exposure and interlabial gap were significantly higher in males of average growth pattern group as compared to males of horizontal growth pattern group. Upper vertical lip thickness

Table 1 Parameters used for classification of growth pattern

S. no.	Parameters		Average	Vertical	Horizontal
1	Jarabak's ratio (Jarabak [10])		63.5 ± 1.5 %	<62 %	>65 %
2	SN-GoGn (Steiner [10])		32° ± 2°	>34°	<30°
3	Lower anterior facial height (McNamara [10])	M	72 ± 2 mm	>74 mm	<70 mm
		F	67 ± 1 mm	>68 mm	<66 mm

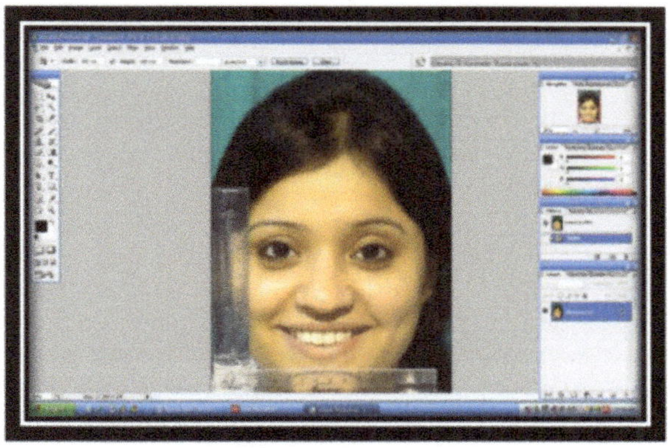

Fig. 5 Standardized photograph in Adobe Photoshop

was significantly higher in males of horizontal growth pattern group.

As seen in Table 6, upper incisor exposure, upper incisor to lower lip distance, interlabial gap, and upper vertical lip thickness were significantly higher in males of vertical growth pattern group as compared to males of average growth pattern group. Buccal corridors left and right and posterior corridors left and right were higher in average growth pattern group.

Table 7 shows upper incisor exposure and interlabial gap were significantly higher in females of average growth pattern group as compared to females of horizontal growth pattern group. Upper vertical lip thickness was significantly higher in females of horizontal growth pattern group.

As shown in Table 8, upper incisor exposure, upper incisor to lower lip distance, and interlabial gap were significantly higher in females of vertical growth pattern group as compared to females of average growth pattern group. Posterior corridors left and right were higher in average growth pattern group.

These results clearly show that the vertical parameters of smile were highest in vertical growth pattern group and least in horizontal growth pattern group in both males and females.

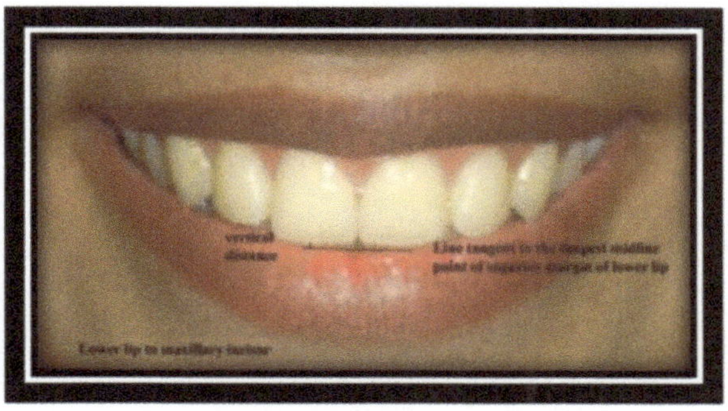

Fig. 7 Lower lip to maxillary incisor

Correlation between smile parameters and skeletal parameters of males in average facial growth pattern group, females in average facial growth pattern group, males in horizontal group, females in horizontal growth pattern group, males in vertical growth pattern group, and females in vertical growth pattern group is in Additional file 1.

Interlabial gap, when correlated with cephalometric parameters, was found to be positively correlated with overjet in average facial growth pattern group of males and was positively correlated with posterior facial height in average facial growth pattern group of females. The interlabial gap was positively correlated with lower anterior facial height in males having horizontal facial growth pattern and no correlations with other cephalometric measurements in females having horizontal facial growth pattern. In the vertical facial growth pattern group, interlabial gap was positively correlated with Y-axis and lower vertical lip length in males but insignificant correlations amongst females.

The incisal edge of the maxillary incisor to lower lip distance was found to be positively correlated with mandibular plane angle in average facial growth pattern group of males and was positively correlated with overjet in average facial growth pattern group of females. It was also positively correlated with palatal plane angle of females in horizontal facial growth pattern group.

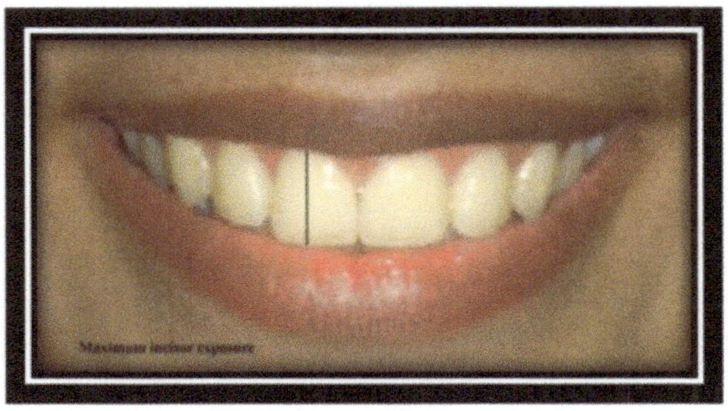

Fig. 6 Maximum incisor exposure

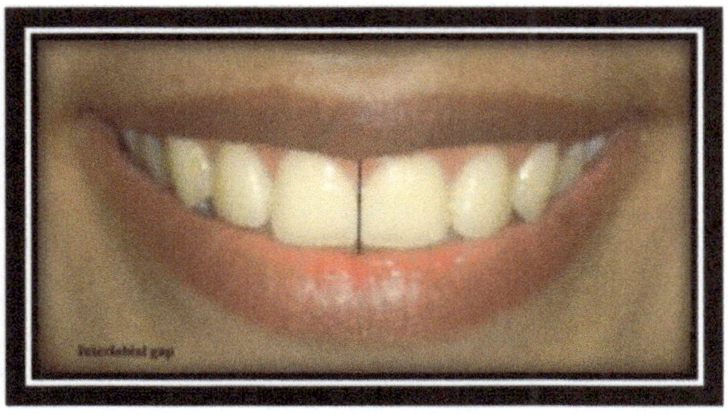

Fig. 8 Interlabial gap

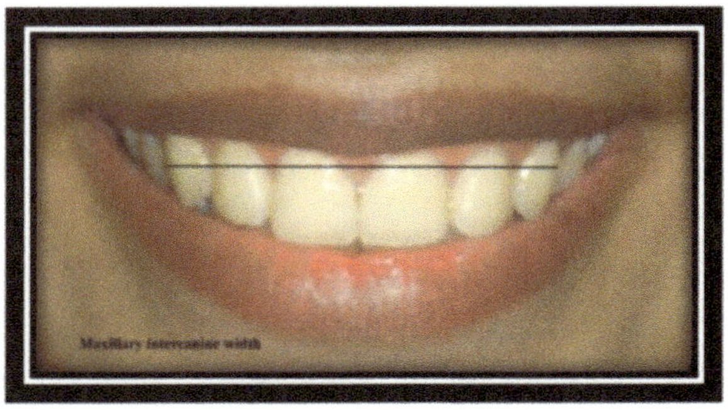

Fig. 9 Maxillary intercanine width

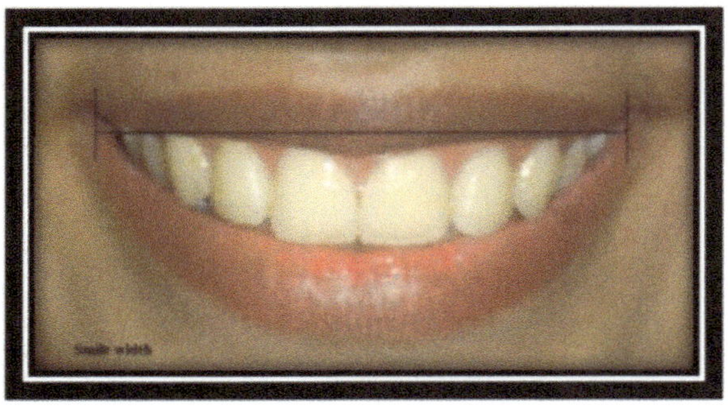

Fig. 11 Smile width

Based on these tables, it can be inferred that saddle angle and lower incisor to NB (angular and linear) was not found to be related to smile parameters and also upper incisor to NA (angular) was found to be positively correlated with upper lip vertical in females of all the three groups.

Discussion

To study a smile beyond static pictures, capturing a dynamic smile [2, 7, 10] was used, thus avoiding the inherent error of a single snapshot. The variables of smile were significantly affected by the facial growth pattern in this study.

Upper incisor exposure

The upper incisor exposure was less in females when compared with males in all three groups and this difference was significant in vertical facial growth pattern group. This is contrary to the findings of Vig and Brundo [11], Peck et al. [12, 13], and Balani et al [14], whereas the above finding is supported by a study done by Weeden et al. [15], where the results demonstrated that males exhibited greater amount of facial movements than females thus increasing the incisal display on smiling.

Incisal display

The incisal display significantly increased from horizontal to average to vertical facial growth pattern, with least incisal display in horizontal facial growth pattern subjects and maximum in vertical facial growth pattern subjects for both males and females. Contrary to this, Mc Namara et al. [16] found that the vertical display on smile of the maxillary right central incisor could not be correlated with the skeletal vertical dimension, as measured from nasion to menton and from anterior nasal spine to menton.

On correlating upper incisor exposure with cephalometric parameters, it was found that the upper incisor display was negatively correlated with posterior facial height and Jaraback's ratio of males in horizontal facial growth pattern group but not in females and it was positively correlated with overjet, Y-axis, and palatal plane angle of males in vertical facial growth pattern group.

Incisal edge to lower lip distance

The incisal edge to lower lip distance was less in females when compared with males in all three groups and this difference was significant in average facial growth pattern group. This is supported by the findings of Vig and Brundo [11] and Peck et al. [12, 13] who found less mandibular tooth exposure in females than males at all ages.

The distance between incisal edge of the maxillary incisor and lower lip was least in horizontal growers and the maximum in vertical growers in both male and female.

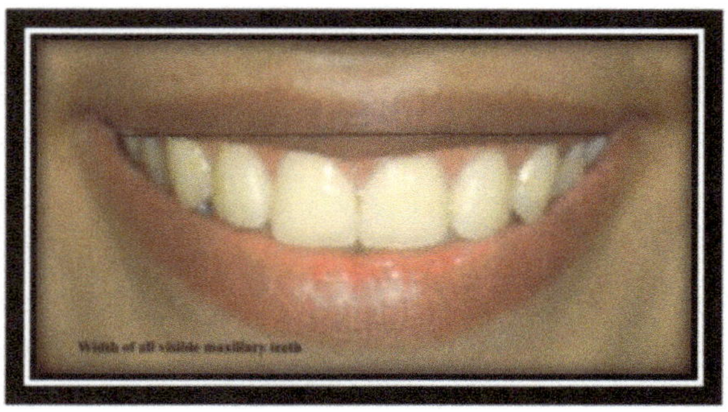

Fig. 10 Width of all visible maxillary teeth

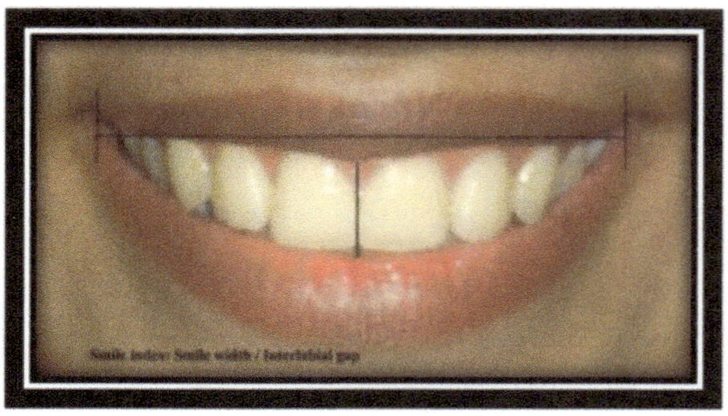

Fig. 12 Smile index

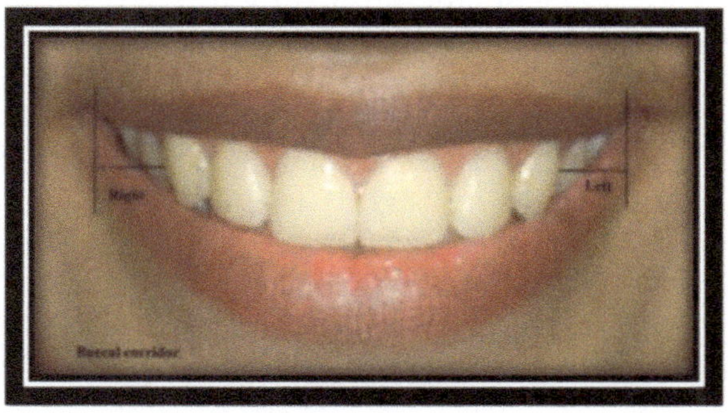

Fig. 13 Right and left buccal corridors

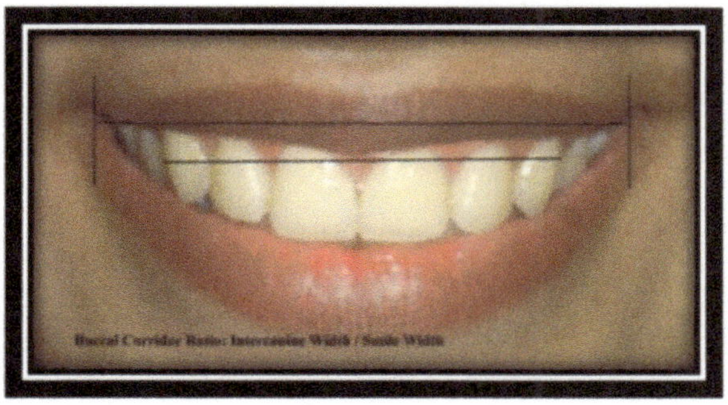

Fig. 15 Buccal corridor ratio

No correlations of distance between incisal edge of the maxillary incisor and lower lip were found with cephalomteric measurements in the vertical facial growth pattern group.

Interlabial gap

The interlabial gap was significantly more in males when compared to that in females in average and vertical facial growth pattern group. This was contrary to Rigsbee et al. [17], Tjan et al. [1], and Jensen et al [18] and is supported by a study done by Weeden et al. [15], where the results demonstrated that males exhibited greater amount of facial movements than females thus increasing the interlabial gap on smiling.

Interlabial gap was significantly found to be maximum in vertical growers, followed by average and least in horizontal growers in both male and female.

Intercanine width

The intercanine width was more in males when compared to that in females in all groups but this difference was statistically significant only in the vertical facial growth pattern group.

Intercanine width was positively correlated with total width of visible maxillary teeth on smile of males in average and vertical facial growth pattern groups but not of males in horizontal growth pattern group. In males and females of vertical growth pattern group, the intercanine width was positively correlated with smile width and total width of visible maxillary teeth on smile.

The intercanine width was found to be least in vertical growers when compared with horizontal and average growers in both male a females. Similar results were found in a study done by Grippaudo et al. [19], in skeletal class II subjects. Changes in upper arch shape with intercanine diameter were proportionately smaller in patients with high angles and larger in low-angle patients.

Total width of all visible maxillary teeth

The total width of all visible maxillary teeth was significantly more in males when compared to that in females in all groups.

The total width of all visible maxillary teeth was negatively correlated with posterior corridor (left and right side) in all the groups indicating that in case of increased visible teeth during smile, the posterior corridor decreased. Due to the same reason, the total width of all visible maxillary teeth was negatively correlated with posterior corridor ratio in all the groups.

Smile width

The smile width was more in males when compared to that in females in all groups, but this difference was statistically significant only in the horizontal facial growth pattern group. This was contrary to the results of Rigsbee et al. [17] and Chetan et al. [20] who found that females

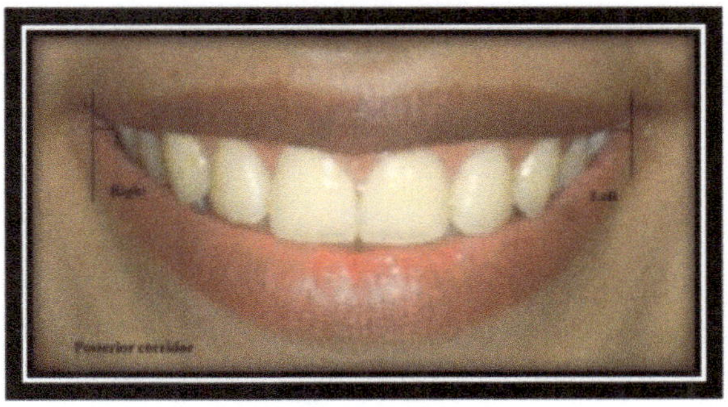

Fig. 14 Right and left posterior corridors

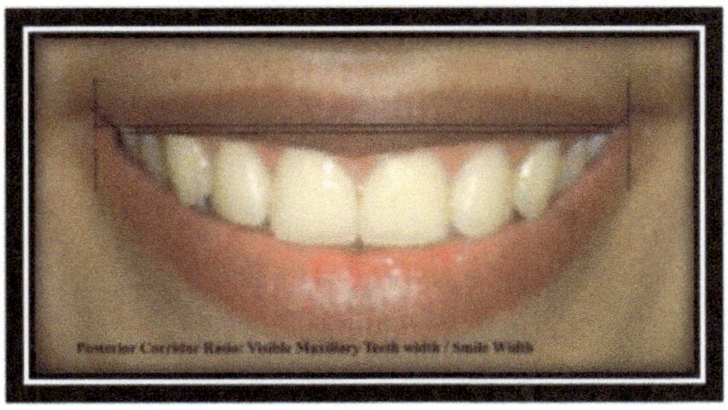

Fig. 16 Posterior corridor ratio

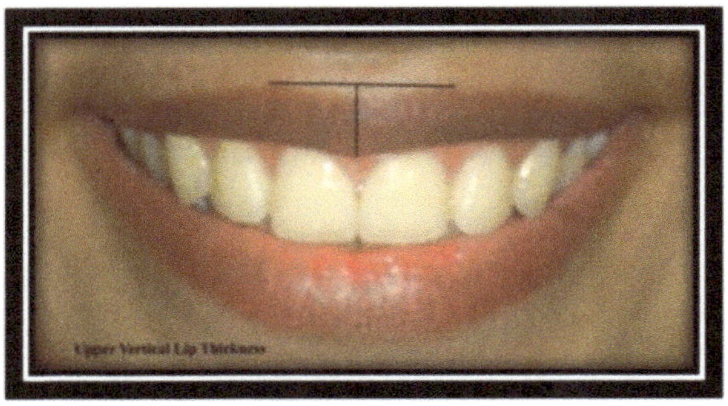

Fig. 17 Upper vertical lip thickness

exhibited more animation as compared to men resulting from a greater degree of upper lip elevation and increased width resulting in an increased display of teeth.

On comparing smile width separately in horizontal and vertical facial growth pattern group with average facial growth pattern group, statistically insignificant difference was found in both males and females in both the facial growth pattern groups.

Buccal corridor

With regard to the buccal corridor of males when compared with females, the mean value was found to be more in case of males in all groups but was significantly more only in males in horizontal facial growth pattern group. A similar finding was reported by Maulik and Nanda [21]who found that females had less buccal corridor space than males.

As regards buccal corridor of the left side when compared with the right side, statistically significant difference was found which demonstrates that the buccal corridor was greater on the left side than on the right side. This finding is supported by the study done by Okamoto et al. [22] where it was found that the displacements of the right and left corners of the mouth during voluntary smile were asymmetric and the left-sided laterality was found.

Buccal corridor of the left side when compared with the right side, in vertical facial growth pattern group

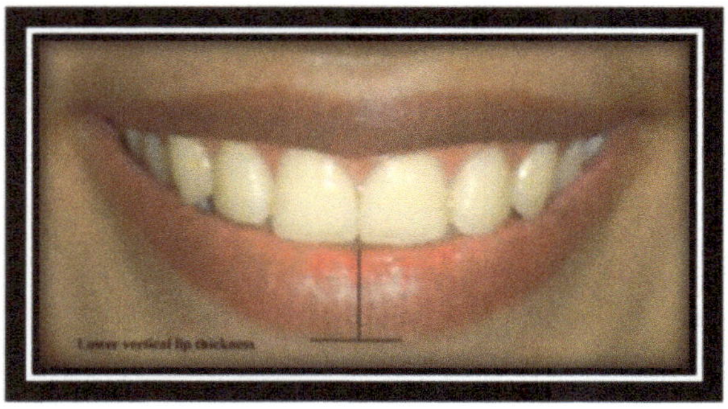

Fig. 18 Lower vertical lip thickness

with average facial growth pattern group, was found to be significantly less in vertical facial growth pattern group in males but not in females. The above findings are supported by the results of Yang et al. [23] who found that FMA and LAFH were negatively correlated with buccal corridor.

The buccal corridors (left and right) were positively correlated to each other indicating that if the buccal corridor was increased on the left side, it would increase on the right side as well, in all the groups irrespective of the age. A similar finding was observed by Krishnan et al. [6] showing a high correlation between the right and left buccal corridor spaces in both men and women. It was also positively correlated with posterior corridor (left and right) indicating that in case of increased buccal corridor, the posterior corridor also increased. No correlation was found between the total anterior facial height and the buccal corridor space similar to the findings of Yang et al [23].

Posterior corridor

Posterior corridor of males, when compared with females, was found to be less in case of males in horizontal and average facial growth pattern groups but was statistically significantly less in males in vertical facial growth pattern group. On comparing posterior corridor of the left and right sides, statistically significant difference was found which indicate that the posterior corridor was greater on the left side than on the right side. This finding is supported by the study done by Okamoto et al. [22] where it was found that the displacements of the right and left corners of the mouth during voluntary smile were asymmetric, and the left-sided laterality was found.

Posterior corridor in vertical facial growth pattern group, when compared with average facial growth pattern group, was found to be significantly less in vertical facial growth pattern group in both males and females. On comparing buccal corridor of left and right sides in horizontal facial growth pattern group with average facial growth pattern group, it was found to be insignificantly different in both males and females.

The posterior corridors (left and right) were positively correlated to each other indicating that if the posterior corridor was increased on the left side, it would increase on the right side as well, in all the groups irrespective of the age.

Upper lip vertical

Upper lip vertical length in males and females demonstrated an insignificant difference in all the groups.

Upper lip vertical length of horizontal facial growth pattern group, when compared with average facial growth pattern group, indicated that upper lip vertical length was

Table 2 Comparison of male and female in average growth pattern (comparison of groups 1 and 2)

Parameter	Males Mean ± SD	Females Mean ± SD	Difference	*t* value	*p* value	Significance
U1 EXP.	8.65 ± 1.04	8.46 ± .85	.192	0.717	.477	NS
LL-U1	.80 ± 0.97	0.14 ± 0.22	.66	3.308	.002	S*
IL GAP	9.71 ± 1.64	8.44 ± 0.82	1.276	3.473	.001	S**
IC WIDTH	40.29 ± 2.39	39.34 ± 1.95	.952	1.544	.129	NS
TW	53.43 ± 3.88	49.66 ± 3.23	3.768	3.736	<0.001	S***
SW	67.39 ± 4.63	65.76 ± 3.42	1.632	1.419	.162	NS
SI	7.16 ± 1.50	7.87 ± 8.87	7.056	−2.02	.049	S*
BC_L	13.89 ± 1.542	13.21 ± 1.97	.68	1.358	.181	NS
BC_R	13.66 ± 2.29	12.68 ± 2.01	.98	1.610	.114	NS
PC_L	7.60 ± 2.38	7.99 ± 2.24	−.392	0.60	.552	NS
PC_R	6.82 ± 2.15	7.42 ± 1.95	−.596	1.03	.310	NS
BC RATIO	6.00 ± 5.16	5.99 ± 4.11	6.49	0.049	.961	NS
PC RATIO	7.95 ± 6.71	7.57 ± 6.07	3.832	2.116	.040	S*
U VERT	5.98 ± 1.27	5.97 ± 1.49	0.012	0.031	.976	NS
L VERT	11.20 ± 1.03	10.33 ± 1.09	.864	2.884	.006	S**

NS $p > 0.05$: insignificant
*$p < 0.05$, significant at 5 % significance level; **$p < 0.01$, significant at 1 % significance level; ***$p < 0.001$, highly significant

more in horizontal and vertical growth pattern group in both males and females and least in average growers.

Lower lip vertical

For lower lip vertical length in males when compared with females, statistically significant difference was found showing increased lower vertical lip length in males in all the three groups.

With regard to the lower lip vertical length in horizontal and vertical facial growth pattern group when compared with average facial growth pattern group, no significant difference was found between the two groups in both males and females. In a study done by Joshi et al. [24], the lip position in relation to various malocclusions was studied which showed a significant difference in the sagittal lip positions in different skeletal

Table 3 Comparison of male and female in horizontal growth pattern (comparison of groups 3 and 4)

Parameter	Males ($n = 25$) Mean ± SD	Females ($n = 25$) Mean ± SD	Difference	*t* value	*p* value	Significance
U1 EXP.	6.93 ± 1.01	7.36 ± 1.14	0.4360	1.43	.160	NS
LL-U1	0.3 ± 0.62	0.15 ± 0.29	0.148	1.081	.285	NS
IL GAP	7.34 ± 1.20	7.4 ± 1.24	0.0560	0.162	.872	NS
IC WIDTH	40.14 ± 1.84	39.58 ± 1.58	0.5560	1.145	.258	NS
TW	52.92 ± 2.83	48.84 ± 3.23	4.0720	4.742	<0.001	S***
SW	68.02 ± 3.59	64.32 ± 4.08	3.708	3.410	.001	S**
SI	9.47 ± 1.38	8.93 ± 1.63	5.34	1.249	0.22	NS
BC_L	14.1 ± 1.72	12.82 ± 2.30	1.2760	2.219	.032	S*
BC_R	13.44 ± 2.18	11.86 ± 1.85	1.5840	2.768	.008	S*
PC_L	7.49 ± 1.55	7.69 ± 1.77	0.2000	0.425	.672	NS
PC_R	7.18 ± 1.54	6.93 ± 1.45	.2440	0.576	.567	NS
BC RATIO	5.91 ± 3.2	6.17 ± 3.85	2.62	−2.62	0.012	S*
PC RATIO	7.78 ± 3.36	7.61 ± 5.09	1.76	1.45	.155	NS
U VERT	6.92 ± 1.61	6.87 ± 1.61	.0520	0.114	.910	NS
L VERT	11.72 ± 1.63	10.42 ± 1.23	1.3000	3.18	.003	S**

NS $p > 0.05$: insignificant
*$p < 0.05$, significant at 5 % significance level; **$p < 0.01$, significant at 1 % significance level; ***$p < 0.001$, highly significant

Table 4 Comparison of male and female in vertical growth pattern (comparison of groups 5 and 6)

Parameter	Males Mean ± SD	Females Mean ± SD	Difference	*t* value	*p* value	Significance
U1 EXP.	10.42 ± 1.28	9.54 ± .93	0.88	2.78	.008	S**
LL-U1	1.82 ± 2.02	1.23 ± 1.25	0.59	1.25	.219	NS
IL GAP	12.95 ± 2.79	11.25 ± 2.03	1.70	2.46	.017	S*
IC WIDTH	39.81 ± 1.85	38.52 ± 2.32	1.29	2.17	.035	S*
TW	54.53 ± 4.22	50.55 ± 3.87	3.98	3.47	.001	S**
SW	65.31 ± 5.24	64.94 ± 5.58	3.72	.24	.809	NS
SI	5.49 ± 1.98	5.91 ± 9.19	4.16	0.96	0.344	NS
BC_L	12.72 ± 2.39	13.04 ± 2.28	0.320	−.49	.63	NS
BC_R	12.39 ± 2.17	12.39 ± 2.23	0.000	.00	1.00	NS
PC_L	5.51 ± 1.63	6.44 ± 1.22	0.924	−2.27	.028	S*
PC_R	5.19 ± 1.70	6.24 ± 1.42	1.05	−2.37	.022	S*
BC RATIO	7.75 ± 8.19	5.96 ± 3.9	1.798	1.09	.278	NS
PC RATIO	1.25 ± 2.05	7.80 ± 4.38	4.678	1.14	.260	NS
U VERT	6.81 ± 1.47	6.32 ± 1.34	0.488	1.23	.226	NS
L VERT	11.23 ± 1.59	9.89 ± 2.05	1.34	2.59	.013	S*

NS $p > 0.05$: insignificant
*$p < 0.05$, significant at 5 % significance level; **$p < 0.01$, significant at 1 % significance level

malocclusions. Thus, it can be inferred vertical as well as the sagittal skeletal features influence the overall soft tissue drape.

To homogenize the sample, only class I subjects were selected. Increasing the sample size randomly followed by categorizing them based on Angle's classification and using regression model to compute additional variables could further improve the study. The use of a three-dimensional methodology [25] can be used for analyzing anthropometric characteristics of soft tissue of face.

Conclusions

From the analysis and obtained results, the following conclusions can be drawn:

Table 5 Comparison of males between average and horizontal facial growth pattern (comparison of groups 1 and 3)

Parameter	Average ($n = 25$)	Horizontal ($n = 25$)	Difference	*t* value	*p* value	Significance
U1 EXP.	8.65 ± 1.04	6.93 ± 1.04	1.72	5.933	0.000	S***
LL-U1	0.80 ± 0.97	0.30 ± 0.62	0.50	2.168	0.035	S*
IL GAP	9.71 ± 1.64	7.34 ± 1.20	2.36	5.814	0.000	S***
IC WIDTH	40.29 ± 2.39	40.14 ± 1.85	0.14	0.245	0.807	NS
TW	53.43 ± 3.88	52.92 ± 2.83	0.50	0.529	0.599	NS
SW	67.39 ± 4.63	68.02 ± 3.59	0.63	0.539	0.592	NS
SI	7.16 ± 1.50	9.47 ± 1.38	2.30	5.646	0.000	S***
BC_L	13.90 ± 1.54	14.10 ± 1.72	0.20	0.441	0.661	NS
BC_R	13.66 ± 2.29	13.44 ± 2.18	0.21	0.342	0.734	NS
PC_L	7.60 ± 2.38	7.50 ± 1.55	0.10	0.176	0.861	NS
PC_R	6.82 ± 2.15	7.18 ± 1.54	0.35	0.672	0.505	NS
BC RATIO	0.60 ± 0.052	0.59 ± 0.032	0.009	0.752	0.456	NS
PC RATIO	0.795 ± 0.067	0.78 ± 0.034	0.016	1.108	0.274	NS
U VERT	5.98 ± 1.27	6.92 ± 1.61	0.944	2.301	0.026	S*
L VERT	11.20 ± 1.03	11.72 ± 1.63	0.52	1.367	0.178	NS

NS $p > 0.05$: insignificant
*$p < 0.05$, significant at 5 % significance level; ***$p < 0.001$, highly significant

Table 6 Comparison of males between average and vertical facial growth pattern (comparison of groups 1 and 5)

Parameter	Average ($n = 25$)	Vertical ($n = 25$)	Difference	t value	p value	Significance
U1 EXP.	8.65 ± 1.04	10.42 ± 1.28	1.77	5.36	0.000	S***
LL-U1	0.80 ± 0.97	1.82 ± 2.02	1.02	2.28	0.027	S*
IL GAP	9.71 ± 1.64	12.94 ± 2.79	3.24	4.99	0.000	S***
IC WIDTH	40.29 ± 2.39	39.80 ± 1.85	0.48	0.79	0.431	NS
TW	53.43 ± 3.88	54.52 ± 4.21	1.10	0.96	0.342	NS
SW	67.39 ± 4.63	65.31 ± 5.23	2.08	1.49	0.143	NS
SI	7.16 ± 1.50	5.49 ± 1.97	1.66	3.36	0.002	S**
BC_L	13.90 ± 1.54	12.72 ± 2.38	1.17	2.07	0.044	S*
BC_R	13.66 ± 2.29	12.39 ± 2.17	1.26	2.01	0.049	S*
PC_L	7.60 ± 2.38	5.51 ± 1.62	2.08	3.61	0.001	S**
PC_R	6.82 ± 2.15	5.18 ± 1.70	1.63	2.97	0.005	S**
BC RATIO	0.60 ± 0.052	0.77 ± 0.81	0.175	1.07	0.291	NS
PC RATIO	0.795 ± 0.067	1.24 ± 2.05	0.452	1.10	0.276	NS
U VERT	5.98 ± 1.27	6.81 ± 1.47	0.83	2.14	0.037	S*
L VERT	11.20 ± 1.03	11.23 ± 1.58	0.036	0.95	0.925	NS

NS $p > 0.05$: insignificant
*$p < 0.05$, significant at 5 % significance level; **$p < 0.01$, significant at 1 % significance level; ***$p < 0.001$, highly significant

1. Smile parameters in males and females were statistically significantly different, with higher mean values for upper incisor exposure, incisal edge to lower lip distance, interlabial gap, intercanine width, total width, smile width, and lower lip vertical length in males than in females.
2. For the horizontal facial growth pattern group when compared to average facial growth pattern group, statistically significant higher mean differences were observed in average growth pattern in upper incisor exposure, incisal edge to lower lip distance, interlabial gap, and upper vertical lip length, irrespective of the sex. The smile index was more and difference was statistically significant in horizontal facial growth pattern group, in both males and females.
3. Vertical facial growth pattern group exhibited statistically significant higher mean difference in

Table 7 Comparison of females between average and horizontal facial growth patterns (comparison of groups 2 and 4)

Parameter	Average ($n = 25$)	Horizontal ($n = 25$)	Difference	t value	p value	Significance
U1 EXP.	8.45 ± 0.84	7.36 ± 1.14	1.09	3.84	0.000	S***
LL-U1	0.14 ± 0.22	0.15 ± 0.29	0.012	0.16	0.870	NS
IL GAP	8.43 ± 0.82	7.40 ± 1.24	1.04	3.47	0.001	S**
IC WIDTH	39.33 ± 1.94	39.58 ± 1.57	0.24	0.49	0.623	NS
TW	49.66 ± 3.22	48.84 ± 3.22	0.81	0.89	0.378	NS
SW	65.76 ± 3.41	64.32 ± 4.08	1.44	1.36	0.181	NS
SI	7.86 ± 0.88	8.93 ± 1.62	1.07	2.88	0.006	S**
BC_L	13.21 ± 1.97	12.82 ± 2.30	0.39	6.46	0.521	NS
BC_R	12.68 ± 2.01	11.86 ± 1.85	0.82	1.50	0.140	NS
PC_L	7.98 ± 2.24	7.69 ± 1.76	0.29	0.51	0.611	NS
PC_R	7.41 1.96	6.93 ± 1.45	0.48	0.99	0.325	NS
BC RATIO	0.59 ± 0.04	0.61 ± 0.038	0.017	1.57	0.122	NS
PC RATIO	0.76 ± 0.06	0.76 ± 0.050	0.004	0.257	0.798	NS
U VERT	5.96 ± 1.50	6.87 ± 1.62	0.90	2.05	0.046	S*
L VERT	10.33 ± 1.08	10.42 ± 1.22	0.092	0.28	0.780	NS

NS $p > 0.05$: insignificant
*$p < 0.05$, significant at 5 % significance level; **$p < 0.01$, significant at 1 % significance level; ***$p < 0.001$, highly significant

Table 8 Comparison of females having average and vertical facial growth pattern (comparison of groups 2 and 6)

Parameter	Average ($n = 25$)	Vertical ($n = 25$)	Difference	t value	p value	Significance
U1 EXP.	8.45 ± 0.84	9.53 ± 0.93	1.08	4.28	0.000	S***
LL-U1	0.14 ± 0.22	1.23 ± 1.24	1.09	4.31	0.000	S***
IL GAP	8.43 ± 0.82	11.24 ± 2.02	2.81	6.42	0.000	S***
IC WIDTH	39.33 ± 1.94	38.52 ± 2.32	0.82	1.35	0.185	NS
TW	49.66 ± 3.22	50.55 ± 3.87	0.89	0.88	0.381	NS
SW	65.76 ± 3.41	64.94 ± 5.58	0.82	0.63	0.534	NS
SI	7.86 ± 0.88	5.90 ± 0.92	1.96	7.66	0.000	S***
BC_L	13.21 ± 1.97	13.04 ± 2.27	0.177	0.29	0.772	NS
BC_R	12.68 ± 2.01	12.39 ± 2.22	0.288	0.48	0.634	NS
PC_L	7.98 ± 2.24	6.43 ± 1.21	1.55	3.04	0.004	S**
PC_R	7.41 1.96	6.23 ± 1.41	1.18	2.45	0.018	S*
BC RATIO	0.59 ± 0.04	0.59 ± 0.03	0.004	0.36	0.723	NS
PC RATIO	0.76 ± 0.06	0.78 ± 0.04	0.023	1.55	0.127	NS
U VERT	5.96 ± 1.50	6.32 ± 1.33	0.356	0.89	0.380	NS
L VERT	10.33 ± 1.08	9.88 ± 2.04	0.444	0.96	0.343	NS

NS $p > 0.05$: insignificant
*$p < 0.05$, significant at 5 % significance level; **$p < 0.01$, significant at 1 % significance level; ***$p < 0.001$, highly significant

upper incisor exposure, incisal edge to lower lip distance, interlabial gap, upper vertical lip length, and occlusal plane angle, than average facial growth pattern group in both males and females; whereas, the smile index and posterior corridor (left and right) were statistically significantly less in vertical facial growth pattern group in both males and females.

4. Intercanine width exhibited positive correlation with total width of all visible teeth during smile in average facial growth pattern group of males and in vertical facial growth pattern group of both males and females.
5. Smile width was positively correlated with posterior corridor (left and right) and buccal corridor (left and right) in all the groups in both males and females.
6. Buccal corridor of the left side was positively correlated with buccal corridor of the right side and posterior corridor of both sides in all the groups in both males and females.
7. Posterior corridor of the left side was positively correlated with posterior corridor of the right side in all the groups in both males and females.
8. Posterior corridor ratio was positively correlated with buccal corridor ratio in all the groups in both males and females.
9. Saddle angle and lower incisor to NB (angular and linear) were not found to be related to smile.
10. Upper incisor to NA (angular) was found to be positively correlated with upper lip vertical in females of all the three groups.

Competing interests
The authors declare that they have no competing interests.

Authors' contributions
NG carried out the entire study and concluded the results. DNK guided the entire approach of the study. SV & PB participated in the sequence alignment and review of the study. All authors read and approved the final manuscript.

Author details
[1]Nora Medical Polyclinics, Tower 4. Marks and Spencer Building, No. 106, Abu Dhabi, United Arab Emirates. [2]Department of Orthodontics, Kothiwal Dental College & Former Dean of Dental Faculty, KGMU, Lucknow, UP, India. [3]Department of Orthodontics, Kothiwal Dental College & Research Centre, Moradabad, UP, India. [4]Department of Orthodontics & Dentofacial Orthopedics, KD Dental College & Hospital, Mathura, UP, India.

References

1. Tjan AHL, Miller GD. Some esthetic factors in a smile. J Prosthet Dent. 1984;51:24–8.
2. Sarver DM, Ackerman MB. Dynamic smile visualization and quantification: part 1. Evolution of the concept and dynamic records for smile capture. Am J Orthod Dentofacial Orthop. 2003;124:4–12.
3. Sarver DM. The importance of incisor positioning in the esthetic smile: the smile arc. Am J Orthod Dentofal Orthop. 2001;120:98–111.

4. Morley J, Eubank J. Macroesthetic elements of smile design. Am Dent Assoc. 2001;132:39–45.
5. Ackerman MB, Ackerman J. Smile analysis and design in the digital era. J Clin Orthod. 2002;36:221–36.
6. Sarver DM, Ackerman MB. Dynamic smile visualization and quantification: Part 2. Smile analysis and treatment strategies. Am J Orthod Dentofac Orthop. 2003;124:116–27.
7. Lundström A, Lundström F, Lebret LM, Moorrees C. Natural head position at natural head orientation: basic considerations in cephalometric analysis and research. Eur J Orthod. 1995;17:111–20.
8. Desai S, Upadhyay M, Nanda R. Dynamic smile analysis: changes with age. Am J Orthod Dentofac Orthop. 2009;136:310.e1–310.e10.
9. Krishnan V, Daniel ST, Lazar D, Asok A. Characterization of posed smile by using visual analog scale, smile arc, buccal corridor measures, and modified smile index. Am J Orthod Dentofac Orthop. 2008;133:515–23.
10. Alexander Jacobson: Radiographic Cephalometry; From Basics to Video-imaging. 1st ed. *Quintessence Publishing Co, Inc.* 1995: 60–62.
11. Vig RG, Brundo GC. The kinetics of anterior tooth display. J Prosthet Dent. 1978;39:502–4.
12. Peck S, Peck L, Kataja M. The gingival line. Angle Orthod. 1992;62(2):91–100.
13. Peck S, Peck L, Kataja M. Vertical lineaments of lip position. Am J Orthod Dentofac Orthop. 1992;101:519–24.
14. Balani R, Jain U, Kallury A, Singh G. Evaluation of smile esthetics in central India. APOS Trends Orthod. 2014;4:162–8.
15. Weeden JC, Trotman CA, Faraway JJ. Three dimensional analysis of facial movement in normal adults: influence of sex and facial shape. Angle Orthod. 2001;71:132–40.
16. McNamara L, McNamara Jr JA, Ackerman MB, Baccetti T. Hard- and soft-tissue contributions to the esthetics of the posed smile in growing patients seeking orthodontic treatment. Am J Orthod Dentofac Orthop. 2008;133:491–9.
17. Rigsbee OH, Sperry TP, BeGole EA. The influence of facial animation on smile characteristics. Int J Adult Orthod Orthognath Surg. 1988;3:233–9.
18. Jensen J, Joss A, Lang NP. The smile line of different Ethnic groups in relation to age and gender. Acta Med Dent Helv. 1999;2(I4):38–46.
19. Grippaudo C, Oliva B, Greco AL, Sferra S, Deli R. Relationship between vertical facial patterns and dental arch form in class II malocclusion. Prog Orthod. 2013;14:43.
20. Chetan P, Tandon P, Singh GK, Nagar A, Prasad V, Chugh VK. Dynamics of a smile in different age groups. Angle Orthod. 2013;83(1):90–6.
21. Maulik C, Nanda R. Dynamic smile analysis in young adults. Am J Orthod Dentofac Orthop. 2007;132:307–15.
22. Okamoto H, Haraguchi S, Takada K. Laterality of asymmetry in movements of the corners of the mouth during voluntary smile. Angle Orthod. 2010;80(2):223–9.
23. Yang H, Nahm DS, Baek SH. Which hard and soft tissue factors relate with the amount of buccal corridor space during smiling? The Angle Orthod. 2007;78(1):5–11.
24. Joshi M, Wu LP, Maharjan S, Raj M. Sagittal lip positions in different skeletal malocclusions: a cephalometric analysis. Prog Orthod. 2015;16:8.
25. Deli R, Galantucci L, Liano A, Gioia E. Three-dimensional methodology for photogrammetric acquisition of the soft tissues of the face: a new clinical-instrumental protocol. Prog Orthod. 2013;14:32.

26

Comparison of two maxillary protraction protocols: tooth-borne versus bone-anchored protraction facemask treatment

Peter Ngan[1*], Benedict Wilmes[2], Dieter Drescher[2], Chris Martin[1], Bryan Weaver[3] and Erdogan Gunel[4]

Abstract

Background: Protraction facemask has been advocated for treatment of class III malocclusion with maxillary deficiency. Studies using tooth-borne rapid palatal expansion (RPE) appliance as anchorage have experienced side effects such as forward movement of the maxillary molars, excessive proclination of the maxillary incisors, and an increase in lower face height. A new Hybrid Hyrax bone-anchored RPE appliance claimed to minimize the side effects of maxillary expansion and protraction. A retrospective study was conducted to compare the skeletal and dentoalveolar changes in patients treated with these two protocols.

Methods: Twenty class III patients (8 males, 12 females, mean age 9.8 ± 1.6 years) who were treated consecutively with the tooth-borne maxillary RPE and protraction device were compared with 20 class III patients (8 males, 12 females, mean age 9.6 ± 1.2 years) who were treated consecutively with the bone-anchored maxillary RPE and protraction appliances. Lateral cephalograms were taken at the start of treatment and at the end of maxillary protraction. A control group of class III patients with no treatment was included to subtract changes due to growth to obtain the true appliance effect. A custom cephalometric analysis based on measurements described by Bjork and Pancherz, McNamara, Tweed, and Steiner analyses was used to determine skeletal and dental changes. Data were analyzed using a one-way analysis of variance.

Results: Significant differences between the two groups were found in 8 out of 29 cephalometric variables ($p < .05$). Subjects in the tooth-borne facemask group had more proclination of maxillary incisors (OLp-Is, Is-SNL), increase in overjet correction, and correction in molar relationship. Subjects in the bone-anchored facemask group had less downward movement of the "A" point, less opening of the mandibular plane (SNL-ML and FH-ML), and more vertical eruption of the maxillary incisors.

Conclusions: The Hybrid Hyrax bone-anchored RPE appliance minimized the side effect encounter by tooth-borne RPE appliance for maxillary expansion and protraction and may serve as an alternative treatment appliance for correcting class III patients with a hyperdivergent growth pattern.

Background

Several studies have recommended early treatment of developing class III malocclusion for growth modification [1–5]. The validity of two-phase treatment is supported by studies that show greater orthopedic response when treatment is started in younger patients [6, 7]. Other studies reported early correction of the malocclusion allows for a favorable growth environment for dentofacial development and may help in preventing development into more severe malocclusion in late adolescence [8]. Early class III treatment using protraction facemask in conjunction with rapid palatal expansion (RPE) appliance has been shown to be successful in correcting skeletal class III malocclusions that are due primarily to deficient maxillary development [9–11]. The protraction facemask generates an anteriorly directed force on the maxilla. The forces act indirectly on the circummaxillary sutures, which are still patent at an early age, and thereby stimulate bone apposition in the suture areas. The goal of combining the RPE with

* Correspondence: pngan@hsc.wvu.edu
[1]Department of Orthodontics, School of Dentistry, West Virginia University, 1073 Health Science Center North, P.O. Box 9480, Morgantown, WV 26506, USA
Full list of author information is available at the end of the article

Table 1 Age distribution for the control, tooth-borne, and bone-anchored protraction facemask groups

	Control			Tooth-borne protraction facemask			Bone-anchored protraction facemask		
	t0	t1	Diff	t1	t2	Diff	T1	T2	Diff
Mean	9.0	9.8	0.8	9.7	10.5	0.8	9.8	10.4	0.6
SD	1.8	1.6	1.6	1.6	1.6	1.6	1.2	1.2	1.2
Min	6.1	6.9		6.90	7.11		8.0	9.0	
Max	12.7	13.2		13.2	14.1		12.0	13.0	

protraction facemask is to provide a more effective protraction of the maxilla by disarticulating the circummaxillary sutures [12, 13].

Conventional protraction facemask therapy, with an indirect application of force to the sutures through tooth-borne anchorage, causes both skeletal and dental changes because the applied force was directed below the center of resistance of the maxilla, resulting in a counterclockwise rotation of the maxilla, backward rotation of the mandible, labial tipping of the maxillary incisors, and lingual tipping of the mandibular incisors. This is usually accompanied by an increase in lower face height and a decrease in overbite [9–12]. The goal of protraction facemask therapy is to obtain pure skeletal changes with minimal undesirable dental effects. Previous studies have shown that tooth-borne protraction facemask therapy have undesirable side effects such as excessive forward movement and extrusion of the maxillary molars, excessive proclination of the maxillary incisors, and an increase in lower face height [14–17]. This is a concern especially in situations in which preservation of arch length is necessary. Attempt has been made in designing an absolute anchorage system for maxillary protraction. These newer treatment modalities include the use of intentionally ankylosed maxillary deciduous canines [18], osseointegrated titanium implants [19, 20], onplants [21], miniscrews, and most recently miniplates [22–33]. Each implant system has strengths and weaknesses. The use of osseointegrated titanium, onplants, and miniplates required invasive surgical procedures. To simplify the placement of bone-anchored devices, Wilmes et al. introduced the Hybrid Hyrax RPE appliance, a tooth- and bone-anchored device [23, 24, 32, 33]. Two mini-implants are placed in the anterior palate, and an expansion device is connected to the mini-implants and the first molars. After expansion, the patient undergoes facemask therapy with elastics attached to the hooks on the Hybrid Hyrax expansion appliance. Several case reports have been published on the application of this device [23, 24, 32, 33]. To date, no literature has been presented comparing the results of the Hybrid Hyrax bone-anchored protraction facemask with the tooth-borne protraction facemask treatment. The purpose of this study is to compare the skeletal and dentoalveolar changes between the two treatment protocols. The null hypothesis is that there is no difference in treatment effects for the sagittal, vertical, and angular changes between the two maxillary protraction protocols.

Methods

This study was approved by the Institutional Review Board of West Virginia University (1401168542). Approval was also granted from one of the authors (B.W.) for the use of orthodontic records from his office. The study groups consisted of 20 patients (8 males, 12 females) who were treated consecutively by the tooth-borne RPE appliance and protraction facemask and 20 patients (8 males, 12 females) who were treated consecutively by the bone-anchored Hybrid Hyrax expansion appliance and protraction facemask. Table 1 shows the age distribution of the two experimental groups. The inclusion criteria for patient selection were class III malocclusion at the time of the initial observation (T1) as defined

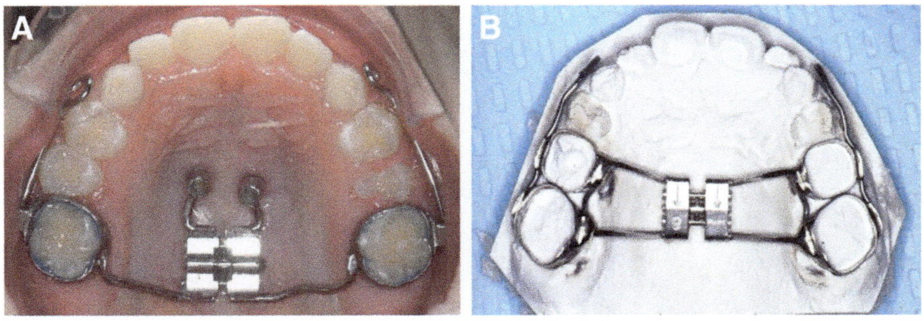

Fig. 1 **a** Bone-anchored Hybrid Hyrax expansion appliance. **b** Tooth-borne Hyrax expansion appliance

by one or more of the following characteristics: anterior crossbite or edge-to-edge incisal relationship; accentuated mesial step or class III permanent molar relationship; a Wits appraisal smaller than −3 mm or an ANB smaller than −2°. The exclusion criteria were no prior orthopedic or orthodontic treatment and no craniofacial syndromes. A sample consisted of 20 class III patients with no treatment who were under observation for class III treatment and matched closely in age and craniofacial morphology with the study groups were used as the control group.

Appliances for class III correction

The tooth-borne RPE was constructed by placing bands on the posterior teeth (Fig. 1a). Bands were fitted on the maxillary primary second molars and permanent first molars. These bands were joined by a heavy wire (.043 in.) to the palatal plate, which had a jack screw in the midline. The appliance was activated twice daily (0.25 mm per turn) by the patient for 1 week. In patients with a constricted maxilla, activation of the expansion screw was applied for 2 weeks. A 0.045-in. wire was soldered bilaterally to the buccal aspects of the molar bands and extended anteriorly to the canine area with a hook for protraction elastics.

The bone-borne Hybrid Hyrax RPE was constructed by placing bands on the permanent first molars (Fig. 1b). Two Benefit micro-implants (2 mm × 9 mm, PSM

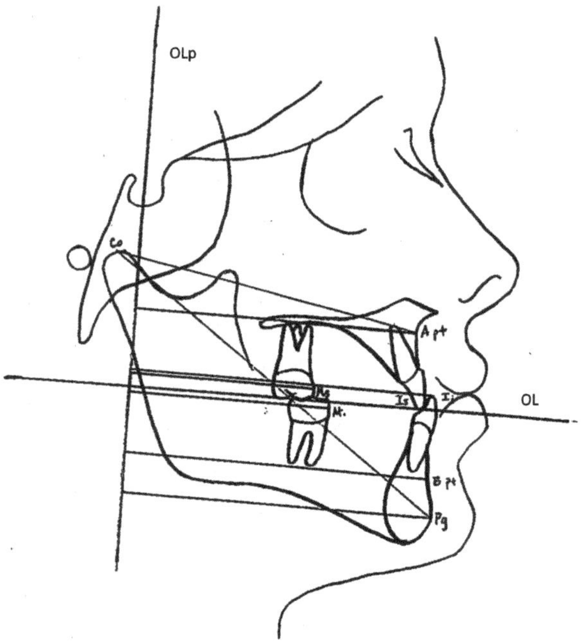

Fig. 2 A reference grid was constructed using occlusal plane (*OL*) and occlusal plane perpendicular (*OLp*). All sagittal measurements were made from the reference grid to the landmarks A point: upper incisal tip (*Is*); lower incisal tip (*Ii*); *B* point; pogonion (*Pg*); mesial buccal cusp of upper molar (*Ms*); and mesial buccal cusp of lower molar (*Mi*)

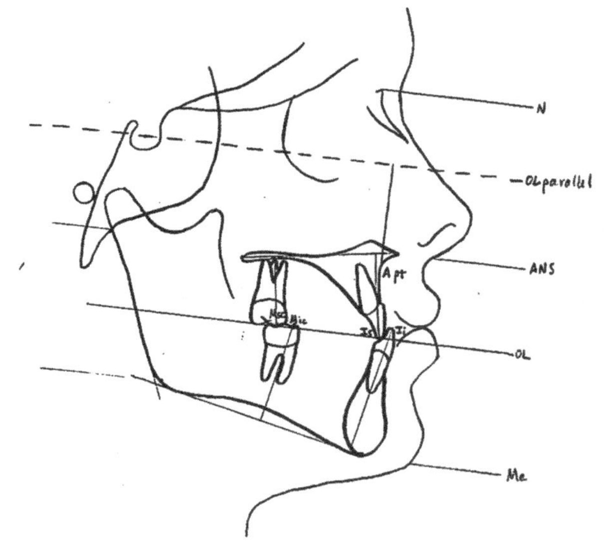

Fig. 3 Landmarks used in vertical measurements. Vertical changes of *A* point was measured from the occlusal plane parallel (*OLp*); maxillary incisal and molar changes were measured from the palatal plane; mandibular incisor and molar changes were measured from the mandibular plane

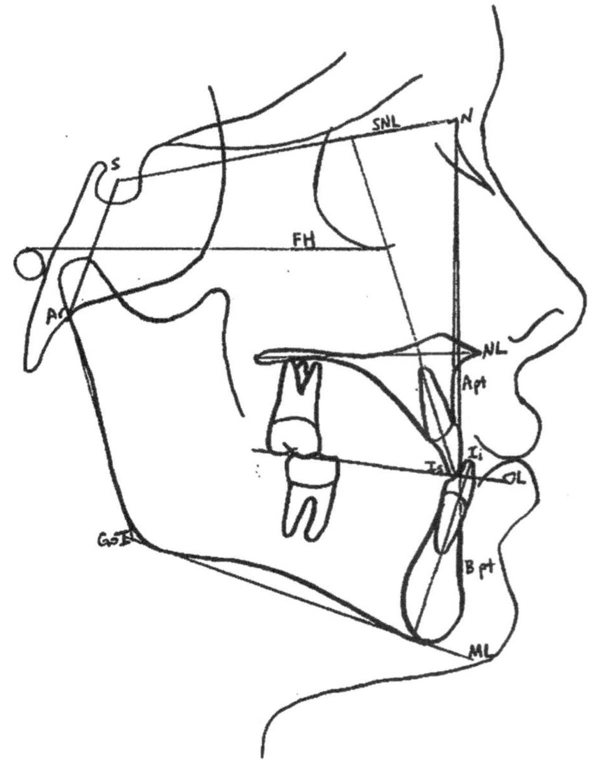

Fig. 4 Landmarks used in angular measurements. Palatal plane, occlusal plane, and mandibular plane were measured with reference to sella nasion plane (*SNL*)

Table 2 Calculation of changes in overjet and molar relationship

Overjet	Molar relationship
Skeletal contribution	Skeletal contribution
1. OLp–A pt.	1. OLp–A pt.
2. OLp–Pg	2. OLp–Pg
Dental contribution	Dental contribution
3. OLp–Is minus OLp–A pt.	3. OLp–Ms minus OLp–A pt.
4. OLp–Ii minus OLp–Pg	4. OLp–Mi minus OLp–Pg
Overjet correction	Molar relationship correction
Sum of 1, 2, 3, and 4	Sum of 1, 2, 3, and 4

Medical Solutions, Tuttlingen, Germany) were placed in the anterior palate, in the area of the third palatal rugae. Transfer caps were added before a silicone impression was taken. Laboratory analogs were placed over the transfer caps, bands were positioned in the impression, and a plaster cast is made. Two standard Benefit abutments were screwed over the laboratory analogs. A Hyrax-type (Trademark of Dentaurum, Inc., Newtown, PA) palatal split screw was welded or soldered to the two anterior abutments and to the molar bands. The jackscrew was activated twice daily (0.25 mm per turn) by the patient for 1 week. In patients with a constricted maxilla, activation of the expansion screw was applied for 2 weeks. Rigid .048-in. stainless steel sectional wires with hooks near the canines are welded or soldered to the buccal sides of the molar bands for the application of orthopedic protraction forces.

Table 3 Sagittal, vertical, and angular measurements in the control group

Variables (mm)	T0				T1				T1 − T0
Sagittal	Mean	SD	Min	Max	Mean	SD	Min	Max	Diff
OLp–A pt.	67.27	3.73	60.19	74.21	68.06	3.90	60.58	75.17	0.80
OLp–B pt.	75.74	4.86	68.45	82.66	76.74	4.96	69.02	83.23	1.00
OLp–Pg	77.11	5.47	69.12	85.54	78.18	5.53	69.60	87.26	1.08
Wits	−8.52	3.10	−13.44	−2.50	−8.26	3.11	−13.63	−2.88	0.27
OLp–Is	74.17	4.68	62.40	80.74	75.49	4.92	63.55	83.90	1.32
OLp–Ii	76.26	4.78	63.94	82.75	77.48	4.95	65.86	85.63	1.22
Overjet	−2.09	0.98	−4.03	0.38	−1.99	0.90	−4.22	0.00	0.11
OLp–Ms	48.05	4.35	40.13	54.82	49.30	4.49	40.99	55.97	1.25
OLp–Mi	51.58	5.68	42.72	60.58	52.80	5.79	42.72	62.21	1.22
Molar relationship	−3.57	2.39	−7.97	0.48	−3.47	2.20	−7.87	−0.58	0.11
Vertical (mm)									
OLparallel–A pt.	20.35	38.78	29.59	5.89	23.81	40.42	31.47	5.62	1.88
Is–NL	20.26	29.86	24.91	2.69	20.64	30.62	25.74	2.61	0.83
Ii–ML	33.60	41.18	37.61	2.14	34.27	43.01	38.28	2.45	0.66
Overbite	0.00	10.46	3.01	2.56	0.00	9.02	3.32	2.36	0.31
Msc–NL	13.25	22.46	18.97	2.05	16.32	22.75	19.44	1.54	0.47
Mic–ML	25.06	30.91	28.32	1.46	26.30	30.62	28.62	1.25	0.30
Angular (°)									
SNA	73.63	81.60	78.57	2.59	73.82	82.75	78.85	2.85	0.29
SNB	73.82	83.04	78.75	2.92	74.02	83.42	79.27	2.76	0.52
ANB	−3.74	3.55	−0.18	2.09	−3.65	3.07	−0.41	2.02	−0.23
SNL–ML	24.00	37.44	32.58	4.54	23.42	38.21	32.09	4.59	−0.49
SNL–OL	12.48	28.80	20.17	5.40	12.58	27.94	19.96	4.99	−0.21
SNL–NL	3.36	12.58	8.62	3.02	1.73	12.38	7.88	3.21	−0.74
Is–SNL	85.73	117.31	100.78	8.62	87.36	116.54	103.17	8.31	2.39
Ii–ML	64.99	100.90	87.30	8.28	68.93	102.72	86.75	9.18	−0.56

The facemask was a one-piece construction with an adjustable anterior wire and hooks to accommodate a downward and forward pull of the maxilla with elastics. The protraction elastics were attached near the maxillary canines with a downward and forward pull of 30° to the occlusal plane. Maxillary protraction generally requires an orthopedic force of 300–600 g per side depending on the age of the patient. In the present study, elastics that delivered 380 g per side as measured by a force gauge were used. The patients were instructed to wear the facemask for 12–14 h a day.

Cephalometric analysis

Pre- and post-treatment lateral cephalograms were digitized and calibrated using the Dolphin Imaging software (Dolphin Imaging, Chatsworth, CA, USA). A customized cephalometric system incorporating measurements from Bjork [35] and Pancherz [36] for the sagittal and vertical variables and Steiner, Tweed, and McNamara analyses for the angular variables were used to determine treatment changes. The landmarks used are shown in Figs. 2, 3, and 4. The magnification factor of the lateral cephalograms was found to be 6 % for both the control and the tooth-borne treatment groups. There was no magnification factor for the digital radiographs of the bone-borne treatment group. The sagittal and vertical variables were reported in millimeters and were recorded to the nearest 0.1 mm. Angular measurements were reported to the nearest 0.1°. Films were printed 1:1 using a Kodak ESP 7250 printer (Kodak, Atlanta, GA, USA) and then traced by one investigator using a 0.5 mm mechanical lead pencil, 3 M Unitek orthodontic protractor (Monrovia, CA), and 0.003 in. matte 3 M Unitek cephalometric acetate tracing film (Monrovia, CA). All radiographs were

Table 4 Sagittal, vertical, and angular measurements for the tooth-borne protraction facemask group

Variables (mm)	T1				T2				T2 – T1
Sagittal	Min	Max	Mean	SD	Min	Max	Mean	SD	Diff
OLp–A pt.	60.58	75.17	68.06	3.90	60.77	75.94	69.59	4.26	1.53
OLp–B pt.	69.02	83.23	76.74	4.96	66.62	82.46	75.41	4.86	−1.33
OLp–Pg	69.60	87.26	78.18	5.53	66.34	85.15	77.14	5.58	−1.05
Wits	−13.63	−2.88	−8.26	3.11	−9.12	1.63	−5.74	3.23	2.52
OLp–Is	63.55	83.90	75.49	4.92	69.98	87.26	78.99	4.46	3.49
OLp–Ii	65.86	85.63	77.48	4.95	66.72	80.83	75.22	4.29	−2.27
Overjet	−4.22	0.00	−1.99	0.90	0.00	8.74	3.77	2.17	5.76
OLp–Ms	40.99	55.97	49.30	4.49	44.74	61.54	51.94	4.86	2.64
OLp–Mi	42.72	62.21	52.80	5.79	43.68	60.67	52.70	5.11	−0.12
Molar relationship	−7.87	−0.58	−3.47	2.20	−5.66	1.73	−0.75	2.06	2.72
Vertical (mm)									
OLparallel–A pt.	23.81	40.42	31.47	5.62	26.11	45.98	34.54	5.24	3.07
Is–NL	20.64	30.62	25.74	2.61	21.02	30.34	26.03	2.52	0.29
Ii–ML	34.27	43.01	38.28	2.45	35.42	42.82	39.02	1.91	0.75
Overbite	0.00	9.02	3.32	2.36	0.00	3.84	2.08	1.07	−1.24
Msc–NL	16.32	22.75	19.44	1.54	17.38	23.33	20.74	1.96	1.30
Mic–ML	26.30	30.62	28.62	1.25	27.07	31.87	29.60	1.47	0.98
Angular (°)									
SNA	73.82	82.75	78.85	2.85	75.36	84.19	79.55	2.78	0.69
SNB	74.02	83.42	79.27	2.76	72.77	81.41	77.54	2.28	−1.73
ANB	−3.65	3.07	−0.41	2.02	−2.59	6.34	2.01	2.54	2.42
SNL–ML	23.42	38.21	32.09	4.59	27.36	41.38	34.43	4.17	2.33
SNL–OL	12.58	27.94	19.96	4.99	11.04	24.10	17.98	4.20	−1.98
SNL–NL	1.73	12.38	7.88	3.21	4.51	12.00	7.89	2.04	0.01
Is–SNL	87.36	116.54	103.17	8.31	94.94	113.47	105.36	6.44	2.19
Ii–ML	68.93	102.72	86.75	9.18	72.96	96.00	81.75	7.09	−4.99

traced by one person (N.D.) who was blinded to the treatment groups to avoid bias to cephalometric tracing. Analysis of the sagittal skeletal and dental changes were recorded along the occlusal plane (OL) and to the occlusal plane perpendicular (OLp) from the first film, this formed the reference grid. The grid was then transferred to a subsequent film by superimposing the tracing on the mid-sagittal cranial structures. The changes in overjet and molar relationship were calculated using the formula depicted in (Table 2) using the formula depicted in Table 3.

Data analysis

The statistical analysis was carried out utilizing the JMP version 90.9 SAS Software (Cary, NC). The starting forms of the control and experimental samples were compared using a two-tailed *t* test. The skeletal and dental changes between the treated and control sample at the two time periods were compared with a two-tailed *t* test. The confidence level was set at 95 %.

Method error

The error in locating, superimposing, and measuring the changes of the landmarks by one examiner was measured on the cephalograms of 10 randomly selected subjects. All cephalograms were recorded twice independently on two separate occasions with a 2-week interval. For all the cephalometric variables, difference between the independent repeated measurements of each individual before/after treatment was recorded. The intraclass correlation coefficient of reliability (*R*) was used to determine the reliability of cephalometric measurements. The *R* value can range from 0 to 1.00 with *R* value greater than 0.90 indicating high reliability. The correlations of all the cephalometric variables ranged from 0.96 to 0.99, with most being above 0.98. The method

Table 5 Sagittal, vertical, and angular measurements for the bone-anchored protraction facemask group

Variables (mm)	T1				T2				T2 − T1
Sagittal	Min	Max	Mean	SD	Min	Max	Mean	SD	Diff
OLp–A pt.	60.0	76.9	66.74	3.93	61.9	78.7	68.28	4.32	1.54
OLp–B pt.	63.5	80.0	71.86	5.13	62.8	80.6	70.57	5.41	−1.29
OLp–Pg	66.7	84.0	73.95	4.70	65.8	84.1	73.82	5.11	−0.13
Wits	−9.6	0.2	−5.12	2.58	−6.9	6.9	−2.54	3.22	2.58
OLp–Is	60.1	79.3	70.28	4.67	60.3	84.4	72.47	5.57	2.19
OLp–Ii	61.9	79.0	71.14	4.67	55.4	80.9	69.88	5.52	−1.26
Overjet	−4.8	2.9	−0.86	2.31	−1.6	5.9	2.6	1.76	3.46
OLp–Ms	40.2	50.7	44.45	3.18	41.1	58.0	46.89	4.27	2.44
OLp–Mi	41.3	55.2	47.52	4.20	42.2	59.1	48.94	4.65	1.42
Molar relationship	−0.6	−7.0	−3.34	1.65	−4.9	0.4	−2.05	1.62	1.29
Vertical (mm)									
OLparallel–A pt.	16.4	38.9	30.14	5.43	16.5	41.3	31.62	6.07	1.48
Is–NL	14.4	27.7	22.41	3.69	19.9	29.0	24.58	2.61	2.17
Ii–ML	27.9	39.9	34.82	3.45	29.7	41.2	36.08	3.11	1.26
Overbite	−1.1	5.9	1.56	2.18	−1.8	4.4	1.42	1.48	−0.14
Msc–NL	9.1	21.9	17.02	3.00	11.8	22.9	18.58	2.73	1.56
Mic–ML	23.3	30.5	26.51	2.06	23.9	32.9	27.7	2.13	1.19
Angular (°)									
SNA	71.9	92.1	80.29	4.74	73.0	91.2	81.88	4.49	1.59
SNB	74.8	90.2	81.2	4.17	71.9	88.8	80.4	4.25	−0.8
ANB	−5.5	3.3	−0.92	2.78	−3.8	6.9	1.48	2.76	2.4
SNL–ML	22.2	44.9	32.62	6.07	21.1	49.5	32.86	7.13	0.24
SNL–OLs	9.0	29.4	18.14	5.89	7.2	32.0	17.31	6.09	−0.83
SNL–NL	2.6	12.9	6.44	3.07	1.1	14.0	6.52	3.68	0.08
Is–SNL	87.2	121.8	103.19	8.23	86.8	114.2	101.16	8.12	−2.03
Ii–ML	78.1	91.9	84.75	3.48	77.8	95.6	83.08	4.54	−1.67

Table 6 Comparison of differences between the tooth-borne and bone-anchored groups after subtracting changes due to growth (control group)

Variables	Tooth-borne protraction facemask		Bone-anchored protraction facemask			
Sagittal	Mean	SD	Mean	SD	*p* value	Sig
OLp-A pt.	0.72	1.29	0.74	1.23	0.98	NS
OLp-B pt.	−2.28	1.43	−2.31	2.15	0.93	NS
OLp-Pg	−2.07	2.11	−1.21	3.05	0.32	NS
Wits	2.19	2.74	2.31	2.40	0.89	NS
OLp-Is	2.12	1.22	0.87	2.43	0.03	*
OLp-Ii	−3.40	2.33	−2.48	2.26	0.23	NS
Overjet	5.53	2.00	3.35	2.45	0.003	*
OLp-Ms	1.35	1.53	1.19	1.78	0.67	NS
OLp-Mi	−1.31	0.55	0.20	2.93	0.06	NS
Molar relationship	2.53	1.55	1.18	1.99	0.02	*
Vertical (mm)						
OLparallel-A pt	1.15	2.00	−0.40	1.40	0.004	*
Is-NL	−0.52	1.50	1.34	2.80	0.01	*
Ii-ML	0.09	2.18	0.60	1.72	0.49	NS
Overbite	−1.49	2.90	−0.45	2.23	0.21	NS
Msc-NL	0.80	1.56	1.09	1.86	0.63	NS
Mic-ML	0.66	1.36	0.89	1.38	0.62	NS
Angular (°)						
SNA	0.39	1.74	1.29	2.13	0.15	NS
SNB	−2.19	1.51	−1.32	1.99	0.13	NS
ANB	2.58	1.80	2.17	2.41	0.95	NS
SNL-ML	2.76	1.39	−0.25	2.90	0.007	*
SNL-OL	−1.73	3.90	−1.04	3.33	0.33	NS
SNL-NL	0.72	2.72	−0.66	2.15	0.87	NS
Is-SNL	−0.19	7.35	−4.42	5.67	0.04	*
Ii-ML	−4.33	7.68	−2.23	3.84	0.09	NS

NS not significantly different
*Significantly different at $p < 0.05$

of cephalometric analysis used in this study was deemed reliable and repeatable.

Results

Cephalometric changes

Changes in cephalometric measurements in the control group and patients treated with the tooth-borne and bone-borne protraction facemask are shown in Tables 3, 4, and 5. The appliance effect was calculated by subtracting the changes due to growth (control group) from the treatment changes (Table 6).

Sagittal and angular differences

Significant differences between the tooth-borne and bone-anchored protraction facemask groups were found in three of the 10 sagittal and angular variables. Figures 5, 6, 7, and 8 summarize the skeletal and dental contributions to the overjet and molar correction from treatment.

For both treatment groups, all subjects were overcorrected to a class I or class II molar relationship. Significant and greater change in overjet was found in the tooth-borne group (5.5 mm) compared to the bone-anchored group (3.4 mm, $p < .001$). This was contributed by similar forward movement of the maxilla (OLp-A pt., 0.7 mm) and backward movement of the mandible (OLp-Pg, 2.2 mm) in both groups, but greater forward movement of the maxillary incisors was found in the tooth-borne group (OLp-Is 2.12 vs. 0.87 mm, $p < .05$).

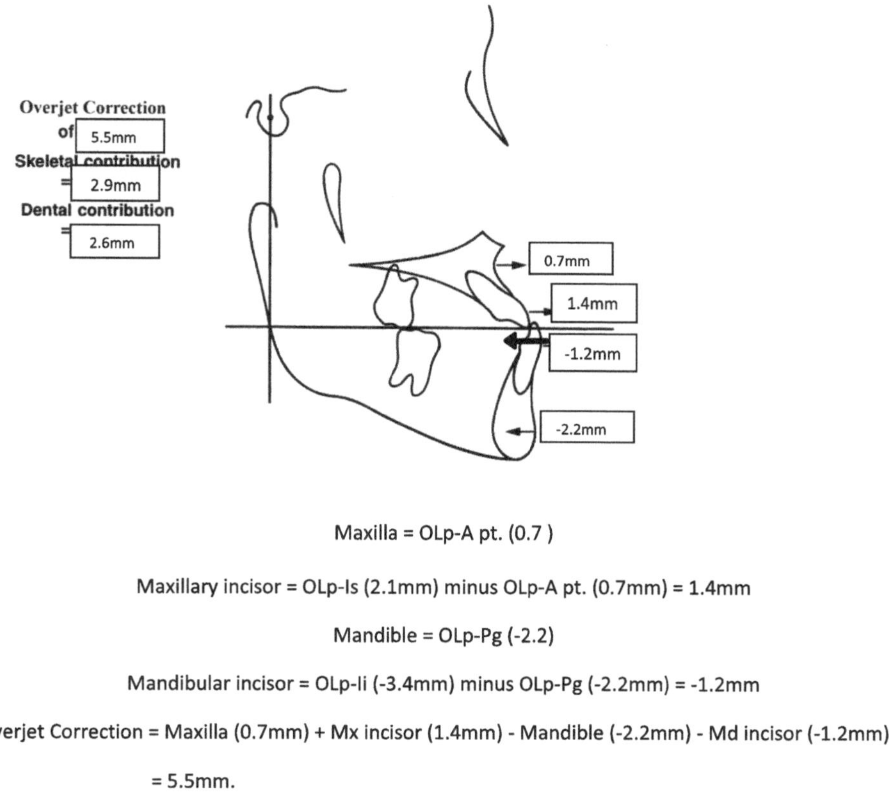

Fig. 5 Skeletal and dental contributions to overjet correction for the tooth-borne protraction facemask group

Significant and greater change in molar relationship was found in the tooth-borne group (2.7 mm) compared to the bone-anchored group (1.1 mm, $p < .05$). This was contributed by similar forward movement of the maxilla and backward movement of the mandible in both groups, but greater differential movement of the maxillary and mandibular molars was found in the tooth-borne protraction facemask group. The mean forward movement of maxillary molars was similar for the tooth-borne (0.6 mm) and bone-anchored protraction facemask groups (0.5 mm).

The anteroposterior jaw relationship was improved in both the tooth-borne group (Wits 2.19 mm, ANB 2.58°) and the bone-anchored group (Wits 2.31 mm, ANB 2.17°).

Vertical and angular differences

Significant differences between the tooth-borne and bone-anchored protraction facemask groups were found in five of the 14 vertical and angular variables. Significantly greater downward movement of the maxilla was found in the tooth-borne (OLparallel–A pt. 1.2 mm) compared to the bone-anchored protraction facemask group (–0.4 mm, $p < .005$). The mandibular plane angle was found to open significantly more in the tooth-borne group (SNL–ML 2.76°) compared to the bone-anchored protraction facemask group (–0.25°, 0.23°, $p < .05$). Significantly greater downward movement and retroclination of the maxillary incisors was found in the bone-anchored group (Is-NL 1.34 mm, Is-SNL –4.42°) compared to the tooth-borne group (–0.55 mm, –0.19°, $p < .05$).

Discussion

Maxillary protraction using both the tooth-borne RPE and RPE reinforced by two mini-implants were able to correct the anterior crossbite and improve the molar relationship in around 6 months. This was contributed by a forward and downward movement of the maxilla, clockwise rotation of the mandible, proclination of the maxillary incisors, and retroclination of the mandibular incisors. The maxilla articulates with nine other bones of the craniofacial complex: frontal, nasal, lacrimal, ethmoid, palatine, vomer, zygoma, inferior nasal concha, opposite maxilla, and occasionally, sphenoid. Palatal expansion may "disarticulate" the maxilla and initiate cellular response in the sutures, allowing a more positive reaction to protraction forces [12, 13, 37]. In this study, the maxilla moved forward an average of 1.5 mm, or 0.7 mm after subtracting changes due to growth, with both the tooth-borne and bone-anchored protraction facemask treatment. This is in line with those reported by Nanda [38], Ishii [39], Merwin [40], and Turley [12].

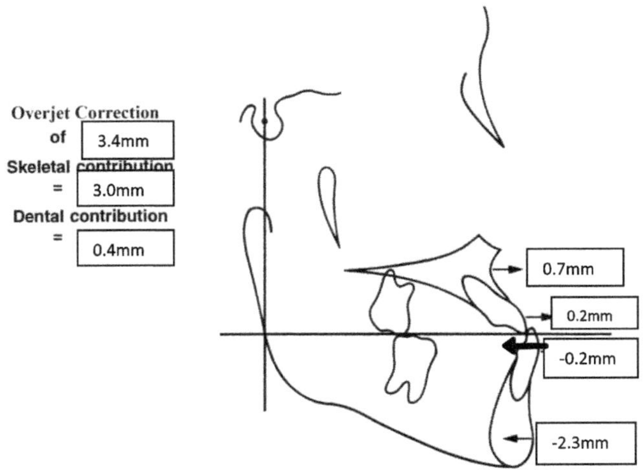

Maxilla = OLp-A pt (0.7mm)

Maxillary incisor= OLp-Is (0.9mm) minus OLp-A pt. (0.7) = 0.2mm

Mandible = OLp-Pg (-2.3mm)

Mandibular incisor= OLp-Ii (-2.5mm) minus OLp-Pg (-2.3mm) = -0.2mm

Overjet Correction= Maxilla (0.7 mm) + Mx incisor (0.2mm) - Mandible (-2.3mm) - Md incisor (-0.2mm)

= 3.4mm.

Fig. 6 Skeletal and dental contributions to overjet correction for the bone-anchored protraction facemask group

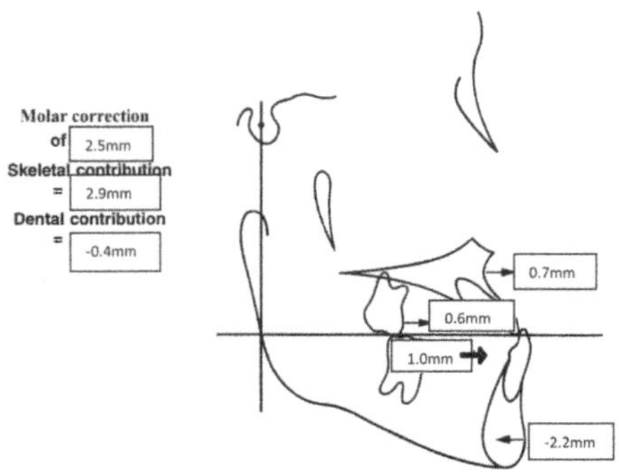

Maxilla = OLp-A pt. (0.7mm)

Maxillary molar= OLp-Ms (1.3mm) minus OLp-A pt. (0.7mm) = 0.6mm

Mandible = OLp-Pg (-2.2mm)

Mandibular molar= OLp-Mi (-1.3mm) minus OLp-Pg (-2.2mm) = 1.0mm

Molar Relationship Correction= Max (0.7) + Mx molar (0.6) – Mand (-2.2) – Md molar(1.0mm)

= 2.5mm.

Fig. 7 Skeletal and dental contributions to molar relationship correction for the tooth-borne protraction facemask group

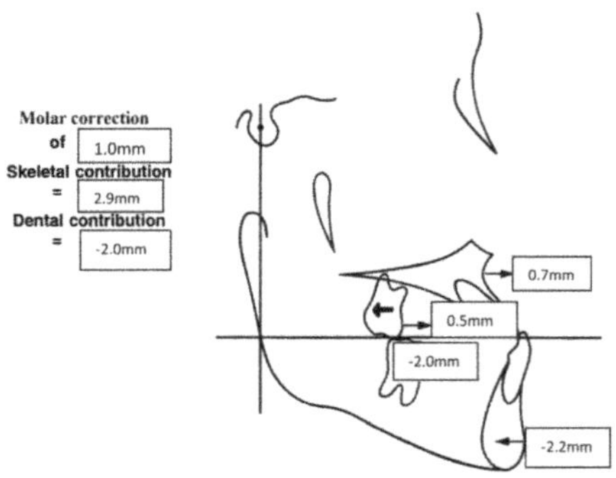

Maxilla = OLp-A pt. (0.7)

Maxillary molar= OLp-Ms (1.2mm) minus OLp-A pt. (0.7mm) = 0.5mm

Mandible = OLp-Pg (-2.2mm)

Mandibular molar= OLp-Mi (0.2mm) minus OLp-Pg (-2.2mm) = 2.4mm

Molar Relationship Correction = Max (0.7) + Mx molar (0.5) – Mand (-2.2) – Md molar (2.4mm)

= 1.0mm.

Fig. 8 Skeletal and dental contributions to molar relationship correction for the bone-anchored protraction facemask group

However, Cevidanes et al. reported larger maxillary advancement with their bone-anchored maxillary protraction (BAMP) compared to conventional RPE [29]. This is probably related to the full-time wear of class III elastics compared to smaller number of hours with the facemask. The maxillary incisors were found to move forward more in the tooth-borne compared to the bone-anchored protraction facemask group, resulting in greater increase in the overjet in the latter group. This may be due to the anchorage provided by the two mini-implants. The maxillary molars were found to move forward an average of 0.6 mm in the bone-anchored groups despite the anchorage provided by the two mini-implants. This is in line with those reported by Wilmes et al. [32, 33] with the Hybrid Hyrax appliance and other investigators that used bone-anchored devices for maxillary protraction [19–21, 27–30]. This small amount of mesial molar movement is probably due to wire bending rather than movement of the mini-implants.

For vertical changes, the mandible was found to move backward in both the tooth-borne and bone-anchored groups (SNB −2.2° and −1.3°, respectively). This, together with the forward movement of the maxilla, contributed to the improvement in the Wits appraisal and ANB changes in both groups. However, the downward movement of the maxilla in the latter group was significantly less. The incorporation of two mini-implants helps in minimizing the downward movement of the maxilla and consequently the clockwise rotation of the mandible in the bone-anchored group (SNL–ML 0.7° for the bone-anchored group vs. SNL–ML 2.9° for the tooth-borne group, $p < .05$). This is also in line with those reported by investigators using bone-anchored devices for maxillary protraction [19–21, 27–33]. In addition, there is more downward movement of the maxillary incisors in the bone-anchored group compared to the tooth-borne group that helps to maintain the overbite in the bone-anchored group.

There are several limitations to the design of this study. This is a retrospective study and the patients were treated by two different operators, one for the tooth-borne patients and one for the bone-borne patients. The radiographs of the two treatment groups were taken from different lateral cephalometric machines but they were adjusted for magnification. The control radiographs were selected from class III patients who were under growth observation, and efforts were made to match the age, sex, and craniofacial morphology as closely as possible. Finally, the results from this study are limited to a short-term observation period immediately after active treatment; long-term studies are needed for the appraisal of the stability of protraction with the Hybrid Hyrax appliance and compared to the long-term results of conventional RPE and facemask treatment [14].

Conclusions

The addition of two mini-implants in the Hybrid Hyrax RPE minimized the side effects encounter by tooth-borne RPE for maxillary protraction such as excessive forward movement of the maxillary molars and incisors, downward movement of the maxilla, and clockwise rotation of the mandible. This appliance may serve as an alternative treatment appliance for correcting class III patients with a hyperdivergent growth pattern.

Competing interests

The authors declared that they have no competing interests.

Authors' contributions

PN designed and edited the manuscript. BW and DD participated in treatment of implant patients used in the study; CM collected the data and prepared for analysis; BW analyzed the data and prepared a draft of the manuscript; EG performed the statistical analysis of the data. All authors read and approved the final manuscript.

Acknowledgement

We would like to acknowledge Dr. Nicole DeShon for her help in the tracing of the cephalometric radiographs.

Author details

[1]Department of Orthodontics, School of Dentistry, West Virginia University, 1073 Health Science Center North, P.O. Box 9480, Morgantown, WV 26506, USA. [2]Department of Orthodontics, University of Düsseldorf, Moorenstrasse, Germany. [3]Department of Oral and Maxillofacial Surgery, School of Dentistry, West Virginia University, Morgantown, USA. [4]Department of Statistics, West Virginia University, Morgantown, USA.

References

1. Chatzoudi MI, Loannidou-Marathiotou L, Papadopoulos MA. Clinical effectiveness of chin cup treatment for the management of class III malocclusion in pre-pubertal patients: a systematic review and meta-analysis. Prog Orthod. 2014;15:62.
2. Tollaro I, Baccetti T, Bassarelli V, Franchi L. Class III malocclusion in the deciduous dentition: a morphological and correlation study. Eur J Orthod. 1994;16:401–8.
3. VanLaecken R, Williams MO, Razmus T, Gunel E, Martin C, Ngan P. Class III correction using an inter-arch spring-loaded module. Prog Orthod. 2014;15:32.
4. Kajiyama K, Murakami T, Suzuki A. Evaluation of the modified maxillary protractor applied to class III malocclusion with retruded maxilla in early mixed dentition. Am J Orthod Dentofac Orthop. 2000;5:549–59.
5. Reed E, Kiebach T, Ngan P, Martin C, Razmus T, Gunel E. Stability of early class III orthopedic treatment in the primary and early mixed dentitions. Sem in Orthod. 2014;20:114–27.
6. Sakamoto T. Effective timing for the application of orthopedic force in the skeletal class III malocclusion. Am J Orthod. 1981;80:411–6.
7. Mermigos J, Full CA, Andreasen G. Protraction of the maxillofacial complex. Am J Orthod Dentofac Orthop. 1990;98:127–33.
8. Benedetti M, Bosch C, Melsen B. Changes occurring during and after treatment of class III malocclusion with rapid palatal expansion and facemask. World J Orthod. 2002;3:199–210.
9. Ngan PW, Hagg U, Yiu C, Wei SHY. Treatment response and long-term dentofacial adaptations to maxillary expansion and protraction. Seminars in Orthod. 1997;4:255–64.
10. Baccetti T, Franchi L, McNamara Jr JA. Treatment and post-treatment craniofacial changes after rapid maxillary expansion and facemask therapy. Am J Orthod Dentofac Orthop. 2000;118:404–13.
11. Saadia M, Torres E. Sagittal changes after maxillary protraction with expansion in class III patients in the primary, mixed and late mixed

dentitions: a longitudinal retrospective study. Am J Orthod Dentofac Orthop. 2000;117:669–80.
12. Nartallo-Turley PE, Turley PK. Cephalometric effects of combined palatal expansion and facemask therapy on class III malocclusion. Angle Orthod. 1998;68(3):217–24.
13. Liou EJ. Effective maxillary orthopedic protraction for growing class III patients: a clinical application simulates distraction osteogenesis. Prog Orthod. 2005;6(2):154–71.
14. Hagg U, Tse A, Bendeus M, Rabie BM. Long-term follow-up of early treatment with reverse headgear. Eur J Orthod. 2003;25:95–102.
15. Lertpitayakun P, Miyajima K, Kanomi R, Sinha PK. Cephalometric changes after long-term early treatment with facemask and maxillary intraoral appliance therapy. Sem in Orthod. 2001;7:169–79.
16. Delaire J. Maxillary development revisited: relevance to the orthopaedic treatment of class III malocclusions. Eur J Orthod. 1997;19:289–311.
17. da Silva Filho OG, Magro AC, Capelozza FL. Early treatment of the class III malocclusion with rapid maxillary expansion and maxillary protraction. Am J Orthod Dentofac Orthop. 1998;113(2):196–203. doi:10.1016/S0889-5406(98)70292-6.
18. Kokich VG, Shapiro PA, Oswald R, Koskinen-Moffett L, Clarren SK. Ankylosed teeth as abutments for maxillary protraction: a case report. Journal Orthod. 1985;88:303–7.
19. Cha B, Choi D, Ngan P, Jost-Brinkmann P, Kim S, Jang I. Maxillary protraction with miniplates providing skeletal anchorage in a growing class III patient. Am J Orthod Dentofac Orthop. 2011;139(1):99–112. doi:10.1016/j.ajodo.2009.06.025.
20. Singer S. Osseointegrated implants as an adjunct to facemask therapy: a case report. Angle Orthod. 2000;70(3):253.
21. Hong H, Ngan P, Han GL, Liu GQ, Wei SHY. Use of onplants as stable anchorage for facemask treatment: a case report. Angle Orthod. 2005;75(3):453–60.
22. Enacar A, Giray B, Pehlivanoglu M, Iplikcioglu H. Facemask therapy with rigid anchorage in a patient with maxillary hypoplasia and severe oligodontia. Am J Orthod Dentofac Orthop. 2003;123(5):571–7.
23. Wilmes B, Nienkemper M, Drescher D. Application and effectiveness of a mini-implant- and tooth-borne rapid palatal expansion device: the hybrid hyrax. World J Orthod. 2010;11(4):323–30.
24. Wilmes B, Drescher D. A miniscrew system with interchangeable abutments. J Clin Orthod. 2008;42(10):574–80.
25. Cha B, Ngan PW. Skeletal anchorage for orthopedic correction of growing class III patients. Semin Orthod. 2011;17(2):124–37. doi:10.1053/j.sodo.2010.12.005.
26. Poletti L, Silvera AA, Ghislanzoni LT. Dentoalveolar class III treatment using retromolar miniscrew anchorage. Prog Orthod. 2013;14:7.
27. Kircelli BH, Pektas ZÖ. Midfacial protraction with skeletally anchored face mask therapy: a novel approach and preliminary results. American Journal of Orthodontics and Dentofacial Orthopedics. 2008;133(3):440–9. doi:10.1016/j.ajodo.2007.06.011.
28. Zhou YH, Ding P, Lin Y, Qui LX. Facemask therapy with miniplate implant anchorage in a patient with maxillary hypoplasia. Chin Med J. 2007;15:1372–5.
29. Cevidanes L, Baccetti T, Franchi L, McNamara Jr JA, De Clerck H. Comparison of two protocols for maxillary protraction: bone anchors versus face mask with rapid maxillary expansion. Angle Orthod. 2010;80(5):799–806.
30. De Clerck H, Cevidanes L, Baccetti T. Dentofacial effects of bone-anchored maxillary protraction: a controlled study of consecutively treated class III patients. American Journal of Orthodontics and Dentofacial Orthopedics. 2010;138(5):577–81. doi:10.1016/j.ajodo.2009.10.037.
31. De Clerck HJ, Cornelis MA, Cevidanes LH, Heymann GC, Tulloch CJF. Orthopedic traction of the maxilla with miniplates: a new perspective for treatment of midface deficiency. Journal of Oral and Maxillofacial Surgery. 2009;67(10):2123–9. doi:10.1016/j.joms.2009.03.007.
32. Wilmes B, Nienkemper M, Ludwig B, Kau CH, Drescher D. Early class III treatment with a hybrid hyrax-mentoplate combination. J Clin Orthod. 2011;45(1):15–21.
33. Ludwig B, Glas B, Bowman SJ, Drescher D, Wilmes B. Miniscrew-supported class III treatment with the hybrid RPE advancer. J Clin Orthod. 2010;44(9):533–9.
34. Şar Ç, Arman-Özçırpıcı A, Uçkan S, Yazıcı AC. Comparative evaluation of maxillary protraction with or without skeletal anchorage. Am J Orthod Dentofac Orthop. 2011;139(5):636–49.
35. Bjork A. The face in profile: an anthoropological x-ray investigation of Swedish children and conscripts. Lund: Berlingska Boktrycheriet 1947;40–58.
36. Pancherz H. The mechanism of class II correction in Herbst appliance treatment. A cephalometric investigation. Am J Orthod Dentofacial Orthop. 1982;82:104–13.
37. Haas AJ. Palatal expansion: just the beginning of dentofacial orthopedics. Am J Orthod. 1970;57:219–55.
38. Nanda R. Biomechanical and clinical considerations of a modified protraction headgear. Am J Orthod Dentofac Orthop. 1980;78:125–39.
39. Ishii H, Morita S, Takeuchi Y, Shinji N. Treatment effects of combined maxillary and chincap appliance in severe skeletal class III cases. Am J Orthod Dentofac Orthop. 1987;92:304–12.
40. Merwin D, Ngan P, Hagg U, Yiu C, Wei SHY. Timing for effective application of anteriorly directed orthopedic force to the maxilla. Am J Orthod Dentofac Orthop. 1997;112:292–9.

27

Effect of non-surgical maxillary expansion on the nasal septum deviation: a systematic review

Tehnia Aziz[1], Kal Ansari[2], Manuel O. Lagravere[1], Michael P. Major[1] and Carlos Flores-Mir[1*]

Abstract

Nasal breathing is a requirement for proper growth and development of the craniofacial complex. Inadequacy of the nasal airway from obstruction such as from nasal septal deviation (NSD) can affect craniofacial development. Further investigation of the possibility of rapid maxillary expansion (RME) correcting NSD would be valuable, considering the undesirable sequelae of NSD on nasal breathing, which can consequently affect craniofacial development. A systematic review of the effect of RME treatment on NSD was conducted. Electronic database searches were conducted until April 2015 using MEDLINE, EMBASE, Web of Science, Cochrane Database of Systematic Reviews (CDSR), Cochrane Central Register of Controlled Trials (CCTR), Cochrane Methodology Register (CMR), Database of Abstracts of Reviews of Effects (DARE), American College of Physicians Journal Club (ACP Journal Club), Health Technology Assessments (HTA), and NHS Economic Evaluation Database (NHSEED). MeSH terms used in database searches were 'nasal septum,' 'palatal expansion,' and 'maxillary expansion,' 'orthodontic device,' and 'palatal expansion technique.' The methodological quality of studies was reviewed using methodological index for non-randomized studies (MINORS). Only two studies were finally selected and reviewed. Both studies had significant methodological limitations. One study reported a significant straightening of the nasal septum in the middle and the inferior third of nasal cavity from RME in children aged 5 to 9 years. The other study reported no positional change in the nasal septum from RME in adolescent orthodontic patients. Thus far, the limited available (moderate risk of bias) evidence suggests a potentially positive effect on the nasal septum asymmetry during childhood, but no significant change in adolescence from RME in patients with NSD. The clinical significance of reported changes could be considered questionable.

Keywords: Maxillary expansion; Nasal septum; Palatal expansion; Systematic review

Introduction

The nasal septum is an important functional and esthetic structure of the nose. It is responsible for regulating airflow through the nose while lending shape and support to the nasal dorsum and caudal aspect of the nose. Within the nasal cavity, a straight septum enables laminar airflow, allowing the inspired air to be warmed, cleaned, and humidified and thus optimized for gas exchange at the alveoli in the lungs. Conversely, a deviated nasal septum can contribute to various degrees of nasal obstruction and altered nasal respiration [1].

Nasal septal deviation (NSD) is defined as deviation of either the bony or the cartilaginous septum or both from the midline. Although, the earliest investigation reported 80 % of humans having some degree of septal deviation [2], more recent numbers in adults range around 65 % [3]. The prevalence range of NSD in neonates has been reported between 1 [4] to roughly 20 % [5]. In school-aged children (6–15 years), it was documented as 20 % when assessed on occipitomental projection radiographs, whereas the clinical diagnosis of NSD was made in approximately 10 % of the same cohort of children [6].

Nasal obstruction from a deviated nasal septum may cause turbulent nasal airflow precipitating in dryness and crusting of the nose, frequent nosebleeds, and recurrent sinusitis [7]. Furthermore, during developmental years, inadequacy of the nasal airway can necessitate chronic mouth breathing, causing moderate to severe maxillary constriction, and a vertical skeletal growth pattern characterized by long anterior lower face height,

* Correspondence: cf1@ualberta.ca
[1]Division of Orthodontics, 5-528 Edmonton Clinic Health Academy, University of Alberta, 11405 87 Ave. NW, Edmonton T6G 1C9, AB, Canada
Full list of author information is available at the end of the article

bilateral maxillary crossbite, high arched palate, low tongue posture, and incompetent lips [8, 9]. In addition, it has been hypothesized that nasal breathing is a requirement for proper growth and development of the craniofacial complex [10]. According to the functional matrix theory, nasal airflow is a continuous stimulus for lowering of the palate and for lateral maxillary growth, indicating a close relationship between nasal breathing and dentofacial morphology.

Rapid maxillary expansion (RME) is routinely used in orthodontic treatment to correct transverse maxillary constriction by opening of the midpalatal suture [11]. It works by separation of the two halves of the palatal bones across the median palatal suture due to a lateral force from the appliance [12]. Both the zygomatic and sphenoid bones of the cranial base are met with resistance during expansion. Therefore, the separation of maxillary bones occurs in a triangular manner, with the apex toward the nasal cavity and the base at the same level as the palatine process [13] resulting in more opening anteriorly than posteriorly [14]. Thus, one can extrapolate that there will be greatest improvement in the caliber of the anterior rate limiting nasal valve area from RME compared to other regions of the nasal cavity. Some studies have reported correction of septal deviation as an incidental finding from RME [15, 16]. To our knowledge, no review of the literature has been conducted to investigate this finding. Therefore, the purpose of this systematic review is to methodically analyze the available literature concerning the effects of RME on nasal septal deviation.

The specific PICOS question to be addressed is "In children or adolescent patients with a deviated nasal septum and a transversally constricted palate, does a nonsurgical palatal expansion produce a simultaneous improvement on the nasal septum position?"

Review

Methods

A review protocol was discussed, but it was not registered online.

Several databases were searched electronically with the help of a senior librarian specializing in health sciences database searches. The searched electronic databases were MEDLINE (from 1966 to the second week of April 2015, OVID), EMBASE (from 1974 to the second week of April 2015, OVID), Web of Science (from 1945 to the second week of April 2015, Thomson Reuters), Cochrane Database of Systematic Review (CDSR), Cochrane Central Register of Controlled Trials (CCTR), Cochrane Methodology Register (CMR), Database of Abstracts of Reviews of Effects (DARE), American College of Physicians Journal Club (ACP Journal Club), Health Technology Assessments (HTA), and NHS Economic Evaluation Database (NHSEED) until the first quarter of 2015.

The MeSH search terms used in database searches were 'nasal septum', 'palatal expansion', and 'maxillary expansion', 'orthodontic device', and 'palatal expansion technique' (see Additional file 1 for specific search terms and their combinations). These combinations of terms were identified with the help of a specialized health science librarian. No language limitation or year of publication limit was set.

Two authors (T.A. and K.A.) independently reviewed the title and abstracts of the database searches. Abstracts from human studies that discussed an orthopedic effect on the nasal septum from nonsurgical palatal expansion were included at the initial selection phase. The full text of all studies that appeared to meet the inclusion criteria were retrieved along with ones that had insufficient information in the abstracts to make a final decision regarding their inclusion. The references of retrieved articles were also manually searched for additional studies that could be included in the systematic review. The authors (T.A. and K.A.) independently assessed full articles obtained for inclusion in the systematic review, and any disagreement was settled through discussion until a consensus was reached.

In summary, the inclusion criterion was any type of clinical trial that evaluated objectively the orthopedic effect on nasal septum from nonsurgical palatal expansion procedures.

The following exclusion criteria were finally applied to the studies after retrieval of full text of articles:

1. No case reports
2. Studies that reported the presence of any concurrent sino-nasal pathology in their patient sample that would preclude visualization of the nasal septum before or after RPE treatment were excluded (examples of such conditions included, but not limited to, were septal perforation, enlarged turbinates and nasal polyps, etc.)
3. Studies that merely reported a visual change in NSD as an incidental finding and did not implement protocols to methodically measure nasal septum pre- and post-expansion were also excluded
4. Surgically assisted palatal expansion

Methodological scoring to assess the quality of included studies was also performed independently by two authors (T.A. and K.A.) through methodological index for non-randomized studies (MINORS) checklist [17]. Any disagreement in individual scores was settled through discussion until the final consensus was reached. Although an overall quality score was tabulated, it was established that the quality assessment would be considered in the discussion and data synthesis mostly through analysis of individual components.

Results

The flow chart of the electronic database searches and the final selection of studies to be included in the systematic review are outlined in Fig. 1 (numbers from the end of May 2014). Online searches resulted in six potential abstracts [15, 16, 18–21] after removal of duplicates that resulted from the overlap of studies between the electronic databases. Four studies [16, 18–20] were later excluded after a full review of the articles, and the reasons for their exclusion are listed in Table 1. This resulted in only two studies [15, 21] to be included in this systematic review. Key details of the included studies are listed in Table 2.

One study [15] reported straightening of the nasal septum by approximately 94 % in the middle and the inferior third of the nasal cavity from RME. Correction in NSD was confirmed by a reduction in the amplitude of septal deviation as measured in millimeters from the mid-sagittal plane. The included sample were 100 children aged 5 to 9 years. RME was accomplished through hyrax activated twice a day for 15 days.

Another study [21] reported no positional change in the nasal septum from RME. In this study, the nasal septal angle was measured in degrees from the midsagittal plane. The sample consisted of 10 children aged 13–17 years with occlusal coverage hyrax appliance. Expansion protocol in this cohort was twice a day hyrax activation for 2–3 weeks.

Results from MINORS [17] are listed in Table 3. Total scores for both studies were the same. Both included studies stated clear objectives (item 1) and assessed outcomes according to the aim of the study (item 4) with appropriate statistical analysis (item 12). Both studies included patients according to predetermined exclusion/inclusion criteria and measurement protocols (items 3, 4). However, unbiased assessment of outcome variable was not fulfilled by either study (item 5). In addition, patients that could have been lost to follow-up were not reported by either study (item 7). Neither study conducted a prospective sample size calculation from effect size (item 8) or had baseline equivalence of control and treatment groups (item 10). One study [21] recruited the control group from data archives; therefore, the criteria of contemporary control and treatment groups were not fulfilled (item 10).

Discussion

Nasal breathing is a prerequisite for proper growth of the craniofacial complex. Moderate to severe nasal septal deviation (NSD) can cause clinically significant nasal obstruction, resulting in irreversible repercussions on the growth and development of craniofacial structures. The purpose of this systematic review was to investigate the effect of rapid maxillary expansion on nasal septal deviation.

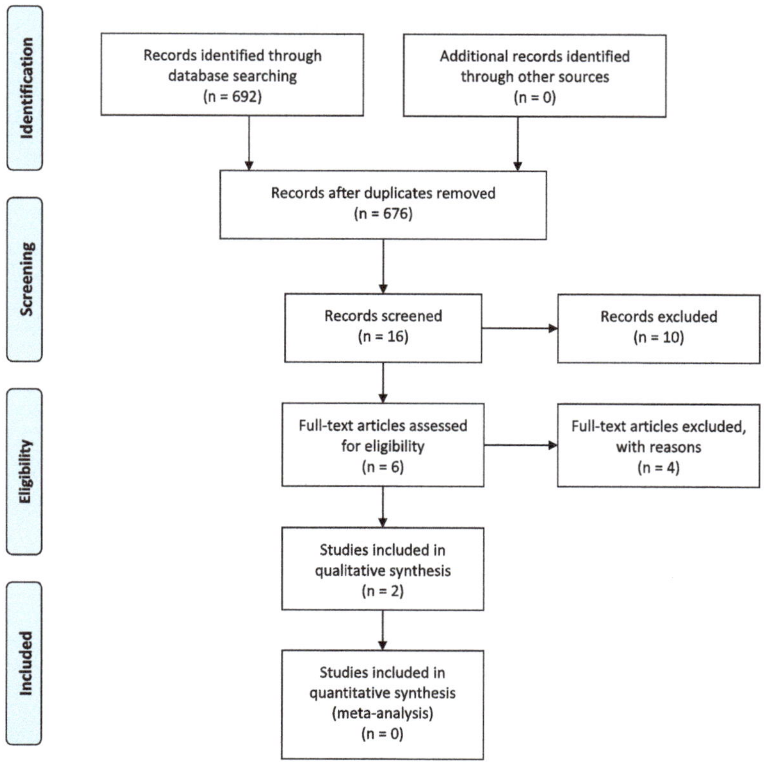

Fig. 1 Flowchart of systematic review selection process

Table 1 Excluded studies and reason for their exclusion

Studies excluded	Reason for exclusion
Baydas et al. [18]	No mention of nasal septum evaluation
Schwarz et al. [19]	Only surgical RME discussed with respect to changes in nasal septum
Gray LP [20]	Reported a visual change in nasal septum from RME without employing methods to measure the change
Gray LP [16]	Reported a visual change in nasal septum from RME without employing methods to measure the change

Historically, RME was believed to primarily affect airway function through changes to nasal volume. For example, Haas [13] reported RME resulted in an increased nasal width of 2–4.5 mm with an expansion protocol of 0.4 to 0.5 mm per day for 12 to 27 days in his patient cohort. It was postulated that the alteration in nasal dimensions following RME is related to the lateral movement of the nasal walls [22], increase in the vertical dimension of the nasal cavity secondary to inferior rotation of the palate [12].

Like Haas, many investigators have focused on changes in nasal volume or the secondary effect of changing nasal airflow resistance after RME. These studies yielded inconclusive findings. Some demonstrated positive nasal changes after RME [23, 24], others found no difference [25], while some found such small differences that the clinical relevance was questioned [26, 27]. However, more clinically directed inquiries, such as subjective patient experience [28, 29] and polysomnography changes with sleep apnea [30], have provided growing support to potential functional airway benefits of RME.

Since changes in nasal volume alone seem inconclusive to account for the effects of RME, alternative explanations are now being explored. One of such hypothesis is the effect of RME on the nasal septum. Data from computational fluid dynamic studies that have modeled nasal septal deviations have been valuable in providing [31, 32] comprehensive information on nasal airflow characteristics. These studies concluded that anterior and inferior septal deviations increase nasal resistance more than posterior and superior septal deviations [31, 32]. Consequently, significant septal deviations in the posterior nasal cavity can occur without significant increase in nasal airway resistance. This is explained due to the fact that in healthy nasal passages, majority of the airflow is at the height of the nasal floor and the area between the inferior and middle turbinates, with less than 15 % of nasal airflow at the superior part of the nasal cavity [31]. Rapid maxillary expansion affects nasal airway because it is considered to modify the nasal valve area, which represents the narrowest nasal cross-sectional area [33]. In other words, nasal valve area is likely the greatest contributor to nasal airway resistance during breathing.

Interestingly, patients with maxillary deficiency in the transverse dimension usually also have small nasal cross-sectional areas [34], which can explain the reason for maxillary expansion having a potentially positive effect on the nasal airway. Further investigation of the possibility of RME correcting NSD would be valuable, considering the undesirable sequelae of NSD on nasal breathing, which can consequently affect craniofacial development. In addition, septal cartilage can act as a growth center in early development; its deviation can cause distortion of the maxillary complex toward the deviated side [15].

Although, there are numerous reports of the effects of RME on the nasal airway, only a few of those studies have hypothesized that RME "straightens" the nasal septum, thereby correcting nasal septal deviation [15, 16, 19, 35].

Table 2 Characteristics of included studies

Study	Baseline characteristics of treatment group	Baseline characteristics of control group	RME protocol	Measurement of the nasal septum	Results
Farronato et al. [15]	$N = 100$ Ages 5–9 years (mean = 7.62 years, SD = 0.7) Nasal septal deviation (NSD) of more than 1 mm as seen on PA radiographs (amplitude of deviation)	$N = 40$ Ages 5–9 years (mean = 7.62, SD = 0.7) Not treated with RME Not clear if they presented with NSD	Hyrax expander1 turn (0.25 mm) twice a day for 15 days	Amplitude of NSD measured on frontal/PA cephalograms as millimeter distance between midline axis of symmetry and deviated nasal septum. Measurements taken before appliance insertion (T0), at appliance removal (T1) and 6 months after appliance removal (T2)	94 % reduction in amplitude of NSD from RME in the middle and lower third of the nasal cavity from T0 to T2
Altug-Atac et al. [21]	$N = 10$ Ages 13–17 years (mean = 15 years) Nasal septal angle (from midsagittal plane = 1.05° (SD = 0.91))	$N = 10$ Ages 13–17 years (mean = 15 years) Not treated with RME Nasal septal angle 0.78 (SD = 1.23)	Occlusal coverage, Hyrax type expander with 2 turns a day for 2–3 weeks	Measured in degrees as angle between the nasal septum midsagittal plane on frontal/PA cephalograms. Measurements taken prior to appliance insertion and after 12 weeks active expansion	No significant positional change in nasal septum from RME

Table 3 Methodological quality assessment of included studies by MINORS

Methodological item	Farronato et al. [15]	Ss score	Altug-Atac et al. [21]	Score
1. A clearly stated aim	Yes	1	Yes	1
2. Inclusion of consecutive patients	Yes	1	Yes	1
3. Prospective collection of data	Yes	1	Yes	1
4. Endpoints appropriate to the aim of the study	Yes	1	Yes	1
5. Unbiased assessment of the study endpoint	No	0	No	0
6. Follow-up period appropriate for the aim of the study	Yes	1	Yes	1
7. Loss to follow-up less than 5 %	Unclear	0.5	Unclear	0.5
8. Prospective calculation of study size	No	0	No	0
9. An adequate control group	No	0	Unclear	0.5
10. Contemporary groups	Yes	1	No	0
11. Baseline equivalence of groups	No	0	Unclear	0.5
12. Adequate statistical analysis	Yes	1	Yes	1
Total score		7.5		7.5

Score key: yes = 1, no = 0, unclear = 0.5

The earliest indication of the potential effect of palatal expansion over the nasal septum anatomy came from Gray [20]. While evaluating 140 cases (mostly between 3 and 14 years of age), he noted a significant improvement in the nasal airway (84 % of the cases), diminution of allergic symptoms (65–70 % of the cases), and infections (87 % of the cases). In addition, a positive psychological benefit (25 % of the cases), as well as dental changes, was noted. The issue with this study was that it is not clear if nasal septum anatomy was assessed after the expansion process. Listed quantified outcomes did not include such assessment. It was implied that the septum deviation was corrected. No specific data analysis was available differentiating changes in children from adolescents.

Another early finding of this effect came also from Gray [16], whereby he noted an improvement in the "curve" of the deviated nasal septum after RME treatment from subjective visualization of posterior anterior radiographs. The sample size in this study consisted of 310 patients ranging from 4 to 24 years of age with majority (86 %) of the patients under the ages of 12. It is not clear, although is likely the case, if the 140 cases from the previous publication [20] were included. Subjective improvement of the nasal airway was reported in these patients with improvement stable at 6 months post expansion. Approximately 80 % of patients reported switching from mouth to nasal breathing post expansion with a significant reduction (roughly 60 %) in colds, sore throats, ear infections, and nasal allergies. No specific data analysis was available differentiating changes in children from adolescents. It was hypothesized that improvement of nasal ventilation from RME prevented dryness and crusting of the nasal mucosa thereby reducing recurrent upper airway infections. Improved ciliary function and normal nasal cycle function were among other benefits purported from increased nasal airflow resulting from RME. However, this study was excluded from our systematic review since the conclusions were based on visual and subjective assessment of X-rays without any objective quantification of change or appropriate statistical analysis. The issue again with this study was that although it is stated that nasal septum improvement was visually assessed, a percentage of correction was not stated.

Finally, Schwarz et al. reported [19] in nine adult patients that underwent surgically assisted maxillary expansion without including nasal septum sectioning failed to notice any nasal septum anatomical change. Coronal tomograms were used to quantify the before and after nasal septum symmetry.

Only two studies [15, 21] were finally included in this systematic review after conducting electronic searches of several databases. Both analyzed the change in nasal septal deviation from RME in two-dimensional coronal views from posterior anterior cephalograms. Farronato et al. [15] recruited 100 growing patients (ages 5–9 years, average 7.62 ± 0.7) presenting with transverse maxillary constriction and measured an increase of 2.3 mm in the width of the nasal cavity and reported 94 % reduction in the septal deviation from RME. The NSD correction was noted in the inferior and middle half of the nasal cavity when compared to a non-expansion control group. Septal correction in this study was measured by placing points on superior, middle, and inferior segments of the septum as visualized from pre and post expansion PA cephalograms. Distances between these landmarks were measured along with maximum amplitude of deviation from an imaginary midline in coronal view. The resulting change was quantified in millimeters and as a percentage. Patient sample in this study had septal deviation of at least

1 mm in the middle/inferior third of the septum as visualized as a deflection in the vertical path from superior to inferior on PA (coronal view) X-rays. However, the results from the other included paper [21] were contradictory to the aforementioned study. The latter study reported no change in NSD from RME in an older cohort of patients (ages 13–17 years).

It has been documented that RME efficacy is greater when done before the growth spurt (2.3 mm) versus at or after the peak growth (1.5 mm) [9]. Incomplete calcification of the midpalatal suture in growing patients translates into ease of displacement of the lateral walls of the nasal cavity [9]. Rapid maxillary expansion treatment in mixed dentition, i.e., prior to midpalatal suture closure has greater improvement in nasal airway resistance due to greater likelihood of skeletal change (nearly 50 %) as opposed to during adolescence when the change is mostly dental. However, to our knowledge, no study has investigated the effect of slow or semi-rapid expansion on nasal airway or structures.

Methodological quality of studies included in this systematic review was analyzed using MINORS checklist. Although, both studies had similar total scores (7.5/12) suggesting moderate level of evidence, there were a few methodological flaws. Both stated clear objectives and assessed outcomes according to the aim of the study; however, the outcome assessor was not blinded, and the reasons for lack of blinding were not mentioned. There was also no prospective sample size calculation, and the reasoning behind this was not elucidated. It is ambiguous whether the baseline characteristics of the control and treatment groups were equivalent. Farronato et al. [15] included a "control" group having no septal deviation and without RME. It would be difficult to ascertain the effect of an intervention such as RME, without a comparable baseline nasal septal deviation in control and treatment groups. Although, the Altug-Atac et al. [21] did report including an age-matched untreated control group, the comparison was historical because the control group was recruited from archived patient database. Furthermore, it is unclear whether the control group and RME group had similar baseline nasal septal deviation for accurate comparison.

Due to lack of literature in this area, it would be beneficial to plan future studies in a preadolescent patient population presenting with transverse maxillary deficiency. The aim of the aforementioned study would be to methodically measure NSD in a three-dimensional view at set landmarks instead of an isolated pre- and post-PA cephalogram image.

Limitations

The question of whether RME is beneficial in reducing the effect of nasal obstruction from a deviated nasal septum in growing patients has not been intensively investigated.

Except from the hand-search of the references of the identified articles during the phase 1 selection process, no further gray literature was searched. Studies that may have been published in common non-indexed electronic databases may have been missed.

Conclusions

Thus far, the limited available (moderate risk of bias) evidence suggests a potentially positive effect on the nasal septum asymmetry during childhood, but no significant change in adolescence from RME in patients with NSD. The clinical significance of reported changes in children could be considered questionable.

Abbreviations

ACP Journal Club: American College of Physicians Journal Club; CBCT: Cone-beam computed tomography; CCTR: Cochrane Central Register of Controlled Trials; CDSR: Cochrane Database of Systematic Review; CMR: Cochrane Methodology Register; DARE: Database of Abstracts of Reviews of Effects; HTA: Health Technology Assessments; MINORS: Methodological index for non-randomized studies; NHSEED: NHS Economic Evaluation Database; NSD: Nasal septal deviation; RME: Rapid maxillary expansion.

Competing interest

The authors declare that they have no competing interests.

Authors' contributions

TA, KA and CF conceptualized the manuscript. TA and KA completed the data collection. All authors read and approved the final manuscript.

Author details

[1]Division of Orthodontics, 5-528 Edmonton Clinic Health Academy, University of Alberta, 11405 87 Ave. NW, Edmonton T6G 1C9, AB, Canada. [2]Division of Otolaryngology, 4071 Grey Nuns Hospital, Edmonton T6L 5X8AB, Canada.

References

1. Flint PW, Haughey BH, Lund VJ, Niparko JK, Richardson MA, Robbins KT, and Thomas JR.. Cummings Otolaryngology - Head and Neck Surgery. 5th ed. Mosby, 2015.
2. Gray LP. Deviated nasal septum. Incidence and etiology. Ann Otol Rhinol Laryngol. 1978;87(3 Pt 3 Suppl 50):3–20.
3. Stallman JS, Lobo JN, Som PM. The incidence of concha bullosa and its relationship to nasal septal deviation and paranasal sinus disease. Am J Neuroradiol. 2004;25(9):1613–8.
4. Podoshin L, Gertner R, Fradis M, Berger A. Incidence and treatment of deviation of nasal septum in newborns. Ear Nose Throat J. 1991;70(8):485–7.
5. Kawalski H, Spiewak P. How septum deformations in newborns occur. Int J Pediatr Otorhinolaryngol. 1998;44(1):23–30.
6. Haapaniemi JJ, Suonpaa JT, Salmivalli AJ, Tuominen J. Prevalence of septal deviations in school-aged children. Rhinology. 1995;33(1):1–3.
7. Sooknundun M, Kacker SK, Bhatia R, Deka RC. Nasal septal deviation: effective intervention and long term follow-up. Int J Pediatr Otorhinolaryngol. 1986;12(1):65–72.
8. Laptook T. Conductive hearing loss and rapid maxillary expansion. Report of a case. Am J Orthod. 1981;80(3):325–31.

9. Baccetti T, Franchi L, Cameron CG, McNamara Jr JA. Treatment timing for rapid maxillary expansion. Angle Orthod. 2001;71(5):343–50.
10. Moss-Salentijn L, Melvin L. Moss and the functional matrix. J Dent Res. 1997;76(12):1814–7.
11. Haas AJ. The treatment of maxillary deficiency by opening of the midpalatal suture. Angle Orthod. 1965;35:200–17.
12. Haas AJ. Palatal expansion: just the beginning of dentofacial orthopedics. Am J Orthod. 1970;57(3):219–55.
13. Haas AJ. Rapid expansion of the maxillary dental arch and nasal cavity by opening the midpalatal suture. Angle Orthod. 1961;31(2):73–90.
14. Enoki C, Valera FC, Lessa FC, Elias AM, Matsumoto MA, Anselmo-Lima WT. Effect of rapid maxillary expansion on the dimension of the nasal cavity and on nasal air resistance. Int J Pediatr Otorhinolaryngol. 2006;70(7):1225–30.
15. Farronato G, Giannini L, Galbiati G, Maspero C. RME: influences on the nasal septum. Minerva Stomatol. 2012;61(4):125–34.
16. Gray LP. Results of 310 cases of rapid maxillary expansion selected for medical reasons. J Laryngol Otol. 1975;89(6):601–14.
17. Slim K, Nini E, Forestier D, Kwiatkowski F, Panis Y, Chipponi J. Methodological index for non-randomized studies (minors): development and validation of a new instrument. ANZ J Surg. 2003;73(9):712–6.
18. Baydas B, Yavuz I, Uslu H, Dagsuyu IM, Ceylan I. Nonsurgical rapid maxillary expansion effects on craniofacial structures in young adult females. A bone scintigraphy study. Angle Orthod. 2006;76(5):759–67.
19. Schwarz GM, Thrash J, Byrd DL, Jacobs JD. Tomographic assessment of nasal septal changes following surgical-orthodontic rapid maxillary expansion. Am J Orthod. 1985;87(1):39–45.
20. Gray LP, Brogan WF. Septal deformity malocclusion and rapid maxillary expansion. Orthodontist. 1972;4(1):2–14.
21. Altug-Atac AT, Atac MS, Kurt G, Karasud HA. Changes in nasal structures following orthopaedic and surgically assisted rapid maxillary expansion. Int J Oral Maxillofac Surg. 2010;39(2):129–35.
22. Perillo L, De Rosa A, Iaselli F, d'Apuzzo F, Grassia V, Cappabianca S. Comparison between rapid and mixed maxillary expansion through an assessment of dento-skeletal effects on posteroanterior cephalometry. Prog Orthod. 2014;15(1):46.
23. Baratieri C, Alves Jr M, de Souza MM, de Souza Araujo MT, Maia LC. Does rapid maxillary expansion have long-term effects on airway dimensions and breathing? Am J Orthod Dentofacial Orthop. 2011;140(2):146–56.
24. Smith T, Ghoneima A, Stewart K, Liu S, Eckert G, Halum S, et al. Three-dimensional computed tomography analysis of airway volume changes after rapid maxillary expansion. Am J Orthod Dentofacial Orthop. 2012;141(5):618–26.
25. Gordon JM, Rosenblatt M, Witmans M, Carey JP, Heo G, Major PW, et al. Rapid palatal expansion effects on nasal airway dimensions as measured by acoustic rhinometry. A systematic review. Angle Orthod. 2009;79(5):1000–7.
26. Ceroni Compadretti G, Tasca I, Alessandri-Bonetti G, Peri S, D'Addario A. Acoustic rhinometric measurements in children undergoing rapid maxillary expansion. Int J Pediatr Otorhinolaryngol. 2006;70(1):27–34.
27. Marcus CL, Brooks LJ, Draper KA, Gozal D, Halbower AC, Jones J, et al. Diagnosis and management of childhood obstructive sleep apnea syndrome. Pediatrics. 2012;130(3):e714–55.
28. Doruk C, Sokucu O, Sezer H, Canbay EI. Evaluation of nasal airway resistance during rapid maxillary expansion using acoustic rhinometry. Eur J Orthod. 2004;26(4):397–401.
29. Oliveira De Felippe NL, Da Silveira AC, Viana G, Kusnoto B, Smith B, Evans CA. Relationship between rapid maxillary expansion and nasal cavity size and airway resistance: short- and long-term effects. Am J Orthod Dentofacial Orthop. 2008;134(3):370–82.
30. Guilleminault C, Monteyrol PJ, Huynh NT, Pirelli P, Quo S, Li K. Adeno-tonsillectomy and rapid maxillary distraction in pre-pubertal children, a pilot study. Sleep Breathing. 2011;15(2):173–7.
31. Garcia GJ, Rhee JS, Senior BA, Kimbell JS. Septal deviation and nasal resistance: an investigation using virtual surgery and computational fluid dynamics. Am J Rhinol Allergy. 2010;24(1):e46–53.
32. Liu T, Han D, Wang J, Tan J, Zang H, Wang T, et al. Effects of septal deviation on the airflow characteristics: using computational fluid dynamics models. Acta Otolaryngol. 2012;132(3):290–8.
33. MacGinnis M, Chu H, Youssef G, Wu KW, Machado AW, Moon W. The effects of micro-implant assisted rapid palatal expansion (MARPE) on the nasomaxillary complex—a finite element method (FEM) analysis. Prog Otrhod. 2014;15(1):52.
34. Baraldi CE, Pretto SM, Puricelli E. Evaluation of surgically assisted maxillary expansion using acoustic rhinometry and postero-anterior cephalometry. Int J Oral Maxillofacial Surg. 2007;36(4):305–9.
35. Bicakci AA, Agar U, Sokucu O, Babacan H, Doruk C. Nasal airway changes due to rapid maxillary expansion timing. Angle Orthod. 2005;75(1):1–6.

28

Rapid palatal expansion effects on mandibular transverse dimensions in unilateral posterior crossbite patients: a three-dimensional digital imaging study

Alessandro Ugolini[1,2*], Tiziana Doldo[1], Luis T. Huanca Ghislanzoni[2], Andrea Mapelli[2], Roberto Giorgetti[1] and Chiarella Sforza[2]

Abstract

Background: The purpose of this controlled study was to investigate indirect effects on mandibular arch dimensions, 1 year after rapid palatal expansion (RPE) therapy.

Methods: Thirty-three patients in mixed dentition (mean age 8.8 years) showing unilateral posterior crossbite and maxillary deficiency were treated with a RPE (Haas type) cemented on the first permanent molars. Treatment protocol consisted of two turns per day until slight overcorrection of the molar transverse relationship occurred. The Haas expander was kept on the teeth as a passive retainer for an average of 6 months. Study models were taken prior (T1) and 15 months on average (T2) after expansion. A control group of 15 untreated subjects with maxillary deficiency (mean age 8.3 years) was also recorded with a 12-month interval. Stone casts were digitized with a 3D scanner (3Shape, DK).

Results: In the treated group, both mandibular intermolar distance (+1.9 mm) and mandibular molar angulation (+9°) increased. Mandibular incisor angulation showed an increase of 1.9°. There was little effect on intercanine distance and canine angulation. Controls showed a reduction in transverse arch dimension and a decrease in molar and canine angulation values.

Conclusions: RPE protocol has indirect widening effects on the mandibular incisors and first molars.

Keywords: Palatal expansion, Mandibular arch, 3D digital models

Background

Posterior crossbite is one of the most prevalent malocclusions in the primary and early mixed dentition, and it is reported to occur in 8 to 22 % of the cases [1, 2]. It occurs when the maxillary back teeth bite inside the mandibular back teeth. Posterior crossbite may develop or improve at any time from when the deciduous teeth come into the mouth to when the permanent teeth come through. If the crossbite affects one side of the mouth only, the mandible may need to move asymmetrically to allow the posterior teeth to meet together. This movement may have long-term effects on the growth of the teeth and jaws. The subsequent neuromuscular adaptation to the acquired mandibular position can cause asymmetric mandibular growth, facial disharmony, and several functional changes in the masticatory muscles and temporomandibular joint (TMJ) [3]. It is unclear what causes posterior crossbites, but they may be due to skeletal, soft tissue, dental, or respiratory factors or develop as the result of a habit, e.g., thumb-sucking or some pathology. For this reason, several treatments have been recommended to correct posterior crossbite.

McNamara has speculated that the position of the mandibular dentition might be influenced more by

* Correspondence: alexugolini@yahoo.it
[1]Department of Orthodontics, University of Siena, Siena, Italy
[2]Functional Anatomy Research Center (FARC), Laboratorio di Anatomia Funzionale dell'Apparato Stomatognatico (LAFAS), Dipartimento di Scienze Biomediche per la Salute, Facoltà di Medicina e Chirurgia, Università degli Studi di Milano, Milan, Italy

maxillary skeletal morphology than by the size and shape of the mandible [4]. This hypothesis could explain why some mandibular arch decompensation happened during rapid maxillary expansion therapy, but very few published researches support this thesis [5–10]. While some recent investigations reviewed the palatal expansion and its effects on the palatal vault and the lower third of the face in a three-dimensional perspective, an evaluation of the effects on the mandible with a 3D noninvasive analysis is still missing [11, 12].

The primary focus of the current study was the assessment of the spontaneous mandibular response after rapid palatal expansion (RPE) therapy, in patients with unilateral crossbite, as measured from three-dimensional digital dental models.

Methods

Subjects

Forty-eight patients with posterior crossbite were consecutively selected. The patients were treated at the Department of Orthodontics, University of Siena (Italy) and were selected according to the following criteria:

- Early or mid mixed dentition stage
- Cervical vertebral stage 1 through 3 (CVS methods 1–3) [13]
- Unilateral posterior crossbite
- Angle Class I or Class II malocclusion
- Underwent RPE banded (Haas type) therapy (RPE, treated group) or to be submitted to RPE banded (Haas type) therapy (control group)
- No subsequent comprehensive orthodontic treatment implemented in either the maxilla or the mandible

The exclusion criteria for selection were as follows:

- Angle Class III malocclusion
- Previous orthodontic treatment
- Hypodontia in any quadrant excluding third molars
- Hormonal imbalances
- TMJ signs and/or symptoms
- Craniofacial abnormalities (e.g., cleft lip and palate)
- Arthritis

The RPE group consisted of 18 girls and 15 boys; average age at T1 was 8.8 years (sd 1.1 years). The control group consisted of 8 girls and 7 boys; average age at T1 was 8.3 (sd 1.2 years). These patients were matched for age, sex, and skeletal maturity with the RPE groups but did not receive any orthodontic treatment, and their dental casts were taken a second time after approximately 12 months.

In the RPE group, the records included pre-treatment (T1, immediately before the cementation of the appliance) and post-treatment dental casts (T2, after the appliance was removed and replaced by a removal plate, 15 months interval on average).

All palatal expanders (tooth-tissue supported, Haas type) were manufactured, cemented, and activated according to the following protocol: at initial activation, the appliances received two quarter turns (0.4 mm). Thereafter, the appliance was activated one quarter turn in the morning and one quarter turn in the evening. The subjects were seen at weekly intervals for approximately 3 weeks. When the desired overcorrection for each patient was achieved, the appliance was stabilized. Expansion was considered adequate when the occlusal aspect of the maxillary lingual cusp of upper first molars contacted the occlusal aspect of the facial cusp of the mandibular lower first molars. The expander was in situ during the expansion and stabilization period for a mean time of 7 months (range 5–9 months). After the removal of the expander, a loose, removable acrylic plate was placed within 48 h. Generally, each patient wore the acrylic plate for a variable amount of time (minimum 8 h/day).

Cast analysis

The sample consisted of 96 cast models which were scanned by a 3SHAPE D640 SCANNER (3Shape, Copenhagen, DK) 3D digital model (*.stl) were thus obtained.

3D digital model processing and cast analysis were accomplished with a multi-step procedure. The first step consisted of landmark digitization on each model through VAM application version 2.8.3 (Canfield Scientific Inc., Fairfield-NJ, USA). The protocol developed by Huanca Ghislanzoni et al. [14] was followed. Dental landmarks were taken on screen on the scanned mandibular dental casts by the principal investigator (A.U.). When either the deciduous teeth were missing or the permanent teeth were not fully erupted, the measurements for that variable were eliminated. For each patient, a total of 15 mandibular landmarks were digitized (two landmarks each for the first molars, canines, and central incisors; plus 3 landmarks as reference plane). Two landmarks per teeth allowed to trace the facial axis of the clinical crown (FACC) of the first permanent molars, deciduous canines, and permanent central incisors, at T1 and at T2, respectively. Mandibular reference planes were computed between the incisive papilla and the intersections of lingual sulci of the first permanent molars with the gingival margin (Fig. 1a, b). Lingual measurements for mandibular intermolar width were obtained at the point of the intersection of the lingual groove with the cervical gingival margin, according to McDougall et al. [15] The occlusal intermolar width was measured as the distance between the mesiobuccal cusp tips of the first permanent molars bilaterally; the

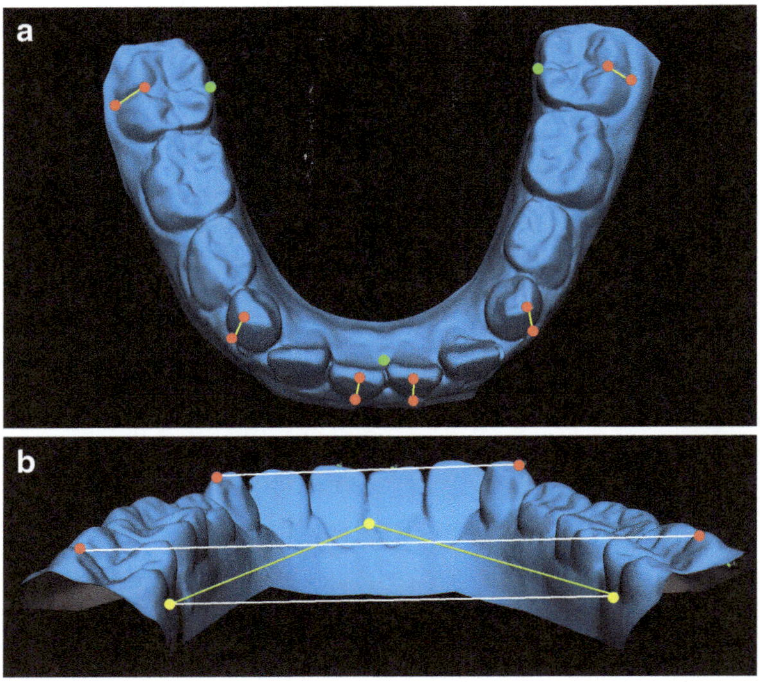

Fig. 1 a, b. Digital model of the mandible with markers: dental markers in *red*, reference plane markers in *green*. **a** FACC, used to calculate angulation, in *yellow*. **b** Intercanine and intermolar (lingual and vestibular) distances in *white*

intercanine width was the distance between cusp tips bilaterally. Mandibular first molar, canine, and incisor angulations were calculated as the angle of projection of the FACC on the reference plane.

The whole set of landmarks was exported into a .txt file. The .txt file was imported into an Excel matrix, and x, y, and z coordinates were divided into three columns.

The 3D point set was re-orientated putting the reference lingual plane parallel to the X plane. Finally, the data set was analyzed with a custom excel procedure for 3D arch analysis. The process was repeated for each mandibular arch cast (Fig. 1a, b).

Method error

Intraclass correlation coefficients were calculated to compare within-subjects variability to between-subjects variability; all values were larger than 0.93. Standard deviations between repeated measurements were found to be in the range of 0.08 to 0.17 mm for linear measurements and in the range of 0.5° to 1.9° for angular measurements. Overall, the method error was considered negligible.

Statistical analysis

Descriptive statistics were computed for all analyzed variables: occlusal and lingual intermolar distances; intercanine distance; left and right molar, canine, and central incisor angulation values; and molar, canine, and incisors mean (right and left average angulation values).

Shapiro-Wilk's test showed that data were normally distributed, and parametric statistics were applied. Patient (RPE group) data were compared with the data collected from the untreated group using Student's *t* tests. Probabilities of less than 0.05 were accepted as significant in all statistical analyses. Sample size was calculated a priori to obtain a statistical power of the study greater than 0.85 at an alpha of 0.05, using the mean values and standard deviations of mandibular molar expansion after RPE therapy found by Lima et al. [7].

The effects size (ES) coefficient was also calculated [16]. The ES coefficient is the ratio of the difference between the recordings of two different groups (within the same recording condition) or two recording conditions (within the same group) divided by the within-subject standard deviation (sd), and it was calculated as follows:

$$\mathrm{ES} = \frac{m_a - m_b}{\sqrt{[(\mathrm{sd}_a^2 \mathrm{x}\ n_a + \mathrm{sd}_b^2\ \mathrm{x}\ n_b)/\mathrm{sd}_a + \mathrm{sd}_b]}}$$

where, m_a and m_b are the means for the generic group/ recording conditions A and B; sd_a and sd_b are the corresponding standard deviations; n_a and n_b are the corresponding sample sizes. For Cohen's *d*, an effect size of 0.2 to 0.3 might be a "small" effect; around 0.5, a "medium" effect; and 0.8 to infinity, a "large" effect.

A linear regression model was employed to assess correlations between treatment duration (months of therapy, MOT) and mandibular dental angulation values.

Results

Descriptive analyses of the mandibular variables at two assessment stages for all 48 subjects are shown in Tables 1 and 2 and Fig. 2. It was possible to measure only fully erupted teeth (permanent or deciduous). Therefore, for some measurements, a reduced number of subjects were analyzed (Table 1). No differences between groups were found at T1. At T2, all patients had their crossbite corrected. No self-crossbite corrections were observed in the control group.

The net changes of the T1-T2 interval are reported in Table 2. In treated (RPE group) subjects, mandibular intermolar distance significantly increased 1.9 mm on the vestibular side and 0.7 mm on the lingual side. Mandibular molar angulation increased 9°. There was a significant but little effect on mandibular incisor angulation (+1.9°), intercanine distance (+1.0 mm), and on canine angulation (+5.1°). Control subjects showed a tendency towards contraction of the transverse dimensions and a decrease in molar, canine, and inferior incisor angulation values.

ES coefficients were also calculated and are listed in Table 2. These variables (36–46 occlusal, 36–46 lingual, 33–43, molar angulation, canine angulation, incisor angulation) were characterized by a significant, medium or large, effect size.

Linear regression between MOT and mandibular first molar angulation showed a significant correlation ($p = 0.02$; $y = 0.529x - 2.050$, $R^2 = 0.441$), while no correlations between MOT and mandibular central incisor and canine angulations were found.

Table 1 Descriptive statistics and comparisons between groups at T1

		Control group			RPE group		
		$n = 15$ (7 M; 8 F)			$n = 33$ (15 M; 18 F)		
Variable	Unit	*N*	Mean	sd	*N*	Mean	sd
Age	years	15	8.3	1.2	33	8.8	1.1
T1-T2	months	15	12	2.4	33	15	2.4
36–46 (occlusal)	mm	15	46.9	2.4	33	47.1	2.9
36–46 (lingual)	mm	15	33.7	1.7	33	33.5	2.4
33–43	mm	14	27.0	1.5	16	26.5	2.0
36 angulation	°	15	−44.7	6.8	33	−47.6	8.8
46 angulation	°	15	−44.7	10.7	33	−48.4	6.9
33 angulation	°	13	−13.7	6.8	20	−15.8	6.8
43 angulation	°	13	−16.3	8.9	20	−17.1	12.0
31 angulation	°	15	−8.1	4.8	25	−9.0	6.2
41 angulation	°	15	−7.7	5.4	25	−8.7	7.6

All comparisons were not significant ($p > 0.05$, Student's *t* test for independent samples)

Discussion

All subjects were selected before the pubertal peak (CVS 1–3), because Baccetti et al. showed that in these three stages, RPE patients exhibit significant and more effective long-term changes at the skeletal level in both maxillary and circummaxillary structures [13, 17]. A control group of untreated patients with the same malocclusion was also used to identify confounding factors such as natural craniofacial growth and development during the study period.

A few data were found in biomedical literature about the RPE effects on mandibular molar, canine, and incisor angulation [10]. Otherwise, no data about changes in mandibular arch angulation in untreated unilateral crossbite malocclusion were reported in previous studies. In the current investigation, normal transversal arch growth was modified by crossbite malocclusion: the patients showed a tendency towards contraction of the transverse mandibular dimension and a decrease in molar, canine, and incisor angulation values. Previous longitudinal investigations found a slight but continued decrease in the intercanine width (0.5–1.5 mm) during the maturation of the permanent dentition [18–20]. Moorrees and Reed showed the intercanine width does not change from the age of 8 to 10 years, and the mandibular intermolar width increases 3–4 mm from 6 to 17 years of age [21].

Two long-term retrospective trials, by Geran et al. and O'Grady et al., reported the changes in untreated (Class I or Class II malocclusion but not crossbite) control groups [8, 9]. They found a reduction in mandibular arch perimeter, mainly related to the exfoliation of the mandibular second deciduous molars; a slight decrease in intercanine width and a very little or no increase in molar width. Unfortunately, the time interval (T1-T2) for decrements reported by Geran et al. for their control group was 5 years, and it cannot be directly compared to our time interval [8].

The current data allow to extend the information about longitudinal modifications in mandibular teeth angulation in untreated crossbite subjects. We found that the decrease in intercanine and intermolar width and part of arch perimeter reduction were mainly caused by the decrease in mandibular teeth angulation value.

When compared to the untreated group, the present RPE group showed significant net increases of intermolar width from pre-expansion (T1) to follow-up (T2): 1.9 mm, occlusal value, and 0.7 mm, lingual value. These increases were greater than some of the mandibular intermolar widths (occlusal) previously reported. Several authors reported an increase in mandibular molar width

Table 2 Mean and standard deviation (sd) of the differences between T2 and T1 values for each patient

		Control group		RPE group		Diff T2-T1	*t* test	Effect size	
	Unit	Mean	sd	Mean	sd		*p* value	*d* value	ES
36–46 (occlusal)	mm	−0.8	0.8	1.1	1.5	1.9	0.00	0.6	Large
36–46 (lingual)	mm	−0.1	0.4	0.6	1.2	0.7	0.00	0.8	Large
33–43	mm	−0.6	0.8	0.4	1.6	1.0	0.01	0.4	Medium
36 angulation	°	−3.3	5.2	6.2	5.8	9.5	0.00		
33 angulation	°	−6.0	5.0	0.7	5.5	6.7	0.00		
43 angulation	°	−2.7	6.6	0.7	7.4	3.4	ns		
46 angulation	°	−3.8	5.7	4.3	6.8	8.1	0.00		
31 angulation	°	−2.5	4.0	2.0	4.1	4.4	0.00		
41 angulation	°	−2.4	3.5	1.8	3.1	4.2	0.00		
Molar angulation (mean)	°	−3.5	5.5	5.2	6.3	8.8	0.00	0.6	Large
Canine angulation (mean)	°	−4.4	5.8	0.7	6.4	5.1	0.01	0.4	Medium
Incisor angulation (mean)	°	−2.4	3.7	1.9	3.6	4.3	0.00	0.5	Medium

Diff. T2-T1 mean differences between RPE and control groups; *ns* not significant, $p > 0.05$
d Cohen's effect size value, *ES* effect size

ranging from 0.24 to 2.8 mm [5, 6, 22, 23]. Wertz evaluated 48 patients for mandibular intermolar width changes after 3–4 months of RPE therapy (plus stabilization) and found 35 patients of 48 with no change, 12 of 48 with increases of 0.5 to 2.0 mm, and 1 of 48 with a decrease of 1.0 mm, but that study included children, teenagers, and adults [22]. Moussa et al. and Sandstrom et al. evaluated mandibular intermolar width change after RPE, but their patients also underwent fixed appliance therapy, and they are not directly comparable to our study [5, 23].

From T1 to T2, both the abovementioned increases suggest a slight first molar uprighting. This hypothesis is confirmed by the angulation values. From T1 to T2, the inferior first molar angulation was significantly increased, +8.8°. In a recent study, Lima et al., found that mandibular intermolar arch width increased significantly after RPE with a Haas-type expansion appliance and that the increase was followed by a slight decrease of the occlusal value, whereas the lingual value was maintained, thus suggesting a tendency to lingual angulation in the long term. [7]. For intercanine width (occlusal value), we found a little effect on intercanine distance (+1.0 mm) but not on canine angulation. Similar results were reported by Lima et al. [7]. Haas reported no change for intercanine width in 5 of 10 analyzed subjects; however, the age range was significant higher than in the present study [24]. All short-term and long-term studies, as

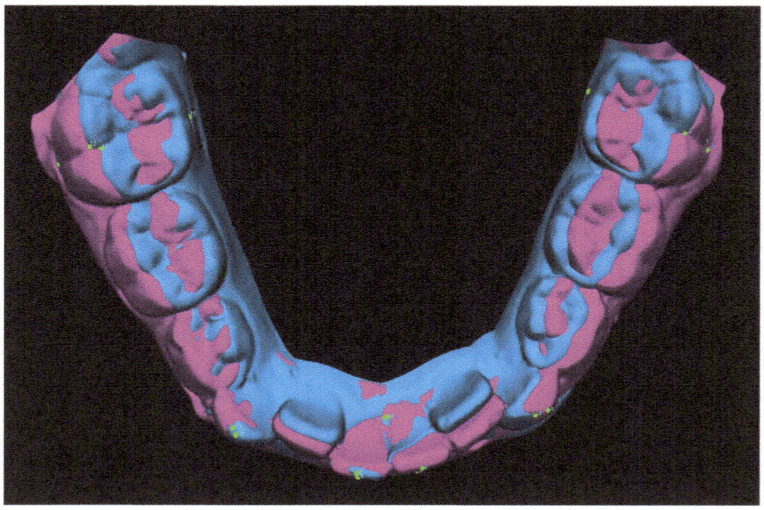

Fig. 2 Superimposition of pre- and post-treatment digital models of the mandible shown as example of mandibular response to RPE treatment

reviewed by Lima et al., showed very different value for intercanine width increases, ranging from 0.5 to 5 mm, which might be attributed to differences in sample selection criteria [7]. Lagravere et al. reported that most of the mandibular intermolar increments noted immediately after RPE were not statistically significant [25].

Baysal et al. evaluated the post RPE changes in mandibular arch widths and buccolingual inclinations of mandibular posterior teeth by using cone beam computed tomography (CBCT) images. They measured linear and angular changes in mandibular posterior region and after 6 months found an increase of the axial inclinations of all mandibular posterior teeth and of the mandibular transversal dimension [10]. There is a good accord between the current and the study by Baysal et al., and data are directly comparable, due to the similar 3D measurement. Although the radiation dose of a CBCT scan is lower than that of a CT scan, CBCT is not considered suitable for all orthodontic growing patients, and it is questionable whether it is appropriate to perform more than one CBCT scan per year. Thanks to our 3D cast analysis system, we can record the same variables using noninvasive procedures.

In the present study, RPE therapy allowed an increment in mandibular arch transversal dimensions and an increase in molar, canine, and incisor angulations. Angulation increase may result from two different biomechanical effects, postulated by Haas [24]. The first is an occlusal change. The direction of occlusal forces is altered by the maxillary expansion, so that the resultant force vector acting on the mandibular teeth (especially molars) is more vestibularly directed, because the occlusal aspect of the lingual cusp of upper first molars contacts the occlusal aspect of the facial cusp of the lower first molars. The second is a "lip bumper effect": the lateral movement of the maxillae widened the area of attachment of the buccal musculature [10]. These theses were indirectly supported by the correlation between molar angulation increase and months of therapy. Instead, the lack of correlation between MOT and incisor angulation could be related to a different tongue postural control in some patients (a possible swallowing disorder).

Although long-term longitudinal data are needed, the present study's sample size, along with the significant effect size of the difference in the decompensation of mandibular arch, enforces the statistical significance of the outcomes.

Conclusions

Mandibular intermolar arch width increased significantly in early mixed dentition patients with unilateral posterior crossbite after RPE (Haas-type) therapy. This increase was followed by a significant increase of molar angulation. There was a significant but little effect on intercanine distance and on canine and incisor angulations. The outcomes in spontaneous mandibular arch response to RPE showed a remarkable and positive clinical effect in mandibular arch-width dimensions in patients treated only with RPE. The molar angulation value increase was also correlated with the months of RPE therapy.

The RPE protocol has widening indirect effects on the mandibular first molars, canines, and incisors, 15 months after RPE therapy. The values of Cohen's of effect size confirmed the clinical indirect effects of RPE on mandibular arch in early mixed dentition patients with unilateral crossbite.

Competing interests

The authors declare that they have no competing interests.

Authors' contributions

AU has undertaken the clinical part of the study and wrote the manuscript. CS, TD, and RG have contributed to the design of the study and have revised the manuscript for submission. AM and LHG have made contributions to the acquisition and analysis of data and performed the statistical analysis and interpretation of data. All authors read and approved the final manuscript.

References

1. Agostino P, Ugolini A, Signori A, Silvestrini-Biavati A, Harrison JE, Riley P. Orthodontic treatment for posterior crossbites. Cochrane Database Syst Rev. 2014;8:8. doi:10.1002/14651858.CD000979.pub2. CD000979.
2. Egermark-Eriksson I, Carlsson GE, Magnusson T, Thilander B. A longitudinal study on malocclusion in relation to signs and symptoms of cranio-mandibular disorders in children and adolescents. Eur J Orthod. 1990;12:399–407.
3. Bishara SE, Burkey PS, Kharouf JG. Dental and facial asymmetries: a review. Angle Orthod. 1994;64:89–98.
4. McNamara JA. Maxillary transverse deficiency. Am J Orthod Dentofacial Orthop. 2000;117:567–70.
5. Moussa R, O'Reilly MT, Close JM. Long-term stability of rapid palatal expander treatment and edgewise mechanotherapy. Am J Orthod Dentofacial Orthop. 1995;108:478–88.
6. Basciftci FA, Karaman AI. Effects of a modified acrylic bonded rapid maxillary expansion appliance and vertical chin cap on dentofacial structures. Angle Orthod. 2002;72:61–71.
7. Lima AC, Lima AL, Filho RM, Oyen OJ. Spontaneous mandibular arch response after rapid palatal expansion: a long-term study on Class I malocclusion. Am J Orthod Dentofacial Orthop. 2004;26:576–82.
8. Geran RG, McNamara Jr JA, Baccetti T, Franchi L, Shapiro LM. A prospective long-term study on the effects of rapid maxillary expansion in the early mixed dentition. Am J Orthod Dentofacial Orthop. 2006;129:631–40.
9. O'Grady PW, McNamara JA, Baccetti T, Franchi L. A long-term evaluation of the mandibular Schwarz appliance and the acrylic splint expander in early mixed dentition patients. Am J Orthod Dentofacial Orthop. 2006;130:202–13.
10. Baysal A, Veli I, Ucar FI, Eruz M, Ozer T, Uysal T. Changes in mandibular transversal arch dimensions after rapid maxillary expansion procedure assessed through cone-beam computed tomography. Korean J Orthod. 2011;41:200–10.
11. Primožič J, Richmond S, Kau C H, Zhurov A, Ovsenik M. Three-dimensional evaluation of early crossbite correction: a longitudinal study. Eur J Orthod. 2011;a. doi:10.1093/ejo/cjq198
12. Primožič J, Baccetti T, Franchi L, Richmond S, Farčnik F, Ovsenik M. Three-dimensional assessment of palatal change in a controlled study of unilateral posterior crossbite correction in the primary dentition. Eur J Orthod. 2011; b. doi:10.1093/ejo/cjr125
13. Baccetti T, Franchi L, McNamara JA. The cervical vertebral maturation (CVM) method for the assessment of optimal treatment timing in dentofacial orthopedics. Seminar in Orthodontics. 2005;11:119–29.

14. Huanca Ghislanzoni LT, Lineberger M, Cevidanes LH, Mapelli A, Sforza C, McNamara Jr JA. Evaluation of tip and torque on virtual study models: a validation study. Prog Orthod. 2013;26:14–9.
15. McDougall PD, McNamara JA, Dierkes JM. Arch width development in Class II patients treated with the Fränkel appliance. Am J Orthod. 1982;82:10–22.
16. Cohen J. A power primer. Psychological Bullettin. 1992;112:155–9.
17. Baccetti T, Franchi L, Cameron CG, McNamara JA. Treatment timing for rapid maxillary expansion. Angle Orthod. 2001;71:343–50.
18. Barrow GV, White JR. Developmental changes of the maxillary and mandibular dental arches. Angle Orthod. 1952;22:41–6.
19. Sillman JH. Dimensional changes of the dental arches: longitudinal study from birth to 25 years. Am J Orthod. 1964;50:824–41.
20. Bishara SE, Jakobsen JR, Treder J, Nowak A. Arch width changes from 6 weeks to 45 years of age. Am J Orthod Dentofacial Orthop. 1997;111:401–9.
21. Moorrees CF, Reed RB. Changes in dental arch dimensions expressed on the basis of tooth eruption as a measure of biologic age. J Dent Res. 1965;44:129–41.
22. Wertz RA. Skeletal and dental changes accompanying rapid midpalatal suture opening. Am J Orthod. 1970;58:41–66.
23. Sandstrom RA, Klapper L, Papaconstantinou S. Expansion of the lower arch concurrent with rapid maxillary expansion. Am J Orthod Dentofacial Orthop. 1988;94:296–302.
24. Haas AJ. Rapid expansion of the maxillary dental arch and nasal cavity by opening the midpalatal suture. Angle Orthod. 1961;31:73–90.
25. Lagravère MO, Heo G, Major PW, Flores-Mir C. Meta-analysis of immediate changes with rapid maxillary expansion treatment. J Am Dent Assoc. 2006;137:44–53.

29

A retrospective analysis of factors influencing the success of autotransplanted posterior teeth

Mirco F. Ronchetti[1*], Silvio Valdec[2], Nikolaos Pandis[3], Michael Locher[2] and Hubertus van Waes[1]

Abstract

Background: Survival and success rates of tooth transplantations even after long follow-up periods have been shown to be very high. Nevertheless, it is important to analyse factors potentially influencing these rates. The aim of this study was to assess the influence on success of potential factors.

Methods: The research was based on a retrospective analysis of clinical and radiological data from a sample of 59 subjects (75 transplanted teeth). The follow-up period varied from 0.44 to 12.28 years (mean 3.95 years). Success rates were calculated and depicted with Kaplan-Meier plots. Log-rank tests were used to analyse the effect of root development stage, apex width, the use of enamel matrix proteins or the surgeon on success of transplantations.

Results: Results for success of premolar transplantations were comparable with already published data, while molars performed worse than shown in other studies. The surgeon performing the transplantation ($p = 0.001$) and tooth type ($p \leq 0.001$) were significantly associated with transplantation success. Use of enamel matrix proteins ($p = 0.10$), root development stage ($p = 0.13$), the recipient area ($p = 0.48$) and apex width ($p = 0.59$) were not significantly associated with success.

Conclusions: Molar transplantations were not as successful as premolar transplantations; however, success rates varied greatly depending on the surgeon's experience. The use of enamel matrix proteins as well as root development stage, the recipient area and apex width did not show significant associations with success of tooth transplantations.

Keywords: Tooth transplantation, Survival, Success factors

Background

The first documented case report of a homoplastic tooth transplantation was described by Fauchard in 1728 in his book *Le Chirurgien Dentiste* [1]. This procedure of tooth autotransplantation is defined as the transfer of a donor tooth to a recipient area in the same individual with the latter being either an extraction site or a surgically prepared socket. Starting from the 1970s and the publications of Slagsvold and Bjercke [2–4] and later with the studies of Andreasen and Paulsen [5–8], the autotransplantation of premolars has become a well-accepted and reliable procedure to replace either missing incisors or premolars. Survival of transplanted premolars has been shown to be high even decades after the surgery. Czochrowska showed a 90 % survival and a 79 % success rate after a mean observation period of 26.4 years post transplantation, indicating that some transplants were kept in situ over long periods of time despite clinical or radiographic signs of failure (no success). Autotransplantation also compared favourably with other procedures for replacement of missing teeth. Furthermore, when comparing clinical parameters of transplanted to non-transplanted teeth, no clinical or radiographic difference except for pulp obliteration was evident [9]. The advantage of autotransplantation compared to osseointegrated implants is the capacity of transplants for functional adaptation, potentially continuous eruption and therefore superior ridge preservation

* Correspondence: mirco.ronchetti@gmx.ch
[1]Clinic of Orthodontics and Paediatric Dentistry, Center of Dental Medicine, Faculty of Medicine, University of Zürich, Zürich, Switzerland
Full list of author information is available at the end of the article

[7–11]. In addition, transplantation of molars, if well selected, has been shown by several authors to be a good treatment option for missing teeth with success ranging from 79 to 100 % [12–14].

Prior studies analysing transplantations have claimed three fourths root length as being the ideal development stage for transplantation [5, 15].

Treatment with enamel matrix proteins like Emdogain® (Biora, Malmö, Sweden; incorporated into Straumann Biologic Division since 2004) has been shown to exhibit an activating effect on periodontal cells [16–20]. Positive effects were also shown for the treatment of infrabony defects [21] as well as for prevention of ankyloses or root resorptions after intentional transplantation or treatment of avulsed teeth [22, 23]. Those findings however have been questioned by other investigators [24–26].

Although the published findings indicate very high success (tooth in situ without any clinical or radiographic sign of failure) and survival rates (tooth in situ with or without presence of clinical or radiographic signs of failure like ankylosis, periodontal issues, root resorption or crown/root ratio >1), it is important to identify all factors determining success and survival rates of tooth transplantations. These factors are the key to higher clinical success and to prevention of unnecessary failures.

The aim of this study was to record success rates of tooth transplantations and to examine parameters which may be associated with success.

Methods

This research project was reviewed and approved by the ethics committee of the canton of Zurich, Switzerland.

All consecutive patients from the dental clinic of the University of Zürich who had undergone one or more tooth transplantations were included in order to minimize selection bias. The search was performed by a computer specialist on the patients' database system, where all transplantations had been registered. The database was introduced in January 2000, and all registered transplantation cases up to 31 December 2012 were included. Before the year 2000, no complete patient database was available.

The following information was extracted from the retrieved files: date of birth; date of transplantation; age at transplantation; numeric number of the transplanted tooth; recipient area; root length in millimetres (measured on single X-rays) and development stage at transplantation according to Moorrees et al. [27]; apex width in millimetres grouped into ≥2 or <2 mm; post treatment development, namely root canal obliteration, root resorption, ankylosis and endodontic issues with subsequent root canal treatment including the dates of these events; and surgeon performing the surgery. Transplantations were performed by three surgeons with different levels of experience. Surgeon 1 is the clinical director

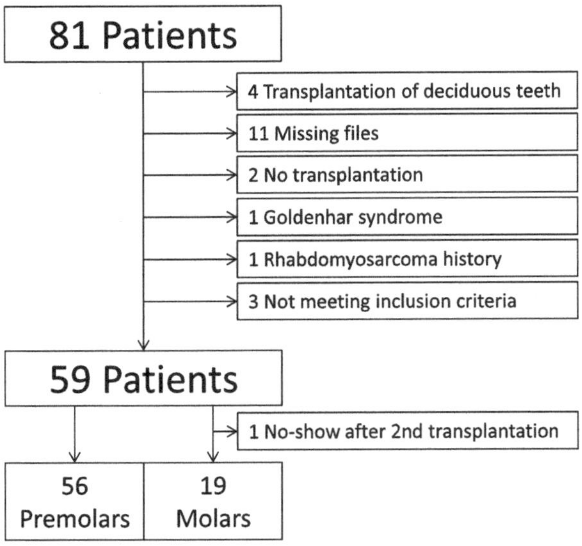

Fig. 1 Patient flow chart

of the Clinic of Paediatric Dentistry with long experience in transplantations; surgeon 2 was a postgraduate student at the Clinic of Paediatric Dentistry; and surgeon 3 was the former director of the Clinic of Oral Surgery with broad surgical experience.

The individual success period of each transplanted tooth was defined as the time period from the transplantation to the latest exam appointment where the tooth was in situ with no clinical signs of failure. Progressive root resorption, periodontal problems, ankylosis and crown to root ratio greater than 1.0 were considered to be failures [9, 28], whereas endodontic treatment was not rated as a failure.

The radiographic evaluation was carried out by two researchers independently. Results were subsequently discussed until consensus was reached.

Data were coded in Excel (version 14.0.6112.5000, Redmond, WA, USA) and analysed using STATA statistical

Table 1 Distribution of transplantations per location, use of enamel matrix proteins and surgeon

	All teeth (75)	Premolars (56)	Molars (19)
Recipient area			
Maxilla	10 (13.5 %)	5 (8.9 %)	5 (26.3 %)
Mandible	65 (86.7 %)	51 (91.1 %)	14 (73.7 %)
Enamel matrix proteins			
Yes	34 (45.3 %)	27 (48.2 %)	7 (36.8 %)
No	41 (64.7 %)	29 (51.8 %)	12 (63.2 %)
Surgeon			
1	31 (41.3 %)	28 (50.0 %)	3 (15.9 %)
2	22 (29.3 %)	13 (23.2 %)	9 (47.4 %)
3	22 (29.3 %)	15 (26.8 %)	7 (36.8 %)

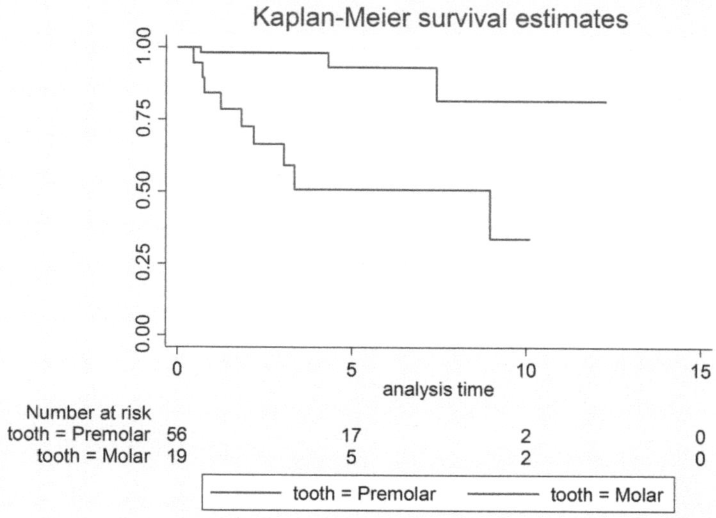

Fig. 2 Kaplan-Meier plot comparing success of premolars and molars

software (version 14.0, STATA Corp, College Station, TX, USA). Descriptive statistics such as mean, median, standard deviation and absolute and relative frequencies were computed. Kaplan-Meier plots were produced, and association between success and root development stages, application of enamel matrix proteins, apex width, recipient area and surgeon were examined using the log-rank test. The root development stage according to Moorrees [27] was grouped into shorter than three fourths (corresponding to Moorrees' levels 1 and 2), three fourths (corresponding to Moorrees' level 3) and longer than three fourths (corresponding to Moorrees' levels 4–6) while apex width at transplantation was divided into $x < 2$ mm and $x \geq 2$ mm. Results of statistical analyses with p values smaller than 0.05 were considered to be statistically significant.

Results

Initially, 81 patients were identified, and after exclusions, 59 patients with 75 transplanted teeth (56 premolars, 19 molars) were included. Data of the latter were analysed in this study. Fourteen patients had undergone a transplantation of molars (wisdom teeth) and 53 of premolars. Reasons for drop outs can be seen in Fig. 1. Overall mean age at transplantation was 13.53 years (SD 2.67), the mean age for premolar transplantation being 12.38 years (SD 1.33) and for molars being 16.91 years (SD 2.78). Mean observation time for premolars was 4.06 years (SD 2.44, range 0.64–12.28 years), while for molars the mean was 3.63 years (SD 3.00, range 0.44–10.10 years). Mean observation time for all included teeth was 3.95 years (SD 2.58, range 0.44–12.28 years). Table 1 displays the distribution of transplantations per location, use of enamel matrix proteins and surgeon. Kaplan-Meier cumulative success rate estimation at 10 years for all teeth was 59.6 %. When success was computed for each tooth type separately, premolars showed a 10-year success rate of 81.6 %, whereas molars showed 33.8 % for the same time period, the difference being highly significant ($p < 0.001$) (Fig. 2). No significant evidence of association was observed between success and root development stage ($p = 0.13$), use of enamel matrix proteins ($p = 0.10$), apex width ($p = 0.59$) or the recipient area ($p = 0.48$). However, strong associations between success and surgeon ($p = 0.001$) and success and tooth type ($p < 0.001$) were identified (Table 2). Kaplan-Meier plots for root development, use of enamel matrix proteins, apex width and surgeon are shown in Figs. 3, 4, 5, 6 and 7.

Discussion

Our sample showed a vast range of observation periods. This can be explained by the fact that failures, when they happened, often occurred at an early stage

Table 2 Analysis of associations between success and potentially influencing factors using the log-rank test. p values <0.05 were considered to be statistically significant

Success	p value
Tooth type (premolars/molars)	<0.001
Root development (<3/4, 3/4, >3/4)	0.13
Enamel matrix protein use (yes/no)	0.10
Apex width (>2/<2 mm)	0.59
Recipient area (maxilla/mandible)	0.48
Surgeon (1, 2, 3)	0.001

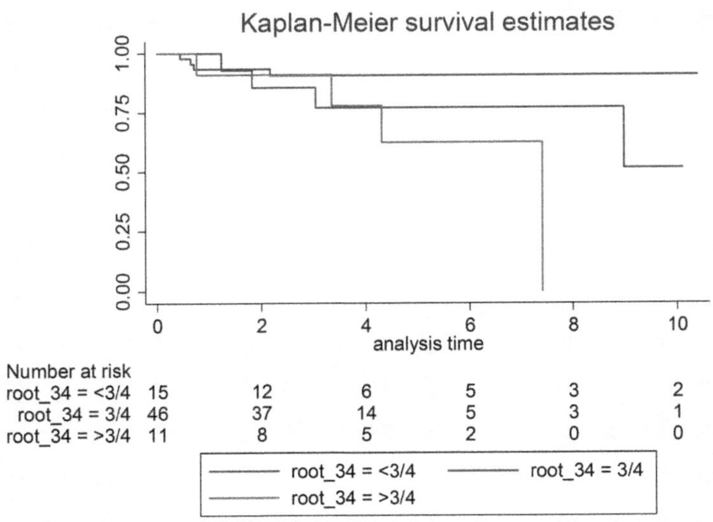

Fig. 3 Kaplan-Meier plot comparing success of three grouped root development stages

after transplantation. In contrary, some teeth had been observed over a long period of time for protocol reasons (consecutive patients). Since only few successful transplantations had observation times shorter than 1 year and by analysing censored data using Kaplan-Meier and log-rank tests with failure as the event, results account for the wide range of observation periods.

Several factors are likely to be associated with survival and success of tooth transplantations. We examined the effect of tooth type, root development stage, recipient area, surgical trauma (surgical skill) and use of intraoperative drugs on success of tooth transplantations.

Premolars with an estimated 10-year success rate of 81.6 % compared favourably to molars with an estimated 10-year success rate of 33.8 %. Thus, while our results for premolars were comparable with most published studies [29], molars in other studies with similar observation periods showed better outcomes [12–14]. However, it should be noted that the first and only failure for molar transplantations conducted by surgeon 3 (most experienced surgeon) occurred after an observation time of 8.97 years while 4 failures out of 9 molar transplantations were seen for surgeon 2 (least experienced surgeon) within a 3.35-year period. Thus, the

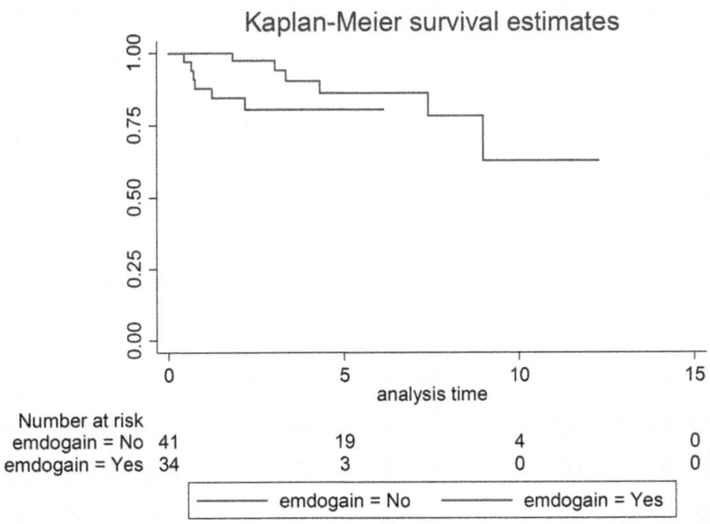

Fig. 4 Kaplan-Meier plot comparing success of transplantations with or without use of enamel matrix proteins

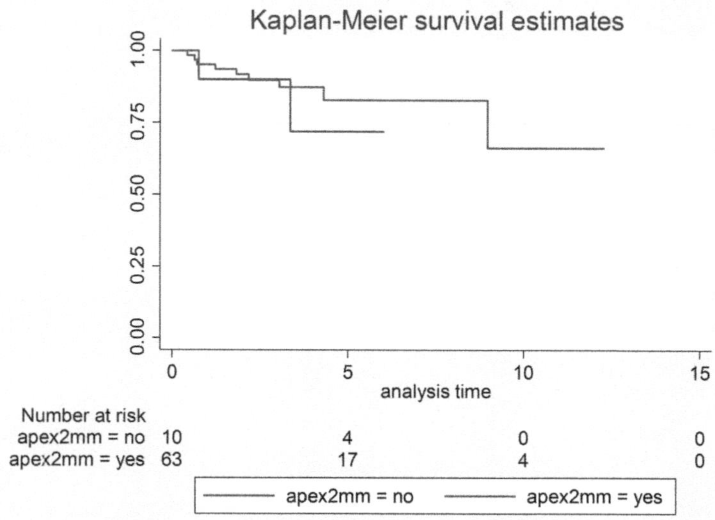

Fig. 5 Kaplan-Meier plot comparing success of teeth with apex larger or smaller than 2 mm

lower success and survival rates might also reflect the individual surgical skill, learning curve or capacity of case selection of the corresponding surgeon. This interpretation is also underlined by combining the highly significant difference between surgeons ($p = 0.001$) when analysed with the log-rank test (Table 2) with the curves on Fig. 7. While surgeons 1 and 2 (experienced surgeons) seem to perform equally well, surgeon 2 (least experienced surgeon) performed consistently worse. The higher failure rate of molar transplantations compared to premolar transplantations can also be related to more complex root anatomy, potentially leading to more tissue trauma as has been suggested by Denys [15].

The use of enamel matrix proteins did not improve success in our sample. However, because of the small number of events, results should be interpreted with caution. Nevertheless, since prior studies without use of enamel matrix proteins performed equally well for premolars and better than our sample for molars [6, 12, 30], it is still uncertain whether the use of this agent for tooth transplantations is beneficial and the higher cost justified [26, 31–33]. It is also noteworthy to mention

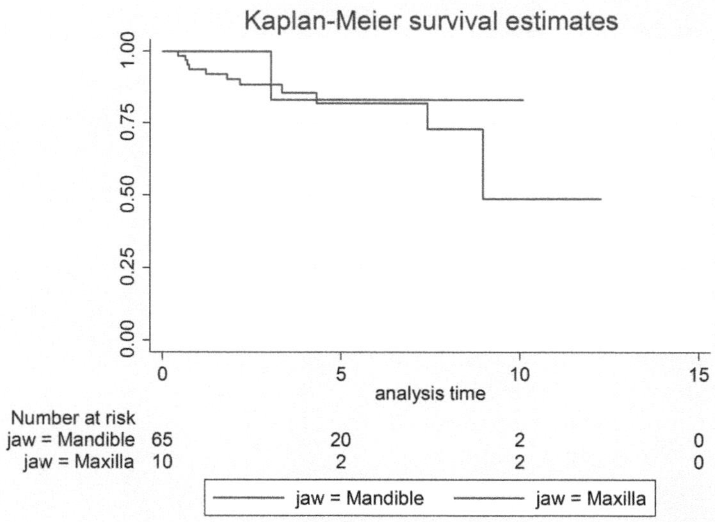

Fig. 6 Kaplan-Meier plot comparing success of the recipient sites (mandible/maxilla)

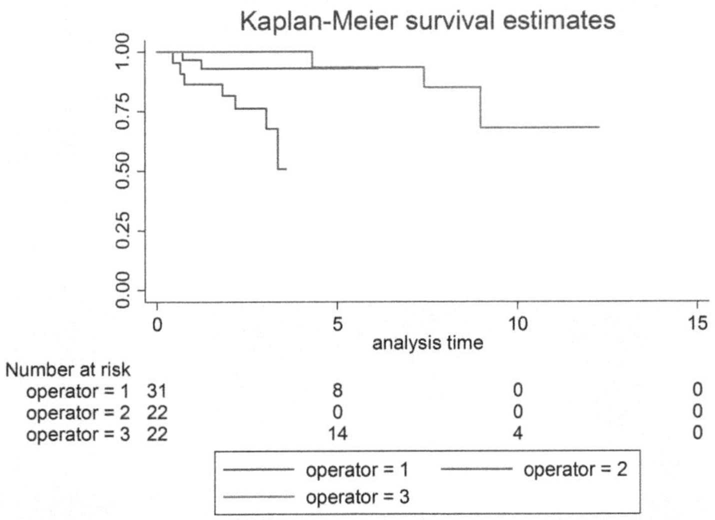

Fig. 7 Kaplan-Meier plot comparing success of the three surgeons

that in Fig. 4 cases where the agent was used seemed to perform worse, though no significance was reached. Nevertheless, some investigators have suggested the use of enamel matrix proteins when treating ankylosed teeth [22, 34]. Therefore, the effect of this substance remains uncertain, and large and well-designed randomized clinical trials should be considered.

Our study found no significant associations between success and root development; however, it is a common clinical practice at our clinic to avoid transplantation of teeth with complete root formation, and thus, to reach a significant level of association as shown in two recent studies [15, 28] was difficult. Nevertheless, on the Kaplan-Meier plot, a tendency of root development greater than three fourths for worse success could be seen, though results were not significant (Fig. 3).

Limitations

Since the study was retrospective, it is susceptible to limitations interconnected with this type of investigation. By defining endodontic treatment as not being a failure, a potential bias may arise since endodontically treated teeth can develop complications which can lead to necessity for extraction or such rated as failure according to the applied grading system. Nevertheless, in a study by Andreasen [6], teeth receiving endodontic treatment within 4 weeks from transplantation showed a 4-year survival rate of 95 %; therefore, endodontic treatment was not judged as a failure. We made an effort to include all cases to minimize selection bias; however, confounding was difficult to adjust for the given small number of events which gave unstable results in the multivariable analyses that were omitted. The sample size especially for molars and the number of events were small which suggests caution when interpreting the results. However, this exploratory study has value in terms of suggesting areas of focus for future studies.

Conclusions

Molar transplantations were not as successful as premolar transplantations; however, success rates also varied greatly depending on the surgeon's experience. In our sample, the use of enamel matrix proteins as well as root development stage, the recipient area and apex width did not show significant associations with success of tooth transplantations.

Competing interests

The authors declare that they have no competing interests.

Authors' contributions

MR: Was involved in the design, coordination, data collection, statistical analysis and interpretation of the study and drafting of the manuscript. SV: Was involved in data collection, analysis of data and critically reviewed the manuscript. NP: Was involved in statistical analysis, interpretation and drafting of the manuscript. ML: Was involved in data collection and critically reviewed the manuscript. HvW: Was involved in the design, data collection and interpretation, critically reviewed the manuscript and was one of the surgeons performing the transplantations. All authors read and approved the final manuscript.

Author details

[1]Clinic of Orthodontics and Paediatric Dentistry, Center of Dental Medicine, Faculty of Medicine, University of Zürich, Zürich, Switzerland. [2]Clinic of Oral Surgery, Center of Dental Medicine, Faculty of Medicine, University of Zürich, Zürich, Switzerland. [3]Department of Orthodontics and Dentofacial Orthopedics, Dental School/Medical Faculty, University of Bern, Bern, Switzerland.

References

1. Pape HD, Heiss R. History of tooth transplantation. Fortschr Kiefer Gesichtschir. 1976;20:121–5.
2. Slagsvold O, Bjercke B. Autotransplantation of premolars with partly formed roots. A radiographic study of root growth. Am J Orthod. 1974;66(4):355–66.
3. Slagsvold O, Bjercke B. Applicability of autotransplantation in cases of missing upper anterior teeth. Am J Orthod. 1978;74(4):410–21.
4. Slagsvold O, Bjercke B. Indications for autotransplantation in cases of missing premolars. Am J Orthod. 1978;74(3):241–57.
5. Andreasen JO, Paulsen HU, Yu Z, Ahlquist R, Bayer T, Schwartz O. A long-term study of 370 autotransplanted premolars. Part I. Surgical procedures and standardized techniques for monitoring healing. Eur J Orthod. 1990;12(1):3–13.
6. Andreasen JO, Paulsen HU, Yu Z, Bayer T, Schwartz O. A long-term study of 370 autotransplanted premolars. Part II. Tooth survival and pulp healing subsequent to transplantation. Eur J Orthod. 1990;12(1):14–24.
7. Andreasen JO, Paulsen HU, Yu Z, Schwartz O. A long-term study of 370 autotransplanted premolars. Part III. Periodontal healing subsequent to transplantation. Eur J Orthod. 1990;12(1):25–37.
8. Andreasen JO, Paulsen HU, Yu Z, Bayer T. A long-term study of 370 autotransplanted premolars. Part IV. Root development subsequent to transplantation. Eur J Orthod. 1990;12(1):38–50.
9. Czochrowska EM, Stenvik A, Bjercke B, Zachrisson BU. Outcome of tooth transplantation: survival and success rates 17–41 years posttreatment. Am J Orthod Dentofacial Orthop. 2002;121(2):110–9. quiz 93.
10. Tsukiboshi M. Autotransplantation of teeth: requirements for predictable success. Dent Traumatol. 2002;18(4):157–80.
11. Zachrisson BU, Stenvik A, Haanaes HR. Management of missing maxillary anterior teeth with emphasis on autotransplantation. Am J Orthod Dentofacial Orthop. 2004;126(3):284–8. doi:10.1016/S0889540604005244.
12. Andreasen JO, Hjorting-Hansen E, Jolst O. A clinical and radiographic study of 76 autotransplanted third molars. Scand J Dent Res. 1970;78(6):512–23.
13. Bauss O, Engelke W, Fenske C, Schilke R, Schwestka-Polly R. Autotransplantation of immature third molars into edentulous and atrophied jaw sections. Int J Oral Maxillofac Surg. 2004;33(6):558–63. doi:10.1016/j.ijom.2003.10.008.
14. Schutz S, Beck I, Kuhl S, Filippi A. Results after wisdom tooth transplantation. A retrospective study. Schweiz Monatsschr Zahnmed. 2013;123(4):303–13.
15. Denys D, Shahbazian M, Jacobs R, Laenen A, Wyatt J, Vinckier F, et al. Importance of root development in autotransplantations: a retrospective study of 137 teeth with a follow-up period varying from 1 week to 14 years. Eur J Orthod. 2013;35(5):680–8. doi:10.1093/ejo/cjs112.
16. Palioto DB, Rodrigues TL, Marchesan JT, Beloti MM, de Oliveira PT, Rosa AL. Effects of enamel matrix derivative and transforming growth factor-beta1 on human osteoblastic cells. Head Face Med. 2011;7:13. doi:10.1186/1746-160X-7-13.
17. Rodrigues TL, Marchesan JT, Coletta RD, Novaes Jr AB, Grisi MF, Souza SL, et al. Effects of enamel matrix derivative and transforming growth factor-beta1 on human periodontal ligament fibroblasts. J Clin Periodontol. 2007;34(6):514–22. doi:10.1111/j.1600-051X.2007.01090.x.
18. Takayanagi K, Osawa G, Nakaya H, Cochran DL, Kamoi K, Oates TW. Effects of enamel matrix derivative on bone-related mRNA expression in human periodontal ligament cells in vitro. J Periodontol. 2006;77(5):891–8. doi:10.1902/jop.2006.050244.
19. Zeldich E, Koren R, Dard M, Weinberg E, Weinreb M, Nemcovsky CE. Enamel matrix derivative induces the expression of tissue inhibitor of matrix metalloproteinase-3 in human gingival fibroblasts via extracellular signal-regulated kinase. J Periodontal Res. 2010;45(2):200–6. doi:10.1111/j.1600-0765.2009.01218.x.
20. Zeldich E, Koren R, Nemcovsky C, Weinreb M. Enamel matrix derivative stimulates human gingival fibroblast proliferation via ERK. J Dent Res. 2007;86(1):41–6.
21. Sculean A, Schwarz F, Becker J, Brecx M. The application of an enamel matrix protein derivative (Emdogain) in regenerative periodontal therapy: a review. Med Princ Pract. 2007;16(3):167–80. doi:10.1159/000100386.
22. Filippi A, Pohl Y, von Arx T. Treatment of replacement resorption with Emdogain—a prospective clinical study. Dent Traumatol. 2002;18(3):138–43.
23. von Buren A, Krastl G, Kuhl S, Filippi A. Management of avulsions in Switzerland 2007–2010. Dent Traumatol. 2014;30(3):176–81. doi:10.1111/edt.12080.
24. Esposito M, Grusovin MG, Coulthard P, Worthington HV. Enamel matrix derivative (Emdogain) for periodontal tissue regeneration in intrabony defects. Cochrane Database Syst Rev. 2005;4:CD003875. doi:10.1002/14651858.CD003875.pub2.
25. Zanatta FB, de Souza FG, Pinto TM, Antoniazzi RP, Rosing CK. Do the clinical effects of enamel matrix derivatives in infrabony defects decrease overtime? A systematic review and meta-analysis. Braz Dent J. 2013;24(5):446–55. doi:10.1590/0103-6440201302192.
26. Schjott M, Andreasen JO. Emdogain does not prevent progressive root resorption after replantation of avulsed teeth: a clinical study. Dent Traumatol. 2005;21(1):46–50. doi:10.1111/j.1600-9657.2004.00295.x.
27. Moorrees CF, Fanning EA, Hunt Jr EE. Age variation of formation stages for ten permanent teeth. J Dent Res. 1963;42:1490–502.
28. Kallu R, Vinckier F, Politis C, Mwalili S, Willems G. Tooth transplantations: a descriptive retrospective study. Int J Oral Maxillofac Surg. 2005;34(7):745–55. doi:10.1016/j.ijom.2005.03.009.
29. Cross D, El-Angbawi A, McLaughlin P, Keightley A, Brocklebank L, Whitters J, et al. Developments in autotransplantation of teeth. Surgeon. 2013;11(1):49–55. doi:10.1016/j.surge.2012.10.003.
30. Lundberg T, Isaksson S. A clinical follow-up study of 278 autotransplanted teeth. Br J Oral Maxillofac Surg. 1996;34(2):181–5.
31. Ferreira MMFB, Lina C, Barbara O, Palmeirao CE. The effect of Emdogain gel on periodontal regeneration in autogenous transplanted dog's teeth. Indian J Dent Res. 2014;25(5):589–93.
32. Iqbal MK, Bamaas N. Effect of enamel matrix derivative (EMDOGAIN) upon periodontal healing after replantation of permanent incisors in beagle dogs. Dent Traumatol. 2001;17(1):36–45.
33. Wiegand A, Attin T. Efficacy of enamel matrix derivatives (Emdogain) in treatment of replanted teeth—a systematic review based on animal studies. Dent Traumatol. 2008;24(5):498–502. doi:10.1111/j.1600-9657.2008.00662.x.
34. Filippi A, Pohl Y, von Arx T. Treatment of replacement resorption by intentional replantation, resection of the ankylosed sites, and Emdogain—results of a 6-year survey. Dent Traumatol. 2006;22(6):307–11. doi:10.1111/j.1600-9657.2005.00363.x.

30

Optical properties of orthodontic aligners—spectrophotometry analysis of three types before and after aging

Luca Lombardo[1], Angela Arreghini[1*], Roberta Maccarrone[1], Anna Bianchi[2], Santo Scalia[2] and Giuseppe Siciliani[1]

Abstract

Background: The aim was to assess and compare absorbance and transmittance values of three types of clear orthodontic aligners before and after two cycles of in vitro aging.

Methods: Nine samples of orthodontic aligners from three different manufacturers (*Invisalign*, Align Technology, Santa Clara, CA, USA; *All-In*, Micerium, Avegno, GE, Italy; *F22 Aligner*, Sweden & Martina, Due Carrare, PD, Italy) were selected, and each sample was subjected to spectrophotometry analysis of both its transmittance and absorbance a total of 27 times. Samples were subsequently aged in vitro at a constant temperature in artificial saliva supplemented with food colouring for two cycles of 14 days each. The spectrophotometry protocol was then repeated, and the resulting data were analysed and compared by means of ANOVA ($p < 0.05$).

Results: All types of aligners tested yielded lower transmittance and higher absorbance values after aging, but the difference was not significant in any case. That being said, the F22 aligners were found to be most transparent, both before and after aging, followed by Invisalign and All-In, and these differences were statistically significant.

Conclusions: Commercial aligners possess significantly different optical, and therefore aesthetic, properties, both as delivered and following aging.

Keywords: Orthodontic aligners, Transparency, Spectrophotometry, F22 Aligner

Background

The rising demand among adult patients for "invisible" orthodontic treatment has led to an exponential growth in the clear aligner market [1]. Indeed, these aligners have low aesthetic impact [2–4], as well as being able to effectively and progressively guide the teeth into their programmed positions. They are also removable and therefore do not hamper oral hygiene maintenance, in turn reducing the risk of white spots, caries, gingivitis and periodontal disease. Being manufactured sequentially to specification from digital malocclusion set-ups and delivered direct from the factory, they are also convenient for the orthodontist, who has to deal with none of the bracket- and archwire-related issues that plague fixed appliances [5].

* Correspondence: angela_arreghini@yahoo.com
[1]Postgraduate School of Orthodontics, University of Ferrara, Via Montebello 31, 44100 Ferrara, Italy
Full list of author information is available at the end of the article

Although clear aligners designed on manual set-ups had long been in use [6], it was only with the advent of Align Technology's entirely digital Invisalign process—exploiting digital scans of patients' models, CAD–CAM technology and 3D printing—that they became an accepted orthodontic technique [7–9]. Upon expiry of the Invisalign patent, a profusion of other aligner manufacturers sprang up, offering products based on different scanning technologies, set-up software, material, thickness, transparency and finishing quality and technique. In general, aligner materials are resin polymers, which, not being inert, are subject to changes in the warmth, humidity, mastication forces and prolonged contact with salivary enzymes in the oral environment [10]. The first aligners were made out of single-layer rigid polyurethane (from methylene diphenyl diisocyanate and 1,6-hexanediol) sheets. Although polyurethane is not inert, and is therefore subject to alteration in vivo, it does seem to be relatively stable in saliva, even though its hydrophilic tendencies will depend on the chemical bonds within it [11].

Nevertheless, Align Technology issued first Exceed-30 (EX30), a flexible material with improved transparency and fracture resistance, and then, in 2012, after 8 years of experimentation, a newly patented material called SmartTrack®. This is a thermoplastic polyurethane with an integrated elastomer that the firm maintains which is able to apply continuous light forces to the teeth and whose greater elasticity should guarantee greater predictability in terms of orthodontic movements [8–12]. At the present time, however, the other manufacturers make greater use of polyethylene terephthalate glycol (PeT-G) [13], followed by polypropylene (PP), polycarbonate (PC), thermoplastic polyurethanes (TPU), ethylene vinyl acetate (EVA) and many more. Aligner thickness tends to vary between 0.50 and 1.5 mm [14].

A relative newcomer to the market, the F22 Aligner, has been designed and manufactured by the Postgraduate School of Orthodontics at the University of Ferrara, Italy. Fruit of long years of experience in the field, it is made out of a chemically inert rigid polyurethane that possesses excellent properties such as transparency, ductility and resistance to stress [15, 16].

Although the mechanical (force release, rigidity, dimensional stability and wear) and chemical (stability) properties of such aligners have been extensively investigated [11, 17, 18], no scientific, reproducible studies into their transparency, i.e. the ability of light to pass through their constituent material, have yet been conducted [19]. Nevertheless, the transparency of these aligners is the major key to their success. Not all materials possess the same chemical characteristics, either before or after wear, and it therefore follows that the optical properties, alongside their mechanical properties, of different aligners will be affected differently by the masticatory stress, salivary enzymes, food colourings, etc. that they are exposed to in the oral environment during their 14 consecutive days of wear (at least 22 h per day, according to the manufacturers' recommendations) [11]. Hence, we set out to compare the transmittance and absorbance of various samples of clear aligners, both as received and after two 14-day cycles of in vitro aging, to determine whether they present any differences in terms of colour stability and aesthetic properties over time.

Methods

Three identical samples of three different aligners from three different manufacturers were selected: three from Invisalign (Align Technology, Santa Clara, CA, USA), three from All-In (Micerium, Avegno, GE, Italy) and three from F22 (Sweden & Martina, Due Carrare, PD, Italy), designed for patients with well-aligned incisors and similar arch forms and dimensions (Fig. 1).

The optical properties (absorbance and transmittance) of each sample of each aligner were assessed by means of spectrophotometry (Jasco UV–vis V630PC, Tokyo, Japan) (Fig. 2). The spectrophotometer in question has the following features: double beam, single monochromator, deuterium light source for UV range and halogen lamp for visible range, and a detector positioned 1 cm behind the detection window. The visible spectrum of light, i.e. of wavelength 400–700 nm, was considered, and the absorbance and transmittance of each sample were automatically recorded by the spectrophotometer. The *transmittance* is the fraction of incident light, at an established wavelength, that passes through the material; the greater the transmittance, the more transparent the material. Conversely, the greater the *absorbance*—the logarithmic inverse of the transmittance—the less transparent the material [20].

Before these measurements were made, each aligner was sectioned from canine to canine with a rotating saw to remove the lingual portion and thereby expose the labial wall. Each aligner was cleaned by running under a jet of distilled water and dried with a jet of air. Each sample was then placed in a specially designed support, 35 mm in height, used to standardize the position of the aligner inside the spectrophotometer with respect to the detection window. The aligners were positioned so that the labial surface of the lower incisors was vertical and in contact with the incident light collection window (Fig. 3). Each sample was measured three times consecutively, varying the inclination of the aligner with respect to the light beam slightly, giving a total of 27 absorbance measurements and 27 transmittance measurements.

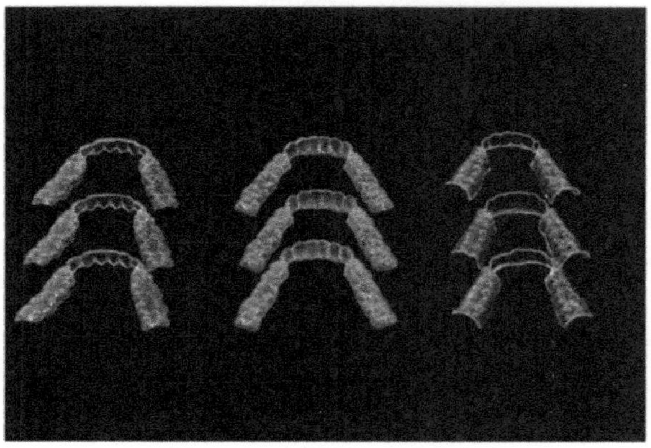

Fig. 1 The nine aligner samples used in the experiment

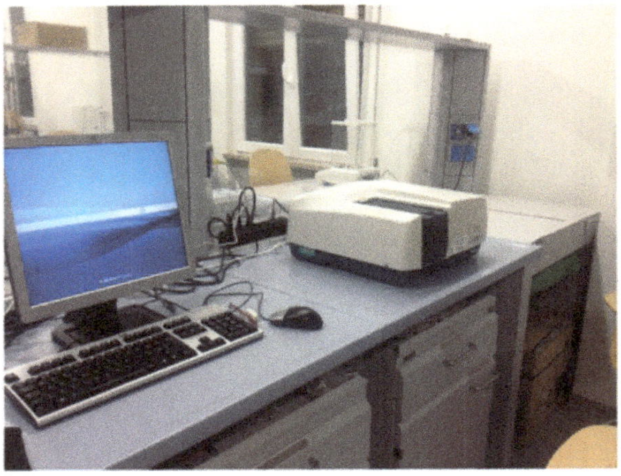

Fig. 2 The UV–vis Jasco mod.V630PC spectrophotometer

The spectrophotometer was calibrated by means of the white light spectrum before each measurement.

The values yielded by the three aligner types as received were then compared via Spectra Manager II software (Jasco, Tokyo, Japan), which was used to plot an average curve (±SD) of the nine measurements made for each type.

The same nine aligners were then immersed in a glass container measuring 30 cm × 17 cm × 14 cm filled with Oral Balance artificial saliva (Biotène Oral Balance, Biopharm Sas, Peschiera Borromeo, Italy), i.e. 250 ml of gel diluted in 1 L of water, to which brown food colouring was added in a 1:1 ratio. The saliva bath was kept at a constant temperature via an immersion heat source connected to a thermostat set at 37 °C ± 1 °C, and the aligners were left in situ for 14 consecutive days. As per previously published aging protocols (Fig. 4a, b) [11], this procedure was repeated, this time with yellow rather than brown food colouring, thereby subjecting the aligners to a total of two 14-day aging cycles.

After aging, the aligners were rinsed with distilled water, dried with an air jet and then subjected once again to the above-described spectrophotometry protocol. Transmittance and absorbance curves generated

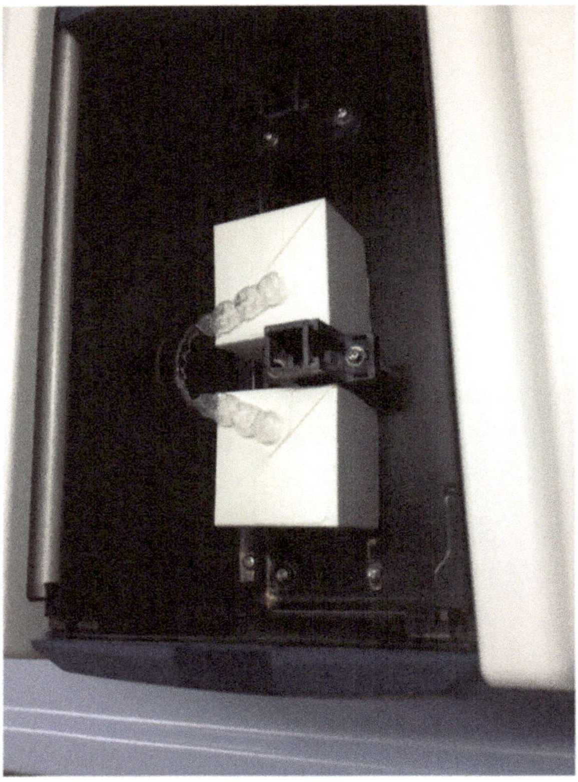

Fig. 3 Positioning the samples in the spectrophotometer

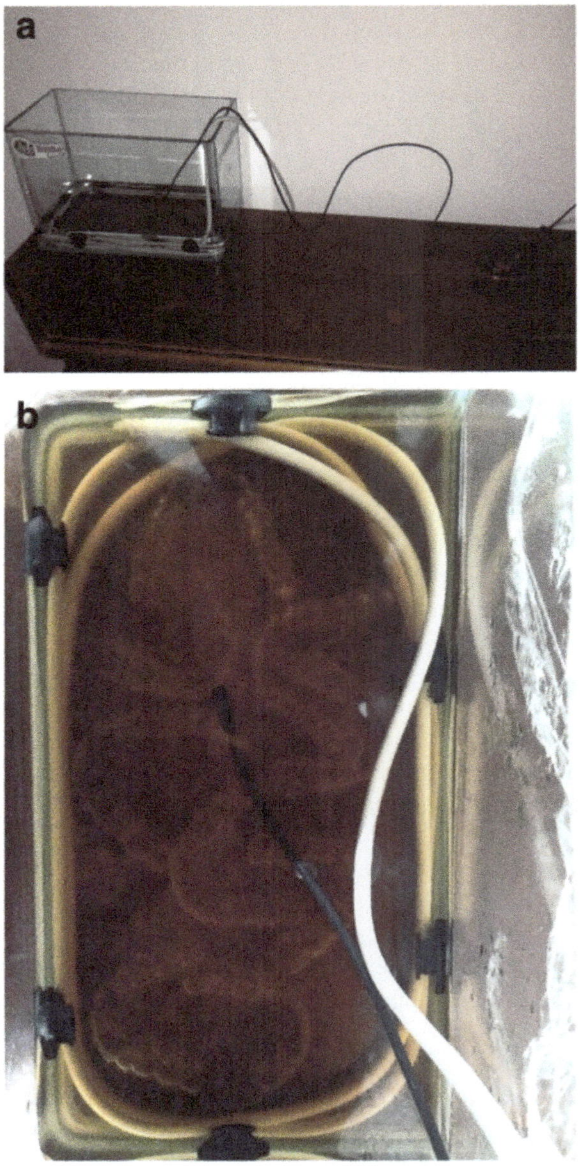

Fig. 4 a Saliva bath used to age the samples. **b** Aging protocol

Table 1 Absorbance values of the three aligners before and after in vitro aging

Aligner	Absorbance at 400 nm (±SD)			Absorbance at 700 nm (±SD)		
	As received	After aging	Significance	As received	After aging	Significance
All-In	0.265 ± 0.036	0.278 ± 0.011	N.S.	0.209 ± 0.030	0.215 ± 0.008	N.S.
Invisalign	0.172 ± 0.004	0.190 ± 0.03	N.S.	0.143 ± 0.004	0.155 ± 0.023	N.S.
F22	0.107 ± 0.023	0.104 ± 0.003	N.S.	0.090 ± 0.024	0.081 ± 0.004	N.S.

N.S. not significant variation

before and after aging were compared, and ANOVA (Graph Pad) was used to statistically analyse the data ($p < 0.05$).

Results

The absorbance data recorded by the spectrophotometer (Tables 1 and 2) at 400 nm and 700 nm—selected as the limits of the measurement range—were used to generate average curves for each aligner type, before and after aging. The absorbance curves of the All-In aligners before and after aging (Fig. 5) are both homogeneous, with mean values at wavelength 400 and 700 nm, respectively, of 0.265 ± 0.036 and 0.209 ± 0.030 for the former and 0.278 ± 0.011 and 0.215 ± 0.008 for the latter. Similarly, homogeneous absorbance curves were obtained for the Invisalign appliances (Fig. 6), but the mean absorbance at 400 nm and 700 nm were, respectively, 0.172 ± 0.004 and 0.143 ± 0.004 as supplied and 0.190 ± 0.027 and 0.155 ± 0.023 after aging. The before and after aging absorbance curves yielded by the F22 appliance (Fig. 7) were also homogeneous and almost superimposable. Indeed, before aging, the absorbance values at 400 and 700 nm, respectively, were 0.107 ± 0.023 and 0.090 ± 0.024 falling little after two aging cycles to 0.104 ± 0.003 and 0.081 ± 0.004.

Comparison of the three curves generated before aging (Fig. 8) reveals that the F22 absorbance values were lower than those produced by Invisalign and that All-In values were always the highest recorded. According to ANOVA, these differences were significant at all wavelengths of visible light (Table 3). The same trend was seen after aging (Fig. 9), and in this case too the differences between aligners were significant (Table 4).

A corresponding inverse pattern was seen in transmittance values (Figs. 10, 11, 12, 13 and 14) and, once again, the F22 aligner provided significantly better optical properties (higher transmittance) at all wavelengths than its competitors (Tables 5 and 6). Differences between each aligner type in absorbance and transmittance before and after aging (Tables 1 and 2) were not, however, significant, although it is interesting to note that the smallest percentage variations in optical properties (Table 7) were recorded for the F22 aligners, indicating their greater stability under these experimental conditions (Figs. 15 and 16).

Discussion

To our knowledge, only one previous study has investigated aligner transparency using spectrophotometry, but in that case only the absorbance of one brand (Invisalign) was measured [11]. Our spectrophotometry results showed that, of the three types tested, F22 had significantly lower absorbance and significantly higher transmittance than All-In and Invisalign, respectively. The difference in optical properties between the three brands was found both as received and after aging, indicating that the F22 aligners remain more transparent throughout treatment, although the chromatic stability of all sample types deteriorated during the aging process. This is in line with findings by Gracco et al. that both in vitro aging (artificial saliva) and in vivo wear increase the absorbance after 14 days. We show that this variation in absorbance, and, inversely, transmittance, was more pronounced with the All-In and Invisalign aligners (even more so) with respect to the F22 appliance. However, the differences between before and after aging measurements were not significant in any case, and we can therefore state that all three aligners tested maintain

Table 2 Transmittance values of the three aligners before and after in vitro aging

Aligner	Transmittance at 400 nm ± SD			Transmittance at 700 nm ± SD		
	As received	After aging	Significance	As received	After aging	Significance
All-In	53.58 ± 4.1	51.08 ± 2.6	N.S.	60.72 ± 2.9	59.60 ± 2.6	N.S.
Invisalign	68.65 ± 1.1	63.38 ± 3.0	N.S.	72.66 ± 1.1	69.27 ± 2.4	N.S.
F22	79.29 ± 5.0	78.25 ± 1.2	N.S.	82.45 ± 4.6	82.45 ± 1.7	N.S.

N.S. not significant variation

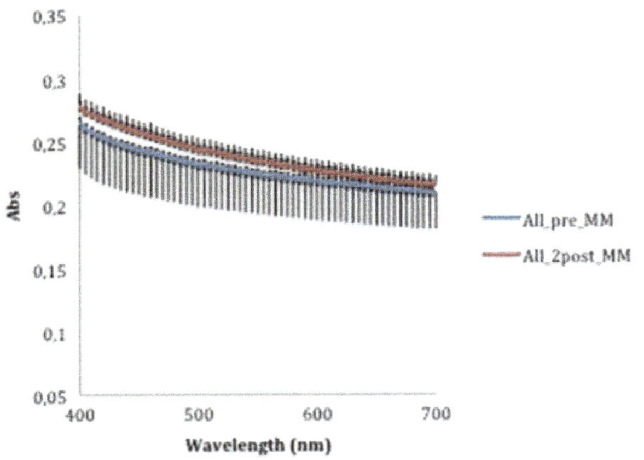

Fig. 5 Comparison of absorbance values of the All-In aligner before and after aging. The *curves* are the average of nine spectrophotometry measurements ± SD

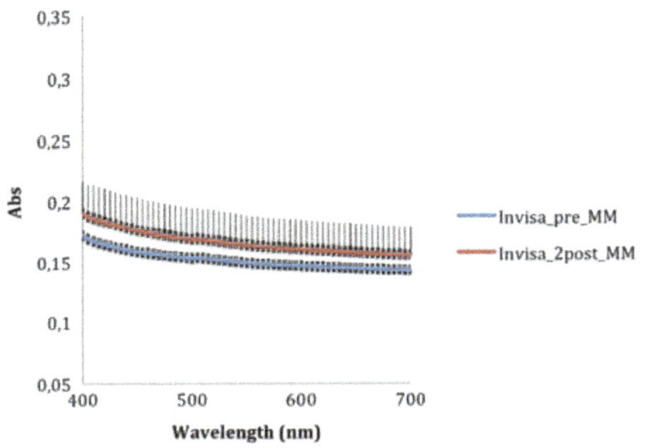

Fig. 6 Comparison of absorbance values of the Invisalign aligner before and after aging. The *curves* are the average of nine spectrophotometry measurements ± SD

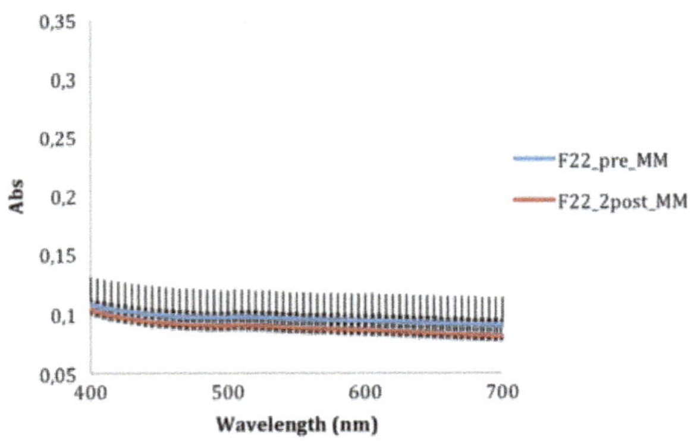

Fig. 7 Comparison of absorbance values of the F22 aligner before and after aging. The *curves* are the average of nine spectrophotometry measurements ± SD

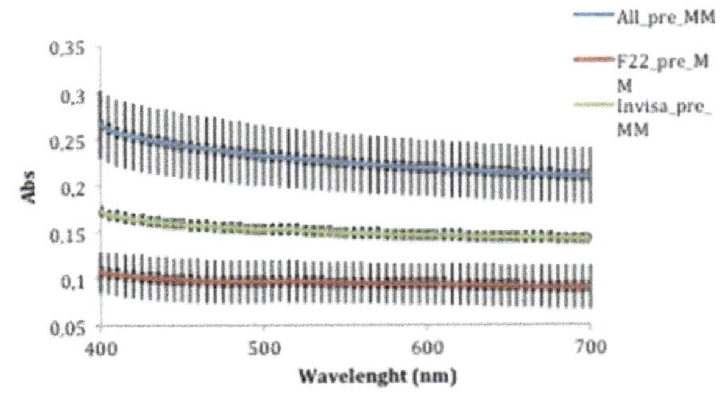

Fig. 8 Absorbance curves ± SD of the three aligners before aging

Table 3 Pre-aging absorbance values of the three aligners

Wavelength (nm)	All-In	Invisalign	F22	*p* value
400	0.265 ± 0.036	0.172 ± 0.004	0.107 ± 0.023	<0.0007
450	0.242 ± 0.035	0.158 ± 0.003	0.098 ± 0.024	<0.0012
500	0.230 ± 0.033	0.152 ± 0.003	0.096 ± 0.023	<0.0012
550	0.223 ± 0.031	0.148 ± 0.003	0.094 ± 0.022	<0.0013
600	0.217 ± 0.030	0.146 ± 0.003	0.093 ± 0.022	<0.0012
650	0.212 ± 0.030	0.144 ± 0.003	0.091 ± 0.023	<0.0015
700	0.209 ± 0.030	0.143 ± 0.004	0.090 ± 0.024	<0.0015

Significance level $p < 0.05$

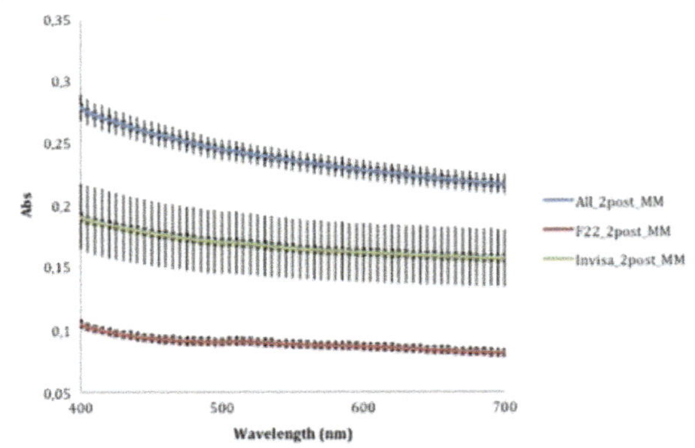

Fig. 9 Absorbance curves ± SD of the three aligners after aging

Table 4 Post-aging absorbance values of the three aligners

Wavelength (nm)	All-In	Invisalign	F22	*p* value
400	0.278 ± 0.011	0.190 ± 0.03	0.104 ± 0.003	<0.001
450	0.257 ± 0.010	0.176 ± 0.03	0.092 ± 0.003	<0.001
500	0.243 ± 0.009	0.168 ± 0.03	0.089 ± 0.003	<0.001
550	0.234 ± 0.009	0.163 ± 0.02	0.087 ± 0.003	<0.001
600	0.226 ± 0.008	0.160 ± 0.02	0.086 ± 0.003	<0.001
650	0.219 ± 0.008	0.157 ± 0.02	0.083 ± 0.004	<0.001
700	0.214 ± 0.008	0.155 ± 0.02	0.080 ± 0.004	<0.001

Significance level $p < 0.05$

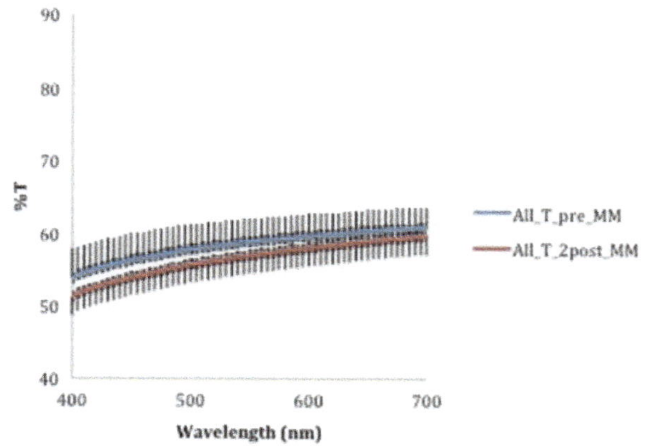

Fig. 10 Comparison of transmittance values of the All-In aligner before and after aging. The *curves* are the average of nine spectrophotometry measurements ± SD

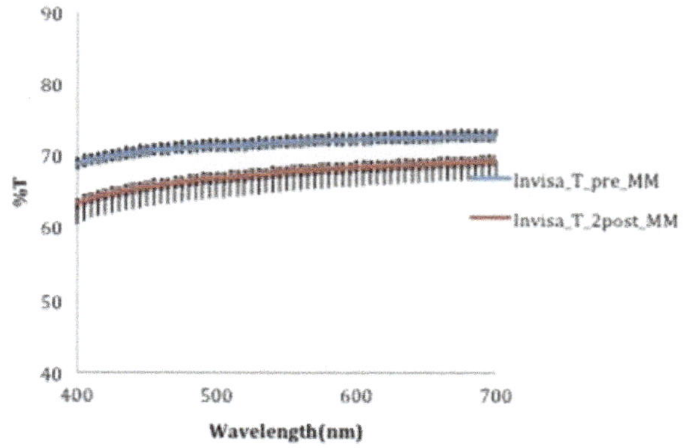

Fig. 11 Comparison of transmittance values of the Invisalign aligner before and after aging. The *curves* are the average of nine spectrophotometry measurements ± SD

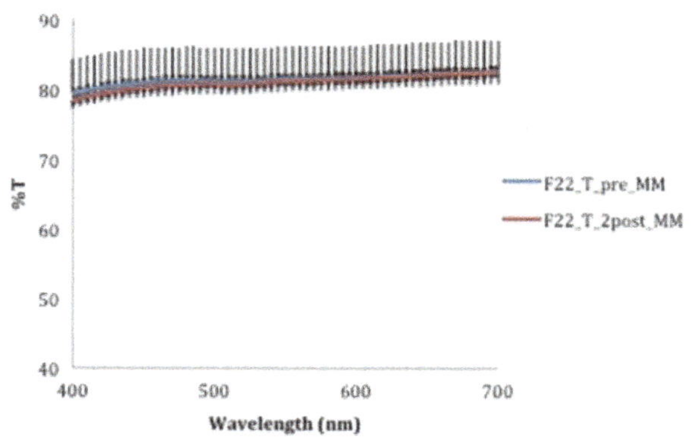

Fig. 12 Comparison of absorbance values of the F22 aligner before and after aging. The *curves* are the average of nine spectrophotometry measurements ± SD

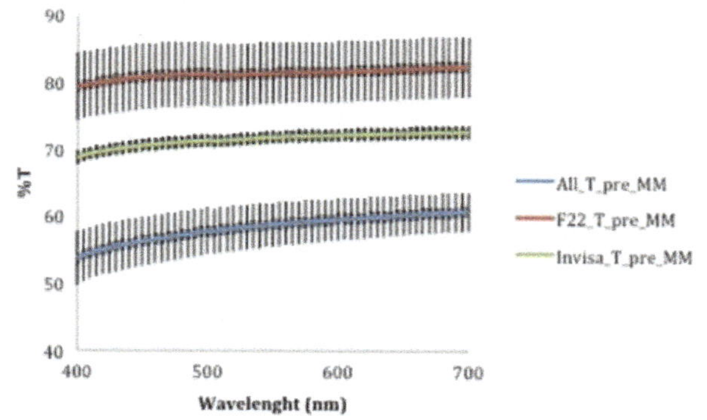

Fig. 13 Transmittance curves ± SD of the three aligners before aging

their optical properties in the presence of artificial saliva for at least 14 days (the recommended period of use). That being said, being tested in vitro, our samples were not subjected to any additional chemical (e.g. acidic drinks and oral enzymes) or mechanical stress (e.g. chewing, bruxism, removal and reinsertion), so we are unable to state to what extent their optical performance would change in vivo. Indeed, other studies [11] tell us that the optical properties of aligners deteriorate still further when worn for the same period in the mouth [21–23].

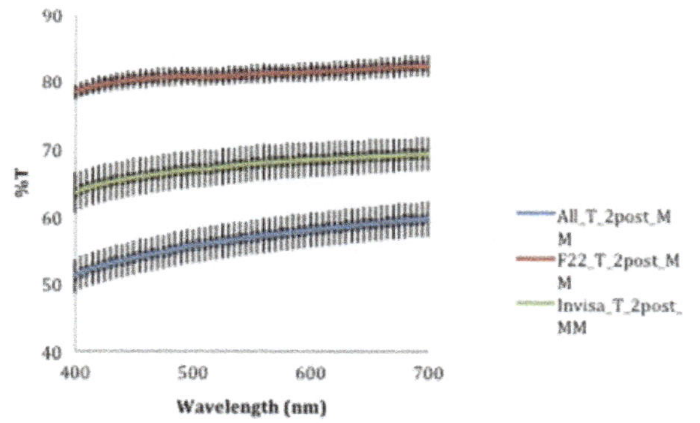

Fig. 14 Transmittance curves ± SD of the three aligners after aging

Table 5 Pre-aging transmittance values of the three aligners

Wavelength (nm)	All-In	Invisalign	F22	*p* value
400	53.58 ± 4.1	68.65 ± 1.1	79.29 ± 5.0	<0.0005
450	56.20 ± 3.7	70.51 ± 1.0	80.82 ± 5.0	<0.0005
500	57.74 ± 3.5	71.29 ± 1.0	81.21 ± 4.7	<0.0005
550	58.73 ± 3.3	71.80 ± 1.0	81.43 ± 4.6	<0.0005
600	59.55 ± 3.1	72.16 ± 1.0	81.67 ± 4.5	<0.0005
650	60.21 ± 3.0	72.44 ± 1.1	82.08 ± 4.6	<0.0005
700	60.72 ± 2.9	72.66 ± 1.1	82.45 ± 4.6	<0.0005

Significance level $p < 0.05$

Table 6 Post-aging transmittance values of the three aligners

Wavelength (nm)	All-In	Invisalign	F22	*p* value
400	51.08 ± 2.6	63.38 ± 3.0	78.25 ± 1.2	<0.001
450	53.84 ± 2.5	65.74 ± 2.8	80.21 ± 1.5	<0.001
500	55.64 ± 2.5	66.96 ± 2.8	80.76 ± 1.5	<0.001
550	56.87 ± 2.6	67.80 ± 2.7	81.10 ± 1.5	<0.001
600	57.94 ± 2.6	68.39 ± 2.6	81.45 ± 1.5	<0.001
650	58.85 ± 2.6	68.87 ± 2.5	81.97 ± 1.6	<0.001
700	59.60 ± 2.6	69.27 ± 2.4	82.45 ± 1.7	<0.001

Significance level $p < 0.05$

Table 7 Percentage variations in aligner absorbance and transmittance after in vitro aging

	% variation at 400 nm		% variation at 700 nm	
Aligner	Absorbance	Transmittance	Absorbance	Transmittance
All-In	+5.77	−4.53	+3.86	−1.83
F22	−0.74	−1.09	−6.55	+0.14
Invisalign	+10.46	−7.70	+8.73	−4.68

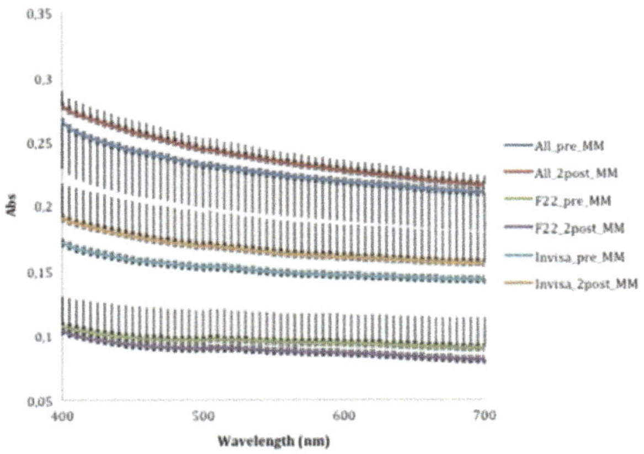

Fig. 15 Comparison of absorbance values of the three aligners before and after aging

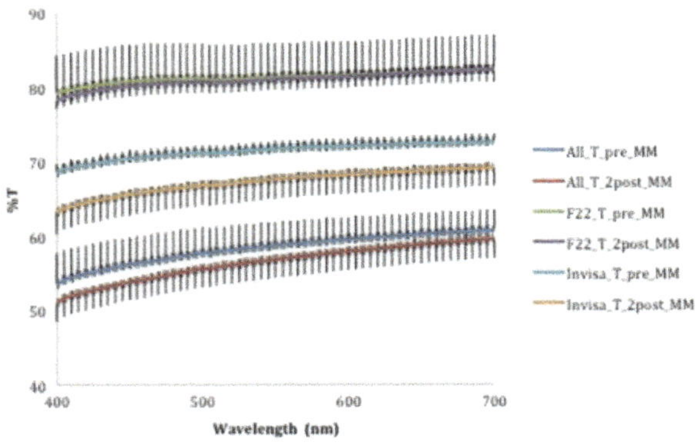

Fig. 16 Comparison of transmittance values of the three aligners before and after aging

Another study has previously attempted to accelerate the aging process by means of a more aggressive treatment (a solution of 75 % ethanol and 25 % water for 2 weeks at 23 °C), but even this was unable to truly replicate the oral conditions [24]. Hence, we elected to age our samples in artificial saliva, the focus being on standardizing the stress to which the aligners were exposed and therefore the changes observed. Nevertheless, only a similar study conducted in vivo will confirm whether or not the differences in transparency between the aligners are also significant after 2 weeks in the oral environment.

Conclusions

The optical properties of orthodontic aligners appear to vary between brands and constituent materials but deteriorate with in vitro aging in all cases. Of those tested, both before and after aging, F22 was significantly more transparent than All-In and Invisalign, whose optical properties were most changed by the process. Further studies will be required to measure the absorbance and transmittance of aligners after a cycle of wear in vivo, as in vitro testing conditions are unable to accurately reproduce the conditions in the oral environment.

Competing interests
The authors declare that they have no competing interests.

Authors' contributions

LL and GS planned the study. AA partecipated the optical tests and drafted the manuscript. RM and AB carried out the optical tests. SS supervised the spettrophotometry analysis. All Authors read and approved the final manuscript.

Acknowledgements
We would like to thank the University of Ferrara and Department of Chemical and Pharmaceutical Sciences Ferrara, where the experiments were performed, for kind use of their spectrophotometer.

Author details
[1]Postgraduate School of Orthodontics, University of Ferrara, Via Montebello 31, 44100 Ferrara, Italy. [2]Department of Chemical and Pharmaceutical Sciences, University of Ferrara, Via Fossato di Mortara 17/19, 44121 Ferrara, Italy.

References

1. Rosvall MD, Field HW, Ziuchkovski J, Rosenstiel SF, Johnston WM. Attractiveness, acceptability, and value of orthodontic appliances. Am J Orthod Dentofacial Orthop. 2009;135:276–88.
2. Boyd R, Miller RJ, Vlaskalic V. The Invisalign system in adult orthodontics: mild crowding and space closure cases. J Clin Orthod. 2000;34:13–5.
3. Kim TW, Echarri P. Clear aligner: an efficient, esthetic, and comfortable option for an adult patient. World J Orthod. 2007;8:13–8.
4. Kohda N, Iijima M, Muguruma T, Brantley WA, Ahluwalia KS, Mizoguchi I. Effects of mechanical properties of thermoplastic materials on the initial force of thermoplastic appliances. Angle Orthod. 2013;83(3):476–83.

5. Lingenbrink JC, King G, Bollen AM, Hujoel P, Huang G, Orsini-Alcalde G. Quality of life comparison between clear removable and conventional orthodontics. J Dent Res. 2002;81:463.
6. Kesling H. The philosophy of the tooth positioning appliance. Am J Orthod. 1945;31:297–304.
7. Align Technology Inc. The Invisalign reference guide. Santa Clara: Invisalign; 2002
8. Align Technology Inc. Material safety data sheet. MSDS Aligner EX203040 Customer support. Santa Clara: Invisalign; 2003.
9. Wong BH. Invisalign A, to Z. Am J Orthod Dentofacial Orthop. 2002;121:540–1.
10. Eliades T, Eliades G, Watts DC. Structural conformation of in vitro and in vivo aged orthodontic elastomeric modules. EurJ Orthod. 1999;21:649–58.
11. Gracco A, Mazzoli A, Favoni O, Conti C, Ferraris P, Tosi G, et al. Short-term chemical and physical changes in Invisalign appliances. Aust Orthod J. 2009;25(1):34–40.
12. Huget EF, Patrick KS, Nunez LJ. Observations on the elastic behavior of a synthetic orthodontic elastomer. J Dent Res. 1990;69:496–501.
13. Dupaix RB, Boyce MC. Finite strain behavior of poly(ethylene terephthalate) (PET) and poly(ethylene terephthalate)-glycol (PETG). Polymer. 2005;46:4827–38.
14. Guarneri MP, Lombardo L, Gracco A, Siciliani G. Lo stato dell'arte del trattamento con allineatori. Bologna, Italy: Martina ED; 2013.
15. Frick A, Rochman A. Characterization of TPU-elastomers by thermal analysis (DSC). Polym Test. 2004;23:413–7.
16. Lu QW, Macosko CW. Comparing the compatibility of various functionalized polypropylenes with thermoplastic polyurethane (TPU). Polymer. 2004;45:1981–91.
17. Fang D, Zhang N, Chen H, Bai Y. Dynamic stress relaxation of orthodontic thermoplastic materials in a simulated oral environment. Dent Mater J. 2013;32(6):946–51.
18. Zhang N, Bai Y, Ding X, Zhang Y. Preparation and characterization of thermoplastic materials for invisible orthodontics. Dent Mater J. 2011. [Epub ahead of print]
19. Watts DC, Cash AJ. Analysis of optical transmission by 400–500 nm visible light into aesthetic dental biomaterials. J Dent. 1994;22(2):112–7.
20. Martens H, Nielsen JP, Balling Engelsen S. Light scattering and light absorbance separated by extended multiplicative signal correction. Application to near-infrared transmission analysis of powder mixtures. Anal Chem. 2003;75(3):394–404.
21. Leininger RI, Hutson T, Jakobsen R. Spectroscopic approaches to the investigation of interactions between artificial surfaces and protein. Ann N Y Acad Sci. 1987;516:173–83.
22. Phua SK, Castillo E, Anderson JM, Hiltner A. Biodegradation of a polyurethane in vitro. J Biomed Mater Res. 1987;21:231–46.
23. Schollenberger CS, Stewart FD. Thermoplastic polyurethane hydrolysis stability. J Elastoplast. 1971;3:28–56.
24. Schuster S, Eliades G, Zinelis S, Eliades T, Bradley TG. Structural conformation and leaching from in vitro aged and retrieved Invisalign appliances. Am J Orthod Dentofacial Orthop. 2004;126(6):725–8.

31

Exploring the association between feeding habits, non-nutritive sucking habits, and malocclusions in the deciduous dentition

Gabriela Mesquita Lopes-Freire[1*], Abel Belizario Cahuana Cárdenas[2], José Enrique Espasa Suarez de Deza[1], Josep Maria Ustrell-Torrent[3], Luciana Butini Oliveira[4] and Joan Ramon Boj Quesada JR[1]

Abstract

Background: This study aimed to explore the association between feeding habits, non-nutritive sucking habits, and malocclusions in deciduous dentition.

Methods: A cross-sectional observational survey was carried out in 275 children aged 3 to 6 years and included clinical evaluations of malocclusions and structured interviews. Statistical significance for the association between feeding habits and the development of malocclusion was determined using chi-square and Fisher's exact tests. In addition, odds ratio (OR) calculations were used for intergroup comparisons. Controlling for confounders was adjusted by excluding children with non-nutritive sucking habits.

Results: The results indicated that there were no significant relationships between exclusive breastfeeding or bottlefeeding and the presence of any type of malocclusion ($p > 0.05$). There was also no significant association between breastfeeding or bottlefeeding duration and malocclusion ($p > 0.05$). In addition, it was observed that exclusive breastfeeding had a protective effect and diminished the risk of acquiring non-nutritive sucking habits ($p = 0.001$).

Conclusions: There was no association between feeding habits and malocclusions in the deciduous dentition in this sample of children. Exclusive breastfeeding reduced the risk of acquiring non-nutritive sucking habits.

Keywords: Breastfeeding, Bottlefeeding, Malocclusion

Background

The sucking habits of infants are described in the literature as being of two types: non-nutritive and nutritive. Finger sucking, thumb sucking, and sucking on a pacifier (dummy, comforter) are considered non-nutritive sucking habits. Breastfeeding and bottlefeeding are considered nutritive sucking habits.

Several studies reported the association between feeding habits (breastfeeding and/or bottlefeeding), non-nutritive habits, and malocclusion [1–8]. The findings on associations between types and duration of feeding habits and malocclusion are conflicting. Moreover, confounder variables (presence of non-nutritive habits) were not performed in many previous studies.

The advantages afforded by breastfeeding have been reported in the literature and include the well-established immunological and psychological benefits, adequate weight gain for the baby, and the correct development of the oral structures involved in the action of sucking. A prospective birth cohort study from Brazil concluded that breastfeeding is associated with improved performance in intelligence tests 30 years later, and might have an important effect in real life, by increasing educational attainment and income in adulthood [9]. Previous studies showed that prolonged breastfeeding may have a protective effect on the development of malocclusions [1–7]. However, a recent systematic review of cohort studies concluded that the scientific evidence could not confirm the types of malocclusion associated with bottlefeeding or a proper period for breastfeeding in order to protect against malocclusion [10].

Observational surveys provide important information about the feeding practices and malocclusion status and contribute to the development of awareness among professionals as well as among the target population. It is

* Correspondence: gabimlopes@gmail.com
[1]Department of Paediatric Dentistry, Faculty of Dentistry, University of Barcelona Hospitalet de Llobregat, Barcelona, Spain
Full list of author information is available at the end of the article

important to investigate the presence of malocclusion in deciduous dentition because it is a public dental health problem in children in Spain. In addition, current recommendations for discontinuing non-nutritive sucking habits may be optimal in preventing habit-related malocclusions at the end of the primary dentition stage [11, 12].

Therefore, the aim of this study was to explore the association between feeding habits, non-nutritive sucking habits, and malocclusions in the deciduous dentition in a population of Spanish children.

Methods

This study was approved by the Research Ethics Committee of the University of Barcelona and the Children Hospital of Barcelona and conducted in a day care center, CAP, Montcada i Reixac. The participants' legal guardians gave positive consent on the day of the clinical examination.

A cross-sectional observational survey was carried out on boys and girls aged 3 to 6 years and included clinical evaluations of malocclusions and structured interviews.

All the children in the study met the inclusion criteria which included children of both genders aged 3 to 6 years; children exclusively in the deciduous dentition phase; agreement to participate in the clinical exam; all the normal numbers, sizes, and shapes of deciduous teeth; no major tooth destruction or reconstruction; children with no systemic diseases and/or neurological diseases; and parental questionnaires about the child's habits.

Children were excluded from the study if their parents did not agree to their participation, they have syndromes or systemic problems affecting craniofacial growth, they have the presence of at least one permanent tooth, they have loss of mesial-distal diameter due to caries, and they have previous orthodontic treatment.

All clinical exams were performed by an experienced examiner, a PhD student (GMLF) who had previous experience in cross-sectional data. The child remained seated on a chair in front of the examiner. The examinations were performed under artificial light, using latex gloves and a disposable spatula. The clinical exam was performed with the aid of a disposable tongue depressor source. To ensure that natural occlusion was evaluated, the child was asked to open and close his/her mouth several times and to swallow saliva before the examination began. When necessary, the mandible was gently guided towards centric occlusion by the examiner.

The outcomes related to the children's dental arch characteristics were examined in the three dimensions with the following criteria.

The transverse relation was measured by direct inspection in the presence of posterior crossbite or if the absence was considered normal occlusion. One of five separate relationships was recorded considering the following categories: normal relationship; posterior unilateral crossbite left side; posterior unilateral crossbite right side; bilateral posterior crossbite—both hemi-arches; and just one tooth was crossed. Posterior crossbite is considered present when, in occlusion, one or more of the maxillary deciduous canine or molars occluded lingual to the buccal cusps of the opposing mandibular teeth. Upper midline shift was registered if the midline was displaced by at least 1 mm. In addition, midline deviation data was also collected and the distance between the upper and lower midlines in the frontal plane was considered.

The vertical relation (relationship of incisors) was measured by direct inspection: one of three separate relationships was recorded in normal, anterior open bite, and overbite. Overbite was obtained by measuring the vertical distance between the upper and lower central incisor edges with the teeth in occlusion [13]. This distance was considered normal when the upper incisor covered the lower up to 3 mm and overbite for values greater than 3 mm. When there was no overlap between the upper and lower incisors, with a minimum space of 1 mm between both incisal edges, it was considered anterior open bite [14].

The sagittal interarch relationship was classified according to the deciduous canine relationship as angle class I, class II, or class III, with class I considered normal occlusion, class I canine and molars bilateral, or class I canine and molars unilateral, and class II or class III considered altered: class II bilateral, class II 1 (increased overjet), class II 2 (without overjet), class II subdivision (I o III), class II unilateral, others with no classification, and class III or anterior crossbite.

A questionnaire in the form of a structured interview was applied with mothers or guardians in order to find out about nutritive sucking habits (breastfeeding and bottlefeeding), non-nutritive sucking habits (pacifiers and finger sucking), and the presence of malocclusions. The data collected included the presence and the duration of non-nutritive sucking habits and, if the child had sucking, any type of non-nutritive sucking habits: pacifier-sucking habit and digit sucking.

Data analyses were performed using SPSS software 22.0. Data analysis included descriptive statistics (frequency distribution). Statistical significance for the association between the non-nutritive sucking habits and the development of malocclusion was determined using chi-square, and Fisher's exact tests with odds ratio (OR) calculations were used for intergroup comparisons. Children with non-nutritive sucking habits were excluded from the analysis. The level of significance was set at 5 %.

Results

The sample consisted of 275 children aged 3 to 6 years; 144 (52.4 %) were males and 131 (47.6 %) were females. Of 275 children, only 28 children were exclusively breastfeeding, and 247 children were breastfeeding/bottlefeeding. The presence of non-nutritive sucking habits was observed in 224 children (81.5 %).

The results presented in Table 1 indicated that there was no significant relationship between exclusive breastfeeding and the presence of any type of malocclusion OR 1.37 (confidence interval (CI) 0.34–5.51, $p = 0.739$). The results also indicated that there was no significant relationship between bottlefeeding and the presence of any type of malocclusion OR 1.35 (CI 0.31–5.96, $p = 0.716$) (Table 2). In addition, there was no significant association between breastfeeding or bottlefeeding duration and malocclusion (Tables 3 and 4).

It was observed in Table 5 that exclusive breastfeeding had a protective effect and diminished the risk of acquiring non-nutritive sucking habits OR 0.18 (CI 0.07–0.40, $p = 0.001$). Exclusive breastfeeding may have reduced the risk of pacifier use OR 0.24 (CI 0.11–0.52, $p = 0.001$). However, there was no significant association between exclusive breastfeeding and finger-sucking habit ($p = 0.374$). In addition, there was no significant association with intensity and duration of non-nutritive sucking habits.

Discussion

The results in the present study indicated that there was no significant relationship between exclusive breastfeeding and the presence of any type of malocclusion. The results also indicated that there was no significant relationship between bottlefeeding and the presence of any type of malocclusion. However, it was observed that exclusive breastfeeding had a protective effect and diminished the risk of acquiring non-nutritive sucking habits.

At present, there is no consensus related to the association between feeding habits and malocclusion. Previous studies have reported that there was influence of feeding patterns on the development of malocclusion [1–8, 15–20]. According to some authors, breastfeeding and bottlefeeding involve different orofacial muscles, which possible have different effects on the harmonic growth of maxilla and dental arches. Meanwhile, breathing, swallowing, and mastication should be developed in harmony, and differences exist in the learning of the coordinated movement between breastfeeding and bottlefeeding children [18].

On the other hand, some studies did not found this association [11, 21, 22]. Some authors observed among children with minimal non-nutritive habits that those who breastfed had similar dental arch parameters and occlusal characteristics as those with shorter duration of breastfeeding or no breastfeeding [11]. A possible explanation is that the effects of breastfeeding on dental arch development are difficult to assess because it is not easy to separate these effects from those non-nutritive sucking behaviors. This result is because most breastfed children also engaged in at least some non-nutritive sucking.

The finding that exclusive breastfeeding had a protective effect and diminished the risk of acquiring non-nutritive sucking habits is in agreement with previous studies [6, 23–26]. In this investigation, thumb sucking has the same result with breastfeeding and bottlefeeding but the use of a pacifier was more utilized for bottlefeeding children. It is important to emphasize that breastfeeding

Table 1 Relationship between exclusive breastfeeding and malocclusion

		Exclusive breastfeeding						
		No		Yes				
		N	%	*N*	%	OR	CI 95 %	*p* value
Transversal relationship	Malocclusion in transversal relationship	3	8.1	0	0.0	Infinity	NA	0.552
	Normal	34	91.9	14	100.0			
	Total	37	100.0	14	100.0			
Midline deviation	Malocclusion in midline	4	11.1	1	7.1	0.54	0.11–2.76	0.662
	Normal	32	88.9	13	92.9			
	Total	36	100.0	14	100.0			
Vertical relationship	Malocclusion in vertical relationship	6	16.2	3	21.4	0.71	0.15–3.33	0.692
	Normal	31	83.8	11	78.6			
	Total	37	100.0	14	100.0			
Sagittal relationship	Malocclusion in sagittal relationship	10	30.3	2	16.7	2.17	0.401–11.76	0.466
	Normal	23	69.7	10	83.3			
	Total	33	100.0	12	100.0			
Presence of malocclusion	Any type of malocclusion	13	40.6	4	33.3	1.37	0.34–5.51	0.739
	Normal	19	59.4	8	66.7			
	Total	32	100.0	12	100.0			

Table 2 Relationship between exclusive bottlefeeding and malocclusion

		Exclusive bottlefeeding						
		Yes		No				
		N	%	*N*	%	OR	CI 95 %	*p* value
Transversal relationship	Malocclusion in transversal relationship	1	7.7	2	5.3	1.50	0.12–18.05	1.00
	Normal	12	92.3	36	94.7			
	Total	13	100.0	38	100.0			
Midline deviation	Malocclusion in midline	1	8.3	4	10.5	0.77	0.08–7.66	1.00
	Normal	11	91.7	34	89.5			
	Total	12	100.0	38	100.0			
Vertical relationship	Malocclusion in vertical relationship	1	7.7	8	21.1	0.31	0.04–2.78	0.42
	Normal	12	92.3	30	78.9			
	Total	13	100.0	38	100.0			
Sagittal relationship	Malocclusion in sagittal relationship	3	30.0	9	25.7	1.24	0.26–5.84	1.00
	Normal	7	70.0	26	74.3			
	Total	10	100.0	35	100.0			
Presence of malocclusion	Any type of malocclusion	4	44.4	13	37.1	1.35	0.31–5.96	0.716
	Normal	5	55.6	22	62.9			
	Total	9	100.0	35	100.0			

seems to have non-nutritive protective impact. If the parents refuse to give the pacifier, the result may be different and thumb-sucking habit is something that children choose or need to do without the factor of parents giving the artifact to stimulate non-nutritive sucking.

A previous study investigated the influence of thumb sucking and pacifier use on breastfeeding patterns in exclusively breastfed infants, on the duration of exclusive breastfeeding, and on the total breastfeeding duration. The authors concluded that thumb sucking was clearly not related to the negative effects on the pattern and duration of breastfeeding. The possible negative effects of pacifier use on breastfeeding pattern and duration were related to frequency. In addition, occasional pacifier use was not found to have any negative effect on breastfeeding duration [27].

Table 3 Relationship between bottlefeeding duration and malocclusion

		Bottlefeeding duration						
		>6–12 months		>12 months				
		N	%	*N*	%	OR	CI 95 %	*p* value
Transversal relationship	Malocclusion in transversal relationship	0	0.0	3	10.0	0	NA	1.00
	Normal	4	100.0	27	90.0			
	Total	4	100.0	30	100.0			
Midline deviation	Malocclusion in midline	1	33.3	3	10.0	4.5	0.31–65.67	0.33
	Normal	2	66.7	27	90.0			
	Total	3	100.0	30	100.0			
Vertical relationship	Malocclusion in vertical relationship	1	25.0	5	16.7	1.67	0.14–19.48	1.00
	Normal	3	75.0	25	83.3			
	Total	4	100.0	30	100.0			
Sagittal relationship	Malocclusion in sagittal relationship	2	50.0	8	30.8	2.25	0.27–18.93	0.584
	Normal	2	50.0	18	69.2			
	Total	4	100.0	26	100.0			
Presence of malocclusion	Any type of malocclusion	2	66.7	11	42.3	2.73	0.23–34.01	0.573
	Normal	1	33.3	15	57.7			
	Total	3	100.0	26	100.0			

Table 4 Relationship between breastfeeding duration and malocclusion

		Breastfeeding duration						
		<6 months		>12 months				
		N	%	*N*	%	OR	CI 95 %	*p* value
Transversal relationship	Malocclusion in transversal relationship	2	11.1	0	0.0	Infinity	NA	0.229
	Normal	16	88.9	19	100.0			
	Total	18	100.0	19	100.0			
Midline deviation	Malocclusion in midline	2	11.1	2	10.5	1.06	0.13–8.47	1.00
	Normal	16	88.9	17	89.5			
	Total	18	100.0	19	100.0			
Vertical relationship	Malocclusion in vertical relationship	4	22.2	4	21.1	1.07	0.22–5.13	1.00
	Normal	14	77.8	15	78.9			
	Total	18	100.0	19	100.0			
Sagittal relationship	Malocclusion in sagittal relationship	5	27.8	4	25.0	1.15	0.25–5.33	1.00
	Normal	13	72.2	12	75.0			
	Total	18	100.0	16	100.0			
Presence of malocclusion	Any type of malocclusion	6	33.3	7	43.8	0.64	0.16–2.58	0.725
	Normal	12	66.7	9	56.3			
	Total	18	100.0	16	100.0			

In offering an explanation for the relationships between breastfeeding and the risk of acquiring non-nutritive sucking habits, some potential limitations of this study should be taken into account. First, no cause-effect relationship can be deduced from a cross-sectional design study such as this one. Longitudinal designs (cohort studies) would increase the knowledge on this subject.

Moreover, there is much controversy surrounding the issue of diagnosis of malocclusions due to the inexistence of a universally accepted index. Comparisons between studies should be interpreted with caution due to the lack of uniformity in sample selection, diagnostic criteria, and classifications and age groups.

A positive attribute of this study was that children with non-nutritive sucking habits were excluded from the analysis. Recently, a systematic review also reported that substantial methodological and clinical heterogeneity was found among the studies in this issue. The

Table 5 Relationship between exclusive breastfeeding and non-nutritive sucking habits

		Exclusive breastfeeding								
		Yes		No		Total				
		N	%	*N*	%	*N*	%	OR	CI 95 %	*p* value
Pacifier	Yes	14	50.0	200	81.0	214	77.8	0.24	0.11–0.52	0.001
	No	14	50.0	47	19.0	61	22.2			
	Total	28	100.0	247	100.0	275	100.0			
Finger sucking	Yes	0	0.0	14	5.7	14	5.1	0	NA	0.374
	No	28	100.0	233	94.3	261	94.9			
	Total	28	100.0	247	100.0	275	100.0			
Duration	>12 months	14	100.0	204	97.1	218	97.3	Infinity	NA	1
	<12 months	0	0.0	6	2.9	6	2.7			
	Total	14	100.0	210	100.0	224	100.0			
Intensity	Moderate or high use	5	41.7	132	64.4	137	63.1	0.39	0.12–1.29	0.131
	Low use	7	58.3	73	35.6	80	36.9			
Non-nutritive sucking habits	Yes	14	50.0	210	85.0	224	81.5	0.18	0.07–0.40	0.001
	No	14	50.0	37	15.0	51	18.5			
	Total	28	100.0	247	100.0	275	100.0			

major limitation is the failure to report controlling for confounder variables. Pacifier use and thumb sucking are confounder variables, since it is not possible to determine whether malocclusion was caused by bottlefeeding or pacifier/thumb sucking. The absence of controlling for confounders may have led to bias results in previous studies [10].

Some authors emphasized that breastfeeding alone seems not to be directly associated with malocclusions, but it may have a synergetic effect with parafunctional oral habits on the development of occlusofacial problems [28]. They also reinforced the arguments for the prevention of bad oral habits, especially among children who have not been fed at their mother's breast or were breastfed for a short period.

Despite the multiple benefits of maternal breastfeeding, artificial feeding is widely used and may have contributed to the high rates of pacifier use and other harmful habits. Exclusive breastfeeding for at least 6 months of age is still the best recommendation to benefit children regarding their systemic health and harmonic craniofacial growth [10].

Conclusions

In conclusion, there was no association between feeding habits and malocclusions in the deciduous dentition in this sample of children. Exclusive breastfeeding reduced the risk of acquiring non-nutritive sucking habits.

Competing interest

The authors declare that they have no competing interests.

Authors' contributions

GMLF participated in all phases of the study and drafting the manuscript. ABCC participated in the data collection. JEESD, JMUT, and JRBQ participated in the design, compiled the results, and supervised the research. LBO collaborated with the writing and reviewing of the text. All the authors read and approved the final manuscript.

Acknowledgements

The authors also thank the University of Barcelona, the Children Hospital of Barcelona, CAP, Montcada i Reixac, and the children and their mothers for their cooperation in carrying out this study.

Author details

[1]Department of Paediatric Dentistry, Faculty of Dentistry, University of Barcelona Hospitalet de Llobregat, Barcelona, Spain. [2]Pediatric Dentistry and Orthodontic Service, Hospital Sant Joan de Déu, Barcelona, Spain. [3]Department of Orthodontics, Oral Health and Masticatory System Group (Bellvitge Biomedical Research Institute) IDIBELL, Faculty of Dentistry, L'Hospitalet, Barcelona, Spain. [4]Department of Pediatric Dentistry, School of Dentistry, Faculdade São Leopoldo Mandic, Campinas, SP, Brazil.

References

1. Peres KG, Barros AJ, Peres MA, Victora CG. Effects of breastfeeding and sucking habits on malocclusion in a birth cohort study. Rev Saude Publica. 2007;41(3):343–50.
2. Kobayashi HM, Scavone Jr H, Ferreira RI, Garib DG. Relationship between breastfeeding duration and prevalence of posterior crossbite in the deciduous dentition. Am J Orthod Dentofacial Orthop. 2010;137(1):54–8.
3. Sanchez-Molins M, Grau Carbó J, Lischeid Gaig C, Ustrell Torrent JM. Comparative study of the craniofacial growth depending on the type of lactation received. Eur J Paediatr Dent. 2010;11(2):87–92.
4. Romero CC, Scavone-Junior H, Garib DG, Cotrim-Ferreira FA, Ferreira RI. Breastfeeding and non-nutritive sucking patterns related to the prevalence of anterior open bite in primary dentition. J Appl Oral Sci. 2011;19(2):161–8.
5. Caramez da Silva F, Justo Giugliani ER, Capsi Pires S. Duration of breastfeeding and distoclusion in the deciduous dentition. Breastfeed Med. 2012;7(6):464–8.
6. Narbutyte I, Narbutyte A, Linkevičienė L. Relationship between breastfeeding, bottle-feeding and development of malocclusion. Stomatologija. 2013;15(3):67–72.
7. Moimaz SA, Garbin AJ, Lima AM, Lolli LF, Saliba O, Garbin CA. Longitudinal study of habits leading to malocclusion development in childhood. BMC Oral Health. 2014;14:96.
8. Agarwal SS, Nehra K, Sharma M, Jayan B, Poonia A, Bhattal H. Association between breastfeeding duration, non-nutritive sucking habits and dental arch dimensions in deciduous dentition: a cross-sectional study. Progress in Orthod. 2014;15:59.
9. Victora CG, Horta BL, de Mola CL, Quevedo L, Pinheiro RT, Gigante DP, et al. Association between breastfeeding and intelligence, educational attainment, and income at 30 years of age: a prospective birth cohort study from Brazil. The Lancet Global Health. 2015;3(4):199–205.
10. Hermont AP, Martins CC, Zina LG, Auad SM, Paiva SM, Pordeus IA. Breastfeeding, bottle feeding practices and malocclusion in the primary dentition: a systematic review of cohort studies. Int J Environ Res Public Health. 2015;12(3):3133–51.
11. Warren JJ, Bishara SE. Duration of nutritive and nonnutritive sucking behaviors and their effects on the dental arches in the primary dentition. Am J Orthod Dentofacial Orthop. 2002;121(4):347–56.
12. Warren JJ, Slayton RL, Bishara SE, Levy SM, Yonezu T, Kanellis MJ. Effects of nonnutritive sucking habits on occlusal characteristics in the mixed dentition. Pediatr Dent. 2005;27(6):445–50.
13. Warren JJ, Bishara SE, Steinbock KL, Yonezu T, Nowak AJ. Effects of oral habits' duration on dental characteristics in the primary dentition. J Am Dent Assoc. 2001;132(12):1685–93.
14. Bhat SS, Rao HA, Hegde KS, Kumar BK. Characteristics of primary dentition occlusion in preschool children: an epidemiological study. Int J Clin Pediatr Dent. 2012;5(2):93–7.
15. Karjalainen S, Rönning O, Lapinleimu H, Simell O. Association between early meaning, non-nutritive sucking habits and occlusal anomalies in 3-year-old Finnish children. Int J Paediatr Dent. 1999;9(3):169–73.
16. Luz CL, Garib DG, Arouca R. Association between breastfeeding duration and mandibular retrusion: a cross-sectional study of children in the mixed dentition. Am J Orthod Dentofacial Orthop. 2006;130(4):531–4.
17. Vázquez-Nava F, Quezada-Castillo JA, Oviedo-Trevino S, Saldivar-González AH, Sánchez-Nuncio HR, Beltrán-Guzmán FJ, et al. Association between allergic rhinitis, bottle feeding, non-nutritive sucking habits and malocclusion in the primary dentition. Arch Dis Child. 2006;91(10):836–40.
18. Wang XT, Ge LH. Influence of feeding patterns on the development of teeth, dentition and jaw in children. Beijing Da Xue Bao. 2015;47(1):191–5.
19. Sum FH, Zhang L, Ling HT, Yeung CP, Li KY, Wong HM, et al. Association of breastfeeding and three-dimension dental arch relationships in primary dentition. BMC Oral Health. 2015;15(1):30.
20. Limeira AB, Aguiar CM, de Lima Bezerra NS, Câmara AC. Association between breast-feeding duration and posterior crossbites. J Dent Child (Chic). 2015;81(3):122–7.
21. Aznar T, Galán AF, Marín I, Domínguez A. Dental arch diameters and relationships to oral habits. Angle Orthod. 2006;76(3):441–5.
22. Ogaard B, Larsson E, Lindsten R. The effect of sucking habits, cohort, sex, intercanine arch, widths, and breast or bottle feeding on posterior crossbite in Norwegian and Swedish 3-year-old children. Am J Orthod Dentofacial Orthop. 1994;106(2):161–6.
23. Serra-Negra JMC, Pordeus IA, Rocha Júnior JF. Study of the relationship between infant feeding methods, oral habits, and malocclusion. Rev Odontol Univ São Paulo. 1997;11(2):79–86.
24. Freire GLM, Ferrari JCL, Percinoto C. Association between maternal breastfeeding and the development of non-nutritive sucking habits. RGO, Rev Gaúch Odontol. 2015;63(2):139-44.
25. Albuquerque SSL, Duarte RC, Cavalcanti AL, Beltrão EM. The influence of feeding methods in the development of nonnutritive sucking habits in childhood. Cien Saude Colet. 2010;15(2):371–8.

26. Ferreira FV, Marchionatti AM, Oliveira MDM, Praetzel JR. Association between duration of breastfeeding and its influence upon the development of harmful oral habits. Rev Sul-Bras Odontol. 2010;7(1):35–40.
27. Aarts C, Hörnell A, Kylberg E, Hofvander Y, Gebre-Medhin M. Breastfeeding patterns in relation to thumb sucking and pacifier use. Pediatrics. 1999;104(4):e50.
28. Thomaz EB, Cangussu MC, Assis AM. Maternal breastfeeding, parafunctional oral habits and malocclusion in adolescents: a multivariate analysis. Int J Pediatr Otorhinolaryngol. 2012;76(4):500–6.

32

Predicting changes in mandibular length and total anterior facial height using IGF-1, cervical stage, skeletal classification, and gender

Mohamed I Masoud[1,2], Hussain Y A Marghalani[2,3], Mohamed Bamashmous[4,5], Najlaa M Alamoudi[6], Douaa El Derwi[6,7], Ibrahim M Masoud[8], Veerasathpurush Allareddy[9*] and Nour F Gowharji[10]

Abstract

Background: The purpose of this study was to predict the annual growth rate of the mandible and total anterior facial height using IGF-1 levels together with cervical stage, skeletal classification, and gender.

Methods: Twenty-five orthodontic patients (12 females and 13 males) had their cervical stages, blood-spot IGF-1 levels, and cephalometric parameters measured at 1-year intervals. The number of years each patient was followed up varied between 1 and 5 years resulting in 43 12-month intervals collected from 77 observations. Descriptive, bivariate, and regression analyses were used to analyze this data.

Results: The linear regression model for predicting the annual mandibular growth rate was significant at $p < 0.01$ with an R-square value of 0.52. We found that the average IGF-1 level for the interval, the change in IGF-1 level, and the presence of a skeletal class III pattern were statistically significant predictors of mandibular growth. The regression model for predicting the annual change in anterior facial height was significant at $p < 0.01$ with an R-square value of 0.42. We found that the change in IGF-1 level was the only statistically significant predictor of this outcome.

Conclusions: The proposed method which combines IGF-1 levels with information that is readily available to clinicians can be used to predict the timing and intensity of the growth spurt. These factors together explain more of the observed individual variation in growth rate than any of the factors used in isolation.

Keywords: Mandible; IGF-1; Vertical dimension; Craniofacial biology; Developmental biology; Growth factors; Growth prediction

Background

Currently, several methods for predicting facial growth are in vogue [1-5]. The frequently used methods include skeletal maturation indicators (SMIs) developed by Fishman and cervical vertebral maturation (CVM) derived from hand-wrist radiographs [1-5]. IGF-1 is a mediator for growth hormone that has been shown to exhibit local and systemic influences in stimulating longitudinal bone growth [6-8]. In earlier studies, we had cross-sectionally related IGF-1 levels to both cervical stages and hand-wrist radiograph stages, with the highest IGF-1 levels being observed in the late pubertal stages [9-11]. Our prior research has shown that there is a significant positive correlation between longitudinal changes in IGF-1 levels and changes in mandibular length with significantly greater mandibular growth occurring when IGF-1 levels showed an ascending pattern and averaged over 250 μg/L over two consecutive observations [11]. To date, the simultaneous interaction between IGF-1, cervical stage, gender, and skeletal classification has not been longitudinally studied, and no method has been proposed to predict the timing and intensity of facial growth using IGF-1 controlling for these factors.

The purpose of the present study was to use linear regression models that use IGF-1 levels to predict the annual growth rate of anterior facial height as well as

* Correspondence: sathpurush@gmail.com
[9]Department of Orthodontics, College of Dentistry and Dental Clinics, The University of Iowa, 801 Newton Road, Iowa City 52242, IA, USA
Full list of author information is available at the end of the article

mandibular length while controlling for the effects of cervical stage, skeletal classification, and gender. We hypothesized that IGF-1 levels will be associated with increases in anterior facial height and mandibular length.

Methods

Institutional review board approval

The study protocol was approved by the institutional review board (IRB) of the Harvard Medical School and the ethical committee of King Abdulaziz University.

Study sample and informed consent

This prospective longitudinal sample consisted of 25 subjects (13 males and 12 females). Inclusion criteria were patients who were to begin orthodontic treatment, in active treatment, or in post-treatment follow-up. Since the study involved radiographic exposure, non-orthodontic patients were not included for ethical reasons. Exclusion criteria included patients who had systemic diseases, growth abnormalities, bleeding disorders, or growth modification as part of their orthodontic treatment. Patients who satisfied the inclusion criteria and agreed to participate in the study were all included without further selection. The subjects were all mostly Mediterranean Caucasians, but interracial marriages are common in the population that was sampled. The objectives of the study were explained to the subjects, and consent forms were signed by those who agreed to participate. The study was conducted following informed consent and IRB approval.

Sample size estimation and power analysis

A power analysis at the beginning of this study showed that we needed over 95 1-year intervals to be able to reject our null hypothesis if a negative result was found. Each 1-year interval required an observation at the beginning and end of the year for the interval to qualify. The original study sample, attrition rate, and the reasons for attrition are described in greater detail in our earlier studies [9-11]. In summary, our original sample comprised 87 subjects with the intent of following them up every 12 months (±2 months) until we collected 95 1-year intervals with the hope that even with attrition, our sample would be collected within 3 to 5 years. However, only 25 subjects showed up for the second observation, so the remaining 62 subjects were eliminated from our longitudinal sample. The sample continued to experience gradual attrition with only 6 subjects agreeing to attend their sixth observation which marked 5 years of follow-up and the end of the study. Any 1-year interval with missing data or non-diagnostic records at the beginning or end of the interval was eliminated from the study. At the end of the study, we had 43 qualifying 1-year intervals (17 female and 26 male intervals) from 77 observations with several observations serving as the end of one interval and the beginning of the next one. This meant that our sample would allow us to accept positive results but that negative results could not prove the absence of a relationship and could not be accepted.

Patient records

As a part of the patients' standard orthodontic records, lateral cephalometric radiographs were obtained and a questionnaire about age, puberty, and history of blood disorders was completed. Each patient had his or her lateral cephalometric radiograph, height, and weight measurements, as well as a blood-spot sample obtained within 1 week of each other for each observation. The blood-spot samples were collected using kits donated by ZRT Laboratory (Beaverton, OR, USA) and were stored in sealed plastic bags in a freezer (−18°C) for no more than 6 months. The samples were sent to ZRT Laboratory and assayed by radioimmunoassay. The patients' cephalometric radiographs were traced using VistaDent OC (version 4.2.28, GAC TechnoCenter Orthodontic Software Solutions, Birmingham, AL, USA). Calibration was performed using a metal ruler that was positioned at the top right corner of the film and exposed together with the patient. The mandibular length was measured from the condylion to the gnathion, the total anterior facial height was measured from the nasion to the menton, and the mandibular plane was measured from the gonion to the gnathion. The skeletal classification was evaluated using the ANB angle [12]. Measurements between 0° and 4° were considered skeletal class I, measurements above 4° were considered skeletal class II, and measurements below 0° were considered skeletal class III. One examiner performed all the measurements. Although the subjects were all orthodontic patients, none of them had growth modification during the observation period and many of them were in pre- or post-treatment follow-up. To evaluate the possible effect of orthodontic treatment on the total anterior facial height, a paired *t*-test was conducted, and this showed that there was no significant change in the mandibular plane angle during the intervals ($p = 0.582$) with a mean change of −0.18° and a standard error of 0.32.

Cervical vertebral staging

The cervical vertebrae were staged using the six stages described by Baccetti et al. [5]. Curvatures were initially called if they were equal to or greater than 1 mm deep. However, when that was done, several patients skipped stages within the 1-year follow-up period. The criteria for calling curvatures were then changed so that any curvature equal to or greater than 0.5 mm would be considered. Skipping stages were almost completely eliminated when that was done. The six cervical stages described by Baccetti et al. [5] were grouped into three groups based on the annual growth rates observed in the year following their appearance [9]: group A which included cervical stages 1 and 2 and was considered to be the pre-pubertal group; group B which included cervical stage 3 and was considered the pubertal group; and group C which included cervical stages 4, 5, and 6 and was considered to be the post-pubertal group. Both the laboratory that measured the IGF-I levels and the individual evaluating the radiographs were blinded to each other's results to eliminate bias.

Outcome and independent variables

The primary outcome variable of interest in the present study was annual growth rate of anterior facial height, and the secondary outcome variable was annual growth rate of the mandible. The independent (predictor) variables were average IGF-1 level and change in IGF-1 level.

Statistical approach

The data was entered in SPSS (SPSS Version 22.0 for Windows, IBM Corp., Armonk, NY, USA) and was analyzed using the same software as well as SAS (SAS Version 9.3 for Windows, SAS Institute Inc., Cary, NC, USA). Two different multivariable linear regression models were used to predict the annual growth rate of total anterior facial height and that of the mandible. The effects of cervical stage, gender, skeletal classification, and initial length variables were adjusted in the multivariable regression models. The changes in outcomes for each one unit change in IGF-1 levels were predicted in the regression models. The total amount of variance explained by all the independent variables in the regression models was computed. Ordinary least squares approach was used to fit the multivariable linear regression models. All statistical tests were two-sided, and a p value of <0.05 was deemed to be statistically significant.

Results

The final study sample comprised 13 male and 12 female subjects. The age of the study subjects ranged from 9.2 to 17.4 years. The cervical stages of the study sample at the initial encounter (T0) included stage 1 (16%), stage 2 (28%), stage 3 (12%), stage 4 (32%), and stage 5 (12%). Skeletal classifications included class I (20%), class II (64%), and class III (16%). A total of 43 1-year time intervals were available.

Results of the multivariable linear regression model examining annual mandibular growth are summarized in Table 1. Following adjustment for multiple factors including gender (male), initial mandibular length, skeletal pattern, and cervical group, the average IGF-1 levels and IGF-1 changes were significantly associated with increase in annual mandibular length. Each one unit increase in the average IGF-1 level was associated with 0.01203 unit increase in mandibular length ($p = 0.02$). Each one unit increase in the IGF-1 change was associated with 0.00864 unit increase in mandibular length ($p = 0.01$). About 52% of the total variance in the mandibular growth was explained by this multivariable regression model. Skeletal class III pattern was associated with 3.08 unit increase in mandibular length when compared to the skeletal class I group ($p = 0.006$). None of the other factors were significantly associated with increase in mandibular length. The following formula can be generated from this regression model:

The annual mandibular growth rate in mm/year = −4.23 + (Average IGF-1 (in μg/L) × 0.012) + (Change in IGF-1 (in μg/L) × 0.009) + (Initial mandibular length in mm × 0.028) + (0 if the patient is a female, 0.917 if the patient is a male) + (0 if the patient is in skeletal class I, −0.265

Table 1 Results of regression analysis to predict annual change in mandibular length

Independent variables	Parameter estimate	Error	*p* value
Intercept	−4.27893	6.06406	0.48
Average IGF-1 in μg/L	0.01203	0.00479	*0.02*
IGF-1 change in μg/L	0.00864	0.00316	*0.01*
Initial mandibular length in mm	0.02822	0.06394	0.66
Male gender (female is the reference group)	0.91686	0.75568	0.23
Skeletal class I (reference group)	Reference	-	-
Skeletal class II	−0.26483	0.79831	0.74
Skeletal class III	3.08272	1.06271	*0.006*
Cervical group A	0.16312	0.86144	0.85
Cervical group B	1.73768	1.10008	0.1235
Cervical group C (reference group)	Reference	-	-

R-square: 0.5215. *p* value for the model: 0.0007.

if the patient is in skeletal class II, and 3.083 if the patient is in skeletal class III) + (0 if the patient is in cervical group C, 0.163 if the patient is in cervical group A, and 1.738 if the patient is in cervical group B).

Results of the multivariable linear regression model for predicting annual change in the total anterior face height are summarized in Table 2. Following adjustment for all available factors, each one unit IGF-1 change was associated with 0.01033 unit increase in total anterior face height ($p = 0.02$). None of the other factors were significantly associated with changes in total anterior face height. About 42% of the total variance in the changes in annual total face height was explained by this multivariable regression model. The following formula can be generated from the regression model:

The annual total anterior facial height growth rate in mm/year = 6.08452 + (Average IGF-1 (in μg/L) × 0.00929) + (Change in IGF-1 (in μg/L) × 0.01033) + (Initial anterior facial height × −0.06665) + (0 if the patient is a female, 1.75912 if the patient is a male) + (0 if the patient is in skeletal class I, 0.30974 if the patient is in skeletal class II, and 1.89292 if the patient is in skeletal class III) + (0 if the patient is in cervical group C, −0.88972 if the patient is in cervical group A, and 2.45562 if the patient is in cervical group B).

The gonial angle, the *y*-axis, and the mandibular plane angle were not included in the multivariable regression models since they were not found to have a statistically significant impact on the outcomes.

Discussion

The multivariable prediction equations derived in the present study can be used to predict the total anterior facial height and annual growth rate of the mandible. The change in IGF-1 establishes a pattern and gives information about whether the patient is pre- or post-pubertal. In an earlier study, we had demonstrated that patients with IGF-1 levels following an ascending pattern have significantly greater mandibular growth per year than patients with descending IGF levels [11]. However, this information can be misleading if used in isolation since IGF-1 values could show no change on a patient that is a very young, or very old, or a patient with an extended growth spurt. Each of those situations would have little or no change in IGF-1 level but would actually be in completely different stages of their development. The average IGF-1 level supplements that information since it allows us to distinguish the patients who are at or around their peak. Including the cervical stage, information was also found to add to the equations' accuracy and variance in predicting facial growth, especially total anterior facial height. With the addition of gender and skeletal classification, we were able to increase the amount of variability in our models with the presence of a class III skeletal pattern being a statistically significant factor in predicting the mandibular growth rate. The variation in size was taken into consideration by adding the initial mandibular length and the initial total anterior facial height to the factors considered in each of their regression models. Despite our small sample size, we can be confident in accepting our positive results as being significant contributors to the equations since the statistics account for possible type I errors (false positive).

Franchi and Baccetti found that aside from the cervical stage, a patient's gonial angle was the only cephalometric measurement that could predict how well a patient responded to functional appliance therapy [13]. Our results found that none of the cephalometric parameters evaluated including the gonial angle, mandibular plane, and *y*-axis significantly added to the ability of our regression models to predict the annual growth rate of the mandible or the anterior facial height. This, however,

Table 2 Results of regression analysis to predict annual change in total anterior face height

Independent variables	Parameter estimate	Error	*p* value
Intercept	6.08452	8.35131	0.47
Average IGF-1 in μg/L	0.00929	0.0061	0.14
IGF-1 change in μg/L	0.01033	0.00437	*0.02*
Initial total anterior facial height in mm	−0.06665	0.07285	0.37
Male (female is the reference group)	1.75912	0.97007	0.08
Skeletal class I (reference group)	Reference		
Skeletal class II	0.30974	1.00557	0.76
Skeletal class III	1.89294	1.46272	0.20
Cervical group A	−0.88972	1.22983	0.47
Cervical group B	2.45562	1.42716	0.09
Cervical group C (reference group)	Reference		

R-square: 0.4228. *p* value for the model: 0.0095.

does not necessarily mean that there is no relationship between these measurements and a patient's growth rate or pattern since our sample size was too small to rule out a type II statistical error (false negative).

Combining IGF-1 with the other factors improved the accuracy of the regression models and accounted for about half the observed variability. Facial growth is influenced by a variety of genetic and environmental factors and regulated by multiple local and system processes. Finding a group of factors that can account for that much of the variability is a significant step towards customizing our treatment plan decision to our individual patients and taking their biological differences into consideration.

The fact that our records were taken annually should be considered while interpreting the study results since the change in IGF-1 levels and average IGF-1 levels could be misleading if the peak in IGF-1 levels happened to occur during a 12-month interval. One would expect IGF-1 measurements taken 3 to 6 months apart to be sufficient to establish a pattern of change and should be able to give a more accurate assessment of the patient's IGF-1 pattern and average level.

Jain and colleagues examined the association between IGF-1 levels and cervical maturation stages and found that amongst a cohort of 45 male subjects, there were highly significant associations between the two variables [4]. Ishaq and colleagues examined 120 subjects (60 males and 60 females) to correlate the levels of IGF-1 to cervical maturation stage and concluded that IGF-1 serum levels are reliable maturation indicators [14]. Our study results are consistent with these findings and further substantiate that IGF-1 levels could serve as a good diagnostic method for determining the optimal time for commencing orthodontic treatment.

All the study subjects in the present study received orthodontic treatment. Due to ethical considerations, it would be impossible to get institutional review board approval to perform a growth study involving radiographic exposure on an untreated population. Prior research has shown that fixed orthodontic appliances even with intermaxillary elastics have clinically insignificant effects on facial growth, and our findings described above are consistent with that [15,16].

The present study has several limitations, and the study results and conclusions should be interpreted keeping these in perspective. The present study used 2-D lateral cephalometric radiographs. The limitations of using 2-D images are well documented [17]. Any errors in landmark identification could yield biased estimates. The nature of the study design precludes us from clearly establishing a cause and effect relationship between the predictor and outcome variables. Only a well-designed randomized controlled trial will enable us to establish this relationship [18]. Only one biological factor was examined which accounts for the moderate correlation coefficient. However, it is still impressive that a single biological factor could account for the amount of variability explained by the multivariable regression models. Despite the fact that none of these patients had growth modification during the follow-up period, many of them were undergoing orthodontic treatment with full fixed appliances which could arguably have had an influence on their growth. As mentioned earlier, the study sample is not representative, and hence, the generalizability and external validity of the findings are questionable. The present study could have benefitted by an increased sample size and examining several more variables that could confound growth. Owing to the practical limitations on recruiting more patients to participate, we were unable to increase the sample size. This is a major limitation of the study. Finally, the prediction equations derived in the present study accounted for 52% of variance in mandibular growth and 42% of variance in anterior facial height. It is clear that a large amount of variance is explained by the predictors. Nevertheless, there could be other variables that are not captured in the models that can play a significant role in determining growth. These should be kept in perspective while treatment planning orthodontic cases.

Conclusions

1. Linear regression models derived from the present study could help in the prediction of the timing and intensity of patients' facial growth spurt using IGF-1 levels while controlling for cervical stage, gender, and skeletal classification.
2. Average IGF-1 for an observation period, change in IGF-1 level, and the presence of a skeletal class III pattern were statistically significant factors in the regression model for predicting changes in mandibular length.
3. Change in IGF-1 level was the only statistically significant factor in the regression model for predicting changes in total anterior facial height.

Competing interests

The authors declare that they have no competing interests.

Authors' contributions

MIM, HYAM, MB, and NFG contributed to the study idea and study design. MIM and MB analyzed the data MIM, MB, and VA interpreted the data. MIM, HYAM, MB, NMA, DED, IMM, NFG, and VA drafted the manuscript. All authors gave the final approval of the manuscript.

Acknowledgements

The authors would like to acknowledge Deanship for Scientific Research, Faculty of Dentistry, King Abdulaziz University for facilitating the conduct of this work.

Author details
[1]Department of Developmental Biology, Harvard School of Dental Medicine, 188 Longwood Avenue, Boston, MA 02115, USA. [2]Orthodontics Department - Faculty of Dentistry, King Abdulaziz University, Abdullah Sulayman st, Jeddah 22254, Saudi Arabia. [3]Department of Orthodontics, University of Buffalo, 140 Squire Hall, Buffalo, NY 14214, USA. [4]Department of Dental Public Health, King Abdulaziz University, Abdullah Sulayman st, Jeddah 22254, Saudi Arabia. [5]Henry M. Goldman School of Dental Medicine, Boston University, 100 East Newton Street, Boston, MA 02118, USA. [6]Pediatric Dentistry Department, Faculty of Dentistry, King Abdulaziz University, Abdullah Sulayman st, Jeddah 22254, Saudi Arabia. [7]Public Health and Community Medicine Department, Faculty of Medicine, Cairo University, Al Kasr st, Kasralainy, Cairo, 11562, Egypt. [8]Dr. Ibrahim Masoud's Dental Specialty Clinic, Jeddah, Saudi Arabia, Falasteen Street, Jeddah 21426, Saudi Arabia. [9]Department of Orthodontics, College of Dentistry and Dental Clinics, The University of Iowa, 801 Newton Road, Iowa City 52242, IA, USA. [10]Department of Pediatric Dentistry, Tufts School of Dental Medicine, 1 Kneeland St, Boston, MA 02111, USA.

References

1. Ricketts RM. A principle of arcial growth of the mandible. Angle Orthod. 1972;42:368–86.
2. Turchetta BJ, Fishman LS, Subtelny JD. Facial growth prediction: a comparison of methodologies. Am J Orthod Dentofacial Orthop. 2007;132:439–49.
3. Fishman LS. Radiographic evaluation of skeletal maturation. A clinically oriented method based on hand-wrist films. Angle Orthod. 1982;52:88–112.
4. Jain S, Jain S, Deoskar A, Prasad VS. Serum IGF-1 levels as a clinical tool for optimizing orthodontic treatment timing. Prog Orthod. 2013;14:46. doi:10.1186/2196-1042-14-46.
5. Baccetti T, Franchi L, McNamara Jr JA. The cervical vertebral maturation (CVM) method for the assessment of optimal treatment timing in dentofacial orthopedics. Sem Orthod. 2005;11:119–29.
6. Isaksson OG, Jansson JO, Gause IA. Growth hormone stimulates longitudinal bone growth directly. Science. 1982;216:1237–9.
7. Shoshana Y, Liu JL, Le Roith D. Growth hormone/insulin-like growth factor-I system: implications for organ growth and development. Pediatr Nephrol. 2000;14(7):544–9.
8. Yakar S. Circulating levels of IGF-1 directly regulate bone growth and density. J Clin Invest. 2002;110(6):771–81.
9. Masoud M, Masoud I, Kent Jr RL, Gowharji N, Cohen LE. Assessing skeletal maturity by using blood-spot insulin-like growth factor I (IGF-I) testing. Am J Orthod Dentofacial Orthop. 2008;134(2):209–16.
10. Masoud MI, Masoud I, Kent Jr RL, Gowharji N, Hassan AH, Cohen LE. Relationship between blood-spot insulin-like growth factor 1 levels and hand-wrist assessment of skeletal maturity. Am J Orthod Dentofacial Orthop. 2009;136(1):59–64.
11. Masoud MI, Marghalani HY, Masoud IM, Gowharji NF. Prospective longitudinal evaluation of the relationship between changes in mandibular length and blood-spot IGF-1 measurements. Am J OrthodDentofacia-lOrthop. 2012;141(6):694–704.
12. Steiner CC. Cephalometrics for you and me. Am J Orthodont. 1953;39:729–55.
13. Franchi L, Baccetti T. Prediction of individual mandibular changes induced by functional jaw orthopedics followed by fixed appliances in Class II patients. Angle Orthod. 2006;76(6):950–4.
14. Ishaq RA, Soliman SA, Foda MY, Fayed MM. Insulin-like growth factor I: a biologic maturation indicator. Am J Orthod Dentofacial Orthop. 2012;142(5):654–61.
15. Alkumru P, Erdem D, Altug-Atac AT. Evaluation of changes in the vertical facial dimension with different anchorage systems in extraction and non-extraction subjects treated by Begg fixed appliances: a retrospective study. Eur J Orthod. 2007;29(5):508–16.
16. Edwards JG. Orthopedic effects with "conventional" fixed orthodontic appliances: a preliminary report. Am J Orthod. 1983;84(4):275–91.
17. Durão AR, Pittayapat P, Rockenbach MI, Olszewski R, Ng S, Ferreira AP, et al. Validity of 2D lateral cephalometry in orthodontics: a systematic review. Prog Orthod. 2013;14:31.
18. Kiriakou J, Pandis N, Madianos P, Polychronopoulou A. Developing evidence-based dentistry skills: how to interpret randomized clinical trials and systematic reviews. Prog Orthod. 2014;15:58.

33

Association between tooth size and interarch relationships in children with operated complete unilateral cleft lip and palate

Patrícia Bittencourt Dutra dos Santos[1*], Daniela Gamba Garib[2], Guilherme Janson[3] and Vivian Helena Assis[4]

Abstract

Background: To evaluate mesiodistal tooth width of patients with UCLP comparing tooth size in different Goslon Yardstick scores and between cleft and noncleft sides.

Methods: The Department of Orthodontics at Bauru Dental School and Hospital of Rehabilitation of Craniofacial Anomalies – University of Sao Paulo. Hundred forty-four pairs of dental casts of patients with UCLP. These dental casts were divided into 3 groups: group I (patients with Goslon rating of 1 and 2), group II (Goslon rating of 3) and group III (Goslon rating of 4 and 5). The control group consisted of 40 pairs of dental casts of noncleft Class I patients at the same age range. Mesiodistal width of maxillary permanent central incisors, lateral incisors and first molars were measured using a digital caliper. Intergroup comparisons were performed using ANOVA followed by Tukey tests. T tests were used to compare tooth size between cleft and noncleft sides ($p < 0.05$).

Results: Differences for tooth size were observed between individuals with different Goslon Yardstik scores. Mesiodistal widths of maxillary central incisors in subjects of Group III were significantly smaller compared to Group I and to the control group. The lateral incisors at the cleft side were smaller than the antimere.

Conclusions: Mesiodistal tooth size was smaller in poor Goslon yardstick scores. Cleft and noncleft sides demonstrated similar maxillary tooth size except for the lateral incisor.

Keywords: Cleft lip; Cleft palate; Tooth size

Background

Cleft patients have considerably more dental anomalies than non-cleft patients [1]. Certain key genetic disturbances have been implicated in both dental anomalies and clefting, suggesting a shared genetic etiology in some cases [2,3]. Among many dental anomalies reported in CLP patients, small tooth size is frequently reported [3-6]. Besides reduced crown size, cleft patients demonstrated simplified crown morphology and malformed teeth [3]. Sabóia et al. [7] hypothesize that tooth size reductions may be part of the oral cleft phenotypic spectrum.

Foster and Lavelle [8] reported that most permanent teeth are smaller in cleft patients compared with non-cleft individuals. On the other hand, the investigation of Peterka and Mullerova [9] revealed no significant dimensional differences between mesiodistal widths of individuals with cleft lip and palate (CLP, isolated cleft palate and complete unilateral cleft lip and palate (UCLP)) and non-cleft subjects, with the exception of central incisors for males and second molars for females which were smaller in individuals with CLP [10]. Sabóia et al. [7] found smaller tooth size for canines, second premolars and first molars in the maxillary arch, and for incisors and second premolars in the mandibular arch. However, these previous studies' samples included all types of clefts (cleft lip (CL), cleft lip and palate (CLP), and cleft palate (CP)). Considering that CL/CLP and CP have different etiological background, it is important to evaluate tooth size in each type of cleft separately. Additionally, no previous study investigated whether crown size can affect interarch sagittal relationship in patients with UCLP.

* Correspondence: pati_bittencourt@hotmail.com
[1]Department of Orthodontics, State University of Rio Grande do Norte, Caicó, RN, Brazil
Full list of author information is available at the end of the article

Therefore, the aim of this study was to evaluate mesiodistal tooth width of permanent teeth in patients with complete unilateral cleft lip and palate, by comparing tooth size in different GOSLON Yardstick scores and between cleft and non-cleft sides.

Methods

The sample size for each group was calculated based on an alpha significance level of 0.05 and a beta of 0.2 to achieve 80% of power to detect a mean difference of 0.94 mm in central incisor size with a 0.6 mm of estimated standard deviation [10]. The sample size calculation showed that 7 patients in each group were needed, and to increase the power even more, it was decided to select 32 patients for groups at least.

This project was approved by the Ethical Committee of the Bauru Dental School. Patient records were anonymized and de-identified prior to analysis. A study sample of 104 Brazilian-Caucasian patients with unilateral complete cleft lip and palate rehabilitated in a single center was retrospectively selected at Hospital of Rehabilitation of Craniofacial Anomalies. A control group of 40 dental casts of non-cleft Class I patients was selected from the growth study center at Bauru Dental School, matched by age and sex with the study sample. The inclusion criteria of the study sample were patients with complete unilateral cleft lip and palate filed at the Hospital from 1999 to 2011, without associated syndromes, with adequate dental casts taken between 8 and 10 years of age available, history of lip repair performed in the first year of life, and palate repair within the second year of life. The primary surgeries had been carried out by five different surgeons using the Millard technique for lip repair and the Van Langenbeck technique for palate repair.

The study sample was divided into three groups according to the GOSLON Yardstick index by a single examiner:

Group I: 35 patients with GOSLON Yardstick index of 1 and 2 (13 females and 22 males);
Group II: 32 patients with GOSLON Yardstick index of 3 (8 females and 24 males);
Group III: 37 patients with GOSLON Yardstick index of 4 and 5 (11 females and 26 males).

Mesiodistal crown width of maxillary permanent central incisors, lateral incisors, and first molars on both arch sides were measured using a digital caliper (Mitutoyo Corporation, Tokyo, Japan) directly on the dental casts by a single examiner (Figure 1). On the cleft side, only the maxillary lateral incisor distal to the cleft was measured. Teeth with interproximal caries or restorations were not considered.

Error study

In order to assess the study error, measurements of 30 dental casts were repeated by the same operator, one month after the first evaluation. Random and systematic errors were assessed using Dahlberg's formula and dependent *t*-tests, respectively.

Statistical analyses

Normal distribution was evaluated with Kolmogorov-Smirnov tests. Comparisons between male and female and between cleft and non-cleft sides were performed with *t*-tests. Comparison between the experimental groups and the control group was performed with one-way analysis of variance (ANOVA), followed by Tukey tests. Results were considered significant at $P < 0.05$. The statistical tests were

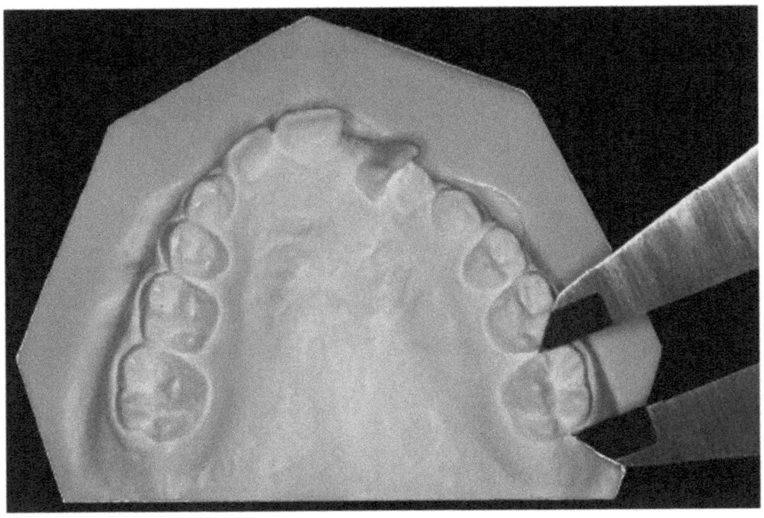

Figure 1 Measurements of crown size in the maxillary arch.

Table 1 Systematic and casual errors (dependent *t*-tests and Dahlberg's formula)

Mesiodistal crown diameter	First measurement		Second measurement		*P*	Dahlberg
	n = 30		*n* = 30			
	Mean	SD	Mean	SD		
Right central incisor	8.39	0.81	8.46	0.85	0.067	0.13
Left central incisor	8.32	0.01	8.37	0.55	0.090	0.10
Right lateral incisor	6,83	0.68	6.90	0.74	0.469	0.22
Left lateral incisor	6.46	00.1	6.44	0,64	0.667	1.16
Right first molar	10.12	00.1	10.07	0.68	0.540	0.29
Left first molar	9.92	00.1	10.00	0.62	0.240	0.26

performed with SPSS 7.0 for Windows (SPSS Inc., Chicago, IL, USA).

Results

Results of the error study are shown in Table 1. There were no statistically significant systematic errors and the random errors were within acceptable range.

In patients with UCLP, there was no difference in tooth size between males and females (Table 2). Crown width of the maxillary central incisors in subjects of Group III was significantly smaller than that of Group I and the control group (Table 3).

The maxillary lateral incisor was smaller on the cleft side (Table 4).

Discussion

It is recognized that poor growth of the maxillary region is related to the effects of primary repair surgery [11], and this is of particular concern for the orthodontist who must correct dentofacial discrepancies during early adolescence. Although those patients who have displayed favorable facial growth may require only relatively routine orthodontic treatment, patients with unfavorable facial growth often need orthognathic surgery for complete correction of dentofacial discrepancies [11]. In our study, all primary plastic surgeries were performed using the same surgical protocol regarding techniques, timing, and sequence. It is important once anteroposterior relationship can be influenced not only by surgery but by surgeon too [12,13].

Table 2 Intergroup comparison between mesiodistal widths of permanent teeth between the female and male cleft patients (*t* test)

Mesiodistal crown diameter	Female cleft Mean (SD)	Male cleft Mean (SD)	*P*
Central incisor	8.39 (0.75)	8.54 (0.65)	0.089
Lateral incisor	6.52 (0.71)	6.57 (0.65)	0.615
Molar	9.97 (0.56)	10.06 (0.62)	0.246

Table 3 Intergroup comparison of maxillary tooth size between cleft and non-cleft groups (ANOVA followed by Tukey tests)

Mesiodistal crown diameter	Group I	Group II	Group III	Control group	*P*
	(*n* = 35)	(*n* = 32)	(*n* = 37)	(*n* = 40)	
	Mean (SD)	Mean (SD)	Mean (SD)	Mean (SD)	
Central incisor	8.63 (0.77)A	8.39 (0.62)AB	8.27 (0.72)B	8.60 (0.60)A	0.004*
Lateral incisor	6.64 (0.75)	6.44 (0.87)	6.31 (0.80)	6.61 (0.52)	0.190
Molars	9.99 (0.54)	10.10 (0.62)	9.95 (0.61)	10.07 (0.63)	0.486

*Statistically significant at $P < 0.05$. Different letters represent statistically significant differences.

The GOSLON Yardstick has been shown to be a robust measurement tool with a high degree of reliability and reproducibility and has proven useful for longitudinal assessment of dental arch relationship [14]. Application of the Yardstick is simple and fast, requiring no specialized or expensive equipment. It does not involve application of precise and detailed criteria but relies on a simple method of judgment. The simplicity is its inherent strength, and its longitudinal robustness makes it a valuable tool. The Yardstick considers clinically important variables in all three planes of space and allows ranking of dental casts in order of difficulty to achieve a favorable outcome [15-17]. For this reason, GOSLON Yardstick was used in this study.

No significant intersex difference was found for tooth size in patients with UCLP (Table 2). Previous reports have shown no differences for tooth dimensions between males and females in patients without oral clefts [10,18-20]. Conversely, some authors reported larger teeth in males [7,21-23] as well as in females with oral clefts [8]. Saboia et al. [7] reported that combined mesiodistal widths were consistently smaller in females with oral cleft when compared to males. However, this last study included all types of clefts (CL, CLP, and CP). Rawashdeh et al. [23] found larger teeth in males with UCLP when compared to females, except for maxillary second premolar and mandibular first premolar on the cleft side.

To our knowledge, this study is the first attempt to evaluate mesiodistal tooth size in patients with UCLP

Table 4 Intergroup comparison between mesiodistal widths of permanent teeth between the cleft and non-cleft sides in the UCLP patients (ANOVA followed by Tukey tests)

Mesiodistal crown diameter	Cleft side Mean (SD)	Non-cleft side Mean (SD)	Control group Mean (SD)	*P*
Central incisor	8.36 (0.66)	8.45 (0.79)	8.60 (0.60)	0.088
Lateral incisor	5.68 (0.51)A	6.84 (0.65)B	6.61 (0.52)B	0.000*
Molar	10.04 (0.61)	9.99 (0.58)	10.07 (0.63)	0.676

*Statistically significant at $P < 0.05$. Different letters represent statistically significant differences.

with different GOSLON Yardstick scores. The hypothesis is that tooth size could be associated with interarch sagittal relationship. Differences were found for tooth size between patients with different GOSLON Yardistick scores (Table 3). This confirms that the maxillomandibular anteroposterior discrepancy is not the only factor related to GOSLON Yardstick scores. Mesiodistal sizes of maxillary teeth were different in extreme GOSLON Yardstick scores.

The findings indicated that the maxillary central incisors were smaller in Group III as compared to Group I and to the control group (Table 3). The difference indicated a tendency for smaller tooth size in patients with UCLP compared to non-cleft patients and patients with a mild GOSLON score. Foster and Lavelle [8] found that the maxillary teeth of complete UCLP patients were significantly smaller compared to non-cleft controls. On the other hand, Peterka and Mullerova [9] found no differences between mesiodistal tooth widths of individuals with UCLP and a control group. Another study including all cleft types (CL, CLP, and CP) found that maxillary canines and first molars were significantly reduced in size in CLP and CP groups compared to non-cleft subjects [7]. It seems that despite some controversy in this issue, the tendency is for cleft patients to present smaller mesiodistal tooth sizes.

When cleft and non-cleft sides were compared, no differences were observed for permanent central incisors and maxillary first molars. Nevertheless, the maxillary lateral incisor mesiodistal dimension was 1.2 mm smaller on the cleft side compared to the non-cleft side (Table 4). This result is comparable to the published data of Rawashdeh and Bakir [23] showing that the maxillary lateral incisor was statistically significantly smaller on the cleft side. Sofaer [24] and Werner and Harris [3] also demonstrated statistically significant levels of asymmetry occurring between the cleft and non-cleft sides for mesiodistal size of maxillary lateral and central incisors, respectively. According to Sofaer [24], this generalized developmental instability can, to some extent, be genetically controlled, because patients with positive family histories showed some signs of greater asymmetry than those with negative family histories.

Boehn [25] found significant antimere differences in the size of the maxillary permanent incisors in patients with cleft lip and palate [23], suggesting that cleft had a local influence on tooth size. The reason for smaller maxillary lateral incisor on the cleft side in complete UCLP is probably its double embryonic origin [25-28]. Lateral incisor located distal to the alveolar cleft is in fact 'half of a tooth' [25-28].

Because patients with poor GOSLON Yardstick scores seem to have reduced tooth size, the orthodontist may leave spaces for composite rehabilitation, to improve sagittal relationship correction. Individual tooth dimensions are important in the clinical assessment of proportions and ratios. Orthodontists aim for an esthetically pleasing dental and facial appearance with a good functional occlusion. To reach these clinical goals, the dentition has to be in proportion; this is important not only from an esthetic standpoint but also occlusally [29].

Conclusions

Maxillary mesiodistal tooth size was inversely associated with GOSLON Yardstick scores. Similar tooth sizes were found for maxillary teeth at the cleft and non-cleft sides with the exception for the maxillary lateral incisor that was smaller on the cleft side.

Competing interests
The authors declare that they have no competing interests.

Authors' contributions
PBDS: selected patients, made measurements, participated in the design of the study, performed the statistical analysis and drafted the manuscript. DGG: conceived of the study and participated in its design and coordination and helped to draft the manuscript. GJ: helped to draft the manuscript, revising it critically for important intellectual content. VHA: selected patients and made measurements. All authors read and approved the final manuscript.

Author details
[1]Department of Orthodontics, State University of Rio Grande do Norte, Caicó, RN, Brazil. [2]Department of Orthodontics, Hospital of Rehabilitation of Craniofacial Anomalies, Bauru Dental School, University of São Paulo, Bauru, São Paulo, Brazil. [3]Department of Orthodontics, Bauru Dental School, University of São Paulo, Bauru, São Paulo, Brazil. [4]Hospital of Rehabilitation of Craniofacial Anomalies, Bauru Dental School, Bauru, São Paulo, Brazil.

References
1. Letra A, Menezes R, Granjeiro JM, Vieira AR. Defining subphenotypes for oral clefts based on dental development. J Dent Res. 2007;86(10):986–91.
2. Dentino KM, Peck S, Garib DG. Is missing maxillary lateral incisor in complete cleft lip and palate a product of genetics or local environment? Angle Orthod. 2012;82(6):959–63. doi:10.2319/012012-49.1.
3. Werner SP, Harris EF. Odontometrics of the permanent teeth in cleft lip and palate: systemic size reduction and amplified asymmetry. Cleft Palate J. 1989;26(1):36–41.
4. Wangsrimongkol T, Manosudprasit M, Pisek P, Chittiwatanapong N. Prevalence and types of dental anomaly in a Thai non-syndromic oral cleft sample. J Med Assoc Thail. 2013;96 Suppl 4:S25–35.
5. Al Jamal GA, Hazza'a AM, Rawashdeh MA. Prevalence of dental anomalies in a population of cleft lip and palate patients. Cleft Palate Craniofac J. 2010;47(4):413–20. doi:10.1597/08-275.1.
6. Eslami N, Majidi MR, Aliakbarian M, Hasanzadeh N. Prevalence of dental anomalies in patients with cleft lip and palate. J Craniofac Surg. 2013;24(5):1695–8. doi:10.1097/SCS.0b013e3182801bc8.
7. de Saboia TM, Kuchler EC, Tannure PN, Rey AC, Granjeiro JM, de Castro CM, et al. Mesio-distal and buccal-lingual tooth dimensions are part of the cleft spectrum: a pilot for future genetic studies. Cleft Palate Craniofac J. 2013;50(6):678–83. doi:10.1597/11-228.
8. Foster TD, Lavelle CL. The size of the dentition in complete cleft lip and palate. Cleft Palate J. 1971;8:177–84.
9. Peterka M, Mullerova Z. Tooth size in children with cleft lip and palate. Cleft Palate J. 1983;20(4):307–13.
10. Lewis BR, Stern MR, Willmot DR. Maxillary anterior tooth size and arch dimensions in unilateral cleft lip and palate. Cleft Palate Craniofac J. 2008;45(6):639–46. doi:10.1597/07-078.1.

11. Mars M, Houston WJ. A preliminary study of facial growth and morphology in unoperated male unilateral cleft lip and palate subjects over 13 years of age. Cleft Palate J. 1990;27(1):7–10.
12. Ross RB. The clinical implications of facial growth in cleft lip and palate. Cleft Palate J. 1970;7:37–47.
13. Normando AD, da Silva Filho OG, Capelozza FL. Influence of surgery on maxillary growth in cleft lip and/or palate patients. J Craniomaxillofac Surg. 1992;20(3):111–8.
14. Mars M, Plint DA, Houston WJ, Bergland O, Semb G. The Goslon Yardstick: a new system of assessing dental arch relationships in children with unilateral clefts of the lip and palate. Cleft Palate J. 1987;24(4):314–22.
15. Chan KT, Hayes C, Shusterman S, Mulliken JB, Will LA. The effects of active infant orthopedics on occlusal relationships in unilateral complete cleft lip and palate. Cleft Palate Craniofac J. 2003;40(5):511–7. doi:10.1597/1545-1569(2003)040<0511:TEOAIO>2.0.CO;2.
16. Mars M, Batra P, Worrell E. Complete unilateral cleft lip and palate: validity of the five-year index and the Goslon yardstick in predicting long-term dental arch relationships. Cleft Palate Craniofac J. 2006;43(5):557–62. doi:10.1597/05-074.
17. Garib DG, Santos PB, Janson G, Assis VH, de Paula Leite Battisti M. Association between dental arch widths and interarch relationships in children with operated unilateral complete cleft lip and palate. Cleft Palate Craniofac J. 2013. doi:10.1597/12-171.
18. Araujo E, Souki M. Bolton anterior tooth size discrepancies among different malocclusion groups. Angle Orthod. 2003;73(3):307–13. doi:10.1043/0003-3219(2003)073<0307:BATSDA>2.0.CO;2.
19. Basaran G, Selek M, Hamamci O, Akkus Z. Intermaxillary bolton tooth size discrepancies among different malocclusion groups. Angle Orthod. 2006;76(1):26–30. doi:10.1043/0003-3219(2006)076[0026:IBTSDA]2.0.CO;2.
20. Nie Q, Lin J. Comparison of intermaxillary tooth size discrepancies among different malocclusion groups. Am J Orthod Dentofacial Orthop. 1999;116(5):539–44.
21. Lavelle CL. Maxillary and mandibular tooth size in different racial groups and in different occlusal categories. Am J Orthod. 1972;61(1):29–37.
22. Bishara SE, Jakobsen JR, Treder JE, Stasi MJ. Changes in the maxillary and mandibular tooth size-arch length relationship from early adolescence to early adulthood. A longitudinal study. Am J Orthod Dentofacial Orthop. 1989;95(1):46–59.
23. Rawashdeh MA, Bakir IF. The crown size and sexual dimorphism of permanent teeth in Jordanian cleft lip and palate patients. Cleft Palate Craniofac J. 2007;44(2):155–62. doi:10.1597/05-197.1.
24. Sofaer JA. Human tooth-size asymmetry in cleft lip with or without cleft palate. Arch Oral Biol. 1979;24(2):141–6.
25. Boehn A. Dental anomalies in harelip and cleft palate. Acta Odontol Scand. 1963;21(SUPPL38):1–109.
26. Hovorakova M, Lesot H, Peterkova R, Peterka M. Origin of the deciduous upper lateral incisor and its clinical aspects. J Dent Res. 2006;85(2):167–71.
27. Yatabe MS, Garib DG, Janson G, Poletto RS, Ozawa TO. Is the presence of Simonart's band in patients with complete unilateral cleft lip and palate associated with the prevalence of missing maxillary lateral incisors? Am J Orthod Dentofacial Orthop. 2013;144(5):649–53. doi:10.1016/j.ajodo.2013.06.018.
28. Sulik K. Orofacial embryogenesis: a framework for understanding clefting sites. In: Fonseca RJMR, Turvey TA, editors. Oral and maxillofacial surgery. Philadelphia: Saunders; 2009. p. 711.
29. Bolton W. The clinical application of a tooth-size analysis. Am J Orthod Dentofacial Orthop. 1962;48:504–29.

Permissions

 Every chapter published in this book has been scrutinized by our experts. Their significance has been extensively debated. The topics covered herein carry significant findings which will fuel the growth of the discipline. They may even be implemented as practical applications or may be referred to as a beginning point for another development.

The contributors of this book come from diverse backgrounds, making this book a truly international effort. This book will bring forth new frontiers with its revolutionizing research information and detailed analysis of the nascent developments around the world.

We would like to thank all the contributing authors for lending their expertise to make the book truly unique. They have played a crucial role in the development of this book. Without their invaluable contributions this book wouldn't have been possible. They have made vital efforts to compile up to date information on the varied aspects of this subject to make this book a valuable addition to the collection of many professionals and students.

This book was conceptualized with the vision of imparting up-to-date information and advanced data in this field. To ensure the same, a matchless editorial board was set up. Every individual on the board went through rigorous rounds of assessment to prove their worth. After which they invested a large part of their time researching and compiling the most relevant data for our readers.

The editorial board has been involved in producing this book since its inception. They have spent rigorous hours researching and exploring the diverse topics which have resulted in the successful publishing of this book. They have passed on their knowledge of decades through this book. To expedite this challenging task, the publisher supported the team at every step. A small team of assistant editors was also appointed to further simplify the editing procedure and attain best results for the readers.

Apart from the editorial board, the designing team has also invested a significant amount of their time in understanding the subject and creating the most relevant covers. They scrutinized every image to scout for the most suitable representation of the subject and create an appropriate cover for the book.

The publishing team has been an ardent support to the editorial, designing and production team. Their endless efforts to recruit the best for this project, has resulted in the accomplishment of this book. They are a veteran in the field of academics and their pool of knowledge is as vast as their experience in printing. Their expertise and guidance has proved useful at every step. Their uncompromising quality standards have made this book an exceptional effort. Their encouragement from time to time has been an inspiration for everyone.

The publisher and the editorial board hope that this book will prove to be a valuable piece of knowledge for researchers, students, practitioners and scholars across the globe.

List of Contributors

Stefan Baumgartner and Theodore Eliades
Clinic for Orthodontics and Paediatric Dentistry, Center of Dental Medicine,University of Zurich, Plattenstr. 11, 8032 Zürich, Switzerland

Anna Iliadi and George Eliades
Department of Dental Biomaterials, School of Dentistry, University of Athens, 2 Thivon Str, 115 27, Goudi, Athens, Greece

Georgios Kanavakis, Moonyoung B Lee and Caroll-Ann Trotman
Department of Orthodontics and Dentofacial Orthopedics, Tufts University, School of Dental Medicine, 1 Kneeland Street DHS#1145, Boston, MA 02111, USA

Karen M Curran, Kevin C Wiseman and Nicholas P Barone
Private Practice, Boston, USA

Matthew D Finkelman
Department of Academic Services, Tufts University School of Dental Medicine, Boston, MA, USA

Sreedevi Srinivasan
Department of Orthodontics, University of Iowa, Iowa City, IA, USA

Abdul Razzak A. Ghazal and Rabab Al-Sabbagh
Department of Orthodontics, University of Hama Dental School, Hama, Syria

Mohammad Y. Hajeer
Department of Orthodontics, University of Damascus Dental School, Damascus, Syria

Ibrahim Alghoraibi
Nano Technology Lab, Physics Department, Faculty of Sciences, University of Damascus, Damascus, Syria

Ahmad Aldiry
Modern Chemistry Lab, Faculty of Veterinary, University of Hama, Hama, Syria

Rahul Trivedi, Amit Bhattacharya, Falguni Mehta, Harshik Parekh and Vaibhav Gandhi
Department of Orthodontics, Government Dental College and Hospital, Asarva, Ahmedabad, 380016, Gujarat, India

Dolly Patel
AMC Dental College, Ahmedabad, 380008, Gujarat, India

Matina V Angelopoulou
Division of Pediatric Dentistry, School of Dentistry, Marquette University, 1801 W Wisconsin Ave, 53233 Milwaukee, WI, USA

Despina Koletsi and Demetrios J Halazonetis
Department of Orthodontics, School of Dentistry, National and Kapodistrian University of Athens, 2 Thivon Str., 11527 Athens, Greece

George Vadiakas
Department of Paediatric Dentistry, School of Dentistry, National and Kapodistrian University of Athens, 2 Thivon Str., 11527 Athens, Greece

Matheus Melo Pithon
Av. Otavio Santos, 395 sala 705, Centro Odontomédico Dr. Altamirando da Costa Lima, Vitoria da Conquista, Bahia 45020750, Brazil

Matheus Melo Pithon, Dauro Douglas Oliveira and Raildo da Silva Coqueiro
Southwest Bahia State University UESB, Jequié, Bahia, Brazil

Daniel Santos Fonseca Figueiredo
Pontifical Catholic University of Minas Gerais, Belo Horizonte, Brazil

Won Moon, Kimberley W. Wu, Matthew MacGinnis, Jay Sung and Howard Chu
UCLA Section of Orthodontics, UCLA School of Dentistry, 10833 Le Conte Avenue, CHS - Box 951668, Los Angeles, CA 90095-1668, USA

George Youssef
Mechanical Engineering Department, California State University, Northridge, 18111 Nordhoff Street, Northridge, CA 91330, USA

Andre Machado
Section of Orthodontics, Federal University of Bahia, Salvador, Bahia, Brazil

Vikrum Nanda, Ehab Bar, Sotirios Tetradis, Aldons J Lusis, Eleazar Eskin and Won Moon
UCLA, California, USA

Boris Gutman
USC, California, USA

Suha Alghamdi
University of Connecticut, California, USA

Rosa Carrieri Rossi
Division of Pediatric Otolaryngology, Federal University of Sao Paulo- UNIFESP Brasil, Rua Botucatu 740, 4 andar, V. Clementino, São Paulo CEP:04023-062, Brazil

Nelson José Rossi and Nelson José Carrieri Rossi
2Educational Association of Brazil- FUNORTE/SOEBRAS, Rua Tijuco Preto 1694, Sao Paulo, Tatuapé CEP:03316-000, Brazil

Hélio Kiitiro Yamashita
Department of Diagnostic Imaging, Division of Otolaryngology and Head and Neck Imaging, Federal University of Sao Paulo- UNIFESP, Rua Botucatu 740, 4 andar, V. Clementino, São Paulo CEP:04023-062, Brazil

Shirley Shizue Nagata Pignatari
Department of Otolaryngology and Head and Neck Surgery, Division of Pediatric Otolaryngology, Federal University of Sao Paulo- UNIFESP, Rua Botucatu 740, 4 andar, V. Clementino, São Paulo CEP:04023-062, Brazil

Vincenzo Grassia, Fabrizia d'Apuzzo and Felice Femiano
Multidisciplinary Department of Medical-Surgical and Dental Specialties, Second University of Naples, Via Luigi De Crecchio 6, 80138 Napoli, Italy

Abdolreza Jamilian
Department of Orthodontics, Dental Branch, Craniomaxillofacial Center Islamic Azad University, No.2713, Vali Asr St, Tehran, Iran

Lorenzo Favero
Department of Neurosciences, University of Padua, Via Giustiniani 2, 35128 Padova, Italy

Letizia Perillo
Multidisciplinary Department of medical-Surgery and Dental Specialties, Second University of Naples; Post-Graduate Orthodontics Programme and Operative Unit, Via Luigi De Crecchio 6, 80138 Napoli, Italy

Mona A Montasser and Mahasen Taha
Orthodontic Department, Faculty of Dentistry 35516, Mansoura University, Mansoura, Egypt

Noha A El-Wassefy
Dental Biomaterials Department, Faculty of Dentistry 35516, Mansoura University, Mansoura, Egypt

Marieke G. Hobbelink, Yan He, Jia Xu, Huixu Xie, Richard Stoll and Qingsong Ye
Orthodontic Department, College of Medicine and Dentistry, James Cook University, Cairns, Australia

Marieke G. Hobbelink
School of Dentistry, University Medical Centre Groningen, Groningen, The Netherlands

Yan He
School and Hospital of Stomatology, Wenzhou Medical University, Wenzhou, China

Hooman Zarif Najafi, Parisa Salehi and Neda Babanouri
Orthodontic Research Center, Orthodontics Department, School of Dentistry, Shiraz University of Medical Sciences, Shiraz, Iran

Morteza Oshagh
Private Practice, Tehran, Iran

Sepideh Torkan
Orthodontics Department, University of Washington, Seattle, WA, USA

Farhad Sobouti
Department of Orthodontics, Dental Faculty, Mazandaran University of Medical Sciences, Sari, Iran

Maziar Khatami
Department of Periodontics, Dental Faculty, Mazandaran University of Medical Sciences, Sari, Iran

Nasim Chiniforush
Laser Research Center of Dentistry, Dental Research Institute, Tehran University of Medical Sciences, Tehran, Iran

Vahid Rakhshan
Iranian Tissue Bank and Research Center, Tehran University of Medical Sciences, Tehran, Iran
Department of Dental Anatomy and Morphology, Dental Branch, Islamic Azad University, Tehran, Iran

Mahsa Shariati
Craniomaxillofacial Surgery Research Center, Shariati Hospital, Tehran University of Medical Sciences, Postal Code: 14174North Kargar Ave., 16 Azar ST, Tehran, Iran

Arti Patel, Syed Mohammed Shamsul Islam and Mithran S. Goonewardene
Department of Orthodontics, School of Dentistry, The University of Western Australia, 35, Stirling Hwy, Crawley, Western Australia 6009, Australia

Kevin Murray
School of Mathematics and Statistics, The University of Western Australia, 35, Stirling Hwy, Crawley, Western Australia 6009, Australia

Abdolreza Jamilian
Department of Orthodontics, Dental Branch, Craniomaxillofacial Center Islamic Azad University, No 2713, Vali Asr St., Tehran 1966843133, Iran

Letizia Perillo
Post Graduate Orthodontic Program, Department of Orthodontics, Second University of Naples, Via bellini, 44 80135, Naples, Italy

Marco Rosa
Post-graduate School in Orthodontics, Insubria University, P.za della Mostra, 19 38122, Trento, Italy

Cinzia Maspero, Guido Galbiati and Lucia Giannini
U.O.C. Chirurgia Maxillo-facciale ed Odontostomatologia (dir: AB. Giannì) Fondazione Cà Granda IRCCS Ospedale Maggiore Policlinico, University of Milan, 20122 Milan, Italy

Giampietro Farronato
Maxillo-Facial and Odontostomatology Unit Fondazione Cà Granda IRCCS Ospedale Maggiore Policlinico, University of Milan, 20122 Milan, Italy

UOC Chirurgia Maxillofacciale e Odontostomatologia, Fondazione IRCCS Cà Granda - Ospedale Maggiore Policlinico, University of Milan, Commenda 10, Milano 20122, Italy

Varun Pratap Singh
Department of Orthodontics and Dentofacial Orthopedics, Nobel Medical College and Teaching Hospital, Kanchanbari, Biratnagar 56700, Nepal

Timothy P Moss
Department of Health Psychology, University of the West of England, Frenchary Campus, cold Harbour Lane, Bristol BS161QY, UK

Ahmed Ghoneima and Katherine Kula
Department of Orthodontics and Oral Facial Genetics, Indiana University School Dentistry, 1121 West Michigan Street, Indianapolis, IN 46202, USA

Ahmed Ghoneima
Department of Orthodontics, Faculty of Dental Medicine, Al-Azhar University, Cairo, Egypt

Sahar AlBarakati
Department of Pediatric Dentistry and Orthodontics, College of Dentistry, King Saud University, Riyadh, Saudi Arabia

Feifei Jiang and Tamer Wasfy
Department of Mechanical Engineering, Indiana University School of Engineering, Indianapolis, IN, USA

Merina Joshi and Li Peng Wu
Department of Stomatology, College of Stomatology, Jiamusi University, Street no. 522, Hongqi street, Jiamusi 154004, Republic of China

Surendra Maharjan and Mukunda Raj Regmi
Department of Health Services, Teku, Kathmandu 44600, Nepal

Giampietro Farronato, Lucia Giannini, Guido Galbiati, Santo Andrea Stabilini, Michele Sarcina and Cinzia Maspero
Maxillo-Facial and Odontostomatology Unit (Head: prof. AB. Giannì), Fondazione Cà Granda IRCCS Ospedale Maggiore Policlinico, Milan, Italy

Sabrina Mutinelli
Private practice, via Brennero 260/B, 38121 Trento, Italy

Mario Manfredi
Private practice, via Monte Cauriol 10, 38068 Rovereto, Italy

Antonio Guiducci
Private practice, viale Stazione 94, 54100 Massa, Italy

Gloria Denotti
University of Cagliari Department of Pedodontics and Interceptive Orthodontics, via Ospedale 54, 09123 Cagliari, Italy

Mauro Cozzani
University of Cagliari School of Dental Medicine, IRCCS "G. Gaslini" and Hospital "Galliera" (Genova), Via Fontevivo 21 N, 19125 La Spezia, Italy

Maryam Fathimani
Orthodontic Department, School of Dentistry, University of Alberta, Edmonton, AB, Canada

Jason P Carey, Garrett W Melenka and Roger W Toogood
Department of Mechanical Engineering, University of Alberta, Edmonton, AB, Canada

Dan L Romanyk and Giseon Heo
School of Dentistry, University of Alberta, Edmonton, AB, Canada

Paul W Major
Faculty of Medicine and Dentistry, 5-478, Edmonton Clinic Health Academy (ECHA), University of Alberta, 11405-87 Avenue NW, Edmonton, AB T6G 1C9, Canada
Luca Lombardo, Alessandro Perri, Angela Arreghini, Michele Latini and Giuseppe Siciliani
Department of Orthodontics, University of Ferrara, Via montebello, 31, Ferrara 44100, Italy

Neha Grover
Nora Medical Polyclinics, Tower 4. Marks and Spencer Building, No. 106, Abu Dhabi, United Arab Emirates

DN Kapoor
Department of Orthodontics, Kothiwal Dental College & Former Dean of Dental Faculty, KGMU, Lucknow, UP, India

Santosh Verma
Department of Orthodontics, Kothiwal Dental College & Research Centre, Moradabad, UP, India

Preeti Bharadwaj
Department of Orthodontics & Dentofacial Orthopedics, KD Dental College & Hospital, Mathura, UP, India

Peter Ngan and Chris Martin
Department of Orthodontics, School of Dentistry, West Virginia University, 1073 Health Science Center North, P.O. Box 9480, Morgantown, WV 26506, USA

Benedict Wilmes and Dieter Drescher
Department of Orthodontics, University of Düsseldorf, Moorenstrasse, Germany

Bryan Weaver
Department of Oral and Maxillofacial Surgery, School of Dentistry, West Virginia University, Morgantown, USA

Erdogan Gunel
Department of Statistics, West Virginia University, Morgantown, USA

Tehnia Aziz, Manuel O. Lagravere, Michael P. Major and Carlos Flores-Mir
Division of Orthodontics, 5-528 Edmonton Clinic Health Academy, University of Alberta, 11405 87 Ave. NW, Edmonton T6G 1C9, AB, Canada

Kal Ansari
Division of Otolaryngology, 4071 Grey Nuns Hospital, Edmonton T6L 5X8AB, Canada

Alessandro Ugolini, Tiziana Doldo and Roberto Giorgetti
Department of Orthodontics, University of Siena, Siena, Italy

Luis T. Huanca Ghislanzoni, Andrea Mapelli, Alessandro Ugolini and Chiarella Sforza
Functional Anatomy Research Center (FARC), Laboratorio di Anatomia Funzionale dell'Apparato Stomatognatico (LAFAS), Dipartimento di Scienze Biomediche per la Salute, Facoltà di Medicina e Chirurgia, Università degli Studi di Milano, Milan, Italy

Mirco F. Ronchetti and Hubertus van Waes
Clinic of Orthodontics and Paediatric Dentistry, Center of Dental Medicine, Faculty of Medicine, University of Zürich, Zürich, Switzerland

Michael Locher and Silvio Valdec
Clinic of Oral Surgery, Center of Dental Medicine, Faculty of Medicine, University of Zürich, Zürich, Switzerland

Nikolaos Pandis
Department of Orthodontics and Dentofacial Orthopedics, Dental School/Medical Faculty, University of Bern, Bern, Switzerland

Luca Lombardo, Angela Arreghini, Roberta Maccarrone and Giuseppe Siciliani
Postgraduate School of Orthodontics, University of Ferrara, Via Montebello 31, 44100 Ferrara, Italy

Anna Bianchi and Santo Scalia
Department of Chemical and Pharmaceutical Sciences, University of Ferrara, Via Fossato di Mortara 17/19, 44121 Ferrara, Italy

Gabriela Mesquita Lopes-Freire, José Enrique Espasa Suarez de Deza and Joan Ramon Boj Quesada JR
Department of Paediatric Dentistry, Faculty of Dentistry, University of Barcelona Hospitalet de Llobregat, Barcelona, Spain

Abel Belizario Cahuana Cárdenas
Pediatric Dentistry and Orthodontic Service, Hospital Sant Joan de Déu, Barcelona, Spain

Josep Maria Ustrell-Torrent
Department of Orthodontics, Oral Health and Masticatory System Group (Bellvitge Biomedical Research Institute) IDIBELL, Faculty of Dentistry, L'Hospitalet, Barcelona, Spain

Luciana Butini Oliveira
Department of Pediatric Dentistry, School of Dentistry, Faculdade São Leopoldo Mandic, Campinas, SP, Brazil

Mohamed I Masoud
Department of Developmental Biology, Harvard School of Dental Medicine, 188 Longwood Avenue, Boston, MA 02115, USA

Mohamed I Masoud and Hussain Y A Marghalani
Orthodontics Department - Faculty of Dentistry, King Abdulaziz University, Abdullah Sulayman st, Jeddah 22254, Saudi Arabia

Hussain Y A Marghalani
Department of Orthodontics, University of Buffalo, 140 Squire Hall, Buffalo, NY 14214, USA

Mohamed Bamashmous
Department of Dental Public Health, King Abdulaziz University, Abdullah Sulayman st, Jeddah 22254, Saudi Arabia
Henry M. Goldman School of Dental Medicine, Boston University, 100 East Newton Street, Boston, MA 02118, USA

Douaa El Derwi and Najlaa M Alamoudi
Pediatric Dentistry Department, Faculty of Dentistry, King Abdulaziz University, Abdullah Sulayman st, Jeddah 22254, Saudi Arabia

Douaa El Derwi
Public Health and Community Medicine Department, Faculty of Medicine, Cairo University, Al Kasr st, Kasralainy, Cairo, 11562, Egypt

Ibrahim M Masoud
Dr. Ibrahim Masoud's Dental Specialty Clinic, Jeddah, Saudi Arabia, Falasteen Street, Jeddah 21426, Saudi Arabia

Veerasathpurush Allareddy
Department of Orthodontics, College of Dentistry and Dental Clinics, The University of Iowa, 801 Newton Road, Iowa City 52242, IA, USA

Nour F Gowharji
Department of Pediatric Dentistry, Tufts School of Dental Medicine, 1 Kneeland St, Boston, MA 02111, USA

Patrícia Bittencourt Dutra dos Santos
Department of Orthodontics, State University of Rio Grande do Norte, Caicó, RN, Brazil

Daniela Gamba Garib
Department of Orthodontics, Hospital of Rehabilitation of Craniofacial Anomalies, Bauru Dental School, University of São Paulo, Bauru, São Paulo, Brazil

Guilherme Janson
Department of Orthodontics, Bauru Dental School, University of São Paulo, Bauru, São Paulo, Brazil

Vivian Helena Assis
Hospital of Rehabilitation of Craniofacial Anomalies, Bauru Dental School, Bauru, São Paulo, Brazil